DERMATOL(

SECRETS

IN COLOR

Second Edition

DERMATOLOGY SECRETS IN COLOR
Second Edition

JAMES E. FITZPATRICK, M.D.
Associate Professor
Department of Dermatology
University of Colorado Health Sciences Center
Denver, Colorado

JOHN L. AELING, M.D.
Professor
Department of Dermatology
University of Colorado Health Sciences Center
Denver, Colorado

HANLEY & BELFUS, INC./ Philadelphia

Publisher: HANLEY & BELFUS, INC.
               Medical Publishers
               210 South 13th Street
               Philadelphia, PA 19107
               (215) 546-7293; 800-962-1892
               FAX (215) 790-9330
               Web site: http://www.hanleyandbelfus.com

Disclaimer: The opinions and assertions contained in this book are the private views of the authors and are not to be construed as reflecting the view of the Department of the Army or the Department of Defense.

Library of Congress Cataloging-in-Publication Data

Dermatology Secrets / [edited by] James E. Fitzpatrick, John L. Aeling. — 2nd ed.
        p.   cm.   — (The Secrets Series®)
    Includes bibliographical references and index.
    ISBN 1-56053-402-8 (alk. paper)
    1. Dermatology — Miscellanea. 2. Skin — Diseases — Miscellanea. I. Fitzpatrick, James E., 1948–   .
    II. Aeling, John L., 1936–   .   III. Series.
    [DNLM: 1. Skin Diseases — Examination Questions. 2. Skin Diseases — Handbooks. WR
    18.2 D435 2001]
    RL72.D466   2001
    616.5 — dc21
                                                    00-039654

Printed in Canada

DERMATOLOGY SECRETS IN COLOR, 2nd edition   ISBN 1-56053-402-8

© 2001 by Hanley & Belfus, Inc. All rights reserved. No part of this book may be reproduced, reused, re-published, or transmitted in any form without written permission of the publisher.

Last digit is the print number: 9 8 7 6 5 4 3 2

CONTENTS

CONTRIBUTORS

John L. Aeling, M.D.
Professor, Department of Dermatology, University of Colorado Health Sciences Center, Denver, Colorado

Syed O. Ali, M.D., CPT, USA
Flight Surgeon, Department of Aviation Medicine, TMC McWethy, Fort Sam Houston, San Antonio, Texas

Scott D. Bennion, M.S., M.D., FACP
Associate Professor of Clinical Dermatology, University of Colorado Health Sciences Center, Denver, Colorado

Paul M. Benson, M.D., COL, MC
Chief, Dermatology Service, Walter Reed Army Medical Center, Washington, D.C.; Associate Professor, Uniformed Services University of the Health Sciences, Bethesda, Maryland

Carl Frederick Bigler, M.D.
Flagstaff Medical Center, Flagstaff, Arizona

Sylvia L. Brice, M.D.
Department of Dermatology, University of Colorado Health Sciences Center, Denver, Colorado

Lisa M. Cohen, M.D.
Clinical Associate Professor, Department of Dermatology, Tufts University School of Medicine, New England Medical Center, Boston, Massachusetts

Donna M. Corvette, M.D.
Assistant Clinical Professor, Department of Dermatology, Medical College of Virginia, Virginia Commonwealth University, Richmond, Virginia

Kathleen M. David-Bajar, M.D., COL, MC
Dermatology Consultant to the Army Surgeon General, Department of Dermatology, Brooke Army Medical Center, San Antonio Uniformed Services Health Education Consortium, Fort Sam Houston, Texas

Carl W. Demidovich, M.D.
Private Practice, Denver, Colorado

Stephen W. Eubanks, M.D.
Department of Dermatology, University Park Medical Center, Denver, Colorado

James E. Fitzpatrick, M.D.
Associate Professor, Department of Dermatology, University of Colorado Health Sciences Center, Denver, Colorado

Brian James Gerondale, M.D.
Private Practice, Ada, Michigan

Martin B. Giandoni, M.D.
Private Practice, Fort Collins, Colorado

Loren E. Golitz, M.D.
Clinical Professor of Dermatology and Pathology, University of Colorado Health Sciences Center, Denver, Colorado

Ronald E. Grimwood, M.D.
Professor and Program Director, Department of Dermatology, University of Texas Health Sciences Center at San Antonio, San Antonio, Texas

Nadja Y. Grammer-West, M.D., LTC, MC
Dermatology Service, HMEDDAC, Germany

Anne R. Halbert, MBBS, FACD
Consultant Dermatologist, Department of Pediatric Dermatology, Princess Margaret Hospital for Children, Perth, Western Australia

Stephen J. Hoffman, M.D., Ph.D.
Assistant Clinical Professor, Department of Dermatology, University of Colorado Health Sciences Center, Denver, Colorado

William D. James, M.D.
Professor of Dermatology, University of Pennsylvania School of Medicine, Philadelphia, Pennsylvania

Martin L. Johnson, M.D., LTC, MC, USAF
Medical Services Flight Commander, 81st Medical Group, Keesler Air Force Base, Mississippi

Richard A. Keller, M.D., COL, MC
Chief of Dermatologic Surgery, Dermatology Service, Walter Reed Army Medical Center, Washington, D.C.; Assistant Professor of Dermatology, Uniformed Services University of the Health Sciences F. Edward Hebert School of Medicine, Bethesda, Maryland

Ann M. Leibold, M.D.
Missouri Baptist Medical Center, St. Louis, Missouri

John G. LeVasseur, M.D., MAJ, USAF
Dermatology Service, Keesler Air Force Base, Mississippi

Lori Lowe, M.D.
Clinical Associate Professor, Departments of Dermatology and Pathology, University of Michigan Medical School, Ann Arbor, Michigan

Thomas W. McGovern, M.D.
Private Practice, Fort Wayne, Indiana

Jeffrey J. Meffert, M.D., COL, MC, USAF
Program Director, Department of Dermatology, San Antonio Uniformed Services Health Education Consortium, Fort Sam Houston, Texas

Julian Ramsey Mellette, M.D.
Professor, Department of Dermatology, University of Colorado Health Sciences Center, Denver, Colorado

Joseph G. Morelli, M.D.
Associate Professor of Dermatology and Pediatrics, Department of Dermatology, University of Colorado Health Sciences Center, Denver, Colorado

Margaret Elizabeth Muldrow, M.D.
Department of Dermatology, University of Colorado Health Sciences Center, Denver, Colorado

Harold S. Nelson, M.D.
Senior Staff Physician, Department of Medicine, National Jewish Center for Immunology and Respiratory Medicine, Denver, Colorado; Professor of Medicine, University of Colorado Health Sciences Center, Denver, Colorado

Scott A. Norton, M.D., M.P.H.
Dermatology Service, Walter Reed Army Medical Center, Washington, D.C

Theresa R. Pacheco, M.D.
Resident, Department of Dermatology, University of Colorado Health Sciences Center, Denver, Colorado

James W. Patterson, M.D.
Professor of Pathology and Dermatology, Department of Pathology, University of Virginia Medical Center, Charlottesville, Virginia

Barbara R. Reed, M.D.
Department of Dermatology, University of Colorado Health Sciences Center, Denver, Colorado

Troy Kent Richey, M.D.
Private Practice, Eugene, Oregon

Curt P. Samlaska, M.D., FACP
Assistant Professor, Department of Medicine, University of Nevada School of Medicine, Las Vegas, Nevada

Clinton Paul Sayers, M.D.
Department of Dermatology, University of Colorado Health Sciences Center, Denver, Colorado

Milton J. Schleve, M.D.
Private Practice, Denver, Colorado

Elizabeth R. Shurnas, M.D.
Private Practice, Denver, Colorado

Stephen T. Spates, M.D.
Department of Dermatology, University of Colorado Health Sciences Center, Denver, Colorado

Leonard C. Sperling, M.D., COL, MC
Professor and Chair, Department of Dermatology, Uniformed Services University of the Health Sciences, Bethesda, Maryland; Dermatology Service, Walter Reed Army Medical Center, National Naval Medical Center, Washington, D.C.

Leslie A. Stewart, M.D.
Clinical Assistant Professor, Department of Dermatology, University of Colorado Health Sciences Center, Denver, Colorado

Alexandra Theriault, M.D.
Assistant Clinical Professor, Department of Dermatology, University of Colorado Health Sciences Center, Denver, Colorado

Paul B. Thompson, M.D.
Clinical Instructor, Department of Dermatology, University of Washington School of Medicine, Seattle, Washington

Jeffrey B. Travers, M.D., Ph.D.
Associate Professor, Departments of Dermatology, Pediatrics, Pharmacology and Toxicology, Indiana University School of Medicine, Indianapolis, Indiana

George W. Turiansky, M.D., LTC, MC
Associate Professor of Clinical Dermatology, Uniformed Services University of the Health Sciences, Bethesda, Maryland; Assistant Chief, Dermatology Service, Walter Reed Army Medical Center, Washington, D.C.

Patrick Walsh, M.D.
Assistant Professor, Department of Dermatology, University of Colorado Health Sciences Center, Denver, Colorado

Karen E. Warschaw, M.D., LTC, MC, USAF
Flight Commander of Dermatology, Chief of Dermatopathology, Wilford Hall Medical Center, San Antonio, Texas

William L. Weston, M.D.
Professor, Departments of Dermatology and Pediatrics, University of Colorado Health Sciences Center, Denver, Colorado

Joseph Yohn, M.D.
Private Practice, Sarasota, Florida

PREFACE

The first edition of *Dermatology Secrets* was published in 1996 in the familiar Socratic method of the Secrets Series® with most of the photographs in black and white. While the first edition was very successful, the editors have always felt that the book could be markedly improved if all of the photographs were in color, which has been accomplished in the second edition. In addition to the usual updating of questions, additions of new questions, and a new chapter (*Special Considerations in Black Skin*), we have paid special attention to improving and increasing the numbers of clinical photographs. Dermatology is after all a visual specialty and there is no substitute for clinical photographs to illustrate cutaneous disease.

A survey taken during a medical meeting of primary care physicians reported that 35% of all the physicians had never taken a dermatology rotation and only 9% characterized their medical school training as being "good or excellent." Many medical schools do not require dermatology training for graduation, yet 1 out of every 13 patients seen in the U.S. will be seen for a skin condition. The importance of adequate dermatologic training is becoming increasingly important as managed care often restricts access to dermatologists, and health care providers find that they must diagnose and treat skin conditions without benefit of consultation. The editors are hopeful that this book will serve to both educate and stimulate interest in this truly fascinating medical specialty.

We would also like to thank our contributing authors, who have taken time out from their busy schedules to prepare their chapters and share their clinical photographs. Finally, the completion of this project would not have been possible without the expertise and devotion of the editorial staff of Hanley & Belfus, who have been very patient with us.

James E. Fitzpatrick, M.D.
John L. Aeling, M.D.

DEDICATION

This book is dedicated to
Edward M. Fitzpatrick (1921–1999)
and Jerry Aeling (1909–2000).

I. General

1. STRUCTURE AND FUNCTION OF THE SKIN

Scott D. Bennion, M.S., M.D., FACP

1. Name the three layers of the skin. What composes them?

The epidermis, dermis, and subcutis (subcutaneous fat). The **epidermis** is the outermost layer and is composed primarily of keratinocytes, or epidermal cells. Beneath the epidermis lies the **dermis,** which is composed primarily of collagen but also contains adnexal structures, including the hair follicles, sebaceous glands, apocrine glands, and eccrine glands. Numerous blood vessels, lymphatics, and nerves also traverse the dermis. Below the dermis lies the **subcutis,** or subcutaneous layer, which consists of adipose tissue, larger blood vessels, and nerves. The subcutis may also contain the base of hair follicles and sweat glands (Fig. 1).

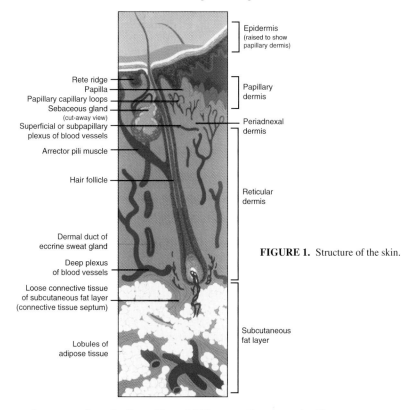

FIGURE 1. Structure of the skin.

2. How many layers are there in the epidermis? How are they organized?

The epidermis has four layers: the basal cell layer, spiny cell layer, granular cell layer, and cornified layer (Fig. 2). The **basal cell layer** (stratum basalis) is composed of columnar or cuboidal cells that are in direct contact with the basement membrane, the structure that separates the dermis from the epidermis. The basal cell layer contains the germinative cells, and for this reason, occasional mitoses may be present.

1

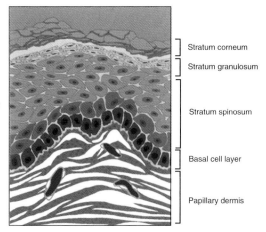

FIGURE 2. Epidermal layers and papillary dermis.

The three layers above the basal cell layer are histologically distinct and demonstrate differentiation of the keratinocytes as they move toward the skin surface and become "cornified." Just above the basal cell layer is the spiny cell layer (**stratum spinosum**), so called because of a high concentration of desmosomes and keratin filaments that give the cells a characteristic "spiny" appearance (Fig. 3A). Above the spiny layer is the granular cell layer (**stratum granulosum**). In this layer, keratohyalin granules are formed and bind to the keratin filaments (tonofilaments) to form large electron-dense masses within the cytoplasm that give this layer its "granular" appearance.

The outermost layer is the cornified layer (**stratum corneum**), where the keratinocytes abruptly lose all of their organelles and nucleus. The keratin filaments and keratohyalin granules form an amorphous mass within the keratinocytes, which become elongated and flattened forming a lamellar array of "corneocytes." The corneocytes are held together by the remnants of the desmosomes (dense bodies) and a "cementing substance" released into the intracellular space from organelles called Odland bodies.

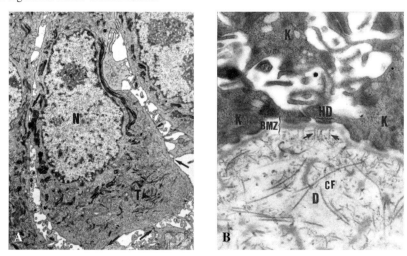

FIGURE 3. *A*, Keratinocyte. An electron micrograph illustrates the ultrastructural components of a typical keratinocyte in the stratum spinosum, including the nucleus (N), tonofilaments (T), and desmosomal intercellular connections (*arrows*) that give this layer its "spiny" appearance. *B*, Basement membrane zone (BMZ). At the interface of the basal keratinocytes (K) of the epidermis and dermis (D) is the BMZ. The keratinocytes are attached to the BMZ by hemidesmosomes (HD). The BMZ is comprised of the lamina lucida, which is the upper clear area, and the lamina densa, which is the dark area just below the lamina lucida. Anchoring fibrils (*arrows*) bind the BMZ to the dermis by intercalating among the collagen fibers (CF) of the dermis.

3. Do other types of cells normally occur in the epidermis?

In addition to keratinocytes, three other cells are normally found in the epidermis. The **melanocyte,** the most common, is a dendritic cell situated in the basal cell layer. There are approximately 36 keratinocytes for each melanocyte. This cell's function is to synthesize and secrete melanin-containing organelles called melanosomes. Melanocytes transfer mature melanosomes to keratinocytes by apocopation. In this process, the tips of the dendritic processes are phagocytized by the keratinocytes.

The next most common cell is the **Langerhans cell,** which is a bone marrow–derived, antigen-presenting cell that has very important immune surveillance functions. On light microscopy, these dendritic cells are primarily distributed in the stratum spinosum. Langerhans cells were first described by Paul Langerhans in 1868, while he was still a medical student.

Also located in the epidermis in small numbers are **Merkel cells.** The function of these cells is not fully established, but they are frequently in contact with nerve fibrils. Ultrastructurally, Merkel cells contain electron-dense bodies that are also found in APUD (amino acid precursor uptake and decarboxylation) cells of endocrine glands.

4. Describe the structure of the basement membrane zone (BMZ).

The BMZ is not normally visible by light microscopy in sections stained with hematoxylin-eosin but can be visualized as a homogeneous band measuring 0.5–1.0 μm thick on periodic acid–Schiff staining. Ultrastructural studies and immunologic mapping demonstrate that the BMZ is an extremely complex structure consisting of many components that function to attach the basal cell layer to the dermis (Fig. 3B). Uppermost in the BMZ are the cytoplasmic tonofilaments of the basal cells which attach to the basal plasma membrane of the cells at the hemidesmosome. The hemidesmosome is attached to the lamina lucida and lamina densa of the BMZ via anchoring filaments. The BMZ, in turn, is anchored to the dermis by anchoring fibrils that intercalate between the collagen fibers of the dermis and secure the BMZ to the dermis. The importance of these structures in maintaining skin integrity is demonstrated by diseases such as epidermolysis bullosa, in which they are congenitally missing or damaged.

5. How is the structure of the epidermis related to its functions?

The three most important functions of the epidermis are protection from environmental insult (barrier function), prevention of desiccation, and immune surveillance. The stratum corneum is an especially important cutaneous barrier that protects the body from toxins and desiccation. Although many **toxins** are nonpolar compounds that can move relatively easily through the lipid-rich intracellular spaces of the cornified layer, the tortuous route between cells in this layer and the layers below effectively forms a barrier to environmental toxins. **Ultraviolet light,** another environmental source of damage to living cells, is effectively blocked in the stratum corneum and the melanosomes. The melanosomes are concentrated above the nucleus of the keratinocytes in an umbrella-like fashion, providing photoprotection for both epidermal nuclear DNA and the dermis.

The prevention of **desiccation** is another extremely important function, as extensive loss of epidermis is often fatal (e.g., toxic epidermal necrolysis). In the normal epidermis, the water content decreases as one moves from the basal layer to the surface, comprising 70–75% of weight at the base and decreasing to 10–15% at the bottom of the stratum corneum.

Immune surveillance against foreign antigens is a function of the Langerhans cells that are dispersed among the keratinocytes. Langerhans cells internalize external antigens and process these antigens for presentation to T lymphocytes in the lymph nodes. Inflammatory cells (i.e., neutrophils, eosinophils, lymphocytes) are also capable of intercepting and destroying microorganisms in the epidermis.

6. What structural components of the epidermis are involved in blistering diseases?

In the epidermis, the keratinocytes are bound to each other by desmosomal complex. These complexes consist of the desmosome and the tonofilaments of the cytoplasm that are made of cytokeratins. In the upper stratum spinosum, the tonofilaments are composed mainly of keratins 1 and 10. Congenital abnormalities in these keratins produce structural weakness between keratinocytes, producing a disease called **congenital bullous ichthyosiform erythroderma** (epidermolytic hyperkeratosis). Abnormalities in keratin types 5 and 14 in the basal cell layers lead to a mild blistering disease named **epidermolysis bullosa simplex** (EBS). **Pemphigus** is an acquired group of blistering diseases of the epidermis in which autoantibodies directed against antidesmosomal proteins produce damage of the desmosomes.

The skin diseases associated with antibodies and damage to the desmosomes and their characteristics are listed in the following table:

DISEASE	CLINICAL APPEARANCE AND LOCATION	MAIN DESMOSOMAL MOLECULES INVOLVED
Pemphigus vulgaris	Oral and diffuse superficial flaccid blisters with ulcers	Desmoglein 3 and plakoglobin
Pemphigus foliaceus	Diffuse superficial blisters and crusting	Desmoglein 1
Pemphigus vegetans	Vegetating, weeping lesions in the intertriginous areas	Desmoglein 3
Pemphigus erythematosus	Butterfly erruption with blistering in malar areas	Desmoglein 3
Paraneoplastic pemphigus	Diffuse erythema multiforme–like painful erruption	Desmoplakins 1 and 2, BP antigen 1 (BPAG-1), and plectin

7. Are there hereditary diseases of the BMZ and dermis that cause blistering and damage to the skin?

Yes, there is a complex group of inherited diseases in which the skin is friable and bullous lesions occur, often with susequent scarring. The two subgroups within this group are junctional epidermolysis bullosas (JEBs) and dystrophic epidermolysis bullosas (DEBs). Like the EBS diseases that affect the epidermal layers, these diseases occur because the vital structure elements of the BMZ and dermis are missing, causing the skin to separate easily and blister. In JEBs the separation occurs within the lamina lucida (LL) of the BMZ. Decreased amounts or abnormalities in the LL components such as laminins I and V and 19-DEJ-1 protein have been identified in this group.

In the DEB group, separation occurs below the BMZ in the dermal layer and a decreased amount or absence of type VII collagen has been noted. As a rule, the deeper in the skin the separation occurs, the more severe the clinical picture with increased scarring and loss of function. DEB patients typically have severe deforming scars and decreased life span.

8. Are there acquired blistering diseases of the BMZ and dermis?

Yes, there are several diseases in which blistering occurs secondary to disruption of the structures of the BMZ and dermis. As with the epidermal blistering diseases, antibodies to the hemidesmosomes and other structures within the BMZ and dermis cause separation of the skin and blistering. In the uppermost portion of the BMZ, the LL, hemidesmosomes bind the basal keratinocytes to the basement membrane. Bullous pemphigoid (BP) is a classic example of an acquired blistering disease in which anti-hemidesmosomal antibodies are produced and appear to induce inflammation and subsequent damage of the hemidesmosomes, causing a blister to develop between the cells and the basement membrane.

The skin diseases associated with antibodies and damage to the basement membrane structures and dermis are listed in the following table:

DISEASE	CLINICAL APPEARANCE AND LOCATION	BM MOLECULE INVOLVED
Bullous pemphigoid	Tense blisters diffusely	BP antigens 1 and 2
Herpes gestationis	Urticarial blisters with pruritus in late pregnancy	BP antigen 2
Epidermolysis bullosa acquisita	Friable skin and blistering knees, elbows, and sites of increased pressure	Type VII dermal collagen
Bullous lupus erythematosus	Blistering face and trunk with flairs of SLE	Type VII dermal collagen
Linear IgA bullous disease (LIBD)	Tense vesicles in annular and target-like patterns on the trunk	BP antigen 2 and 97 kDa

9. What abnormalities in structural components of the basement membrane are involved in bullous skin diseases?

Structures within the basement membrane can be congenitally absent or decreased in number, or as with the epidermal desmosomes, they can be affected by antibodies directed against them. In the uppermost portion of the BMZ, in the lamina lucida, hemidesmosomes bind the basal keratinocytes to the basement membrane. **Bullous pemphigoid** is an acquired blistering disease in which anti-hemidesmosomal antibodies are produced and appear to induce inflammation and subsequent damage to the hemidesmosomes, causing a blister to develop between the cells and basement membrane.

10. What is the function of the sebaceous gland?

The sebaceous gland is a holocrine gland that is a part of the pilosebaceous unit. Its function is to produce **sebum,** which is a combination of wax esters, squalene, cholesterol esters, and triglycerides. Sebum is secreted through the sebaceous duct into the hair follicle, where it covers the skin surface, possibly as a protectant. Sebum may also have antifungal properties. Sebaceous glands are located everywhere on the skin except the palms and soles.

11. How do the eccrine sweat glands and apocrine sweat glands differ?

Embryologically, **eccrine glands** derive from the epidermis and are not part of the pilosebaceous unit. The eccrine sweat glands function in temperature regulation via secretion of sweat, a combination of mostly water and electrolytes, which evaporates and cools the skin. Their ducts pass through the dermis and epidermis to empty directly onto the skin surface. Eccrine glands are located everywhere on the skin surface except on modified skin areas, such as the lips, nailbeds, and glans penis. Eccrine sweat glands are found only in higher primates and horses.

Apocrine glands originate from the same hair germ that gives rise to the hair follicle and sebaceous gland. The apocrine duct empties into the follicle above the sebaceous gland. Their anachronistic function is to produce scent. They are located primarily in the axillae and perineum, and their activity is sex hormone–dependent. The breast and cerumen glands are both modified apocrine sweat glands.

12. How is the dermis organized?

The dermis is organized into two distinct areas: the papillary dermis and the reticular dermis. The superficial **papillary dermis** is a relatively thin zone beneath the epidermis. On light microscopy, it is composed of thin, delicate collagen fibers and is highly vascularized. The hair follicles are enveloped by a **perifollicular dermis** that is contiguous with, and morphologically resembles, the papillary dermis. Collectively, the papillary dermis and perifollicular dermis are called the **adventitial dermis,** although this term is rarely used in dermatology texts.

The deeper zone is the **reticular dermis,** which composes the bulk of the dermis. It is less vascular than the papillary dermis and demonstrates thick, well-organized collagen bundles.

13. What are the components of the dermis?

The main components of the dermis include **collagen** (70–80%) for resiliency, **elastin** (1–3%) for elasticity, and **proteoglycans** to maintain water within the dermis. The bulk of the collagen within the dermis consists of types I and III and is organized into collagen bundles which mostly run horizontally throughout the dermis. The elastic fibers are interspersed between the collagen fibers. **Oxytalan fibers** are small elastic fibers found primarily in the papillary dermis and are usually oriented perpendicularly to the skin surface. The proteoglycans (primarily hyaluronic acid) compose the amorphous ground substance around the elastic and collagen fibers. The primary cell in the dermis is the fibroblast, which is responsible for making collagen, elastin, and proteoglycans.

14. What are the functions of the dermis?

1. Temperature regulation through control of cutaneous blood flow and sweating, achieved by the dermal vessels and eccrine sweat glands.

2. Mechanical protection of underlying structures, achieved primarily by the collagen and hyaluronic acid.

3. Innervation of the skin that mostly occurs in the dermis and is responsible for cutaneous sensation.

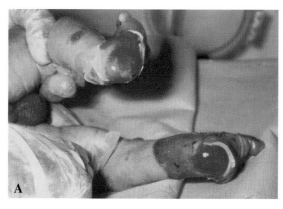

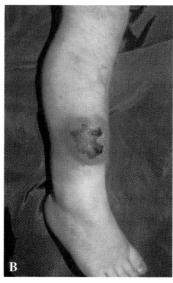

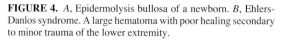

FIGURE 4. *A*, Epidermolysis bullosa of a newborn. *B*, Ehlers-Danlos syndrome. A large hematoma with poor healing secondary to minor trauma of the lower extremity.

15. Which structural component of the dermis is involved in congenital and autoimmune skin diseases?

Collagen. Antibodies against **type VII collagen,** which makes up the anchoring filaments within the dermis, are found in the autoimmune diseases **bullous systemic lupus erythematosus** and **acquired epidermolysis bullosa.** The anchoring filaments function to bind the basement membrane to the dermis, and damage to this collagen results in blister formation below the basement membrane. Clinically, blistering damage beneath the basement membrane causes significant scarring, in contrast to blisters in the epidermis or above the basement membrane that do not cause scarring. **Congenital epidermolysis bullosa** (EB), in which there is a congenital paucity or absence of type VII collagen and anchoring fibers, can result in severe scarring. The most severe form of this disease, recessive dystrophic EB, is associated with "mitten" deformities of the hands and feet, severe scarring of the upper respiratory and gastrointestinal tracts, and early death (Fig. 4A).

Congenital abnormalities in the various collagens in the dermis, especially **types I and III,** are found in several of the **Ehlers-Danlos syndromes.** The cutaneous manifestations of these syndromes are hyperextensibility of the skin, easy bruisability, and poor healing with resultant wide scar formation (Fig. 4B).

16. How does the vasculature of the dermis function in temperature control?

Body temperature is regulated, in part, through control of dermal blood flow. Lowering body temperature is accomplished through increased blood flow in the vascular plexus in the high papillary dermis, allowing heat to be removed through radiation from the skin. The dermal vasculature is composed of a superficial and deep plexus of arterioles and venules that are interconnected by communicating vessels (Fig. 5). The incoming blood flow to the superficial capillary plexus in the upper dermis can be decreased by increased smooth muscle tone in the ascending arterioles, or it can be shunted directly from the arterioles to the venous channels in the deeper plexus systems via glomus bodies, which are modified arterioles surrounded by multiple layers of muscle cells. During cold temperatures, decreased papillary blood flow to the papillary dermis, in essence, shunts the blood away from the skin surface and decreases heat loss from the body.

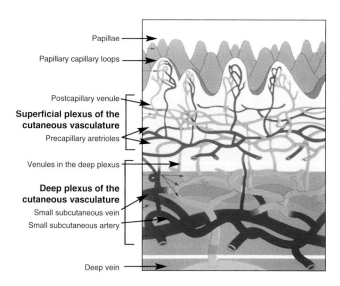

Papillae

Papillary capillary loops

Postcapillary venule

Superficial plexus of the cutaneous vasculature

Precapillary aretrioles

Venules in the deep plexus

Deep plexus of the cutaneous vasculature

Small subcutaneous vein

Small subcutaneous artery

Deep vein

FIGURE 5. Vasculature of the skin.

17. How is the skin innervated?

The innervation of the skin recapitulates the blood flow: large, myelinated, cutaneous branches of the musculocutaneous nerves branch in the subcutaneous tissue to form a deep nerve plexus in the reticular dermis. Nerve fibers from the deep plexus ascend to form a superficial sub-papillary plexus. Nerves from these plexuses innervate the skin as free nerve endings which function as important sensory receptors. They transmit touch, pain, temperature, itch, and mechanical stimuli. These exist in the papillary dermis as individual fibers surrounded by **Schwann cells**.

The other type of receptor in the skin is the corpuscular receptor. There are two types, called the **Meissner's corpuscle** and the **Pacinian corpuscle**, and these serve as mechanoreceptors for pressure and vibration. The distribution of receptors varies according to the body location, with increased numbers on the areola, labia, glans penis, and acral skin.

18. Is loss of cutaneous sensation that serious?

The importance of skin innervation is best illustrated by diseases that destroy cutaneous nerves. The archetypical disease is **Hansen's disease (leprosy)**. This disease attacks and destroys cutaneous nerves, resulting in severe mutilation of the extremities after years of unperceived trauma.

19. How is the subcutis organized?

The subcutis, or subcutaneous fat, is arranged into distinct fat lobules which are divided by fibrous septae composed primarily of collagen. Blood vessels, nerves, and lymphatics are also found in the fibrous septae. In addition to its role as a caloric reserve, the subcutaneous fat serves as a heat insulator and shock absorber.

BIBLIOGRAPHY

1. Arnold H, Odom R, James W (eds): Andrew's Diseases of the Skin, 8th ed. Philadelphia, W.B. Saunders, 1990.
2. Demis DJ (ed): Clinical Dermatology. Philadelphia, J. B. Lippincott, 1994.
3. Fitzpatrick TB, Eisen A, Wolff K, Freedberg I, Austen K (eds): Dermatology in General Medicine, 4th ed. New York, McGraw-Hill, 1993.
4. Goldsmith L (ed): Physiology, Biochemistry, and Molecular Biology of the Skin, 2nd ed. New York, Oxford University Press, 1991.
5. Lever WF, Schaumburg-Lever G: Histopathology of the Skin, 7th ed. Philadelphia, J.B. Lippincott, 1990.

2. MORPHOLOGY OF PRIMARY AND SECONDARY SKIN LESIONS

Donna M. Corvette, M.D.

1. Why do dermatologists use words that no one else understands?

The language of dermatology *is* unique. It encompasses terms that rarely, if ever, are used in other medical specialties. The use of these correct dermatologic terms is important to accurately describe skin lesions to dermatologists during telephone calls and during rounds and teaching. A good description of a skin lesion enables the listener to formulate a series of differential diagnoses, whereas a poor one does not.

2. But why are the descriptions so long?

The goal is similar in all fields of medicine—effective communication. If a cardiologist wants to describe a mitral regurgitation murmur, limiting the description to "a holosystolic murmur" hinders the listener's differential. Adding features of the murmur helps ensure the correct diagnosis: best heard at the apex, radiates to left axillae, and increased with handgrip maneuver.

The same is true in dermatology. Using appropriate terminology and important clues, such as configuration and skin distribution, effectively paints an accurate portrait for the listener. Using vague terms—spot, bump, rash, and lesion—will only inflame your consultant. Such vocabulary is counterproductive to formulating accurate differential diagnoses. "Grouped vesicles on an erythematous base" immediately suggests herpes simplex; "brown, friable 'stuck-on' papules with horn cysts in an elderly patient" accurately describes seborrheic keratoses. "Well-demarcated, erythematous plaques with micaceous, silvery scales located on extensor surfaces" is suggestive of psoriasis. "Violaceous, polygonal papules with Wickham's striae located on flexural surfaces" is consistent with lichen planus. On the other hand, "red, scaly rash on the foot" describes an enormous, nebulous group of disorders.

3. How can I possibly learn the language of dermatology?

First, learn the definitions of the various primary, secondary, and special skin lesions. Each of these groups consists of a short list of terms that specifies basic types. Then, follow this simple template when describing skin lesions:

Size
Color or additional descriptive terms (e.g., pigmentation, shape)
Type of primary, secondary, or special skin lesion (e.g., papule, macule)
Arrangement (e.g., grouped lesions)
Distribution (e.g., truncal, generalized)

The template provides a systematic way to add adjectives to the type of lesion. Repetition is key; practice using the template when describing skin lesions.

4. What is a primary skin lesion?

It is the initial lesion that has not been altered by trauma, manipulation (scratching, scrubbing), or natural regression over time. Examples include:

Macules	Wheals
Papules	Vesicles
Plaques	Bullae
Patches	Pustules
Nodules	Cysts

5. How are each of the primary lesions defined?

Primary Skin Lesions

PRIMARY LESION	DEFINITION	MORPHOLOGY	EXAMPLES
Macule	Flat, circumscribed skin discoloration that lacks surface elevation or depression		Café au lait Vitiligo Freckle Junctional nevi Ink tattoo
Papule	Elevated, solid lesion <0.5 cm in diameter		Acrochordon (skin tag) Basal cell carcinoma Molluscum contagiosum Intradermal nevi
Plaque	Elevated, solid "confluence of papules" (>0.5 cm in diameter) that lacks a deep component		Bowen's disease Mycosis fungoides Psoriasis Eczema Tinea corporis
Patch	Flat, circumscribed skin discoloration; a very large macule		Nevus flammeus Vitiligo
Nodule	Elevated, solid lesion >0.5 cm in diameter; a larger, deeper papule		Rheumatoid nodule Tendon xanthoma Erythema nodosum Lipoma Metastatic carcinoma
Wheal	Firm, edematous plaque that is evanescent and pruritic; a hive		Urticaria Dermographism Urticaria pigmentosa
Vesicle	Papule that contains clear fluid; a blister		Herpes simplex Herpes zoster Dyshidrotic eczema Contact dermatitis
Bulla	Localized fluid collection > 0.5 cm in diameter; a large vesicle		Pemphigus vulgaris Bullous pemphigoid Bullous impetigo

Primary Skin Lesions (continued)

PRIMARY LESION	DEFINITION	MORPHOLOGY	EXAMPLES
Pustule	Papule that contains purulent material		Folliculitis Impetigo Acne Pustular psoriasis
Cyst	Nodule that contains fluid or semisolid material		Acne Epidermal inclusion cyst Pilar cyst

6. How do you determine whether a lesion is flat or raised?

Palpation is the most reliable method, but side-lighting also helps. It can be difficult to distinguish a macule from a papule or a patch from a plaque in a photograph.

7. How does a primary lesion differ from a secondary lesion?

Secondary skin lesions are created by scratching, scrubbing, or infection. They may also develop normally with time. Examples include:

Crusts	Scale
Ulcers	Fissures
Excoriations	Scars
Erosions	

8. How are the secondary skin lesions defined?

Secondary Skin Lesions

SECONDARY LESION	DEFINITION	MORPHOLOGY
Crust	A collection of cellular debris, dried serum, and blood; a scab Antecedent primary lesion is usually a vesicle, bulla, or pustule	
Erosion	A partial focal loss of epidermis; heals without scarring	
Ulcer	A full-thickness, focal loss of epidermis and dermis; heals with scarring	

Secondary Skin Lesions (Continued)

SECONDARY LESION	DEFINITION	MORPHOLOGY
Fissure	Vertical loss of epidermis and dermis with sharply defined walls; crack in skin	
Excoriation	Linear erosion induced by scratching	
Scar	A collection of new connective tissue; may be hypertrophic or atrophic Scar implies dermoepidermal damage	
Scale	Thick stratum corneum that results from hyperproliferation or increased cohesion of keratinocytes	

9. What is a maculopapular eruption?

A dermatitis composed of both macules and papules. Maculopapular eruptions are commonly seen with viral exanthems and drug-induced reactions (see figure below). The cutaneous eruption of measles is an example of a maculopapular eruption.

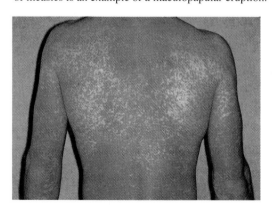

This patient with mononucleosis was exposed to ampicillin and subsequently developed generalized maculopapular eruption.

10. Give some examples of special skin lesions.

Telangiectasias	Purpura
Petechiae	Comedones
Burrows	Target lesions

11. What are telangiectasias?

Telangiectasias are small, dilated, superficial blood vessels (capillaries, arterioles, or venules) that blanch (disappear) with pressure.

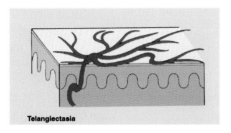

Telangiectasia

12. Are telangiectasias pathognomonic for a certain disease?

No. Telangiectasias may occur in many cutaneous disorders, including collagen vascular diseases such as dermatomyositis, systemic lupus erythematosus, and progressive systemic sclerosis. They are also commonly seen as a consequence of chronic ultraviolet radiation and topical steroid usage. Telangiectasias may also be seen in tumors such as nodulo-ulcerative basal cell carcinoma, which is classically described as a pearly colored papule with telangiectasias and central ulceration.

13. What is a burrow?

An elevated channel in the superficial epidermis produced by a parasite, such as the mite *Sarcoptes scabiei*. Scabies burrows characteristically are located on the wrists and in fingerwebs; the diagnosis is confirmed by demonstrating the mite microscopically in skin scrapings. The human hookworm may also produce a serpiginous burrow; however, demonstrating this organism is much more difficult.

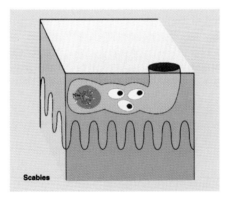

Scabies

14. What is a comedo?

A comedo is a folliculocentric collection of sebum and keratin. Comedonal acne characteristically consists of both open (blackheads) and closed comedones (whiteheads). When the contents of a closed comedo are exposed to air, a chemical reaction occurs, imparting the black color of an open comedo.

15. What is the difference between petechiae and purpura?

The size of the lesion is the major difference. Both petechiae and purpura result from extravasation of red blood cells into the dermis; hence, they do not blanch with pressure. Petechiae, however, are much smaller than purpura; they are < 5 mm in diameter.

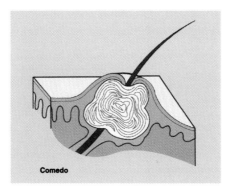

Comedo

16. What are target lesions?

Target lesions typically consist of three zones. The first zone consists of a dark or blistered center (bull's eye) which is surrounded by a second, pale zone. The third zone consists of a rim of erythema. Target lesions classically are found on the palms of a patient with erythema multiforme.

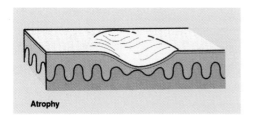

Atrophy

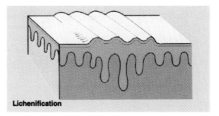

Lichenification

17. List some of the additional descriptive adjectives used in dermatology that refer to color or pigmentation.

- **Depigmented**—Absence of cells that produce melanin (melanocytes); a lack of color. Depigmented macules and patches are commonly found in vitiligo.
- **Hypopigmented**—Lighter than normal skin color; normal number of melanocytes but decreased production of melanin by the melanocytes. The ash-leaf macule of tuberous sclerosis is an example of a hypopigmented macule.
- **Hyperpigmented**—Darker than normal skin color. Junctional nevi and café au lait macules (neurofibromatosis) are hyperpigmented macules.
- **Erythematous**—Redness of the skin.

18. How do atrophy and lichenification differ?

- **Atrophy** is thinning of the epidermis, dermis, or subcutis (fat). Epidermal atrophy leads to a fine cigarette-paper wrinkling of the skin surface, whereas dermal and fat atrophy cause a depression in the skin surface.
- A **lichenified** lesion is a focal area of thickened skin produced by chronic scratching or rubbing. The skin lines are accentuated, resembling a washboard.

19. Do skin diseases have characteristic arrangements or configurations?

Some but not all cutaneous diseases demonstrate characteristic arrangements or configurations of lesions. Commonly used adjectives include:

- **Annular**—Used to describe lesions that are ring-shaped. Annular plaques are typical findings in granuloma annulare, tinea corporis (ringworm), and erythema marginatum.
- **Gyrate**—From the Latin *gyratus,* which means "to turn around in a circle." Gyrate skin le-

sions are rare presentations. Gyrate erythema that resembles wood-grain or topographic maps is seen in erythema gyratum repens, which usually heralds the presence of an internal malignancy.

- **Dermatomal**—Used to describe lesions that follow neurocutaneous dermatomes. The classic example is herpes zoster (shingles), which demonstrates grouped vesicles on an erythematous base in a dermatomal distribution.
- **Linear**—More than 20 diseases may demonstrate linear configurations. One example is allergic contact dermatitis to poison ivy; it characteristically demonstrates linear erythematous papules or vesicles.
- **Grouped**—Papules, pustules, or blisters (oops, vesicles or bullae) may demonstrate grouped configurations. A typical example is herpes simplex, which demonstrates grouped vesicles on an erythematous base.

20. What is the Koebner phenomenon?

Traumatizing the epidermis of a patient with a certain preexisting skin disease will cause the same skin disease to form in the traumatized skin. Noticing this skin finding is helpful when creating a differential diagnosis. Only certain diseases are associated with a Koebner phenomenon: lichen planus, lichen nitidus, and psoriasis are examples.

21. Do skin diseases characteristically occur in certain locations?

Yes. This is the reason that a complete skin examination should be performed on all patients. Seborrheic dermatitis characteristically occurs on the scalp, nasolabial folds, retroauricular areas, eyelids, eyebrows, and presternal areas; it tends to spare the extremities. Psoriasis may resemble seborrheic dermatitis, but it characteristically demonstrates a different distribution, usually involving the extremities (elbows, knees), intergluteal fold, scalp, and nails.

BIBLIOGRAPHY

1. Arnold HL, Odom RB, James WD: Andrew's Diseases of the Skin: Clinical Dermatology, 8th ed. Philadelphia, W.B. Saunders, 1990.
2. Demis DJ: Clinical Dermatology, 22nd ed. Philadelphia, Lippincott-Raven, 1995.
3. Elder D, Elenitsas R, Jaworsky C, Johnson B Jr (eds): Lever's Histopathology of the Skin, 8th ed. Philadelphia, Lippincott-Raven, 1997.
4. Fitzpatrick TB, Eisen AZ, Wolff K, Freedberg IM, Austen KF (eds): Dermatology in General Medicine, 4th ed. New York, McGraw-Hill, 1993.
5. Moschella SL, Hurley HJ: Dermatology, 2nd ed. Philadelphia, W.B. Saunders, 1985.

3. DIAGNOSTIC TECHNIQUES

Stephen T. Spates, M.D.

1. What is the most sensitive office laboratory test for diagnosing dermatophyte infections of the skin?

Microscopic examination of a potassium hydroxide (KOH) preparation of scrapings taken from the affected area is the most sensitive office laboratory test, if performed properly. A study of 220 specimens examined by both KOH and culture demonstrated positive KOH preparations and cultures in 45% of samples, a positive KOH preparation and negative culture in 52% of samples, and a negative KOH preparation and a positive culture in only 3% of samples. Cultures can be useful since other studies have shown a 5–15% increase in positive specimens by culturing all KOH-negative materials. However, it cannot be emphasized enough that the diagnostic accuracy of the KOH preparation depends on the experience and skill of the individual performing the test. A proper KOH preparation and interpretation is an important skill for any health care provider dealing with skin disease.

2. How is a KOH examination performed?

The highest rate of recovery of organisms occurs in specimens taken from the tops of vesicles, the leading edges of annular lesions, or deep scrapings from the nails suspected to be infected with fungi. The site should be swabbed with an alcohol pad or water and scraped with a #15 blade. In some instances, such as the scalp or nail, a curette may be more effective. The moist corneocytes are then easily transferred from the blade to a glass slide. One or two drops of KOH (10–20%) are added, and the specimen is cover-slipped. Alternatively, the cover slip may be applied first and the KOH applied to one edge. The KOH preparation is gently warmed, but not boiled, and then examined under the microscope. It is important to focus back and forth through the material so that the refractile hyphae can be found (Fig. 1). Fungal hyphae can be recognized by their regular cylindrical shapes with branching and presence of septae that may demonstrate a subtle greenish hue. Older lesions may demonstrate numerous rounded spores called arthrospores. A pencil eraser or pen cap gently applied to the surface of the coverslip may enhance keratinocyte breakdown, especially for clumped specimens. If no organisms are observed initially, waiting 10–15 minutes may aid visualization.

An alternative fungal stain to the KOH is the chlorazol black E stain. The specimen is prepared the same way as the KOH; however with this preparation the hyphae take on a subtle gray to gray-black color and are more easily visualized.

3. What laboratory tests are useful for diagnosing tinea capitis?

Fluorescing the affected area with a **Wood's light** is the quickest technique. If the hair fluoresces a yellow-green, then a fungal infection is likely. However, the lack of fluorescence does

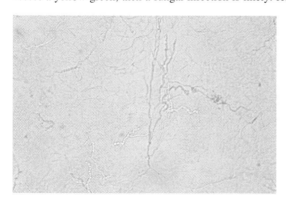

FIGURE 1. Hyphae traversing KOH preparation of skin scraping.

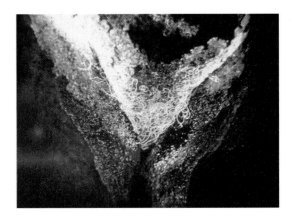

FIGURE 2. Wood's light examination of the groin area demonstrating the characteristic coral red fluorescence associated with erythrasma. (Courtesy of John L. Aeling, MD.)

not exclude tinea capitis, because *Trichophyton tonsurans* accounts for 80–95% of scalp ringworm infections in the United States, and it does not fluoresce.

Examination of **KOH-treated** infected hair is more sensitive and rapidly performed. The best results are obtained when broken-off hairs are examined since these are the ones infected by hyphae and arthrospores. Infection can be immediately apparent on KOH examination if the fungus grows outside the hair shaft (ectothrix). Most dermatophytes, such as *T. tonsurans,* grow within the hair shaft (endothrix), and a few minutes are required to let the KOH break down the hair shaft so that the hyphae and arthrospores can be more easily visualized.

The diagnosis can also be proved by **fungal cultures.** The easily broken, infected hairs are embedded in the media. The specimen can be obtained using a #15 blade, curette, or hemostat. A new toothbrush can also be "brushed" through the affected area of the scalp and then applied to the media.

4. What is a Wood's light or lamp? How is it useful in skin diseases?

A Wood's light produces invisible long-wave ultraviolet radiation, or "black light," at 360 nm. When this light strikes the surface of the skin or urine, fluorescence is produced in some disorders. This fluorescence is best observed in a completely dark room.

The Wood's lamp is useful in diagnosing some cases of tinea capitis (*Microsporum* spp. fluoresce and *Trichophyton* spp. do not), tinea versicolor (dull yellow fluorescence), erythrasma (coral red fluorescence, Fig. 2), and *Pseudomonas* infections of the skin (green fluorescence). It is also useful as a screening test in porphyria cutanea tarda as the urine fluoresces a coral red color (Fig. 3).

The Wood's light may also be used in certain disorders of pigmentation. In patients with hyperpigmentation, it is used to localize the site of the pigment, since it accentuates epidermal pigment, while dermal pigment is unchanged. It is also used in patients with hypopigmentation

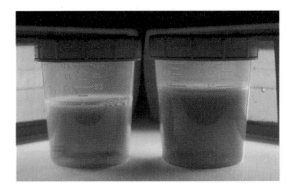

FIGURE 3. Wood's light examination of urine demonstrating characteristic coral red fluorescence in a patient with porphyria cutanea tarda compared to a normal urine specimen. (Courtesy of James E. Fitzpatrick, MD.)

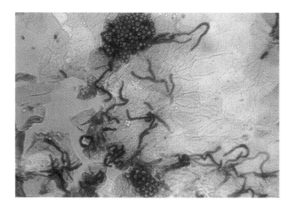

FIGURE 4. A positive cellophane tape preparation of tinea versicolor that has been stained with methylene blue. The characteristic clusters of spores and short hyphae are easily demonstrated. (Courtesy of James E. Fitzpatrick, MD.)

since it can differentiate between depigmentation and hypopigmentation. It is especially helpful in establishing the diagnosis of vitiligo since it demonstrates complete depigmentation. It can also be used to delineate the borders of melanocytic lesions such as lentigo maligna prior to surgery.

5. What are the common culture media used for isolating dermatophytes?

Dermatophyte test media (DTM) and Sabouraud's dextrose agar, with or without antibiotics (e.g., Mycosel agar, Mycobiotic agar), are the two most common types of culture media used. Many dermatologists prefer DTM since it has the advantage of a color indicator that changes the media from yellow to red when a dermatophyte is present. DTM is 95–97% accurate in differentiating dermatophytes from nondermatophytes, usually within the first 2 weeks.

Sabouraud's dextrose agar is a standard in mycology laboratories and also in many dermatologists' offices. It consists of dextrose (energy source), peptone (protein source), and agar (for a firm surface). Antibiotics can be added to suppress bacterial contaminants, and cyclohexamide is added to suppress yeasts and nondermatophytes. Plain Sabouraud's agar is a good culture medium for *Candida albicans*.

6. What is a simple test for tinea versicolor other than a KOH preparation?

Clear **cellophane tape preparations** are an excellent diagnostic test because the organism is found in the upper stratum corneum. First the skin is scraped to make sure there is adequate scale. The tape is applied over the scale and then mounted on a glass slide and examined under the microscope. Clusters of short hyphae and yeasts are seen producing a "spaghetti and meatballs" pattern. Methylene blue may also be added to the slide, selectively staining the organism (Fig. 4). *Malassezia furfur* (*Pityrosporum orbiculare*), the etiologic agent of tinea versicolor, cannot be cultured on any of the routine fungal media kept in most laboratories.

7. What is a Tzanck preparation or smear?

A Tzanck smear is a standard technique for the rapid diagnosis of herpes simplex virus (HSV) or varicella-zoster virus (VZV) infections. It cannot distinguish between these two agents, nor can it distinguish between HSV subtypes (HSV type 1 or 2). It is performed by scraping the base of a fresh blister with a scalpel blade and then spreading the adhering cells and material on a glass slide. The slide is then stained with Giemsa, Wright's, or Sedi stain. The typical multinucleated giant cells or atypical keratinocytes with large nuclei are then sought under the microscope (Fig. 5).

8. How accurate is the Tzanck preparation in diagnosing viral vesicles?

The sensitivity varies with the stage of the viral vesicle. One study reported the Tzanck preparation to be positive in 67% of vesicular lesions, 54% of pustular lesions, and 16% of crusted lesions of HSV. Tzanck preparations were positive in 80% of clinically suggestive cases of VZV.

Accuracy Comparison: Tzanck, PCR, Culture

	HSV	VZV
Tzanck	60%	75%
PCR	83%	97%
Culture	83%	44%

9. What is the best method of diagnosing scabies?

The best method is to scrape a burrow and demonstrate the parasite inside it. A classic burrow appears as an irregular, linear, slightly elevated lesion, best found on the flexor wrists, finger webs, and genitalia. Eighty-five percent of adult male patients with scabies will have mites on the hands or wrists. Occasionally, the mite can be seen with the naked eye as a small dot at one end of the burrow. A sample is collected with a number 15 scalpel blade. Following the application of mineral oil on either the blade or skin, the burrow is scraped vigorously, but not so vigorously as to draw blood. The mineral oil is collected from the skin and transferred to a glass slide, which is then examined under the microscope. The diagnosis is established by identifying either the fecal pellets, eggs, or mite (Fig. 6).

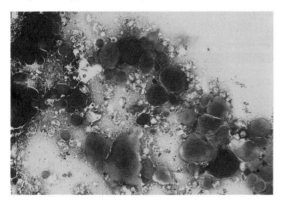

FIGURE 5. A positive Tzanck preparation demonstrating large multinucleated acantholytic keratinocytes. The nuclei of normal keratinocytes are the size of neutrophils, which are also seen in this preparation. (Courtesy of James E. Fitzpatrick, MD.)

10. How do you diagnose mite bites acquired from an animal?

Clinically, patients present with pruritic red bumps, most commonly on the arms, breasts, and abdomen. The most common sources of these animal mites are cats infested with *Cheyletiella* species. This nonburrowing mite exhibits "bite and run" tactics, so it is not likely to be found on the patient's body. The key to making the diagnosis is to have the cat examined by a veterinarian who is familiar with these parasites. The diagnosis is established by a cellophane tape preparation taken from the cat, dog, or rabbit demonstrating either the six-legged larval form or the eight-legged adult. Unlike the scabies mite, *Cheyletiella* has well-developed, claw-like, palpal mouth parts.

11. How do you diagnose lice infestations?

Lice infestation is caused by *Pediculus humanus capitis* (head louse), *P. humanus corporis* (body louse), or *Phthirus pubis* (pubic louse). Lice can be identified by eye or using a hand lens but they can be very difficult to locate. If body lice infestation is suspected, examination of the seams of clothing is more likely to be diagnostic than examining the skin. Lice will appear as brownish-gray specks. Head and pubic lice are more often seen in hairy areas and are often found with their mouthparts embedded in the skin with outstretched claws grasping hairs on either side. Usually more numerous are nits (eggs), which are white-gray oval structures smaller than 1 mm in size that are firmly attached to the hair shaft. Eggs that are near the junction of the hair shaft and the skin are indicative of active or recent infection. Since hair casts are white and may resemble nits, it is sometimes necessary to examine possible nits under the microscope to prove the diagnosis.

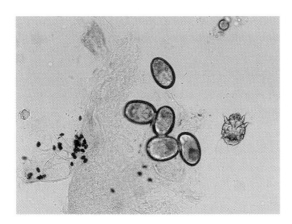

FIGURE 6. A positive scraping for scabies showing an immature mite, eggs, and numerous fecal pellets. (Courtesy of James E. Fitzpatrick, MD.)

12. What is the diagnostic test of choice for a patient presenting with a suspected syphilitic chancre on his penis?

Dark-field examination of the chancre is the most specific test for the diagnosis of syphilis. This test is typically positive unless the patient has applied or ingested antibiotics. In addition to primary syphilis, darkfield microscopy can also be used to diagnose all the mucocutaneous lesions of secondary syphilis. It is less reliable for examining specimens from the mouth or rectum because of the high prevalence of commensal, nonpathogenic treponemes in these locations that may be mistaken for *Treponema pallidum,* the agent of syphilis.

The best specimens for darkfield examination are serous fluid expressed from the bases of the chancre following cleaning with sterile saline and clean gauze. The specimen then should be immediately evaluated for the organism's characteristic corkscrew morphology and flexing, hairpin motility. If a patient is suspected of having a syphilitic chancre and a darkfield is negative, it should be repeated at least once before the diagnosis is excluded. A darkfield examination offers immediate results and is a cheap test. However, it is often not available.

Fluorescent antibody microscopy offers a sensitive alternative and has the advantages that it does not require live organisms and it can be done on fixed slides. This technique utilizes antibodies to *T. pallidum*. It requires less expertise due to the high specificity of the antibody reagents, but this test is not widely available.

13. How is secondary syphilis diagnosed?

As with primary syphilis, the most specific test is darkfield microscopy or by special stains on skin biopsies. More often, screening tests for syphilis such as nontreponemal serologic tests for syphilis, usually a rapid plasma reagin (RPR) or a Venereal Disease Research Laboratory (VDRL) test, is ordered. Nontreponemal serologic tests for syphilis detect antibodies to reagin, a cholesterol-lecithin-cardiolipin antigen that cross-reacts with antibodies present in the sera of patients with syphilis. These antibodies are not specific for syphilis and should always be confirmed by a specific test for syphilis, usually a fluorescent treponemal antibody-absorption (FTA-ABS) or the microhemagglutination-*T. pallidum* (MHA-TP) test.

Nontreponemal serologic tests for syphilis are positive in almost all cases of secondary syphilis. False-negatives sometimes occur in patients with very high antibody titers because of antibody excess; this "prozone reaction" can be overcome by diluting the patient's serum. Adequate treatment causes the titer to decline to low titers or nonreactivity. If a patient with HIV infection gets syphilis, usually the RPR is significantly elevated. Uncommonly, seronegative primary and secondary syphilis have been reported in association with HIV infection.

14. How long do serologic tests for syphilis remain positive?

Nontreponemal test antibody titers (e.g., VDRL) are reported quantitatively in the form of the highest positive titer. This titer correlates with disease activity and treated patients may demonstrate negative results or very low titers. More than 50% of patients will be seronegative 1 year after treatment. A patient with a positive treponemal test (e.g., FTA-ABS) is less likely to revert to negative and only 24% of patients will be seronegative 1 year after treatment. Both treated and untreated patients may demonstrate positive serologic tests for the rest of their lives.

15. In a male patient with symptomatic gonococcal urethritis, how efficacious is a Gram stain of the exudate in comparison to a culture utilizing selective media for gonococcus?

A Gram stain of a urethral discharge in symptomatic males is an excellent method of diagnosing gonorrhea. A positive Gram stain showing multiple neutrophils, some containing clusters of gram-negative diplococci with the sides flattened toward one another, is cited as having a sensitivity of 98%. With such a Gram stain, a culture is expensive and adds little diagnostic yield (about 2%). Cultures are usually done in males with a urethritis and a negative or nondiagnostic Gram stain of the urethral exudate.

In women suspected of having gonorrhea, the site of choice for obtaining specimens is the endocervix. However, Gram-stained smears are relatively insensitive (30–60%), and their interpretation is difficult. A culture on selective media is essential to diagnose gonorrhea in women.

16. What is the best way to diagnose allergic contact dermatitis?

The diagnostic test of choice is a properly applied and correctly interpreted **patch test.** Contact dermatitis is divided into irritant or allergic subtypes. Irritant contact dermatitis is not immunologically mediated and is due to chemical damage of the skin. For example, excessive handwashing or exposure to battery acid will involve almost everyone exposed in such fashion. On the other hand, allergic contact dermatitis is immunologically mediated and is an acquired sensitivity that affects only certain individuals.

17. How are patch tests applied?

The suspected allergen is usually placed in an appropriate vehicle in an appropriate concentration. The patch test allergens are usually purchased in prepared forms, but less common allergens can be prepared individually. The allergens are placed in special wells that are then taped against the skin of the back for 48 hours and then removed. It is important to instruct patients to keep the testing area completely dry. This skin area is then examined 24–72 hours after the patch is removed for a reading. A strong positive reaction has erythema, infiltration, papules, and vesicles. A bullous reaction is extremely positive. Interpretation of patch tests and correlation with the clinical disease are complex and usually performed only by dermatologists.

18. In what diseases is a skin biopsy helpful?

A skin biopsy with routine hematoxylin-eosin staining is the best diagnostic technique for many cutaneous neoplasms that cannot be diagnosed visually. It is also helpful in many inflammatory skin disorders, especially those in which a specific diagnosis cannot be made from clinical examination, blood tests, and scrapings of the skin. The skin is readily available for biopsy, and specimens may also be submitted for immunofluorescence, electron microscopy, special stains, cultures, and polymerase chain reaction studies.

19. When are shave biopsies indicated?

The choice of the biopsy technique requires knowledge of basic dermatology, i.e., where the pathology is likely to be located. A shave biopsy is usually the most superficial of the skin biopsies and particularly useful when the lesion is in or close to the epidermis. A shave biopsy is best for pedunculated, papular, or otherwise exophytic lesions. It is particularly useful for diagnosis of basal cell and squamous cell carcinomas, seborrheic keratoses, warts, intradermal nevi, and pyogenic granulomas. Shave biopsies are usually poor choices for most inflammatory skin conditions. Unlike punch biopsies, shave biopsies only require a clean and not sterile field and do not require sutures.

20. What are the indications for punch biopsies?

A punch biopsy is a round knife that takes a cylinder of tissue including the epidermis, dermis, and sometimes subcutaneous fat. Although punch biopsies from 2–10 mm in diameter can be used, the most common diameter is 4 mm. A 6-mm punch biopsy is particularly useful if the specimen is to be divided for culture or other procedures. When splitting the biopsy, the specimen is cut through the dermal rather than the epidermal side to reduce crush artifact. A 6-mm punch biopsy of the skin is also helpful in the diagnosis of cutaneous T-cell lymphoma and for scalp biopsies, where a good sampling of follicles is sometimes necessary. The surgical defect left by punch biopsies may be allowed to heal in secondarily, but most dermatologists close the defect with a single suture.

21. What are the indications for an excisional or incisional biopsy?

Excisional or incisional biopsies are usually elliptical in shape and typically deeper than punch biopsies. An **excisional biopsy** is the complete removal of a lesion down into the fat, followed by layered closure of the skin. It is particularly helpful in the complete removal of malignancies, such as malignant melanoma, basal cell carcinoma, and squamous cell carcinoma. Excisional biopsies can also be performed when the cosmetic result is felt to be superior to that with a punch biopsy.

An **incisional biopsy** is the incomplete or partial removal of a lesion down into the fat, followed by a layered closure of the skin. If a suspected malignancy is felt to be too large to remove with simple surgery, an incisional biopsy is used to remove the thickest portion for diagnostic pathologic examination. It is also useful for diagnosing panniculitis, sclerotic or atrophic lesions in which it is important to compare normal adjacent skin to that of the lesion (e.g., scleroderma), and lesions with active expanding borders such pyoderma gangrenosum.

22. Define and describe direct immunofluorescence of the skin.

Direct immunofluorescence (DIF) of the skin is a histologic stain for antibodies or other tissue proteins in skin biopsy specimens. A tissue sample (skin) obtained from the patient is immediately frozen in liquid nitrogen or placed in special media to preserve the immunoreactants. Arrangements should be made to ensure proper and timely transport to the immunofluorescence laboratory. Once received, the tissue is sectioned and then incubated with antibodies to human immunoglobulins or complement components that have been tagged with a fluorescent molecule to allow their visualization. The samples are then examined with a fluorescence microscope, where fluorescence indicates that immunoreactants were deposited in the patient's tissue. The specific immunoreactants present, and the pattern and intensity of staining, are used to determine the diseases most likely to be associated with the DIF findings.

23. Name some skin diseases in which DIF is helpful in making a diagnosis.

Many of the immunobullous diseases are associated with specific DIF findings, including bullous pemphigoid, herpes gestationis, cicatricial pemphigoid, epidermolysis bullosa acquisita, dermatitis herpetiformis, linear IgA bullous dermatosis, and the various types of pemphigus. In addition, DIF may be helpful in evaluating cutaneous and systemic lupus erythematosus, other collagen vascular diseases, vasculitis such as Henoch-Schönlein purpura (Fig. 7), and certain porphyrias.

24. How does indirect immunofluorescence of the skin differ from direct immunofluorescence of the skin?

Indirect immunofluorescence studies examine for the presence of circulating autoantibodies in the serum, in contrast to direct immunofluorescence that examines for the presence of autoantibodies deposited in the skin. The serum from the patient is incubated with an appropriate normal substrate such as monkey esophagus, rat bladder, or human skin. The substrate is incubated with fluorescein-labeled antibodies directed against the antibody in the tissue. The specimen is then examined under a fluorescent microscope. By running this test at various dilutions, the amount of circulating antibody can be determined and reported in the form of a titer. Titers are useful in some diseases (e.g., pemphigus vulgaris) in determining the disease activity and treatment.

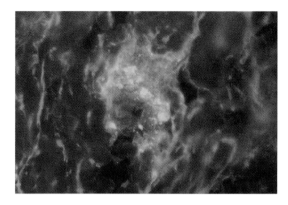

FIGURE 7. Direct immunofluorescent study demonstrating granular deposits of IgA within a blood vessel of a patient with Henoch-Schönlein purpura. (Courtesy of James E. Fitzpatrick, MD.)

25. How are bacterial skin cultures performed and when are they useful?

Bacterial cultures are useful when active infection of the skin is suspected. Bacterial cultures demonstrate high yields in superficial infections such as impetigo, ecthyma, and infected ulcers and low yields in cellulitis. When culturing superficial infections, the involved area should first be cleaned with an alcohol pad and then thoroughly swabbed. A higher concentration of bacteria may be found at the point of maximal inflammation. The best results in cellulitis are obtained when the leading edge is injected with nonbacteriostatic saline using a 20-gauge needle mounted on a tuberculin syringe. The aspirate may be sent for culture while still in the syringe if it can be taken to the laboratory immediately or the aspirated material may be submitted in a bacterial culturette.

BIBLIOGRAPHY

1. Arndt KA: Operative procedures. In Manual of Dermatologic Therapeutics with Essentials of Diagnosis, 4th ed. Boston, Little, Brown and Co., 1989, pp 171–180.
2. Buntin DM, et al: Sexually transmitted diseases: Viruses and ectoparasites. J Am Acad Dermatol 25:527–534, 1991.
3. Dahl MV: Clinical Immunodermatology, 2nd ed. Chicago, Year Book Medical Publishers, 1988.
4. Fisher A: Contact Dermatitis, 3rd ed. Philadelphia, Lea & Febiger, 1986, pp 9–29.
5. Fitzpatrick TB, Bernhard JD: The structure of skin lesions and fundamentals of diagnosis. In Fitzpatrick TB, Eisen AZ, Wolff K, et al (eds): Dermatology in General Medicine, 4th ed. McGraw-Hill, New York, 1993, pp 27–55.
6. Grossman MC, Silvers DN: The Tzanck smear: Can dermatologists accurately interpret it? J Am Acad Dermatol 27:403–405, 1992.
7. Habif TP: Clinical Dermatology: A Color Guide to Diagnosis and Therapy, 3rd ed. St. Louis, Mosby, 1996, pp 242–247.
8. Head E: Laboratory diagnosis of the superficial fungal infections. Dermatol Clin 2:93–108, 1984.
9. Hutchinson CM, Hook EW: Syphilis in adults. Med Clin North Am 74:1389–1416, 1990.
10. Judson FN: Gonorrhea. Med Clin North Am 74:1353–1366, 1990.
11. Lefler E, Haim S, Merzbach D: Evaluation of direct microscopic examination versus culture in the diagnosis of superficial fungal infections. Mykosen 24:102–106, 1981.
12. Lucky AW: Epidemiology, diagnosis, and management of tinea capitis in the 1980s. Pediatr Dermatol 2:226–228, 1985.
13. Martin AG, Kobayashi GS: Yeast infections: Candidiasis, pityriasis (tinea) versicolor. In Fitzpatrick TB, Eisen AZ, Wolff K, et al (eds): Dermatology in General Medicine, 4th ed. New York, McGraw-Hill, 1993, pp 2462–2467.
14. Nahass GT, et al: Comparison of Tzanck smear, viral culture, and DNA diagnostic methods in detection of herpes simplex and varicella-zoster infection. JAMA 268:2541–2544, 1992.
15. Taplin D, Zaias N, Rebell G, Blank H: Isolation and recognition of dermatophytes on a new medium (DTM). Arch Dermatol 99:203–209, 1969.

II. Inherited Disorders

4. DISORDERS OF KERATINIZATION

Ann M. Leibold, M.D.

1. What are the ichthyosiform dermatoses?

The ichthyosiform dermatoses refer to a heterogeneous group of disorders presenting with **excessive scaling of the skin.** The term *ichthyosis* is derived from the Greek root *ichthy*, meaning fish. The inherited forms of the ichthyoses are most common, although the condition can occur secondary to other diseases.

2. What features help differentiate the most common ichthyoses?

Both clinical and pathologic features are helpful in the diagnosis of specific ichthyoses. Onset of symptoms, sites of skin changes, and skin biopsy results can be very helpful data that are easy to obtain.

Ichthyosis vulgaris (Fig. 1, *A–B*) usually develops around puberty, involves the palms and soles with dryness and hyperlinearity, spares the flexural areas, and, on skin biopsy, demonstrates a decreased granular layer associated with moderate hyperkeratosis. Cutaneous involvement resembles mild dry skin with follicular accentuation (keratosis pilaris). One-half of affected patients have atopy or a family history of atopy.

X-linked ichthyosis, in contrast, is present by 1 year of age, spares the palms and soles, affects the posterior neck with "dirty"-appearing scales (Fig. 1, *C*), and demonstrates a normal granular layer with hyperkeratosis on skin biopsy. The skin changes gradually worsen with age, with the neck, face, and trunk ultimately developing thick, brown scales. Hypogonadism and corneal opacities are frequent associations.

Clinical Features of the Major Inherited Ichthyoses

DISORDER	ONSET	TYPE OF SCALE	SITES	HISTOLOGY	OTHER FINDINGS	DEFECT
Ichthyosis vulgaris	Childhood	Fine	Palms, soles, extensors	Diminished granular layer	Atopy, keratosis pilaris	Deficient filaggrin
X-linked ichthyosis	Birth or infancy	Coarse, brown	Neck, face, trunk, flexors	Normal granular layer	Corneal opacities, cryptorchidism	Deficient steroid sulfatase
Epidermolytic hyperkeratosis	Birth	Erosions/bullae coarse, verrucous later	Generalized, esp. flexors	Epidermolytic hyperkeratosis	Foul odor, pyogenic infections	Defect in keratins 1 and 10
Congenital ichthyosiform erythroderma (CIE)	Birth	Fine, white, with erythroderma	Generalized with flexors, palms, soles	Increased granular layer, focal parakeratosis	Ectropion, nail dystrophy, poor growth, alopecia	Unknown
Lamellar ichthyosis	Birth	Platelike, dark, erythroderma	Generalized with flexors, palms, soles	Increased granular layer, hyperkeratosis	Same as CIE	Deficient transglutaminase I
Harlequin fetus	Birth	Massive thick plates	Generalized	Massive compact hyperkeratosis	Ectropion, eclabium, ear and limb deformities	Abnormal lamellar granules (?)

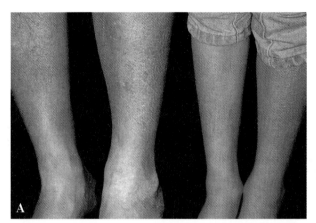

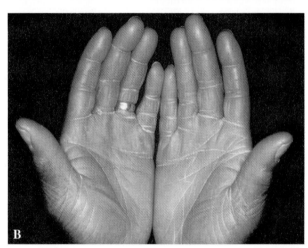

FIGURE 1. *A,* Grandfather and granddaughter with ichthyosis vulgaris. *B,* Palmar hyperkeratosis, a finding often associated with ichthyosis vulgaris. *C,* X-linked ichthyosis, showing characteristic coarse, brown scales. *D,* Young child with congenital ichthyosiform erythroderma demonstrating diffuse erythema and scale. (*A, B,* and *D* courtesy of James E. Fitzpatrick, MD.)

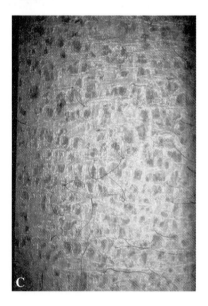

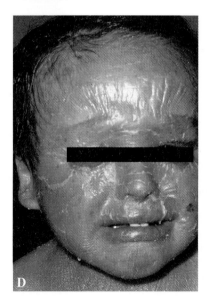

3. Name the hereditary syndromes presenting with ichthyosis as a component.

Hereditary Syndromes with Ichthyosis

SYNDROME	CLINICAL FEATURES	SKIN FINDINGS
Conradi-Hünermann disease (chondrodysplasia punctata)	Chondrodysplasia punctata, limb defects, cataracts, cardiovascular and renal abnormalities, mental retardation	CIE, whorled hyperpigmentation, palmoplantar keratoderma
CHILD syndrome	Hemidysplasia and limb defects with sharp midline demarcation	CIE
Sjögren-Larsson syndrome	Spasticity, mental retardation, retinal degeneration	Lamellar scales
Chanarin-Dorfman syndrome (neutral lipid storage disease)	Fatty liver, myopathy, cataracts, deafness, CNS defects	CIE
Netherton's syndrome	Trichorrhexis invaginata (bamboo hairs), atopy, aminoaciduria	Ichthyosis linearis circumflexa
Refsum's disease	Cerebellar ataxia, peripheral neuropathy, retinitis pigmentosa	Like ichthyosis vulgaris
Rud's syndrome	Hypogonadism, mental retardation, seizures, short stature, polyneuropathy	Like lamellar ichthyosis
Multiple sulfatase deficiency	Metachromatic leukodystrophy, hepatosplenomegaly	Like X-linked ichthyosis
Trichothiodystrophy (PIBIDS)	Photosensitivity, ichthyosis, brittle hair, intellectual impairment, decreased fertility, short stature	CIE
KID syndrome	Keratitis, neurosensory deafness, alopecia	Grainy, spiculated scaling

4. How common are congenital ichthyoses?

Inheritance and Incidence of the Major Congenital Ichthyoses

DISORDER	INHERITANCE	INCIDENCE
Ichthyosis vulgaris	Autosomal dominant	1:250
X-linked ichthyosis	X-linked recessive	1:6,000
Epidermolytic hyperkeratosis	Autosomal dominant	1:300,000
Congenital ichthyosiform erythroderma (CIE)	Autosomal recessive	1:100,000
Lamellar ichthyosis	Autosomal recessive	1:300,000
Harlequin fetus	Autosomal recessive	Rare

5. Which congenital ichthyoses present in the neonatal period?

Although ichthyosis vulgaris and X-linked ichthyosis typically do not cause skin changes until later in infancy or childhood, most other types are evident in the newborn period. The presentation in these infants is variable. A collodion baby is one dramatic presentation. Infants with congenital ichthyosiform erythroderma (CIE) may appear diffusely red with a fine, white scale (Fig. 1, *D*). Epidermolytic hyperkeratosis presents with widespread denuded areas and bullae—hence its older name, bullous CIE; the hyperkeratotic component develops later. The most severely affected infant, the harlequin fetus, is born with massive hyperkeratotic plates associated with limb deformities, rudimentary ears, ectropion, and eclabium. These infants rarely survive beyond the first week.

6. What is a collodion baby?

A collodion baby is a newborn infant whose skin looks like a "baked apple," with a shiny, tough, membranous-like covering. This term describes a phenotype that occurs in several types of ichthyosis. Although CIE is the most common underlying condition, lamellar ichthyosis, Netherton's syndrome, and Conradi's syndrome may also present as a collodion baby. Collodion babies are at increased risk for infections and fluid and electrolyte imbalances due to cutaneous fissures and impaired barrier function of the skin. Treatment in a high humidity environment allows gradual sloughing of the collodion membrane. Manual debridement and keratolytics are not recommended. Topical application of vitamin D analogs, calcipotriene and calcipotriol, may be beneficial. The use of acetreitin in harlequin ichthyosis may be life-saving, although fraught with side effects.

7. Name several conditions associated with acquired ichthyosis.

Dry, scaling skin may have a number of nonhereditary causes, including malignancies, nutritional disorders, metabolic disorders, drug therapy, and other miscellaneous conditions. The pathogenesis of the skin changes associated with malignancies is unknown, although reduced dermal lipid synthesis, malabsorption, and immunologic abnormalities have been identified. Many of the nutritional problems involve abnormal vitamin A metabolism. Chronic renal failure results in hypervitaminosis A which produces rough, scaly skin. Hypovitaminosis A produces follicular hyperkeratosis and dry skin. Medications produce ichthyosis by various mechanisms. Niacin, triparanol, butyrophenones, dixyramine, and nafoxidine alter cholesterol synthesis. Cimetidine and the retinoids are antiandrogenic and reduce sebum secretion.

Conditions Associated with Acquired Ichthyosis

MEDICATIONS	MALIGNANCIES	NUTRITIONAL DISORDERS	METABOLIC DISORDERS	MISCELLANEOUS DISORDERS
Butyrophenones	Non-Hodgkin's lymphoma	Essential fatty acid deficiency	Chronic renal failure	Systemic lupus erythematosus
Cimetidine	Hodgkin's lymphoma	Hypervitaminosis A	Hypothyroidism	Sarcoidosis
Clofazimine	Carcinoma of the breast, lung, cervix, colon	Hypovitaminosis A	Panhypopituitarism	Leprosy
Dixyrazine	Mycosis fungoides	Kwashiorkor		Dermatomyositis
Isoniazid	Leukemia	Pellagra		HIV infection
Nafoxidine	Lymphosarcoma			Polycythemia
Niacin	Rhabdomyosarcoma			Haber's syndrome
Triparanol	Kaposi's sarcoma			
Allopurinol	Leiomyosarcoma			
Retinoids	Multiple myeloma			

8. Are laboratory tests helpful in the diagnosis of ichthyoses?

In general, a widely available laboratory test for the diagnosis of ichthyoses is lacking. Other than skin pathology, **ichthyosis vulgaris** is not diagnosable by laboratory testing. Cultured keratinocytes will demonstrate absent or reduced filaggrin in keratohyalin granules and fail to react to antifilaggrin monoclonal antibodies by light microscopy, but this is not a widely available test. **X-linked ichthyosis** is caused by a deficiency of steroid sulfatase. The enzyme can be assayed in cultured keratinocytes, fibroblasts, leukocytes, or scales. Low levels of cholesterol sulfate in blood can be detected by the increased mobility of low-density lipoproteins on serum protein electrophoresis. Female heterozygotes can be detected by Southern blot hybridization from peripheral blood leukocytes. The gene has been mapped to the short arm of X chromosome (Xp22.3).

Several of the rare ichthyosiform syndromes are associated with enzyme deficiencies detectable in cell cultures. For instance, **Conradi-Hünermann disease** is associated with a peroxisomal enzyme deficiency (dihydroxyacetone phosphate acyltransferase), **Sjögren-Larsson** syndrome involves a deficiency of fatty alcohol:NAD$^+$ oxidoreductase (FAO), and **Refsum's disease** is associated with a deficiency of α-phytanic oxidase. Abnormal fatty acid metabolism in **Chanarin-Dorfman syndrome** results in triglyceride vacuoles identifiable in polymorphonuclear cells and monocytes in peripheral blood smears.

9. Is prenatal diagnosis possible?

Prenatal diagnosis is available for many of the congenital ichthyoses if one is suspected based on family history. **Fetal skin biopsy** performed at 19–21 weeks will demonstrate early development of a thickened stratum corneum, normally not present until 24 weeks. This is useful in lamellar ichthyosis, epidermolytic hyperkeratosis, Sjögren-Larsson syndrome, and harlequin fetus. Lamellar ichthyosis may also be detected via a transglutaminase activity assay from a fetal skin sample. Epidermolytic hyperkeratosis, known to result from mutations in keratins 1 and 10, can be detected by direct gene sequencing done on **chorionic villus sampling** in the second trimester. Cultured chorionic villi cells or amniocytes will demonstrate the enzyme deficiency in X-linked ichthyosis, Sjögren-Larsson syndrome, and Refsum's disease. A high ratio of maternal urinary estrogen precursors in a male fetus also suggests the diagnosis of X-linked ichthyosis. Trichothiodystrophy can be identified by unscheduled DNA synthesis in cultured amniocytes exposed to UV light.

10. How is ichthyosis treated?

Acquired ichthyosis usually improves with treatment of the underlying condition. **Congenital ichthyosis** is difficult to treat, especially in its severe forms. Topical emollients containing glycolic acid, lactic acid, urea, or glycerin may partially improve dryness and scaling. Topical tretinoin (Retin-A) is effective but poorly tolerated due to irritation. Oral retinoids, including isotretinoin, etretinate, and acetretin, are very effective, but relapses after treatment cessation are common. The use of oral retinoids is limited by major side effects including teratogenic effects, and chronic use, which is often required in congenital disorders, is associated with hyperostoses. Blistering may indicate bacterial infection and should be cultured and managed with oral antibiotics. One open study demonstrated oral liarozole fumarate, a cytochrome P-450 inhibitor, to be efficacious and well tolerated in the treatment of several types of ichthyosis. The foul odor present in epidermolytic hyperkeratosis may be due to bacterial colonization and can be improved by the use of an antibacterial soap.

11. What is Hailey-Hailey disease?

Hailey-Hailey disease, also known as benign familial pemphigus, is an autosomal dominant condition characterized histologically by acantholysis (loss of cohesion between keratinocytes) and clinically by patches of minute vesicles that break and form crusted erosions.

12. How does Hailey-Hailey disease present?

Skin changes consisting of localized patches of minute vesicles and erosions start in areas of friction, usually the neck, groin, and axilla (Figs. 2 and 3). Patches spread peripherally with serpiginous borders and show central healing with hyperpigmentation or granular vegetations. Onset of lesions is often delayed until the second or third decade. Associated symptoms include itching, pain, and foul odor.

13. Do any factors exacerbate the skin changes?

Physical trauma and heat or sweating worsen skin lesions of Hailey-Hailey disease. Patients have reported the onset of new lesions within hours of wearing restrictive shirt collars, tight bra straps, and ECG electrodes. Most patients report worsening in the summer.

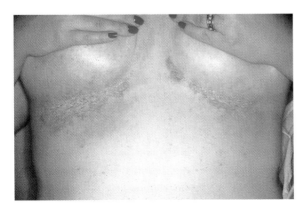

FIGURE 2. Patient with Hailey-Hailey disease demonstrating characteristic involvement of flexural areas of inframammary crease.

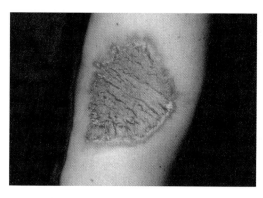

FIGURE 3. Hailey-Hailey disease, showing a patch of minute vesicles, erosions, and crusting in the antecubital fossa.

14. Which diseases may be confused with Hailey-Hailey disease?

Eczema, impetigo, fungal or viral infections, pemphigus vulgaris, pemphigus vegetans, or Darier's disease. The recurring, chronic nature of Hailey-Hailey disease, lack of oral and ocular involvement, and intertriginous predilection help to differentiate these conditions.

15. How is Hailey-Hailey disease treated?

Topical steroids are generally helpful in relieving burning and itching. Both *Staphylococcus aureus* and *Candida albicans* infections may exacerbate lesions, requiring treatment with appropriate antibacterial and antifungal agents. Recalcitrant cases have been treated with carbon dioxide laser, dermabrasion, topical cyclosporine, dapsone, vitamin E, PUVA, methotrexate, thalidomide, and vitamin D analogs, with variable results.

16. What is Darier's disease?

Darier's disease, also known as keratosis follicularis and Darier-White disease, is a dominantly inherited disorder of keratinization that begins in the first or second decade of life. Recent studies suggest that it is due to mutations in chromosome 12q23–q24.1, which encodes a calcium ATPase pump (SERCA2). Microscopically, it is characterized by distinctive changes of both premature keratinization and acantholysis.

17. How do you diagnose Darier's disease?

The diagnosis is based on clinical manifestations and histologic features. The primary lesions are flesh-colored papules that may coalesce into plaques and develop tan, scaly crusts (Fig. 4).

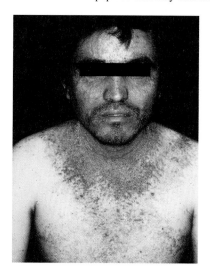

FIGURE 4. Darier's disease. Confluent, crusted papules involving the face, scalp, and chest.

These keratotic papules are located in "seborrheic areas," such as the chest, back, ears, nasolabial folds, scalp, and groin. Thick, foul-smelling, warty masses can develop. Flat, wartlike papules may be seen on the dorsa of distal extremities, and 1–2-mm punctate keratoses may be present on the palms and soles. Oral and rectal mucosal surfaces often demonstrate small, cobblestone-like papules. The diagnosis can be confirmed by skin biopsies that reveal acantholytic dyskeratosis.

18. Are there any nail or hair changes in Darier's disease?

Nails demonstrate longitudinal ridging, as well as red and white longitudinal streaks. Distal nail edges show V-shaped notching and subungual thickening. Rarely, alopecia results from extensive scalp involvement.

19. Is Darier's disease difficult to treat?

Complete clearing of Darier's disease is rare. Soothing moisturizers containing urea or lactic acid reduce scaling and irritation. Salicylic acid in a propylene glycol gel and topical tretinoids are also effective in reducing crusts and scale, although retinoids may need to be initiated on an alternate-day schedule in combination with mid-potency topical steroids to minimize irritation. Aggravating factors such as heat, humidity, sunlight, and lithium should be avoided. Infection should be prevented with antibacterial soaps and treated with antibiotics. Oral retinoids are effective, but toxicity limits their use; intermittent use may be preferable, such as starting the medication before a summer holiday to prevent sun-induced exacerbations. Recalcitrant verrucous lesions have been treated with dermabrasion, carbon dioxide laser vaporization, and surgery.

BIBLIOGRAPHY

1. Akiyama M: Severe congenital ichthyosis of the neonate. Int J Dermatol 37:722–728, 1998.
2. Aoki T: 1-Alpha,24-dihydroxyvitamin D3 (tacalcitol) is effective against Hailey-Hailey disease both in vivo and in vitro. Br J Dermatol 139:897–901, 1998.
3. Burge S: Management of Darier's disease. Clin Exp Dermatol 24:53–56, 1999.
4. Burge SM: Darier-White disease: A review of the clinical features in 163 patients. J Am Acad Dermatol 27:40–50, 1992.
5. Burge SM: Hailey-Hailey disease: The clinical features, response to treatment and prognosis. Br J Dermatol 126:275–282, 1992.
6. Hashimoto K: Harlequin fetus with abnormal lamellar granules and giant mitochondria. J Cutan Pathol 19:247–252, 1992.
7. Homayoun A: Acquired ichthyosis and related conditions. Int J Dermatol 23:458–461, 1984.
8. Jitsukawa K: Topical cyclosporine in chronic benign familial pemphigus. J Am Acad Dermatol 27:625–626, 1992.
9. Kartamaa M: Familial benign chronic pemphigus (Hailey-Hailey disease): Treatment with carbon dioxide laser vaporization. Arch Dermatol 128:646–648, 1992.
10. Kirtschig G: Treatment of Hailey-Hailey disease by dermabrasion. J Am Acad Dermatol 28:784–786, 1993.
11. Lucker GP, Heremans AM, Boegheim PJ, et al: Oral treatment of ichthyosis by the cytochrome P-450 inhibitor liarozole. Br J Dermatol 136:71–75, 1997.
12. McGuire J: The biologic basis of the ichthyoses. Pediatr Dermatol 4:67–78, 1986.
13. Paller A:. Laboratory tests for ichthyosis. Dermatol Clin 12:99–107, 1994.
14. Rizzo WB: Sjögren-Larsson. Semin Dermatol 12:210–218, 1993.
15. Rothnagel JA: Prenatal diagnosis of epidermolytic hyperkeratosis by direct gene sequencing. J Invest Dermatol 102:13–16, 1994.
16. Savary JB: Prenatal diagnosis in a subset of trichothiodystrophy patients defective in DNA repair. Br J Dermatol 127:485–491, 1992.
17. Schachner LA: Pediatric Dermatology, 2nd ed. New York, Churchill Livingstone, 1995.
18. Shwayder T: All about ichthyosis. Pediatr Clin North Am 38:835–857, 1991.
19. Tabsh K: Sjögren-Larsson syndrome: Technique and timing of prenatal diagnosis. Obstet Gynecol 82:700–703, 1993.
20. Williams ML: Genetically transmitted, generalized disorders of cornification. Dermatol Clin 5:155–178, 1987.

5. NEUROCUTANEOUS DISORDERS

Anne R. Halbert, MBBS, FACD

NEUROFIBROMATOSIS

1. What are the two most common forms of neurofibromatosis?

Neurofibromatosis type 1 (NF-1, von Recklinghausen's disease) and neurofibromatosis type 2 (NF-2, central or bilateral acoustic neurofibromatosis). NF-1 accounts for 85–90% of all cases of neurofibromatosis and affects approximately 1 in 3000 individuals. NF-2 is a genetically distinct entity with a prevalence of only 1 in 50,000.

2. Outline the diagnostic criteria for NF-1.

The diagnosis can be made if two or more of the following criteria are present:
- 6 or more café-au-lait macules of > 5 mm in greatest diameter in prepubertal children and > 15 mm diameter in postpubertal individuals
- 2 or more neurofibromas of any type or 1 plexiform neurofibroma
- Freckling in axillary or inguinal regions
- 2 or more Lisch nodules
- Optic glioma
- Distinctive osseous lesion, such as sphenoid dysplasia or thinning of long bone cortex, with or without pseudoarthrosis
- First-degree relative with NF-1

3. What are the diagnostic criteria for NF-2?

The diagnostic criteria are met by an individual who has either of the following:
- Bilateral acoustic neuromas
- First-degree relative with NF-2 and either:
1. Unilateral VIII nerve mass *or*
2. Two of the following: neurofibroma, meningioma, glioma, schwannoma, or juvenile posterior subcapsular lenticular opacity.

4. What is the inheritance of NF-1?

The inheritance is autosomal dominant, with 50% of cases representing new mutations. The NF-1 gene has been localized to chromosome 17. (Neurofibromatosis has 17 letters, the same number as the chromosome.)

5. What is the earliest skin sign of NF-1?

Café-au-lait macules. These sharply defined, light brown patches may be present at birth but more commonly start appearing in the first year of life (Fig. 1). They are noted initially by 4 years or less in all affected children and within the first year in 82% of cases.

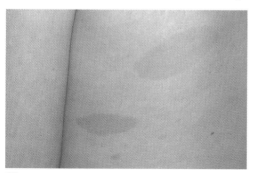

FIGURE 1. Multiple café-au-lait macules of > 5 mm diameter.

6. What is Crowe's sign? When does it develop?

Crowe's sign is diffuse freckling of the axillae or other body folds. It develops in 70% of NF-1 patients, usually in middle childhood.

7. When do peripheral neurofibromas appear in NF-1?

Peripheral neurofibromas usually start to develop during puberty but increase in size and number in early adult life. They are soft, pink or flesh-colored papules, nodules, or tumors mainly distributed over the trunk and limbs (Fig. 2). Multiple neurofibromas can develop or existing neurofibromas may enlarge during pregnancy. This is an important fact that should be discussed during genetic counseling.

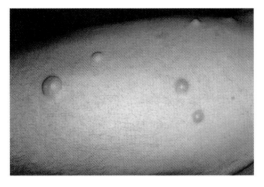

FIGURE 2. Multiple peripheral neurofibromas.

8. What is a plexiform neurofibroma?

It is a diffuse, elongated neurofibroma occurring along the course of a nerve, usually the trigeminal or upper cervical nerves. Mostly present at birth, these lesions may be associated with overlying skin hypertrophy, hyperpigmentation, or increased hair and may cause considerable cosmetic disfigurement (Fig. 3).

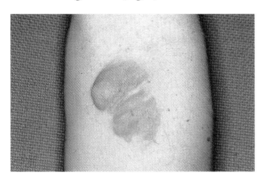

FIGURE 3. Soft bag-like lesion of a plexiform neurofibroma.

9. What are Lisch nodules?

Melanocytic hamartomas of the iris. When multiple, these lesions are pathognomonic of NF-1, occurring in > 90% of patients by the second decade of life. They are best seen on slit-lamp examination.

10. What is the most common CNS tumor occurring in NF-1?

Optic glioma. Other CNS tumors include astrocytomas, schwannomas, and non-neoplastic hamartomas. Epilepsy occurs in 7.5% of patients, frequently due to these underlying focal lesions.

11. How common is intellectual impairment in NF-1?

Nearly 30% of patients have mild intellectual impairment or learning difficulties; 3% have moderate to severe retardation.

12. What are the most common skeletal abnormalities in NF-1?

Macrocephaly	(45%)
Short stature	(34%)
Kyphoscoliosis	(11.5%)
Pseudoarthroses of tibia or fibulae	(1%)

13. Apart from CNS tumors, what other neoplasia occur in NF-1?
The most common malignancy is a neurofibrosarcoma (3–6%), which usually develops in sub-cutaneous or plexiform neurofibromas. Other neoplasia include pheochromocytoma (1%), leukemia, Wilms' tumor, and rhabdomyosarcoma.

14. How frequently should patients with NF-1 be assessed? What should this assessment include?
Children should be assessed every 6 months, and adults annually. The clinical examination should include a blood pressure measurement (hypertension may occur secondary to renovascular stenosis or pheochromocytoma) and a full neurologic examination. Children also require regular surveillance for kyphoscoliosis, signs of precocious puberty or hypogonadism, and periodic developmental assessments. Investigations should be guided by symptoms or physical signs. Acromegaly, Addison's disease, gynecomastia, osteomalacia, and hyperparathyroidism have all been associated with NF-1. Magnetic resonance imaging (MRI) with gadolinium contrast is the most sensitive investigation for intracranial or spinal lesions. Pruritus can be a severe symptom and is probably associated with numerous mast cells present within the tumors. Ketotifen, a mast cell blocker, has been reported to be beneficial in the treatment of this frustrating symptom.

15. What is the most common manifestation of NF-2?
Bilateral acoustic neuromas are the most common manifestation of NF-2 and are present in > 90% of patients. Other neurologic tumors include meningiomas, schwannomas, and spinal cord ependymomas.

16. What is the inheritance of NF-2?
NF-2 has an autosomal dominant inheritance, with the defective gene on chromosome 22.

17. When do symptoms begin in NF-2?
Usually in the second decade of life or later.

18. Do patients with NF-2 have café-au-lait macules or peripheral neurofibromas?
Yes, but fewer than NF-1 patients. Less than six café-au-lait macules are usually present.

19. What is the characteristic ocular sign of NF-2?
Posterior subcapsular cataracts (50%). Unlike in NF-1, Lisch nodules or optic gliomas do not occur.

TUBEROUS SCLEROSIS

20. Tuberous sclerosis is also known as epiloia. What does this term mean?
Epiloia was a term coined from the diagnostic triad of *epi*lepsy, *lo*w *i*ntelligence, and *a*denoma sebaceum.

Triad of Tuberous Sclerosis

Epilepsy	60%
Mental retardation	40–60%
Skin signs	60–70%

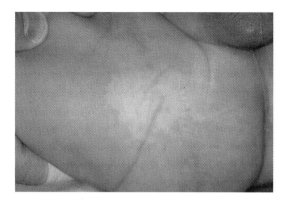

FIGURE 4. Ash-leaf macule in an infant.

21. What is the inheritance of tuberous sclerosis?
Inheritance is autosomal dominant, with high penetrance but variable expression. Up to 60% of cases are said to represent new mutations, but "normal" parents must undergo thorough clinical and radiologic evaluation to exclude subclinical disease.

22. Where are the genetic defects for tuberous sclerosis?
Genetic linkage analysis indicates that about 50% of families show linkage to chromosome 9 and 50% to chromosome 16.

23. What is the earliest skin sign of tuberous sclerosis?
Hypomelanotic macules (Fig. 4). Frequently present at birth or in early infancy, these lesions are a helpful sign in infants with convulsions. Best seen with Wood's lamp examination, they are polygonal or ash-leaf in shape, ranging in size from 1–3 cm and numbering 1–100. Occasionally, they are accompanied by 1–3-mm confetti-like white spots scattered over the trunk and limbs. Melanocytes are present in hypomelanotic macules, but there is abnormal melanin synthesis and impaired melanosome transfer from melanocytes to keratinocytes.

Common Skin Signs of Tuberous Sclerosis

Ash-leaf hypomelanotic macules
Facial angiofibromas
Periungual fibromas (Koenen's tumors)
Shagreen patch
Forehead fibromatous plaque

24. Adenoma sebaceum is a misnomer. What is the correct term for the facial lesions seen in tuberous sclerosis?
Angiofibromas. These lesions consist of hyperplastic blood vessels and collagen and are not tumors of sebaceous glands. Facial angiofibromas appear at 4–9 years of age and increase in size and number during puberty. They are firm, discrete, reddish papules of 1–10 mm, developing initially in the nasolabial folds and frequently progressing over the malar region, forehead, and chin (Fig. 5). Angiofibromas are frequently misdiagnosed as facial acne.

25. What are Koenen's tumors?
Subungual and periungual fibromas. These develop at or after puberty and present as firm, flesh-colored growths 5–10 mm long, projecting from the nailfolds and beneath the nail plate (Fig. 6).

26. What is a shagreen patch?
An irregularly thickened, slightly elevated, flesh-colored plaque consisting of collagen. Seen in tuberous sclerosis, it develops in later childhood or adolescence and is most commonly located over the lumbosacral area.

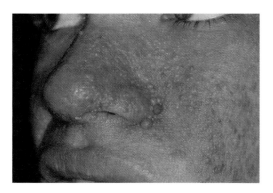

FIGURE 5. Facial angiofibromas in tuberous sclerosis (adenoma sebaceum).

27. Name the other typical sites for fibromatous tumors in tuberous sclerosis.

Firm, fibromatous plaques may develop on the forehead (Fig. 7), and fibromatous tumors are occasionally present on the gums and palate.

28. What are tubers, and where do they occur?

Tubers are potato-like nodules of glial proliferation and are the characteristic CNS lesion of tuberous sclerosis. They may occur anywhere in the cerebral cortex, basal ganglia, and ventricular walls (subependymal nodules), and their number and size correlate with clinical features of seizures and mental retardation. Cortical tubers are often isodense with normal brain tissue and are best detected with MRI. Subependymal nodules may calcify and are readily detectable with computed tomographic (CT) scanning. Fifty percent of plain skull x-rays taken in later childhood also reveal bilateral areas of calcification in the brain.

29. What signs of tuberous sclerosis may be revealed on fundoscopic examination?

Retinal hamartomas (phacomata) occur in 50% of patients. They may be seen as white streaks along vessels of the retina or elevated multinodular lesions near the optic disc.

30. Which cardiac abnormality is characteristic of tuberous sclerosis?

Congenital rhabdomyomas (50%). These tumors are due to abnormal differentiation of embryonic myocardium into atypical Purkinje cells. They are usually multiple and often clinically silent, although ventricular outflow obstruction may occur. They may regress later in childhood.

31. Can renal involvement occur in tuberous sclerosis?

Yes. Angiomyolipomas are common hamartomatous tumors in the kidney, consisting of blood vessels, smooth muscle, fat, and fibrous tissue. They may be multiple and bilateral and are usually asymptomatic. Renal cysts are also common.

32. What is the prognosis for patients with tuberous sclerosis?

The prognosis is variable and depends on the severity of the clinical manifestations. In severe cases, death may occur from epilepsy, infection, cardiac failure, or, rarely, pulmonary fibrosis.

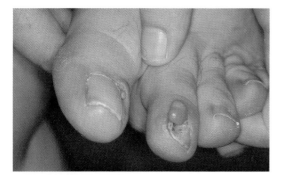

FIGURE 6. Koenen's tumor (periungual fibroma).

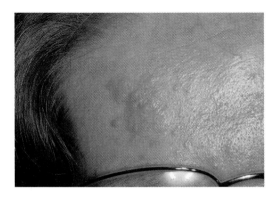

FIGURE 7. Fibromatous plaque on the forehead of a patient with tuberous sclerosis.

STURGE-WEBER SYNDROME

33. Name the two essential components of the Sturge-Weber syndrome.
A facial port wine stain and homolateral leptomeningeal angiomatosis.

34. What is the inheritance of the Sturge-Weber syndrome?
It is not inherited. It is a sporadic developmental malformation of the vasculature of the leptomeninges, facial dermal capillaries, and often, ocular vessels.

35. Where does the port wine stain most commonly occur in Sturge-Weber syndrome?
The port wine stain most commonly involves the areas innervated by the ophthalmic (V1) and maxillary (V2) divisions of the trigeminal nerve. In virtually all cases, some portion of the forehead, upper eyelid, and nasal root is involved (Fig. 8). The port wine stain may be bilateral and may involve nasal or oral mucosa. Port wine stains are present on the extremities or trunk in addition to the face in 40% of cases.

36. What are the complications of leptomeningeal angiomatosis?
The vascular malformation of the cerebral meninges becomes complicated by meningeal artery calcification, calcification of the subjacent cortex, and cerebral atrophy. This results in epilepsy in 75–90% of cases, mental retardation (particularly in those with severe epilepsy), and occasionally, contralateral hemiplegia.

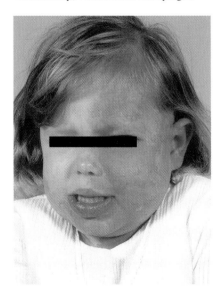

FIGURE 8. Sturge-Weber syndrome. The bilateral port wine stain involves the left V1, V2, and V3 regions and right V3.

37. When does epilepsy usually begin in the Sturge-Weber syndrome?

The onset is usually between the second and seventh months of life, although this is occasionally delayed until later childhood. Initially, partial motor seizures occur, but these tend to become generalized seizures as the child gets older.

38. Can the extent of neurologic involvement be predicted from the size of the facial port wine stain?

No. There is no correlation between extent of facial port wine stain, leptomeningeal angiomatosis, or degree of neurologic impairment.

39. What investigations confirm leptomeningeal angiomatosis?

CT scanning with contrast or MRI localizes the pial vascular anomalies and reveals intracranial calcification early in life. In later childhood (mean age, 7 years), a plain skull x-ray may reveal the typical double contoured, curvilinear, "tram tracks" of calcification.

40. Do ocular complications occur in the Sturge-Weber syndrome?

Ocular complications occur in 30–60% of cases and include capillary malformations of the conjunctiva, iris, and choroid (ipsilateral to the facial port wine stain), glaucoma, and megalocornea. These complications may be associated only with a facial port wine stain involving the V1 distribution and does not necessarily imply CNS involvement. Glaucoma most commonly begins in the first 2 years of life; hence, regular ophthalmologic review from birth is vital in patients with V1 facial port wine stains.

41. How can the facial port wine stain be treated?

The tunable pulsed dye laser (wavelength 577/585 nm) is the most effective treatment modality. Regular laser treatment may result in significant fading and also helps prevent the soft tissue hypertrophy that gradually develops with many port wine stains.

42. In what other neurocutaneous disorder does facial or occipitocervical port wine stain occur?

Von Hippel-Lindau disease. Other features of this autosomal dominant disorder may include bilateral retinal angiomatosis (50%); cerebellar, medullary, or spinal hemangioblastoma (40%); renal cell carcinoma (25%); and occasionally, pheochromocytoma.

ATAXIA-TELANGIECTASIA

43. What is the inheritance of ataxia-telangiectasia?

Autosomal recessive, with the defective gene on regions 22 and 23 of chromosome 11q.

44. What is the earliest clinical sign of ataxia-telangiectasia?

Progressive cerebellar ataxia, due to degeneration of Purkinje cells, is the earliest clinical manifestation and begins at age 12–18 months. Choreoathetoid movements, hypotonia, dysarthria, and abnormal eye movements gradually develop, and intelligence frequently declines.

45. Name the typical skin sign of ataxia-telangiectasia.

Mucocutaneous telangiectases. These begin on the bulbar conjunctiva and ears between 2–6 years of age and may progress to involve the periorbital skin, trunk, extremities, body folds, and other mucosal surfaces.

46. List the two most common causes of death in patients with ataxia-telangiectasia.

Severe respiratory infections and lymphoreticular malignancies. Thymic hypoplasia with humoral and cellular immunodeficiencies predisposes to infection; sinopulmonary infections with bronchiectasis and pneumonia are particularly common. DNA defects with increased spontaneous and x-ray-induced breaks and rearrangements predispose to lymphorecticular malignancies.

ACKNOWLEDGMENT

The clinical photographs were kindly provided by Drs. William Weston and Joseph Morelli.

BIBLIOGRAPHY

1. Dunn DW: Neurofibromatosis in childhood. Curr Probl Pediatr 17:445–497, 1987.
2. Enjolras O, Riche MC, Merland JJ: Facial port wine stains and Sturge-Weber syndrome. Pediatrics 76:48–51, 1985.
3. Huson SM: Recent developments in the diagnosis and management of neurofibromatosis. Arch Dis Child 64:745–749, 1989.
4. Huson SM, Compston DAS, Harper PS: A genetic study of von Recklinghausen neurofibromatosis in south east Wales: II. Guidelines for genetic counseling. J Med Genet 26:712–721, 1989.
5. Kwiatkowski DJ, Short MP: Tuberous sclerosis. Arch Dermatol 130:348–354, 1994.
6. Landau M, Krafchik BR: The diagnostic value of cafe-au-lait macules. J Am Acad Dermatol. 40:877–890, quiz 891–892, 1999.
7. National Institutes of Health Consensus Development Conference: Neurofibromatosis [conference statement]. Arch Neurol 45:575–578, 1988.
8. Novice FM, Collison DW, Burgdorf WHC, Esterly NB: Handbook of Genetic Skin Disorders. Philadelphia, W.B. Saunders, 1994.
9. Paller AS: The Sturge-Weber syndrome. Pediatr Dermatol 4:300–304, 1987.
10. Roach ES, DiMario FJ, Kandt RS, Northrup H: Tuberous Sclerosis Consensus Conference: Recommendations for diagnostic evaluation. National Tuberous Sclerosis Association. J Child Neurol 14:401–407, 1999.
11. Smith LL, Conerly SL: Ataxia-telangiectasia or Louis-Bar syndrome. J Am Acad Dermatol 12:681–696, 1985.
12. Tallman B, Tan OT, Morelli JG, et al: Location of port wine stains and the likelihood of ophthalmic and/or central nervous system complications. Pediatrics 87:323–327, 1991.

6. MECHANOBULLOUS DISORDERS

Ronald E. Grimwood, M.D.

1. What are the mechanobullous disorders?

This group of disorders is characterized by a small blister (vesicle) or large blister (bulla) that forms after trauma to the skin.

2. Does a common friction blister fall into the category of a mechanobullous disorder?

Yes. We all can get a blister from trauma to our skin. The extent of blistering relates to the amount of trauma and susceptibility of the individual's skin to withstand a shearing force. However, there are some inherited disorders that result in large blisters with only minor trauma to the skin.

3. Do all of the blisters in the mechanobullous disorders occur in the same layer within the skin?

No. There are three basic levels of separation within the skin that result in the clinical lesion we call a blister. The two basic layers of skin are the epidermis and dermis. The junction between these two layers contains important structural proteins and is called the dermal-epidermal junction (DEJ) (Fig. 1). Separation due to trauma may occur in any one of these three anatomic sites. In the common friction blister, the separation occurs in the epidermis.

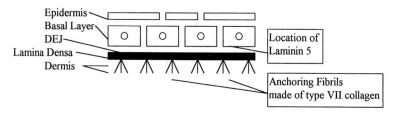

FIGURE 1. Layers of skin.

4. What inherited mechanobullous skin disorders cause blistering with minor trauma to the skin?

Inherited Mechanobullous Disorders

DISORDER	LEVEL OF BLISTER FORMATION	MODE OF INHERITANCE
Epidermolysis bullosa simplex		
Localized	Epidermis (basal layer)	Autosomal dominant
Generalized	Epidermis (basal layer)	Autosomal dominant
Junctional epidermolysis bullosa		
Localized	DEJ	Autosomal recessive
Generalized	DEJ	Autosomal recessive
Dystrophic epidermolysis bullosa		
Generalized	Dermis	Autosomal recessive and dominant forms

5. Describe the clinical findings in epidermolysis bullosa (EB) simplex.

In the common **localized** variety, the presentation is that of easy blistering noted on the hands and feet. These individuals may go undiagnosed until they are placed in a situation that generates increased pressure to these surfaces, such as marching in the military. The **generalized** form may present at birth but usually appears at 6–12 months of age in areas of trauma. The affected areas generally heal without scarring.

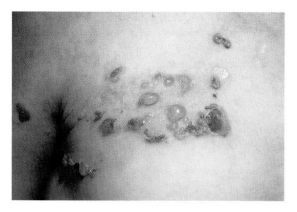

FIGURE 2. Dowling-Meara variant of EB simplex demonstrating generalized truncal blistering.

The term *epidermolysis* is a misnomer; it literally means cytolysis of the epidermis. This is obviously not the case since the defect in some forms of EB is restricted to the DEJ or dermis. Although it has been proposed that this term be dropped for all forms except the epidermal types, the name is firmly entrenched in the literature.

6. Is the cause of EB simplex known?

There is good evidence to suggest that there are gene defects coding for the production of epidermal proteins (keratins). EB simplex is not a single disease but rather a heterogeneous disorder with at least several subtypes. Each subtype probably has a different defect. The defect has been identified in one of the subtypes called the Dowling-Meara variant, with the defect being localized to the keratin 5 and 14 proteins that help form the structural integrity of the epidermal cells (Fig. 2).

7. What are the clinical findings in junctional EB?

At birth, a few blisters may be present over areas of trauma, and it may be impossible to tell this type from EB simplex. However, infants may have oral erosions that are not found in

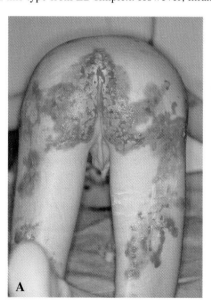
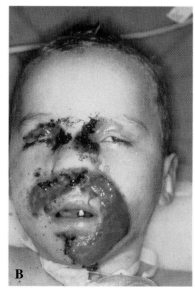

FIGURE 3. *A–B*, Junctional epidermolysis bullosa, Herlitz type. Chronic central erosions are characteristic.

EB simplex. Junctional EB includes localized variants that are not as involved and a severe generalized form (Herlitz, or EB letalis) which is potentially fatal (Fig. 3). As with EB simplex, blisters and erosions over areas of trauma are common. Unlike EB simplex, children with the Herlitz variant of junctional EB have prominent central facial erosions that are difficult to resolve. They also have dental defects, nail dystrophy, and tracheal and bronchiolar involvement producing respiratory distress. There is a high incidence of infection associated with sepsis and potentially death.

8. Is the cause of junctional EB known?

Evidence suggests that one or several structural proteins in the DEJ may be diminished, absent, or structurally altered in junctional EB. The alteration results in a weakened adherence between the epidermis and dermis. One such protein is laminin 5, which was formerly called kallinin or nicein. This protein or group of proteins is abnormally expressed in patients with junctional EB and may be the key to localizing the gene(s) that are responsible for the defect.

9. What are the clinical findings in dystrophic EB?

In the **recessive** form of this condition, hemorrhagic blisters appear at birth or within a few months after birth. The blistered areas heal with scarring that can lead to the loss of functional digits in the hands (Fig. 4). Oral and esophageal involvement causes feeding problems with resultant esophageal stricture. The teeth are malformed, and anemia is common due to chronic blood loss.

The **dominant** form of the disease is less severe and tends to be more localized. Atrophic scarring is still the rule over affected areas. A unique dominant dystrophic form exists (transient bullous dermolysis at the newborn) that is only transient. The blistering tendency decreases with age.

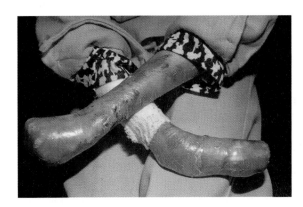

FIGURE 4. Recessive dystrophic epidermolysis bullosa. Severe scarring resulting in loss of functional digits.

10. Is the cause of dystrophic EB known?

The primary defect in dystrophic EB is an absent or structurally altered protein found in the dermis. This protein is type VII collagen, which makes up the anchoring fibrils that connect the basement membrane with the dermal collagen. Recently, mutations in the type VII collagen gene (COL7A1) located on the short arm of chromosome 3 have been found in families with dystrophic EB.

11. Can a definitive diagnosis of the various EB types be made on clinical presentation?

No. In newborns and infants it is virtually impossible to tell these disorders apart. Several techniques can aid in establishing the correct diagnosis, however. One such technique is immunomapping, which involves the use of antibodies directed against known proteins located at specific sites in the skin. The patient's skin is subjected to minor trauma followed by a biopsy. The specimen is then "mapped" with the locating antibodies. This technique locates the actual level of the blister formation in the skin specimen and determines the major category of mechanobullous disorder (i.e., epidermal, junctional, or dystrophic). The diagnosis can be further refined by using monoclonal antibodies that are specific for the missing or altered proteins.

12. Are there any treatments for the mechanobullous disorders?

There are no specific treatments for this group of disorders. The cutaneous lesions are best treated by minimizing trauma to prevent the formation of new blisters. Soft-leather, well-ventilated shoes are helpful in preventing blisters on the feet. Some also recommend low ambient temperatures because there is a perception that most forms of EB are worse at higher temperatures. Emollients are effective in minimizing shearing forces.

In variants with oral manifestations, such as junctional EB and recessive dystrophic EB, meticulous oral hygiene with close dental follow-up is essential. Capping, crowns, and restorations can be helpful. Blenderized food is necessary early on for patients with recessive dystrophic EB to help minimize trauma to the esophagus and prevent esophageal webbing. Hand deformities in dystrophic EB can be surgically corrected but the recurrence rate is high.

13. Is phenytoin a useful treatment?

The anticonvulsant drug phenytoin (Dilantin) is known to inhibit the production of collagenase by fibroblasts. For this reason, it was used in three open clinical trials in the 1980s to treat the recessive form of dystrophic EB, because the defect appears to result in a decrease in type VII collagen. All three studies demonstrated clinical improvement in patients with recessive dystrophic EB. More recently, a larger, multicenter, placebo-controlled, double-blind, crossover trial did not demonstrate a difference between placebo and phenytoin. This treatment has generally fallen out of favor, although older references may still list it for recessive dystrophic EB.

14. Are prenatal diagnostic techniques useful for this group of disorders?

Fetoscopy with fetal skin biopsy has been the primary method of prenatal diagnosis for EB and other inherited skin diseases. Examination of fetal skin by transmission electron microscopy has been, until recently, the only reliable method of diagnosis, and its reliability depends directly on the expertise of the laboratory personnel who process the specimens and the individual who interprets the results. Another technique that has been used with some success is monoclonal antibodies, which can help to exclude the diagnoses of junctional EB or dystrophic EB.

BIBLIOGRAPHY

1. Caldwell-Brown D, Stern RS, Lin AN, et al: Lack of efficacy of phenytoin in recessive dystrophic epidermolysis bullosa. N Engl J Med 327:163–167, 1992.
2. Carter WG, Ryan MC, Gahr PJ: Epiligrin, a new cell adhesion ligand for integrin α3 β1 in epithelial basement membranes. Cell 65:599–610, 1991.
3. Chavanas S, Gache Y, Tadini G, et al: A homozygous in-frame deletion in the collagenous domain of bullous pemphigoid antigen BP180 (type XVII collagen) causes generalized atrophic benign epidermolysis bullosa. J Invest Dermatol 109:74–78, 1997.
4. Christiano AM, Fine JD, Uitto J: Genetic basis of dominantly inherited transient bullous dermolysis of the newborn: A splice site mutation in the type VII collagen gene. J Invest Dermatol 109:811–814, 1997.
5. Domloge-Hultsch N, Gammon WR, Briggaman RA, et al: Epiligrin, the major human keratinocyte integrin ligand, is a target in both an acquired autoimmune and an inherited subepidermal blistering skin disease. J Clin Invest 90:1628–1633, 1992.
6. Fine JD, Bauer EA, Briggaman RA, et al: Revised clinical and laboratory criteria for subtypes of inherited epidermolysis bullosa. J Am Acad Dermatol 24:119–135, 1991.
7. Lin AN, Carter DM (eds): Epidermolysis Bullosa: Basic and Clinical Aspects. New York, Springer, 1992.
8. Marinkovich MP: The molecular genetics of basement membrane diseases. Arch Dermatol 129:1557, 1993.
9. McGrath JA, Gatalica B, Christiano AM, et al: Mutations in the 180-kD bullous pemphigoid antigen (BPAG2), a hemidesmosomal transmembrane collagen (COL17A1), in generalized atrophic benign epidermolysis bullosa. Nat Genet 11:83–86, 1995.
10. Meneguzzi G, Marinkovich MP, Pisani A, et al: Kalinin is abnormally expressed in epithelial basement membranes of Herlitz's junctional epidermolysis bullosa patients. Exp Dermatol 1:221–229, 1992.
11. Verrando P, Schofield O, Ishida-Yamamoto A, et al: Nicein (BM-600) in junctional epidermolysis bullosa: Polyclonal antibodies provide new clues for pathogenic role. J Invest Dermatol 101:738–743, 1993.
12. Vidal F, Aberdam D, Miquel C, et al: Integrin beta 4 mutations associated with junctional epidermolysis bullosa with pyloric atresia. Nat Genet 10:229–234, 1995.
13. Yancey KB: Adhesion molecules II: Interactions of keratinocytes with epidermal basement membrane. Prog Dermatol 28:1–12, 1994.

III. Inflammatory Disorders

7. PAPULOSQUAMOUS SKIN ERUPTIONS

Jeffrey B. Travers, M.D., Ph.D.

1. Name the papulosquamous skin eruptions.

Papulosquamous skin disorders are inflammatory reactions characterized by red or purple papules and plaques with scale. These diseases include psoriasis, pityriasis rubra pilaris, seborrheic dermatitis, pityriasis rosea, pityriasis lichenoides et varioliformis acuta, and parapsoriasis. Lichen planus and lichen nitidus are also considered papulosquamous disorders (see Chapter 12).

2. What is psoriasis? What is its incidence?

Psoriasis is a common, genetically determined, inflammatory and hyperproliferative skin disease. Although there are morphologic variations, the most characteristic lesions consist of chronic, well-demarcated, dull-red plaques with silvery scale found commonly on extensor surfaces and the scalp (Fig. 1). Psoriasis occurs in about 1–2% of the population worldwide. Its incidence varies among population groups, being highest in those of Western Europe and Scandinavia. It is less common in blacks and Chinese and rare in pure Native Americans.

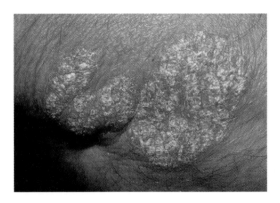

FIGURE 1. Psoriasis vulgaris. Elbow involvement of psoriasis vulgaris, demonstrating typical well-demarcated, red plaques with silvery scale.

3. List the different types of psoriasis.

The different clinical presentations of psoriasis can be separated by morphology or location.

Morphologic Variants	Locational Variants
Chronic plaque psoriasis	Scalp psoriasis
Guttate psoriasis	Palmoplantar psoriasis
Pustular psoriasis	Inverse psoriasis
Erythrodermic psoriasis	Nail psoriasis
	Psoriatic arthritis

4. What is guttate psoriasis?

Guttate psoriasis is a variant of psoriasis usually seen in adolescents and young adults. It is characterized by crops of small, drop-like, psoriasis papules and plaques (Fig. 2A). The word *guttate* is derived from the Latin *gutta,* which means drop. This type of psoriasis is often found in association with streptococcal pharyngitis, and treatment of the pharyngitis with oral antibiotics may improve or even clear the psoriasis.

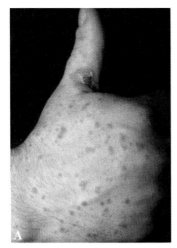 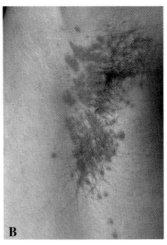

FIGURE 2. *A,* Guttate, or the acute eruptive type of psoriasis, showing widespread drop-like lesions. This type of psoriasis is associated with streptococcal infections, probably through the immune-stimulating effects of exotoxins secreted by the bacteria. *B,* Inverse psoriasis involves intertriginous areas such as the axilla, as shown here. Note the lack of silvery scale seen in psoriasis vulgaris.

5. Does pustular psoriasis refer to psoriasis that is secondarily infected?

The pustular forms are uncommon, less stable variants of psoriasis. Instead of whitish to silvery scales on erythematous plaques seen in other forms, pustular psoriasis is characterized by superficial pustules, often with fine desquamation. Although triggers such as infection can precipitate a flare of pustular psoriasis, the pustules are sterile. Patients often need systemic treatments, such as retinoids, immunosuppressives, or phototherapy, to keep their disease under control.

6. What is inverse psoriasis?

Inverse psoriasis refers to psoriasis that involves intertriginous areas (axillae, groin, umbilicus). This distribution is opposite to the usual extensor distribution of psoriasis vulgaris. Psoriatic lesions with both distributions sometimes can be found in the same patients. Clinically, psoriatic lesions found in these "inverse" distributions often do not have scale, but consist of sharply-demarcated red plaques (Fig. 2B). Treatment of inverse psoriasis usually involves low-potency (nonfluorinated) topical corticosteroids.

7. How is heredity involved in psoriasis?

Although a specific genetic abnormality has not been identified, psoriasis is generally considered to be a genetically determined disease. There are reports of striking family pedigrees that suggest an autosomal dominant inheritance, but with only partial penetrance. Keep in mind that psoriasis is probably not a single disease, but a family of diseases involving epidermal hyperproliferation. The external environment presumably plays a role in the clinical expression. The strongest evidence for the importance of external factors in the expression of psoriasis is seen in acute guttate psoriasis, which often is seen in association with streptococcal pharyngitis.

8. If one of my relatives has psoriasis, what is the chance that I will get psoriasis?

Questionnaire-based studies reveal that almost 5% of first-degree relatives of psoriasis also have psoriasis, compared to 1.2% of relatives of nonpsoriatic spouses of probands. If a sibling has psoriasis, other siblings have a 16% incidence if one parent has psoriasis and a 50% chance if both parents are affected. Twin studies indicate that if one twin has psoriasis, the other twin is similarly affected in 20% of dizygotic pairs and in 73% of monozygotic pairs. The absence of 100% concordance in monozygotic twins (who have identical genetic material) indicates that environmental factors also contribute to the expression of psoriasis.

9. Name the types of psoriatic arthritis.

Although the exact incidence of psoriatic arthritis is unknown, an estimated 5–10% of patients with psoriasis suffer from psoriatic arthritis. The arthritis may precede, accompany, or, more commonly, follow the skin disease. The five types of psoriatic arthritis are:

- Asymmetric (60–70%)
- Symmetric polyarthritis (15%)
- Distal interphalangeal joint (DIP) disease (5%)
- Destructive arthritis (5%)
- Axial arthritis (5%)

10. Describe the clinical features of the psoriatic arthritides.

Asymmetric arthritis, the most common form of psoriatic arthritis, usually involves one or several joints of the fingers or toes. The appearance of this type of arthritis can be similar to subacute gout and include "sausage-like" swelling of a digit due to involvement of the proximal and DIP joints and flexor sheath. **Symmetric polyarthritis** resembles rheumatoid arthritis, but tests for rheumatoid factor are negative and the condition is clinically less severe than rheumatoid arthritis. Although not common, **DIP joint disease** of hands and feet is the most characteristic presentation of arthritis with psoriasis. **Destructive arthritis** (arthritis mutilans) is a severely deforming arthritis involving predominantly fingers and toes. Gross osteolysis of the small bones of the hands and feet can result in shortening, subluxations, and, in severe cases, telescoping of the digits, resulting in an "opera glass" deformity. **Axial arthritis,** resembling idiopathic ankylosing spondylitis, can be seen by itself or with peripheral joint disease.

11. What are the abnormal nail findings seen in psoriasis? Which is most common?

A careful examination of the nails should be part of the cutaneous skin exam, especially when a rash is present that might be psoriasis. Characteristic nail changes are found in 25–50% of psoriatics. These changes include nail pitting, discoloration, onycholysis, subungual hyperkeratosis, and nail deformity. Nail pitting, the most common nail finding in psoriasis, consists of small, discrete, punched-out depressions on the nail surface (Fig. 3). Circular areas of nailbed discoloration that resemble oil drops are often seen under the nail plate (hyponychium). The nail can become thin and brittle at the distal edge with separation from the nailbed (onycholysis) or thickened with subungual debris. Ridges, grooves, or even frank deformity of the nail plate can also be seen.

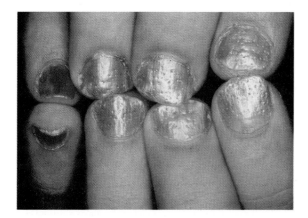

FIGURE 3. Nail pitting is one of the most common changes associated with psoriasis. As demonstrated here, even nail polish often cannot hide these discrete pits.

12. You are working in a dermatology clinic, seeing a patient with a rash that is possibly psoriasis. Outside the room, the attending asks if you noticed any evidence of "Koebner's phenomenon" or an "Auspitz sign" when you examined the patient. What are these?

The isomorphic or **Koebner's phenomenon** is the development of psoriasis at the site of physical trauma (scratch, surgical wound, or sunburn). Other papulosquamous disorders that exhibit Koebner's phenomenon include lichen planus and lichen nitidus. Patients with psoriasis should be warned of this tendency before subjecting themselves to cosmetic procedures involving physical trauma (such as having a tattoo).

The **Auspitz sign** is the presence of small bleeding points seen on a psoriatic lesion when the scales are removed. This bleeding is due to thinning of the epidermis between the elongated rete ridges. Note that it is not a good idea to attempt to elicit these two signs on your psoriatic patients.

13. Name three types of drugs that precipitate or exacerbate psoriasis.

Beta-blocking agents, antimalarials, and lithium. All three can precipitate or exacerbate psoriasis. These medications should be used with caution in psoriatics.

14. What other factors can provoke or exacerbate psoriasis?

Any evidence of skin or other systemic infection (especially streptococcal pharyngitis) should warrant appropriate oral antibiotics.

15. Do systemic corticosteroids help psoriasis?

Although treatment with systemic corticosteroids rapidly clears psoriasis, the disease usually "breaks through," requiring higher doses of corticosteroids. If systemic corticosteriod treatment is withdrawn, the psoriasis usually relapses and may worsen. This "rebound" worsening of psoriasis may even result in erythrodermic (total body) or severe pustular psoriasis.

16. What topical medications are used to treat psoriasis?

Patients with limited disease (usually < 20% of their body surface) can often be managed on topical agents alone. Although systemic corticosteroids probably should never be used, topical and intralesional **corticosteroids** are a first-line treatment. For plaques, medium- to high-potency corticosteroids used daily can result in a rapid response, often controlling the inflammation and itching. Unfortunately, the relief is often temporary, and tolerance can occur. Side effects include atrophy and telangiectasia, especially if high-potency topical preparations are used on the face or intertriginous areas (see also Chapter 54).

Coal tar preparations can also be effective, especially if used with topical corticosteroids. **Anthralin,** a synthetic derivative of chrysarobin, a tree bark extract, is effective in daily, short applications for chronic plaque psoriasis, but its irritant qualities often worsen inflammatory psoriasis. **Calcipotriene** (Dovonex), a vitamin D_3 analog that has been introduced only recently, is an effective treatment for localized psoriasis, but its cost and the possibility of systemic absorption resulting in changes in calcium homeostasis probably preclude its use in extensive disease. Calcipotriene should be limited to a maximum dosage of 100 gm/wk.

17. How is ultraviolet radiation used to treat psoriasis?

It has been known for centuries that sunlight can improve psoriasis. Two forms of ultraviolet radiation are used clinically: ultraviolet B (UVB, 290–320 nm) and ultraviolet A (UVA, 320–400 nm) with an oral psoralen (PUVA). Although not as effective as PUVA, UVB has less incidence of side effects and is often used first in the treatment of light-sensitive psoriasis (see also Chapter 54).

18. What systemic drugs are used to treat psoriasis?

Retinoids (isotretinoin, etretinate), methotrexate, and cyclosporine. Because of the possible side effects of these treatments, their use should not be entered into lightly.

Retinoids are felt to be most effective and are probably one of the treatments of choice for pustular psoriasis (see also Chapter 55).

Methotrexate suppresses DNA synthesis by inhibiting the enzyme dihydrofolate reductase. In addition to its antimitotic effects, methotrexate inhibits neutrophil function. Side effects include bone marrow suppression, stomach upset, and hepatotoxicity. Although the incidence of hepatic fibrosis and cirrhosis is low with cumulative doses < 1.5 gm, liver function tests are not a reliable indicator of methotrexate-induced hepatotoxicity and a liver biopsy is recommended after 1.5 gm and every 1.0–1.5 gm thereafter. Methotrexate should be avoided in psoriatics who either have underlying liver disease or are heavy drinkers.

The antilymphocytic drug **cyclosporine** can be used for severe psoriasis. The doses used, 3–5 mg/kg/day, are usually less than the dosages used to inhibit organ transplant rejection. The most important side effects are hypertension and nephrotoxicity.

19. Describe the rash of pityriasis rubra pilaris.

Pityriasis ruba pilaris (PRP) is a rare disease in which the primary abnormality appears to be hyperproliferation of the epidermis (Fig. 4). Five variants have been described, the most common being type I, the classic adult onset. In this type, the eruption commonly begins on the head and neck as reddish-orange, slightly scaly macules and thin plaques. The rash extends in a cephalo-caudal fashion, and within several weeks, red perifollicular papules with central plugs develop in the lesions. The scalp often has extensive yellowish scale, and the palms and soles become thickened and yellow, resulting in a well-demarcated, very characteristic "PRP sandal." Although total body involvement (erythroderma) is not uncommon, the rash of PRP often has characteristic skip areas of normal skin ("islands of sparing"). Considering that the rash usually looks very impressive, it is surprising that patients often complain of only mild irritation and pruritus.

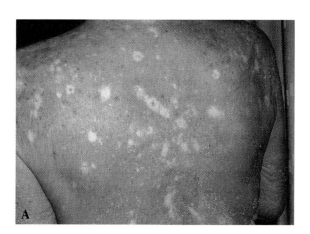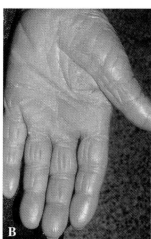

FIGURE 4. Pityriasis rubra pilaris. *A*, Extensive involvement in an adult showing characteristic salmon color and "islands of sparing." *B*, Characteristic thickened yellow palmar changes.

20. Although pityriasis rubra pilaris can occur at any age, in what decades is it most often seen? What is the prognosis?

PRP has a bimodal age distribution, with the highest incidence in the fifth and sixth decades and a smaller peak in childhood. The prognosis is variable, but usually 80% of patients clear spontaneously in several years.

21. How is pityriasis rubra pilaris treated?

Treatment strategies for PRP depend on the extent of involvement and how much the patient is bothered. Lubrication with emollients and topical corticosteroids are rarely helpful. The treatment of choice is oral retinoids, with methotrexate being reserved for retinoid-resistant cases.

22. Describe the distribution of the "seborrheic areas."

Seborrheic areas have a rich supply of sebaceous glands and include the scalp, face, central chest, and intertriginous areas. Skin diseases that can have a "seborrheic distribution" include seborrheic dermatitis, psoriasis, Darier's disease, and pemphigus foliaceus.

23. What does seborrheic dermatitis look like?

Seborrheic dermatitis is a chronic dermatitis, the typical morphologic appearance being red, well-demarcated lesions with greasy yellow scales, distributed in the seborrheic areas. Scalp involvement is almost universal. Facial involvement is common and manifests itself as erythema and scaling on the medial sides of the eyebrows, glabella, and nasolabial folds. Ocular involvement (blepharitis and conjunctivitis) and ear involvement (external auditory canal and posterior auricular scalp) are also frequently seen. Visible scalp desquamation, commonly known as dandruff, is probably the precursor and/or a mild form of seborrheic dermatitis.

24. What causes it?

Seborrheic dermatitis is probably a hypersensitivity response to the common skin yeast, *Pityrosporum ovale*.

25. How can you differentiate between seborrheic dermatitis and psoriasis of the scalp?

The differentiation between these two disorders can be difficult. However, in contrast to seborrheic dermatitis, scalp psoriasis is often patchy, consisting of thicker plaques with silvery scale. The rest of the body should be examined, including the nails, to look for other evidence of psoriasis. The patient should also be questioned about a possible family history of psoriasis.

26. How is seborrheic dermatitis treated?

Although treatment of seborrheic dermatitis is suppressive, it is not curative. The scalp is best treated with medicated shampoos (selenium sulfide, zinc pyrithione, and tar). Patients should be instructed to leave the shampoo on their scalp for at least 5 minutes before rinsing (or two or three songs for patients who are inclined to sing in the shower). Use of a medium- or high-potency topical steroid solution on the scalp is often helpful for patients who experience burning or pruritus or have resistant areas. Facial seborrheic dermatitis is very responsive to low-potency topical corticosteroids (hydrocortisone) or topical antifungals. Oral antibiotics should be given if there is evidence of secondary infection.

27. What is pityriasis rosea? Describe the characteristic rash.

Pityriasis rosea is an acute, benign, self-limiting disorder that affects teenagers and young adults. The eruption has a characteristic pattern, and three-fourths of cases start with a single 2–4-cm, sharply defined, thin oval plaque. Within a few days to weeks, crops of similar-appearing, though usually smaller, lesions follow the initial "herald patch" (Fig. 5). The eruption characteristically involves the trunk and proximal extremities, usually sparing the face, palms, and soles. Lesions on the trunk tend to run parallel to the lines of skin cleavage, resulting in a "Christmas tree" pattern. The lesions usually resolve within several weeks to a month but may persist longer. Except for a mild prodrome, affected patients are usually asymptomatic. The lesions of pityriasis

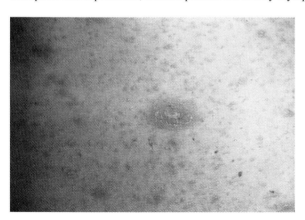

FIGURE 5. Pityriasis rosea. A young patient demonstrates the characteristic thin plaques with scale on his trunk. The larger herald patch can be seen by the left axilla.

rosea oftentimes have "trailing scale" (e.g., collarette of scale that does not extend to the border of the lesion), and papular variants can be seen, especially in children.

Although the etiology of pityriasis rosea is unknown, the occasional prodromal symptoms, characteristic disease course, tendency for life-long immunity, seasonal variance, and reports of epidemics all point to an infectious (viral) agent. Treatment consists of reassurance, emollients, and antipruritic agents for symptomatic patients. Ultraviolet radiation treatment (sunshine or UVB) hastens the disappearance of the eruption. Some studies suggest that human herpesvirus 7 is the causative agent.

28. In the dermatology clinic, a 20-year-old man presents who has been referred from the primary care clinic with a diagnosis of pityriasis rosea. He has a rash that looks like pityriasis rosea, but he complains of fevers, myalgias, and swollen lymph glands. He remembers having an ulcer on his penis several months ago. What test do you recommend?

The eruption of secondary syphilis can mimic pityriasis rosea, though patients often have systemic manifestations. A sexual history should be elicited in such patients, and a rapid plasma reagin (RPR) or Venereal Disease Research Laboratory (VDRL) test should be obtained. Because syphilis is readily treatable, and because untreated syphilis can result in life-threatening cardiovascular and neurologic sequelae, many dermatologists customarily obtain an RPR or VDRL test on every sexually active patient who presents with a pityriasis rosea-like eruption.

29. What are the two major types of parapsoriasis? Why is it important to differentiate between them?

Parapsoriasis is a term often used to describe slowly evolving, asymptomatic, scaly plaques, often found on the trunk and proximal extremities. Parapsoriasis is divided into small plaque (1–5 cm diameter) and large plaque (5–15 cm diameter) forms. The prognosis of the two types differs, and approximately 10% of cases of large-plaque parapsoriasis eventuate in T-cell lymphoma. Parapsoriasis is resistant to most topical treatments but often responds to phototherapy.

30. What is pityriasis lichenoides et varioliformis acuta?

Pityriasis lichenoides et varioliformis acuta (PLEVA or Mucha-Habermann disease) is a rare disease characterized by crops of polymorphous lesions on the trunk, thighs, and upper arms. The eruption consists of red-brown papules that can become purpuric, scaly, and even necrotic. The patients usually are asymptomatic, although itching and low-grade fevers and malaise are not uncommon. Individual lesions resolve in several weeks leaving postinflammatory hyper- or hypopigmentation and occasionally scars. The clinical course of PLEVA often waxes and wanes and can last months to years.

31. How is PLEVA treated?

Oral antibiotics (erythromycin or tetracycline) have been suggested, but no controlled studies exist. Phototherapy and even methotrexate have been used for recalcitrant or severe cases.

BIBLIOGRAPHY

1. Arndt KA, LeBoit PE, Robinson JK, Wintroub BU (eds): Cutaneous Medicine and Surgery. Philadelphia, W.B. Saunders, 1996.
2. Drago F, Ranieri E, Malaguti F, et al: Human herpesvirus 7 in pityriasis rosea. Lancet 349:1367, 1997.
3. Habif TP: Clinical Dermatology: A Color Guide to Diagnosis and Therapy, 3rd ed. St. Louis, Mosby, 1996.
4. Leung DYM, Hauk P, Strickland I, et al: The role of superantigens in human diseases: Therapeutic implications for the treatment of skin diseases. Br J Dermatol 139:17, 1998.
5. Norris DA, Travers JB, Leung DYM: Lymphocyte activation in the pathogenesis of psoriasis. J Invest Dermatol 109:1, 1997.
6. Wolverton SE, Wilkin JK (eds): Systemic Drugs for Skin Diseases, Philadelphia, W.B. Saunders, 1991.

8. DERMATITIS (ECZEMA)

Thomas W. McGovern, M.D.

1. What is dermatitis?

Dermatitis literally means **inflammation of the skin,** but dermatologists use the term to refer to a specific group of inflammatory skin diseases. Clinically, dermatitis presents with pruritic, erythematous lesions with or without distinct margins. Such lesions pass through acute (vesicular), subacute (scaling and crusting), and chronic (acanthotic with thick epidermis) phases. Primary lesions include macules, papules, vesicles, edematous patches, or plaques. Secondary lesions with oozing, crusting, scaling, fissuring, and lichenification frequently follow. The primary histologic event is spongiosis (intercellular epidermal edema) with lymphocytic and/or eosinophilic infiltrates in the epidermis and dermis.

2. What is eczema?

From the Greek meaning "a boiling out," **eczema** has been used as a descriptive term since the sixth century. Unfortunately, there is no clear-cut agreement among dermatologists as to the meaning of the term, and its use is controversial in some circles. Most, but not all, dermatologists use *dermatitis* and *eczema* interchangeably. In general, dermatitis is used more commonly in the U.S., and eczema is used more commonly in Europe.

The difficulty in defining eczema is illustrated by Calnan who stated, "Eczema is like jazz. One assumes that everyone recognizes it, and that this makes any need to define it unnecessary."

3. Why is dermatitis so important?

Up to 25% of all patients presenting with a new skin disease have a form of dermatitis. Patients typically suffer from pruritus that is distracting them from their daily activities, and they are desperate for relief.

4. Name some common diseases classified as dermatitis.

Contact dermatitis (irritant or allergic)   Autosensitization dermatitis (Id reaction)
Atopic dermatitis   Stasis dermatitis (a vascular disorder)
Pompholyx (dyshidrosis)   Lichen simplex chronicus (a psychocutaneous
Nummular dermatitis   disorder)
Seborrheic dermatitis   Generalized exfoliative dermatitis

5. What is atopy?

Coca coined this word in 1923 to mean "out-of-place-ness" or "different." Atopy refers to the predisposition to develop asthma, allergic rhinitis, and an associated skin disease appropriately called "atopic dermatitis" and referred to by many lay people simply as "eczema." Atopic patients typically have blood and tissue eosinophilia, increased IgE responses, increased transepidermal water loss, exquisite sensitivity to pruritic stimuli (e.g., wool sweaters), and immune system dysfunction.

While allergic rhinitis and asthma are associated with the release of histamine, atopic dermatitis is not. In fact, instead of presenting with a type I hypersenstivity reaction (wheals), atopic dermatitis patients present with scaly plaques reminiscent of a type IV hypersensitivity reaction. 70% of patients with atopic dermatitis have a family history of at least one of the three atopic disorders. The incidence of atopic dermatitis has risen from 2% in those born before 1960 to 9–20% in those born after 1970; the reason is unknown. Patients have inherently irritable (sensitive) skin in which scratching is responsible for many objective changes. Psychological, climactic, and immunologic factors may modify these changes.

6. What immunologic aberrations have been described in atopic patients and how do they manifest clinically?

ABERRATIONS	CLINICAL FINDINGS
Increased IgE response to antigens Hyper-releasable basophils and mast cells High-affinity IgE receptors on Langerhans' cells, mast cells, and Th-2 cells Th-1/Th-2 biphasic reversal	Increased IgE levels and "immediate" (prick) test or RAST reactivity to allergens Increased reactivity to nonallergens (e.g., light touch is perceived as itch as with wool fibers) Hyperreactive organ responses: (systemic—anaphylaxis; upper airway—rhinitis; lower airway—asthma; skin—urticaria, atopic dermatitis) Tissue and circulating eosinophilia Increased susceptibility to viral (especially herpes simplex virus), bacterial (especially *Staphylococcus aureus*), and dermatophyte (especially chronic *Trichophyton rubrum*) infections Impaired delayed-type hypersensitivity reactions (e.g., atopic patients have a lower rate of poison ivy allergy than the general population)

7. How is atopic dermatitis diagnosed?

Three of four clinical features must be present to make the diagnosis:
- Pruritus—the primary symptom and even referred to as the "primary lesion" by some
- Typical morphology and distribution of lesions for age
- Chronic or chronically relapsing course
- Personal or family history of asthma, allergic rhinitis, or atopic dermatitis

8. In atopic dermatitis, which comes first: the itch or the rash?

No primary skin lesion has ever been established in atopic dermatitis. Hanifin and Rajka, who established the accepted criteria for diagnosing atopic dermatitis, suspect that all the cutaneous changes of atopic dermatitis may be due to itch-induced scratching. As Beltrani states, "Atopic dermatitis is an itch which when scratched erupts." If there is no scratching, there is no eruption.

9. How does atopic dermatitis present at different ages?

Atopic dermatitis may present at any age, but 60% of patients experience their first outbreak by their first birthday, and 90% by their fifth. Four clinical phases are recognized:
- **Infantile phase** (2 mo–2 yrs): Characterized by intense itching, erythema, papules, vesicles, oozing, and crusting. Patients typically develop eruptions on the cheeks (Fig. 1A), forehead, and scalp, with less involvement of the trunk or extremities. The diaper area is usually spared. Dermatitis clears in half of the patients by 3 years of age.
- **Childhood phase** (3–11 yrs): More chronic, lichenified scaly patches and plaques that may have crusting and oozing. Classic areas include the wrists, ankles, backs of the thighs, buttocks, and antecubital and popliteal fossae, although other areas, including extensors, may be involved in early childhood (Fig. 1B). Two-thirds of patients clear by age 6.
- **Adolescent/young adult phase** (12–20 yrs): Thick, dry, lichenified plaques without weeping, crusting, or oozing that involve the face, neck, upper arms, back, and flexures (Fig. 1C).
- **Adult phase** (> 20 yrs): Most commonly involves the hands, sometimes the face and neck, and rarely diffuse areas. Only 10% of infantile or childhood cases of atopic dermatitis persist into adulthood.

10. What physical findings are associated with atopic dermatitis?
- Dry skin—due to decreased ability to bind and retain water in the skin
- Keratosis pilaris—a keratinizing disorder in which the follicular openings are filled with horny plugs; it is most commonly seen on the posterolateral arms and anterior thighs
- Hyperlinear palm and sole creases that worsen with lubrication
- Allergic "shiners"—symmetric, asymptomatic, bluish discoloration of periorbital skin often associated with chronic nasal congestion

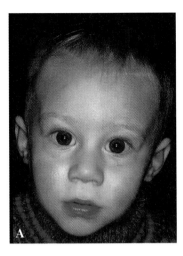

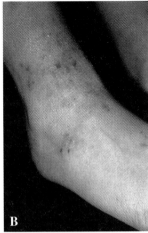

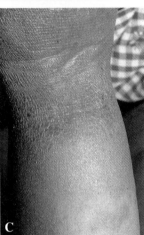

FIGURE 1. Phases of atopic dermatitis. *A,* Infantile phase. Typical erythematous, oozing, and crusted plaques seen on the cheek of an infant with atopic dermatitis. *B,* Childhood phase. A 5-year-old with oozing crusted lesions with secondary excoriations on the thigh and calf. *C,* Adolescent/young adult phase. Characteristic chronic flexural dermatitis in an adolescent. (Panel *C* courtesy of James E. Fitzpatrick, MD.)

- Dennie-Morgan lines—a double infraorbital fold seen in 60–80% of atopic patients; however, it is seen in so many non-atopic patients that it may not represent a true association
- Pityriasis alba - asymptomatic, finely scaly, hypopigmented macules, typically on the face of infants or children that begins with a brief erythematous inflammatory phase
- Exaggerated vertical linear crease of the nasal bridge
- Vascular abnormalities—skin pallor, low finger and toe temperatures, pronounced vasoconstriction on exposure to cold

11. What is Kaposi's varicelliform eruption?

This dramatic and uncommon complication of atopic dermatitis appears after exposure to certain infectious agents. The altered skin barrier allows HSV (eczema herpeticum), vaccinia (eczema vaccinatum), or coxsackie A16 virus (eczema coxsackium) to widely infect the body.

12 What factors provoke or exacerbate atopic dermatitis?

Excessive washing without appropriate skin lubrication is the most common irritant, as repeated water exposure degrades the skin's barrier to external irritants and internal water loss. Important topical irritants include wool, synthetic fabrics, poorly fitting clothes, mineral oils, solvents, sand, and excessive perspiration. Airborne particles, such as tobacco smoke, animal dander, molds, and house dust mites exacerbate disease in some patients, especially infants with severe dermatitis. Secondary infections due to *Staphylococcus aureus* or *Pityrosporum orbiculare* may also aggravate the disease. Although 85% of atopic patients have positive skin prick tests or RAST results for specific IgE in response to food or inhalant allergens, a relationship between allergen presence and skin disease has not been established.

The most common itch-provoking factors in atopic dermatitis are:

Heat and perspiration	96%	Alcohol	44%
Wool	91%	Common cold	36%
Emotional stress	81%	Dust mites	> 35%
Certain foods	49%		

13. Can foods induce atopic dermatitis?

Allergies to milk, eggs, nuts, soybean products, wheat, and seafood have been implicated by some researchers, but their true role in atopic dermatitis remains controversial. Food elimination diets have no proven benefit. Some studies suggest that breastfeeding reduces the incidence of atopic dermatitis in the first year of life, while others have not demonstrated a difference.

14. Can atopic dermatitis be cured?

No, but a variety of measures can control it:

- Avoid provoking factors (scrubbing, too frequent bathing, scented soaps, etc.)
- Reduce dryness and pruritus by applying emollients to moist skin, add moisture, and lubricate. Use mild, unscented soaps only on hairy or oily areas, and water only to bathe other areas. Avoid overbathing and apply moisturizer within 3 minutes of exiting the bath or shower to retain moisture added from bathing. Urea and alpha-hydroxy acid–containing products are especially effective.
- Wear cotton clothing as much as possible, and if the arms and forearms are affected, wear long-sleeved shirts to reduce evaporation from the skin. (This helped me greatly with my atopic dermatitis in high school, and I haven't seen it in any books! TM)
- For acutely inflamed and weeping skin, use open wet-to-dry compresses because they are soothing, antipruritic, cleansing, hydrating, and cooling.
- For subacute or chronic lesions, topical corticosteroids are the mainstay of therapy. Typically, younger patients require less potent steroids and vice versa.
- For resistant or widespread plaques, topical corticosteroids under occlusion may be used (which can increase penetration up to 100-fold!). These should be applied for 8–12 hours/day for 3–7 days.
- Tar preparations are vasoconstrictive, astringent, disinfectant, and antipruritic.
- Oral or topical antipruritic agents may be helpful. Oral antihistamines may help because of their sedating effects, but because histamine does not appear to play a role in the itching of atopic dermatitis, they are not particularly helpful for the pruritus.
- If lesions are secondarily infected, antibiotic therapy for at least 2 weeks should be prescribed. There is some evidence that toxins and/or superantigens produced by *S. aureus* induce dermatitis in some patients and that antibiotics may have a role in atopic patients not responding to standard therapy.
- New medications used to treat atopic dermatitis include the immunomodulators cyclosporin (ineffective topically, effective orally) and tacrolimus (effective topically). Azathioprine, UVB, and PUVA are also effective for more severe cases of atopic dermatitis.
- The primary goal of therapy in atopic dermatitis should be recognizing and avoiding the triggers of each individual patient's pruritus.

15. Should topical steroids be used on lesions that may be infected or colonized with bacteria?

Absolutely. Lesions get infected because the skin defense barrier is broken. The topical steroids allow it to heal and thus the bacteria have greater difficulty infecting the skin. Such bacteria have receptors for fibrin or fibronectin that can be exposed in dermatitic, but not normal, skin.

16. Describe the "two-pajamas treatment."
One especially effective method for applying topical steroids under occlusion is known as the "two-pajamas treatment." It involves taking two pairs of cotton pajamas and soaking one pair in tepid water. At bedtime, a mild- or moderate-strength corticosteroid is applied to the involved skin immediately after bathing. The wet pajamas are then donned, followed by the dry pair. These are worn through the night. In the morning, this treatment can be repeated, or the patient can bathe and immediately apply emollients and clothing. This type of therapy can be modified as the "two-socks," "two-gloves," "two-caps," "two-shirts," or "two-pants" treatment as the distribution of lesions dictates.

17. Is "hand dermatitis" a specific entity?
No. This "lumping" term includes any dermatitis mostly confined to the hands. Irritants, allergens, infection, id reactions, atopic dermatitis, and many other causes may be responsible.

18. What is pompholyx?
Pompholyx, from the Greek word for *bubble,* comprises up to 20% of hand dermatitis cases. It also has been called **dyshidrotic eczema** or **dyshidrotic dermatitis** because of a supposed and unproven association with sweat gland activity. Others reject the term *pompholyx* and instead call this clinical entity "episodic vesiculobullous eczema of the palms and soles" or "hand and foot eczema."

Clinically, one sees crops of clear, deep-seated, tapioca-like vesicles on the palms and sides of the fingers in 80% of cases (Fig. 2). Another 10% also have sole involvement, whereas the remaining 10% have only sole involvement. Although erythema is often absent, heat and prickling sensations may precede attacks. Nails may become dystrophic.

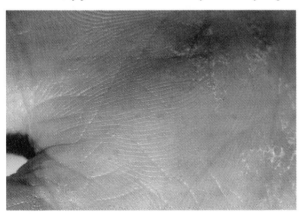

FIGURE 2. Pompholyx. Characteristic "tapioca" or "sago-grain" vesicles on the palms seen in pompholyx.

19. What causes pompholyx?
Nobody knows for sure. Most cases do not have an apparent cause or association. It may represent a palmoplantar manifestation of atopic dermatitis, since epidemiologic studies suggest a high prevalence of atopy in patients with pompholyx. Similar lesions may also be seen in patients with nummular dermatitis, contact dermatitis, oral allergy to metals (especially nickel), infections, and even pemphigus or pemphigoid. Emotional stress may exacerbate, but not cause, pompholyx.

20. How should pompholyx be managed?
Most attacks resolve spontaneously within 1–3 weeks. However, because pompholyx is generally symptomatic, certain measures should be tried. Hand protection, aluminum subacetate (Burow's solution) soaks for debridement when oozing, and bland emollients help. Large blisters can be drained, and systemic antibiotics may be used if infection is suspected. Potent topical corticosteroids can be used with or without occlusion for moderate or severe acute disease. Occasionally oral or intramuscular corticosteroids are required and bring rapid relief to patients. Alternatively, oral methotrexate can be used in severe cases as a steroid-sparing agent. Aluminum chloride (20% solution) may help in cases exacerbated by sweating. If the disease is aggravated

by stress, rest and sedation may help. Chronic and/or hyperkeratotic forms of disease can benefit from keratolytics, tar, ultraviolet B light, or even PUVA (psoralens plus UVA).

21. Describe the typical presentation of nummular dermatitis.

Nummular comes from the Latin *nummulus,* meaning "coin-like." Patients report the rapid onset of tiny papules and papulovesicles that form erythematous, coin-shaped plaques. These lesions range in size from 1–10 cm in diameter, studded by pinpoint vesicles and erosions, and resting on a background of dry skin (Fig. 3). Lesions sometimes clear centrally and resemble tinea corporis. Lesions occur most commonly on the extensor surfaces of the lower extremities, are often bilaterally symmetrical, may recur at sites of previous involvement, and are typically pruritic. Upper extremities and trunk are involved less frequently. When the trunk is involved, the back is usually severely affected while the chest and abdomen are typically spared.

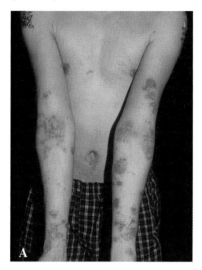 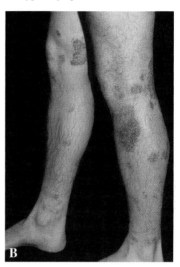

FIGURE 3. Nummular dermatitis. *A,* Typical lower-extremity distribution of coin-shaped lesions in an adult man. *B,* Close-up view of coin-shaped lesions of nummular dermatitis, also known as discoid eczema. Note the peripheral margin studded with pinpoint vesicles and erosions.

22. What is the age of onset for nummular dermatitis?

It mainly affects men and women aged 55–65 years, although there is another peak for incidence in girls and women 15–25 years old. Patients most commonly present in the winter months.

23. What causes nummular dermatitis?

Once again, nobody knows. The disease is related to dry skin but not to atopy. It is aggravated by wool, soaps, frequent bathing, and many over-the-counter topical medications. Up to 95% of patients have *S. aureus* colonizing or infecting lesions. This suggests that nummular dermatitis may be a hypersensitivity reaction to the bacteria. Alcohol abuse has been associated with nummular dermatitis, and it may be that an attenuated immune response makes patients more susceptible to bacterial infection.

24. Is there a cure for nummular dermatitis?

No. However, the disease can be controlled. Many of the same principles apply here that apply to the treatment of atopic dermatitis. Limiting baths and soap exposure, avoiding irritants, frequent use of emollients, topical corticosteroids, avoiding dry environments, and antihistamines all have a role in treatment. Topical corticosteroids are the mainstay of therapy. With the high rate of staphylococcal colonization, many dermatologists routinely prescribe a 2–3-week course of oral antibiotics, such as dicloxacillin or cephalexin. Systemic steroids should be used only for severe cases and limited to a tapered course over 2–3 weeks. Severe chronic cases may also benefit from PUVA.

25. Does nummular dermatitis resolve spontaneously?

Yes, but not often. In a prospective study of patients followed for 2 years, 22% were disease-free. Another 25% were free of lesions for weeks to months, but 53% were free of lesions only with continued local therapy. If there is no clearing within 1 year, the disease tends to persist for many years.

26. How does seborrheic dermatitis present in children?

Seborrheic dermatitis presents in infants between 2–10 weeks of age and clears spontaneously by 8–12 months of age before reappearing at puberty. Distribution in infants includes the scalp (often termed **cradle cap,** Fig. 4A), diaper area (known as **napkin dermatitis**), and other intertriginous folds. The primary lesions are round to oval patches of dry scales or yellowish-brown, greasy crusts with variable erythema.

27. How does seborrheic dermatitis present in adults?

In adults, dandruff—visible desquamation from the scalp—appears to be the precursor lesion. With progression, the scalp may become inflamed and covered with greasy scale (Fig. 4B). Dull or yellowish-red, sharply marginated, nonpruritic lesions covered with greasy scales are seen in areas with a rich supply of sebaceous glands. Characteristically, the medial eyebrows, glabella, nasolabial crease, and eyelid margins (blepharitis) are involved. Postauricular and ear canal lesions are common. The trunk may show presternal or interscapular involvement. Intertriginous areas, such the inframammary crease, umbilicus, and genitocrural folds, also are occasionally involved. Seborrheic dermatitis is one of the most common causes of chronic dermatitis of the anogenital area.

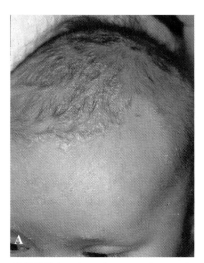
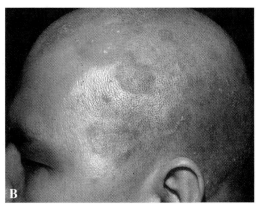

FIGURE 4. Seborrheic dermatitis. A, Infant demonstrating characteristic scalp seborrheic dermatitis commonly known as "cradle cap." B, Adult demonstrating yellowish-red sharply demarcated lesions with greasy scale. (Courtesy of James E. Fitzpatrick, MD.)

28. What is the cause of seborrheic dermatitis?

Unknown. The term *seborrheic dermatitis* may be a misnomer because the pathogenic role of sebum has not been established. The lipophilic yeast *Pityrosporum,* a normal inhabitant of the skin, has been implicated recently. This conclusion is based on the finding of higher than normal numbers of the organisms in seborrheic areas and the response of seborrheic dermatitis to antifungal therapies, such as selenium sulfide and ketoconazole.

An increased incidence and severity of seborrheic dermatitis are seen in persons with Parkinson's disease, facial paralysis, poliomyelitis, syringomyelia, quadriplegia, and emotional stress, suggesting that the CNS may influence seborrheic dermatitis. The mechanism is uncertain but may relate to increased rates of sebum production reported in some neurologic conditions. HIV-infected individuals also frequently demonstrate severe seborrheic dermatitis.

29. Discuss the treatment approaches to seborrheic dermatitis.

First, the patient must realize that there is no permanent cure. Avoid greasy ointments and reduce soap use. Shampoos active against *Pityrosporum orbiculare,* such as selenium sulfide, zinc pyrithione, or ketoconazole, or shampoos containing keratolytics, such as tar, salicylic acid, or sulfur, can control dandruff. For extremely thick scalp lesions that may overlap with psoriasis (sebopsoriasis or seborrhiasis), Baker's P and S Liquid may be left on 8–12 hours before scrubbing to loosen adherent scales, followed by appropriate shampoos. Corticosteroid scalp solutions after washing are excellent for controlling inflammation.

Blepharitis responds to warm water compresses, gentle cleansing with diluted, nonirritating shampoo (such as baby shampoo), and topical sulfacetamide ointment. The face and trunk respond to mild steroid lotions or creams, such as over-the-counter hydrocortisone, or to ketoconazole cream. A short course of ultraviolet B light or oral ketoconazole may be helpful.

30. What is an "id" reaction?

An id reaction, also known as **autosensitization dermatitis**, is immunologically mediated cutaneous inflammation in the absence of locally viable organisms or other locally inciting cause. It typically presents as a secondary, acute, papulovesicular dermatitis distant to an area of primary dermatitis. The eruption most commonly presents in a symmetric distribution on the hands, forearms, flexor aspects of the arms, extensor aspects of the arms and thighs, and, less commonly, on the face and trunk. The papulovesicles frequently coalesce into small plaques with associated red macules or wheals.

Infectious id reactions sometimes occur during cases of tuberculosis, leprosy, candidiasis, scabies, dermatophytosis (Fig. 5), and bacterial infections. The distant lesions often take on the characteristics of the primary cutaneous lesions: granulomatous inflammation in tuberculids and leprosids and pustules in bacterids, candidids, and dermatophytids.

An id reaction typically follows an acute exacerbation of pre-existing dermatitis, such as in stasis dermatitis. A true id reaction has a sudden onset and is not due to direct external contact or infection. Diagnosis requires demonstration of an antigen at some remote site, absence of allergen in the id lesions, and involution of the id reaction as the primary lesion subsides.

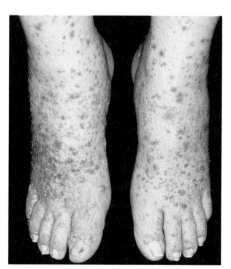

FIGURE 5. Severe papulosquamous id reaction of the lower legs secondary to a severe dermatophyte infection. (Courtesy of James E. Fitzpatrick, MD.)

31. What does an id reaction have to do with Sigmund Freud?

Nothing! In dermatologic usage, *id* derives from a Greek suffix for a father–son relationship or resemblance, as in a tuberculid or syphilid. Freud's *id* derives from a third person Latin pronoun.

32. What causes an id reaction?

One theory proposes that sensitized T-cells from the site of primary dermatitis travel to distant skin sites and stimulate the skin with various cytokines to cause an eruption. Alternatively, skin damage in the primary focus may expose or alter "hidden" skin antigens to which T-cells set up an autoimmune reaction. No one knows why this happens. Id reactions not only occur during infections, but also in noninfectious skin conditions such as burns, stasis dermatitis, and contact dermatitis.

33. How is an id reaction best treated?

The cure lies in treating the primary lesion, because by definition, an id reaction resolves when the primary dermatitis departs. Many id reactions require symptomatic treatment with antipruritics, wet-to-dry soaks, and topical corticosteroids.

34. What do you call a dermatitis that covers virtually the whole cutaneous surface?

This extreme condition is called **exfoliative dermatitis** in the U.S. and **erythroderma** in the U.K. Over 90% of the body surface is red and scaly, and about 20–30 grams of scale are shed daily.

35. Name the most common causes of exfoliative dermatitis.

Idiopathic	30%
Drug allergy	28%
Preexisting skin disease	25%
Atopic dermatitis (10%)	
Psoriasis (8%)	
Lymphoma/leukemia	14%
Contact dermatitis	3%

36. How can you determine the cause of a patient's exfoliative dermatitis?

Patients should be evaluated carefully for the causative factors (see Question 35). History and skin biopsy are the two most helpful aids. Lymph node biopsy helps rule out lymphoma. In many cases, the underlying cause is never established.

37. What general treatment measures are used to treat patients with exfoliative dermatitis?

1. First, treat the underlying disorder, if known.
2. Problems arising from the erythema and exfoliation must be treated empirically. Patients can dehydrate, go into cardiac failure, become hypothermic, have thrombophlebitis, and experience severe skin and lung infections. Fluid intake must be carefully monitored and controlled. Frequent tub baths with lubrication and topical steroids may be helpful.
3. Antihistamines are helpful in reducing pruritus.
4. All nonessential drugs should be discontinued.
5. Systemic corticosteroids should not be used unless the underlying disease is clearly steroid-responsive, because systemic corticosteroids can exacerbate psoriasis into a generalized pustular form.
6. Phototherapy may be helpful in selected patients, particularly if psoriasis is suspected.
7. Oral antibiotics should be used for secondary infections.

BIBLIOGRAPHY

1. Beltrani VS: Atopic dermatitis: The spectrum of disease. J Cut Med Surg 3(Suppl 2):8–15, 1999.
2. Egan CA, Rallis TM, Meadows KP, Krueger GG: Low-dose oral methotrexate treatment for recalcitrant palmoplantar pompholyx. J Am Acad Dermatol 40:612–614, 1999.
3. Fitzharris P, Riley G: House dust mites in atopic dermatitis. Int J Dermatol 38:173–175, 1999.

4. Grunebaum E, Lavi S: The role of food and inhaled allergens in atopic dermatitis. J Cut Med Surg 3(Suppl 2):24–28, 1999.
5. Hebert AA: Laboratory evaluation of the child with recalcitrant eczema. Dermatol Clin 12:109–121, 1994.
6. Kanani AS, Sussman GL: The role of infection in atopic dermatitis. J Cut Med Surg 3(Suppl 2):29–32, 1999.
7. Krafchik BR: Treatment of atopic dermatitis. J Cut Med Surg 3(Suppl 2):16–23, 1999.
8. Magro CM, Crowson AN: A distinctive cutaneous reaction pattern indicative of infection by reaactive arthropathy-associated microbial pathogens: The superantigen ID reaction. J Cutan Pathol 25: 538–544, 1998.
9. Mar A, Marks R: The descriptive epidemiology of atopic dermatitis in the community. Australas J Dermatol 40:73–78, 1999.
10. Rocamora V, Romani J, Puig L, de Moragas JM: Id reaction to molluscum contagiosum. Pediatr Dermatol 13:349–350, 1996.
11. Silva V, Fischman O, de Camargo ZP: Humoral immune response to *Malassezia furfur* (*Pityrosporum orbiculare*) in patients with pityriasis versicolor and seborrheic dermatitis. Mycopathologica 139: 79–85, 1997.
12. Stevens SR, Kang K, Cooper KD: Atopic dermatitis: Introduction and overview. J Cut Med Surg 3(Suppl 2):2–7, 1999.

9. CONTACT DERMATITIS

Leslie A. Stewart, M.D.

1. How common is contact dermatitis?

Contact dermatitis results in approximately 5.7 million physician visits each year, making it one of the most frequent skin complaints seen by doctors.

2. Name the two pathogenic types of contact dermatitis.

Contact dermatitis refers to cutaneous inflammation resulting from the interaction of an external agent and the skin. These reactions occur through one of two mechanisms: a nonimmunologic **irritant contact dermatitis** (ICD) or an **immunologic allergic contact dermatitis** (ACD). ICD accounts for 80% of all reactions, while ACD is responsible for approximately 20%.

3. How do substances produce irritant contact dermatitis?

While over 2800 substances have been identified as contact allergens, almost any substance under the right circumstances can act as an irritant. It is important to note that irritating compounds can be allergenic, and allergenic compounds can be irritating. There is no reliable confirmatory skin test for irritants. Diagnosis is based on the exposure history and clinical picture.

Irritants produce direct toxic injury to the skin. An irritant substance is one that causes an inflammatory reaction in most individuals when applied in sufficient concentration for an adequate length of time. The potential for an individual compound to cause contact dermatitis varies greatly. Factors affecting a cutaneous response include the **substance's** chemical and physical properties, concentration, vehicle, and duration of exposure; **patient** age, area of exposure, underlying dermatitis, and genetic makeup; and **environmental factors** such as humidity and temperature.

4. Name the two subtypes of irritant contact dermatitis, and describe them.

ICD can be divided into acute toxic and cumulative insult subtypes. **Acute toxic eruptions** occur from a single exposure to a strong toxic chemical, such as an acid or alkali, inducing erythema, vesicles, bullae, or skin sloughing. Reactions occur within minutes to hours after exposure, localize to the areas of maximal contact, and have sharp borders. In most cases, healing occurs soon after exposure.

Chronic cumulative insult reactions are the more common type of ICD. These are due to multiple exposures of many low-level irritants, such as soaps and shampoos, over time. This dermatitis may take weeks, months, or even years to appear. It is characterized by erythema, scaling, fissuring, pruritus, lichenification, and poor demarcation from the surrounding skin.

5. Explain the pathogenesis of allergic contact dermatitis (ACD).

ACD is a type IV, delayed, cell-mediated, hypersensitivity reaction. Initially, a low-molecular-weight antigen hapten (< 500 daltons) contacts the skin and forms a hapten–carrier protein complex. This complex then associates itself with an epidermal Langerhans' cell, which presents the complete antigen to a T-helper cell causing the release of various mediators. Subsequently, T-cell expansion occurs in regional lymph nodes, producing specific memory and T-effector lymphocytes which circulate in the general bloodstream. This whole process of sensitization occurs in approximately 5–21 days.

Upon re-exposure to the specific antigen, there is proliferation of activated T cells, mediator release, and migration of cytotoxic T cells, resulting in cutaneous eczematous inflammation at the site of contact. This phase occurs within 48–72 hours after exposure. Because many allergens are irritants, preceding irritation is common and may enhance allergen absorption. In contrast to irritant reactions, relatively small concentrations of an allergen can be enough to elicit an inflammatory reaction.

6. Does allergic contact dermatitis have any subtypes?

ACD can be divided into acute and chronic forms. **Acute ACD** is characterized by erythema, edema, vesicle formation, and pruritus. It frequently spreads beyond the areas of contact and becomes generalized. The classic example is poison ivy dermatitis.

Chronic ACD reactions are pruritic, erythematous, scaly, lichenified, and frequently excoriated. These may mimic chronic ICD.

Comparison of Irritant and Allergic Contact Dermatitis

	IRRITANT	ALLERGIC
Examples	Water, soap	Nickel, fragrance, hair dye
Number of compounds	Many	Fewer
Distribution of reaction	Localized	May spread beyond area of maximal contact and become generalized
Concentration of agent needed to elicit reaction	High	Can be minute
Time course	Immediate to late	Sensitization in 2 wks; elicitation takes 24–72 hrs.
Immunology	Nonspecific	Specific type IV delayed hypersensitivity reaction
Diagnostic test	None	Patch test

7. Can urticarial reactions occur from contact with a substance?

Occasionally, urticarial reactions may occur with certain exposures, instead of the eczematous changes seen with ACD and ICD. **Allergic contact urticaria** involves a specific IgE–mast cell interaction resulting in the release of vasoactive compounds. While urticaria occurs at the site of contact, more generalized symptoms can appear, including angioedema, anaphylaxis, rhinoconjunctivitis, and widespread urticaria. A good example is the latex-glove immediate reaction reported in health care professionals. **Nonimmunologic contact urticaria** occurs when the antigen either induces direct mast cell release of mediators without antibody involvement or produces a direct effect on the cutaneous vasculature. Many agents found in cosmetic products can cause a nonimmunologic contact urticaria. These include sorbic acid, benzoic acid, and cinnamic acid. This may explain the facial burning and stinging that some patients experience using cosmetics.

8. How is contact urticaria diagnosed?

To diagnose contact urticaria, a **prick test** is usually performed. In this test, a small amount of the allergen is placed on the skin, and a needle is used to prick the skin. A urticarial wheal of appropriate size constitutes a positive test, usually developing within 15–20 minutes after allergen administration (Fig. 1).

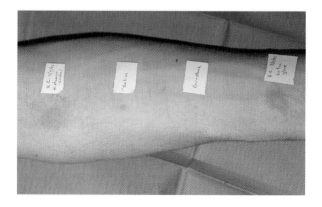

FIGURE 1. Prick test for the diagnosis of contact urticaria.

9. Why is the distribution of a contact dermatitis rash important?

The location and distribution of the dermatitis are vital clues to the underlying culprit. For example, an eczematous dermatitis on the dorsal feet should alert the clinician to the possibility of a shoe dermatitis.

Location of Contact Dermatitis and Suspicious Agents

LOCATION	SUSPICIOUS AGENT
Eyelids	Nail polish, eye makeup, airborne allergens
Earlobes or neck	Metal jewelry
Forehead, scalp margins	Hair dyes
Face	Cosmetic fragrances and preservatives, airborne allergens
Axilla	Deodorants
Hands	Gloves, occupational contacts
Waistband	Elastic
Dorsal feet	Shoes

10. List three common misperceptions regarding the location of a contact dermatitis.

1. A dermatitis has to be bilateral if the exposure is bilateral, i.e., with a shoe or glove allergy. In most cases, contact reactions tend to be patchy and do not have the same intensity at all sites of exposure.

2. The rash of contact dermatitis occurs at the site of maximal contact. Allergens can frequently be spread to distant sites of contact, as when nail polish is transferred to the eyelid, inducing a dermatitis when a sensitized patient rubs her eyelids with her fingernails.

3. Contact dermatitis does not affect the palms and soles because of their thick stratum corneum. Although it is true that other more sensitive areas such as the eyelids, face, and genitalia are more likely to be reactive, contact dermatitis definitely should be considered when dealing with an eczematous dermatitis of the palms or soles.

11. How is patch testing done?

Because ICD and ACD can be indistinguishable both clinically and histologically, patch testing is the only method available to diagnose ACD and differentiate it from ICD. Two patch test methods are currently in widespread use (Fig. 2): the Finn chamber and True test systems.

With the Finn chamber method, a small amount of the allergen, usually in a petrolatum vehicle, is placed into individual aluminum wells affixed to a strip of paper tape. With the True test method, no advance preparation is necessary, as the allergens have already been commercially incorporated into the back of the paper tape strips. Only 24 "screening" allergens are currently available with the True test, while hundreds are available with the Finn chamber method. These strips are applied to the patient's upper back, which is the preferred testing site. After 48 hours, the patches are removed and the initial reading is recorded. Because these allergic reactions are delayed, a second interpretation must be performed at 72 hours, 96 hours, or even at 1 week after the initial test application. Additional readings beyond 48 hours increase the positive patch test yield by 34%.

The classic positive allergic patch test reaction shows spreading erythema, edema, and closely set vesicles that persist after removal of the patch or may appear after 2–7 days. Irritant reactions may have a glazed, scalded, follicular, or pustular appearance that usually fades after the patch is removed.

12. What substances are tested in the standard "screening" patch test?

Usually, patients with a suspected allergic contact dermatitis are patch tested with a "standard" panel of 20–24 allergens to screen for the most common sensitivities. However, this panel only detects 75–80% of the most common allergies. Additional testing with more specialized allergens is frequently warranted. Testing should only be done with known materials in accepted concentrations.

TRUE TEST	FINN CHAMBER	ALLERGEN	SOURCES
–	+	Benzocaine 5%	Topical anesthetic
+	–	Caine mix	Topical anesthetic
+	+	Nickel sulfate 2.5%	Metal jewelry
+	+	Potassium dichromate 0.25%	Leather, cement
+	–	Cobalt	Metal jewelry, paint
+	+	Neomycin sulfate 20%	Topical antibiotics
+	+	p-Phenylenediamine 1%	Hair dye
+	+	Ethylenediamine 1%	Topical medications
–	+	Cinnamaldehyde 1%	Perfume, flavors
+	+	Balsam of Peru 25%	Perfume, medications
+	–	Fragrance mix	Perfume, flavors
+	+	Formaldehyde 1%	Preservative, fabric finishes
+	+	Quaternium-15 2%	Cosmetic and industrial preservative
–	+	Imidazolidinyl urea 2%	Cosmetic preservative
+	–	Paraben mix	Cosmetic preservative
+	–	Thimerosal	Cosmetic and medicament preservative
+	–	Cl⁺Me⁻ Isothiazoline (MCI/MI)	Cosmetic and industrial preservative
+	+	Lanolin alcohol 30%	Topical skin care products
+	+	Epoxy resin 1%	Glues, plastics
+	+	p-tert-butylphenol formaldehyde resin 1%	Glues
+	+	Colophony (resin) 2%	Adhesives, solder flux
+	+	Mercaptobenzothiazole 1%	Rubber, fungicide
+	+	Carba mix 3%	Rubber, fungicide
+	+	Thiuram mix 1%	Rubber, fungicide
+	+	Mercapto mix 1%	Rubber, fungicide
+	+	Black rubber mix 0.6%	Black rubber

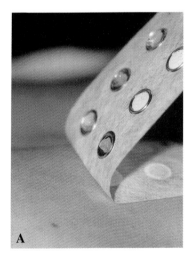

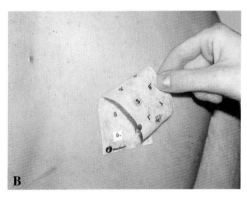

FIGURE 2. *A*, Finn chamber method. *B*, True test method.

13. An astute physician shouldn't need to patch test. Right?

Many clinicians believe that a thorough history and physical exam are sufficient for an accurate diagnosis of ACD. They believe that patch testing is unnecessary because they can tell whether a reaction is ICD or ACD simply by evaluating the dermatitis. Results of several studies, however, show that clinicians are often wrong when guessing whether contact dermatitis is irritant or allergic. In fact, experienced dermatologists may only suspect the true allergen in 50% of cases. Patch testing is the only way to differentiate between the two conditions because clinically and histologically ICD and ACD cannot be reliably differentiated.

14. What is an angry back?

The angry back or excited skin syndrome occurs when a strong positive patch test produces a state of overall skin hyper-reactivity in which other patch test sites become positive (Fig. 3). These additional reactive sites must be retested at a later date because they may be nonreproducible and actually be false-positives. The mechanism of this reaction has not been elucidated but is thought to be more common with the allergens nickel and chromium.

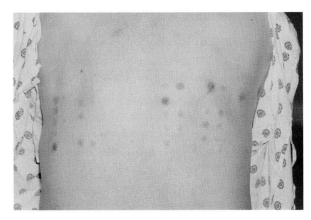

FIGURE 3. Angry back or excited skin syndrome.

15. What is a repeated open application test (ROAT)?

The ROAT, or usage test, is used when patch testing is negative yet there remains a strong clinical suspicion for ACD. Remember, patch testing is a one-time occlusive test that does not always duplicate low-level chronic daily exposure. With the ROAT, patients apply the suspected product to a quarter-sized area on the forearm twice a day for 1 week. If the patient is allergic, a localized dermatitis will occur, confirming the suspected allergy.

16. What is the differential diagnosis of contact dermatitis?

Contact dermatitis, with its scaling, erythema, lichenification, and/or vesicles, belongs in the group of eczematous disorders. Other such conditions—atopic dermatitis, nummular eczema, neurodermatitis, stasis dermatitis, seborrheic dermatitis, photodermatoses, dermatophyte infections, drug eruptions, and dyshidrotic eczema (pompholyx)—should always be considered when evaluating a prospective patient for contact dermatitis. A complete history including previous skin diseases, drug and exposure histories, location and course of the eruption, patch testing, and potassium hydroxide tests should help point to the diagnosis of contact dermatitis.

17. Is pruritus a diagnostic symptom of allergic contact dermatitis?

No. Unfortunately, pruritus is a very nonspecific symptom that occurs in a wide range of cutaneous disorders. While stinging and/or burning symptoms are more indicative of irritation, pruritus can occur with both ICD and ACD.

18. Which is the most common allergen on the standard tray?

The metal **nickel,** found commonly in costume jewelry, is the most common allergen on the standard tray. Approximately 5.8% of the general population in the U.S. is sensitized, while patch test clinics around the country note a prevalence rate of 14% in their dermatitis populations (Fig. 4). The high rate of sensitization is felt to be secondary to ear piercing, which is why this allergy is more common in females. In men, nickel dermatitis is predominantly of occupational origin.

19. Is nickel the most common allergen overall?

Poison ivy is actually the most common type IV allergen, with approximately 50–70% of the general population sensitized.

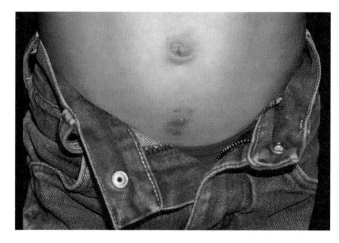

FIGURE 4. Nickel allergic contact dermatitis on the abdomen of a child due to the presence of nickel in the pants' metal snap. The rash had been previously misdiagnosed as a nummular eczema.

20. If a change in a skin care product does not lead to clearing of a patient's rash, does this mean that the original product was not the culprit?

Not necessarily. Many consumer cosmetic and toiletry products contain the same allergens (usually fragrances and preservatives). Moreover, many products contain cross-reacting agents that can exacerbate the original problem. For example, patients who are allergic to the topical anesthetic benzocaine need to avoid PABA-containing sunscreens. Both compounds belong to the *para*-amino group and can cross-react with one another.

21. Can patients develop allergic contact dermatitis to medicines?

Absolutely. Up to 5% of patients with **chronic eczema** become allergic to topical corticosteroids. Sensitization occurs to the steroid moiety by itself or to a vehicle ingredient. It is not uncommon for this population also to react to the moisturizers given for lubrication. In those cases, fragrances and preservative components are the usual culprits. Patients with **stasis dermatitis** are particularly at risk for developing ACD to topical agents, with a reported incidence of 50%. The high level of sensitivity is due to the decrease in cutaneous barrier function in their dermatitic skin, which enhances absorption of allergens and irritants into the skin.

22. Are patients with atopic dermatitis more or less likely to develop a contact dermatitis?

Because patients with atopic dermatitis have a relative T-cell defect (resulting in an increased tendency for herpes viral infections and warts), it has been expected that they should not develop ACD as frequently as normals. Others believe that patients actually may have enhanced sensitization because more allergens are absorbed through the dermatitic skin. Similarly, studies reporting the number of sensitized atopics have been contradictory, with some revealing lower, the same, or higher rates than in the general population. The general consensus, however, is that patients with atopic eczema are probably at least as likely to develop ACD as normals, but are definitely more at risk for ICD due to their decreased skin irritation threshold and increased transepidermal water loss.

Patients with atopic dermatitis and other chronic dermatitis problems should be advised to avoid over-the-counter products that have a high incidence of eliciting ACD, i.e., neomycin, fragrances, benzocaine, and products containing quaternium (Dowicil) as a preservative system. When an ACD is superimposed on a chronic dermatitis, the diagnosis is often delayed and management becomes more difficult.

23. How is contact dermatitis managed?

If the patient has **ACD,** the allergen should be detected by patch testing, and subsequently it should be thoroughly avoided. Sources of the allergen as well as cross-reacting agents should be explained to the patient. An acceptable nonsensitizing substitute should be offered.

For **ICD,** avoidance of as many irritants as possible is key. Frequent water exposure, which desiccates and chaps the skin, should be kept to a minimum. Frequent moisturization and hand protection with gloves, if indicated, are important. With contact dermatitis, systemic steroids should be used only in acute situations. Compresses may be helpful if vesicles are present. When the condition is chronic, topical steroids of appropriate strength and moisturizers are the mainstay of therapy.

BIBLIOGRAPHY

1. Adams R: Occupational Skin Disease, 3rd ed. Philadelphia, W.B. Saunders, 1999.
2. Lammintausta K, Maibach HI: Contact dermatitis due to irritation. In Adams RM (ed): Occupational Skin Disease, 2nd ed. Philadelphia, W. B. Saunders, 1990, pp 1–25.
3. Marks JG, Belsito DV, et al: North American Contact Dermatitis Group standard tray patch test results (1992–1994). Am J Contact Dermatitis l6:160–165, 1995.
4. Marks JG, DeLeo VA: Contact and Occupational Dermatology. St. Louis, Mosby, 1992.
5. Nethercott JR: Occupational skin disorders. In La Dou J (ed): Occupational Medicine. Norwalk, Appleton & Lange, 1990, pp 209–216.
6. Podmore P, Burrows D, Bingham EA: Prediction of patch test results. Contact Dermatitis 11:283–284, 1984.
7. Rietschel R, Fowler J: Fisher's Contact Dermatitis, 4th ed. Baltimore, Williams & Wilkins, 1995.
8. Rietschel RL, Adams RM, Maibach HI, et al: The case for patch test readings beyond day 2. J Am Acad Dermatol 18:42–45, 1988.
9. Rietschel RL, Adams RM, et al: Guidelines of care for contact dermatitis. Dermatol World Jul (suppl): 6–9, 1993.
10. Sherertz EF: Controversies in contact dermatitis. Am J Contact Dermatitis 5:130–135, 1994.
11. Stewart L: Occupational contact dermatitis. Immunol Allergy Clin North Am 12:831–846, 1992.
12. Tucker SB: Occupational skin disease. In Jordan RE (ed): Immunologic Diseases of the Skin. Norwalk, Appleton & Lange, 1991, pp 271–276.

10. VESICULOBULLOUS DISORDERS

Kathleen M. David-Bajar, M.D., COL, MC

1. How are the bullous diseases defined?

Blisters are defined as circumscribed skin lesions containing fluid. They may arise at various depths in the epidermis and dermis and are sometimes classified on the basis of the depth of skin involved. One broad classification divides blisters into those that develop within the epidermis **(intraepidermal)** versus those that develop below the epidermis **(subepidermal)**.

If the blister is ≤ 5 mm in diameter, it is referred to as a **vesicle**; if >5 mm, it becomes a **bulla**. Some require that blisters be 1 cm before using the term bulla.

Intraepidermal blisters	Subepidermal blisters
Allergic contact dermatitis (spongiotic)	Porphyria cutanea tarda
Bullous dermatophyte infection (spongiotic)	Bullous pemphigoid
Herpes simplex (acantholytic)	Cicatricial pemphigoid
Herpes zoster/varicella (intraepidermal acantholytic)	Dermatitis herpetiformis
Bullous impetigo	Linear IgA bullous dermatosis
Miliaria crystallina (subcorneal)	Bullous systemic lupus erythematosus (SLE)
Epidermolysis bullosa simplex (mechanobullous)	Epidermolysis bullosa acquisita
Pemphigus vulgaris (suprabasilar acantholytic)	Dystrophic epidermolysis bullosa
Pemphigus foliaceus (subcorneal acantholytic)	Junctional epidermolysis bullosa
Hailey-Hailey disease (intraepidermal acantholytic)	
Incontinentia pigmenti (spongiotic)	
Bullous congenital erythroderma (mechanobullous)	

2. What sorts of things cause vesicles and bullae?

Blisters of the skin may be induced by a wide variety of external agents and diseases, including trauma, infections, metabolic disorders, genetic deficiencies, and inflammatory diseases. (Infectious causes of blisters are discussed in Chapters 25 [viral] and 27 [bacterial].)

Infections
Bacterial (impetigo, staphylococcal
    scalded skin syndrome)
Viral (herpes simplex, varicella zoster)
Hand, foot, and mouth disease
Fungal (bullous dermatophyte infections)

Inflammatory Diseases
Bullous pemphigoid
Bullous SLE
Cicatricial pemphigoid
Dermatitis herpetiformis
Epidermolysis bullosa acquisita
Herpes gestationis
Linear IgA bullous dermatosis
Pemphigus foliaceus
Pemphigus vulgaris
Friction blisters

External Agents
Allergic contact dermatitis
Arthropod bites
Chemical burns
Heat (secondary burns)
Photo-drug eruptions
Radiation

Metabolic Disorders
Acrodermatitis enteropathica
Bullous diabeticorum
Pellagra
Porphyrias (porphyria cutanea tarda,
    variegate porphyria)
Pseudoporphyria

Genetic Deficiencies
Acrodermatitis enteropathica
Bullous congenital erythroderma
Epidermolysis bullosa
Hailey-Hailey disease
Incontinentia pigmenti

3. How do you approach a patient who presents with an acute onset of a vesiculobullous eruption?

The patient history is very important in the initial evaluation of blisters. If the onset of lesions was acute, exposure to contact allergens, arthropods, phototoxic and other drugs or chemicals, trauma, and infectious agents should be queried. Certain chronic vesiculobullous diseases may have an acute onset but then persist or recur and become chronic.

Acute	Chronic
Allergic contact dermatitis	Bullous pemphigoid
Arthropod bites	Bullous SLE
Drug eruptions (may become chronic if drug is not withdrawn)	Cicatricial pemphigoid
	Dermatitis herpetiformis
Erythema multiforme (may recur, especially if associated with herpes simplex)	Epidermolysis bullosa acquisita
	Linear IgA bullous dermatosis
Hand, foot, and mouth disease	Pemphigus foliaceus
Herpes simplex	Pemphigus vulgaris
Varicella zoster virus infections	Genetic blistering diseases
Impetigo	
Miliaria crystallina	
Physical, thermal, or chemical trauma-induced blisters	
Toxic epidermal necrolysis	

4. Which skin findings are helpful in evaluating a patient with blisters?

Several features of vesiculobullous lesions are important to note, including the distribution symmetry, involvement of mucosal surfaces, and associated lesions (such as erosions, ulcers, and crusts). Additional types of skin lesions, such as urticarial lesions, should be noted. In bullous pemphigoid, urticarial lesions often precede the development of blisters. In some vesiculobullous diseases such as dermatitis herpetiformis, secondary excoriations may be the only lesions visible, with no intact blisters.

The character of the blisters also may provide useful information. Flaccid blisters may indicate a more superficial blistering process than is seen with tense blisters. However, factors other than the depth of the blister are important, including site (blisters on acral skin, which has a thick stratum corneum, are often tense even when superficial) and the specific disease process (in toxic epidermal necrolysis, the blistering is subepidermal, but vesicles and bullae are usually flaccid with large sheets of skin sloughing).

5. Do particular vesiculobullous diseases occur in characteristic distributions?

Disease	Characteristic distribution
Acrodermatitis enteropathica	Acral, periorificial
Allergic contact dermatitis	Reflects pattern of contact; often linear
Bullous dermatophyte infection	Feet, hands
Bullous diabeticorum	Distal extremities
Bullous pemphigoid	Flexural areas, lower extremities
Cicatricial pemphigoid	Eyes, mucous membranes
Dermatitis herpetiformis	Elbows, knees, buttocks
Erythema multiforme	Acral areas, palms, soles, mucosa
Hailey-Hailey disease	Intertriginous areas, neck
Hand, foot, and mouth disease	Mouth, palms, fingers, soles
Herpes zoster	Dermatomal distribution
Linear IgA bullous dermatosis (childhood type)	Groin, buttocks, perineum
Pemphigus vulgaris	Oral mucosa, other sites
Pemphigus foliaceus	Head, neck, trunk

6. Which tests are most useful in evaluating vesiculobullous diseases?

Most of the tests helpful in determining the cause of vesiculobullous eruptions are performed on the blister itself. When infectious causes are being considered, appropriate **cultures** (aerobic bacteria, viruses, fungi) may be obtained, and **smears** from the blisters may be stained for bacteria, dermatophytes, or the multinucleate giant cells of herpes virus infections. For noninfectious vesiculobullous diseases, a skin **biopsy** is often a useful test.

7. How should a skin biopsy of a vesiculobullous eruption be performed?

The lesion for biopsy should be an early lesion, to avoid secondary changes that might make the diagnosis more difficult. A small, intact blister is a good choice, as the entire lesion and some of the surrounding skin can be removed in one piece. If a punch biopsy technique is used, it is important to avoid rupturing the blister. A small excision biopsy is a good choice and minimizes the possibility of rupturing the blister. The specimen should be placed in 10% formalin and processed for routine histologic examination. Clinical information, including the age and sex of the patient, a description of the lesions, associated symptoms, and any exacerbating factors, should be provided, along with a differential diagnosis based on the clinical examination.

8. When are special tests necessary to diagnose blistering diseases of the skin?

In addition to routine histology, a skin biopsy for **direct immunofluorescence** is often helpful in diagnosing the immunobullous diseases. For precise diagnosis of the inherited forms of epidermolysis bullosa, **electron microscopy** studies may be necessary. Other tests are indicated in specific circumstances, such as **urine porphyrin** tests when porphyria cutanea tarda is being considered, and **zinc levels** when acrodermatitis enteropathica is possible.

Disease	Direct immunofluorescence findings
Bullous pemphigoid	Linear C3, IgG at DEJ
Bullous SLE	Linear/granular IgG, other Igs at DEJ
Cicatricial pemphigoid	Linear C3, IgG, IgA at DEJ
Dermatitis herpetiformis	Granular IgA, C3 in upper dermis
Epidermolysis bullosa acquisita	Linear IgG, IgA, other Igs at DEJ
Herpes gestationis	Linear C3, IgG at DEJ
Linear IgA bullous dermatosis	Linear IgA, C3 at DEJ
Pemphigus foliaceus	IgG, C3 in intercellular spaces of epidermis
Pemphigus vulgaris	IgG, C3 in intercellular spaces of epidermis
Porphyria cutanea tarda	Homogenous IgG at DEJ, around vessels

(DEJ, dermal-epidermal junction, Ig=immunoglobulin, C3, third complement component.)

9. How are specimens obtained for direct immunofluorescence?

Generally, this specialized testing would be ordered by a dermatologist, as selection of an appropriate laboratory and proper handling of the tissue are essential to an accurate result. For most immunobullous diseases, tissue for direct immunofluorescence testing is obtained from skin next to a blister, and it is either frozen immediately in liquid nitrogen or placed in a transport medium such as Michel's media. It should *never* be placed in formalin; direct immunofluorescence testing involves identifying immunoglobulins and complement deposited in the skin, molecules that may be altered by formalin.

In some diseases, such as pemphigus vulgaris and bullous pemphigoid, indirect immunofluorescence testing also may be helpful. This procedure identifies antibodies present in the circulation; therefore, serum is submitted for evaluation. Again, only a few laboratories perform this testing routinely, so consultation with the laboratory prior to obtaining the specimen is recommended to ensure appropriate handling of the specimen.

10. Describe the blistering diseases due to external agents.

Allergic contact dermatitis: Direct contact with allergens may cause an acute, pruritic vesicular eruption in the areas of contact. When it is due to plants such as poison ivy, the pattern is often linear, corresponding to areas where the plant brushed by the skin. Diagnosis can usually be made on the basis of history and clinical findings, particularly exposure to the offending agent. Skin biopsy for routine histologic examination may be helpful in difficult cases. (See also Chapter 9.)

Bullous drug eruptions: A number of drugs can produce characteristic vesiculobullous eruptions. (See Question 11. See also Chapter 14).

Miliaria crystallina: Superficial, fragile vesicles develop as eccrine sweat ducts become obstructed. Predisposing factors include high fever and occlusion, as well as sunburn. Clinical findings are usually diagnostic, but routine skin biopsy can be helpful in making a diagnosis.

Trauma-induced blisters: Heat, chemicals, friction, and radiation (second-degree sunburn) may induce blisters. These can generally be identified readily by history and physical examination.

11. Name examples of drugs that can cause vesiculobullous eruptions.

Eruption	Offending Drug(s)
Bullous pemphigoid	Tetracycline
Erythema multiforme	Phenytoin, barbiturates, sulfonamides
Linear IgA bullous dermatosis	Vancomycin, lithium, captopril
Phototoxic drug eruption	Psoralens, thiazides, furosemide
Porphyria-like drug eruption	Furosemide, tetracycline, naproxen
Toxic epidermal necrolysis	Phenytoin, sulfonamides, NSAIDs

12. What is epidermolysis bullosa?

This is a group of diseases with inherited defects in the skin that result in blistering spontaneously or with minor trauma. Many subtypes have been described.

- **Epidermolysis bullosa simplex,** an autosomal dominant trait, begins at birth or early in childhood, with blisters due to mild trauma that heal without scarring. This disease is due to defects in keratins 5 and 14.
- **Junctional epidermolysis bullosa** also typically begins at birth and may present with generalized blistering. The blisters occur at the dermal-epidermal junction and are believed to be due to defects in laminin 5, BPAg2, or α6β4 integrin, molecules involved in anchoring the epidermis to the dermis. This type of epidermolysis bullosa may be inherited as an autosomal recessive trait.
- **Dystrophic epidermolysis bullosa** may be autosomal dominant or recessive in inheritance. It ranges from mild to severe blistering that can be disfiguring. It is due to a defect in the dermal anchoring fibrils.

For all types of epidermolysis bullosa, skin biopsies for routine histology as well as electron microscopy are often required for diagnosis. Referral to a center specializing in epidermolysis bullosa is optimal, and also the National Epidermolysis Bullosa Registry (telephone: 919–966–2007) may be contacted. The mechanobullous diseases are covered in Chapter 6.

13. Describe the other genetic blistering diseases.

Acrodermatitis enteropathica: This condition may be autosomal recessive or acquired and is due to a deficiency of zinc. Cutaneous findings include scaling and vesicles in a periorificial and acral distribution associated with alopecia. Diarrhea is often present. This disorder occurs in infants, especially premature infants, and alcoholics (acquired form) or other patients with impaired gastrointestinal absorption of zinc. Skin biopsy and serum zinc levels are helpful diagnostic tests.

Bullous congenital ichthyosiform erythroderma (epidermolytic hyperkeratosis): This autosomal dominant disease presents with diffuse erythema at birth, with later development of flaccid bullae, and still later with furrowed hyperkeratosis. The defect is in keratins 1 and 10. Diagnosis is by skin biopsy and family history, in addition to clinical findings and course.

Hailey-Hailey disease (benign familial pemphigus): In this autosomal dominant disorder, blisters, erosions, and crusts develop in the intertriginous areas. These may begin early in life or later. The intraepidermal blisters form secondary to a loss of cohesion between keratinocytes (acantholysis). The underlying defect is in ATP2C1, which encodes a calcium pump. Secondary bacterial infections are common. Diagnosis is by routine skin biopsy.

Incontinentia pigmenti: This X-linked disease is seen predominantly in females; affected males usually die in utero. It begins in neonatal life, with vesicles occurring in a whorled pattern. Later, verrucous lesions develop, and finally, hyperpigmented patches appear. Skin biopsy is a helpful diagnostic test.

14. Which vesiculobullous diseases are caused by metabolic disorders?

Bullous diabeticorum: In this disorder, tense bullae arise spontaneously on the distal extremities in patients with both insulin- and noninsulin-dependent diabetes. The course is chronic and recurring. Diagnosis is by clinical findings and skin biopsy. Although routine histologic examination is not specific, it may help to rule out other bullous diseases.

Pellagra: This nutritional disorder is caused by a deficiency of niacin, which results in dermatitis, dementia, and diarrhea. The dermatitis may occur in a photodistribution, consisting of vesicles, papules, erosions, and hyperpigmentation. The diagnosis is by clinical findings, as biopsy is nondiagnostic. In developed countries, patients at risk for pellagra include alcoholics and those on isoniazid therapy.

Porphyria cutanea tarda: In this disorder, skin fragility, tense blisters, scarring, and milia develop in sun-exposed areas, particularly the dorsal hands. The patients have decreased levels of uroporphyrinogen decarboxylase, sometimes due to alcoholic liver disease or to drugs such as estrogen and iron. Hypertrichosis may develop on the face. Diagnosis is by skin biopsy for routine histology, as well as porphyrin studies, including a 24-hour urine collection for uroporphyrins. Other porphyrias, including **variegate porphyria** and **hereditary coproporphyria,** may present with identical cutaneous findings, and should be separated from porphyria cutanea tarda on the basis of associated clinical findings and complete porphyrin studies. Direct immunofluorescence of the skin may be a helpful test for porphyria but does not distinguish one type from another.

Pseudoporphyria: The cutaneous findings are similar to those of porphyria cutanea tarda, but porphyrin studies are normal. It is associated with uremia, hemodialysis, and some drugs, especially NSAIDs. Diagnosis is by routine skin biopsy and negative porphyrin studies.

15. Describe the inflammatory bullous pemphigoid diseases.

Bullous pemphigoid: This chronic bullous disease develops most commonly in older adults and may begin with urticarial plaques, with later development of tense bullae (Fig. 1A). Lesions occur particularly on the flexural surfaces but may be widespread. Blisters form crusts and may heal with pigmentary changes, but not scarring. The oral mucosa is sometimes affected, but lesions in this area are usually minor. Diagnosis is by skin biopsy of an early blister for routine histologic examination, which demonstrates a subepidermal blister with numerous eosinophils. Perilesional skin biopsy for direct immunofluorescence may also be used for diagnosis. In addition, the serum may be examined with indirect immunofluorescence to detect the presence of circulating antibodies directed against the basement membrane.

Cicatricial pemphigoid: Blistering and scarring of mucosal surfaces, especially the ocular mucosa, are seen in this disease. It primarily affects the elderly, with some patients having involvement of the cutaneous surface with blisters. The diagnosis is made from clinical findings, routine histology of lesional skin, direct immunofluorescence of perilesional skin, and indirect immunofluorescence testing of serum.

16. How do pemphigus vulgaris and pemphigus foliaceus differ?

Pemphigus vulgaris is a chronic blistering disease that typically affects adults and usually begins in the oral mucosa. Flaccid vesicles and bullae develop on the face, scalp, neck, chest, groin, and intertriginous areas. These are often tender rather than pruritic. Generalized involvement may occur, and pemphigus vulgaris may be life-threatening.

Pemphigus foliaceus is a more superficial form of pemphigus and is generally not as severe as the vulgaris type. Patients develop very superficial vesicles and bullae, typically on the scalp, face, upper chest, and back. Because the blisters are very superficial, they often rupture, and secondary changes of scale, crust, and erosions may be the only findings present. For both varieties,

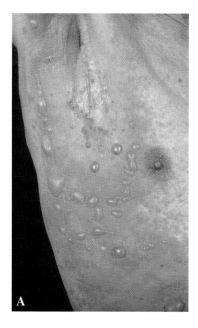
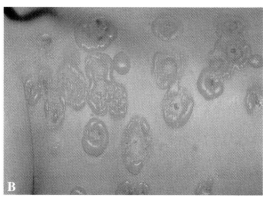

FIGURE 1. *A*, Bullous pemphigoid. Erythematous, urticarial plaques with multiple vesicles and bullae are seen in patients. Many of the blisters are tense. *B*, Linear IgA bullous dermatosis. Tense, circular, "sausage-shaped" bullae in a child.

the diagnosis is made by routine histologic exam of an early blister, as well as by direct immunofluorescence of perilesional skin and indirect immunofluorescence of patient serum.

17. Linear IgA bullous dermatosis occurs in two different clinical situations. What are they?
    One is in **early childhood** and has been termed chronic bullous disease of childhood. Pruritic, urticarial blisters, often sausage-shaped, develop on the buttocks and perianal areas, as well as the trunk and extremities (Fig. 1B). Mucosal lesions are common. The **adult** form often occurs in the elderly and may be associated with drugs such as vancomycin. Skin lesions may resemble bullous pemphigoid or dermatitis herpetiformis. Diagnosis is by routine histologic exam of an early blister, direct immunofluorescence of perilesional skin, or indirect immunofluorescence to detect IgA antibodies directed against the basement membrane zone of skin.

18. Do dermatitis herpetiformis or herpes gestationis have anything to do with herpes viruses?
    No. These are inflammatory bullous diseases and are believed to have an autoimmune etiology. **Dermatitis herpetiformis**, an extremely pruritic condition, most commonly begins in early adult life and typically affects Caucasian males. Symmetrically distributed papules and vesicles develop on the elbows, knees, buttocks, extensor forearms, scalp, and, sometimes, face and palms (Fig. 2). In some patients, the lesions are generalized and severe. Patients may have an associated gluten-sensitive enteropathy, though it is seldom symptomatic. Diagnosis is by routine histologic exam of an early blister and direct immunofluorescence of nonlesional skin (IgA is seen in the dermal papillae). Scratching may destroy all intact blisters for skin biopsy, and thus direct immunofluorescence may be a particularly helpful diagnostic test.
    Herpes gestationis is a rare, pruritic blistering disease seen in pregnant women, typically beginning in the second trimester. Lesions often begin in the periumbilical area and may initially be urticarial. Later, tense vesicles and bullae develop, which may resemble bullous pemphigoid. The disease may flare after delivery and may recur in subsequent pregnancies. The pregnancy should

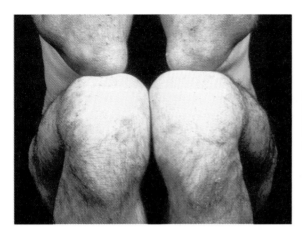

FIGURE 2. Dermatitis herpetiformis. Erythematous, crusted papules are symmetrically distributed on the elbows and knees of this patient. The lesions are extremely pruritic.

be monitored, because premature births as well as small-for-gestational-age infants have occurred in some patients. The diagnosis is made from clinical findings, routine histology of an early blister or urticarial lesion, and direct and indirect immunofluorescence test.

19. What is bullous systemic lupus erythematosus?

Bullous SLE is a rare blistering eruption that has been reported primarily in patients with established SLE. Vesicles and bullae may develop on inflamed or uninflamed skin. In some patients, the lesions may resemble bullous pemphigoid, and in others, epidermolysis bullosa acquisita. The diagnosis is made on the basis of clinical findings, routine histologic exam (which may show findings similar to those seen in dermatitis herpetiformis), and immunofluorescence studies including direct, indirect, and a special split-skin indirect immunofluorescence test.

20. What is epidermolysis bullosa acquisita?

In this disease, vesicles and bullae follow trauma and tend to occur on areas with frictional trauma, such as the fingers, knees, and elbows. Mucosal lesions are common. Like bullous SLE, diagnosis is by clinical findings, routine histology, direct immunofluorescence, indirect immunofluorescence, and split-skin indirect immunofluorescence testing.

BIBLIOGRAPHY

1. Epidermis: Disorders of epidermal cohesion. In Freedberg IM, et al (eds): Fitzpatrick's Dermatology in General Medicine. New York, McGraw-Hill, 1999.
2. Scott JE, Ahmed AR: The blistering diseases. Med Clin North Am 82:1239–1283, 1998.

11. PUSTULAR ERUPTIONS

James E. Fitzpatrick, M.D.

1. How does a pustule differ from a vesicle or bulla?

A pustule is a purulent vesicle or bulla. Whereas a vesicle contains clear or transluscent fluid, a pustule is filled with neutrophils or, less commonly, eosinophils. Pustules are one of the primary lesions in skin. Most pustular eruptions begin as pustules, but others may pass through a transitory stage in which they appear vesicular (vesiculopustules).

2. How are pustules classified?

Pustules may be classified on the basis of where the acute inflammatory cells accumulate (e.g., subcorneal, follicular), pathogenesis (e.g., infectious, autoimmune), predominant inflammatory cells (e.g., neutrophils, eosinophils), and clinical presentation. Pustules may be unilocular or multilocular.

Classification of Pustules

PATHOGENESIS	SITE OF ACCUMULATION
Infectious	
Arthropod reactions	Intraepidermal
Candidiasis	Subcorneal
Furuncle/carbuncle	Follicular
Impetigo	Subcorneal
Hot tub (pseudomonal) folliculitis	Follicular
Kerion (tinea capitis)	Follicular
Vaccinia infection/vaccination	Intraepidermal
Inherited	
Pustular psoriasis	Subcorneal, intraepidermal
Reiter's syndrome	Subcorneal, intraepidermal
Drug eruptions	
Acneiform drug-induced eruptions	Follicular
Toxic erythema with pustules	Subcorneal
Halogenodermas	Intraepidermal
Miscellaneous	
Acne necrotica miliaris	Follicular
Erythema toxicum neonatorum	Follicular
Folliculitis decalvans	Follicular
IgA pemphigus	Subcorneal
Miliaria pustulosa	Sweat duct
Pustular bacterid	Intraepidermal
Rosacea	Follicular
Subcorneal pustular dermatosis	Subcorneal
Transient neonatal pustular dermatosis	Subcorneal
Infantile acropustulosis	Subcorneal, intraepidermal

3. What is the most common pustular skin eruption?

Acne vulgaris, although not all lesions in this condition are pustular (see Chapter 21). The infectious pustular eruptions are also common (see Chapters 24–34).

4. Name the different types of pustular psoriasis. How do they differ?

Pustular psoriasis may be broadly subdivided into localized and generalized forms. **Localized pustular psoriasis** may occur on any site and may also occur within plaques of classic psoriasis. Distinctive variants include acrodermatitis continua of Hallopeau (Fig. 1A), which is characterized by pustules and crusting of the distal fingers and toes, and localized pustular

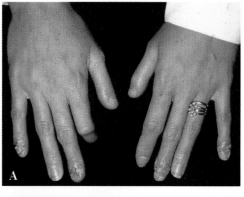

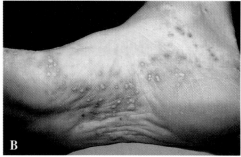

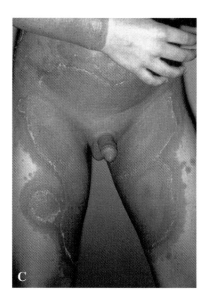

FIGURE 1. Pustular psoriasis. *A*, Acrodermatitis continua of Hallopeau demonstrating extensive crusting and nail dystrophy. *B*, Chronic pustular eruption of the sole of the foot. *C*, Patient with generalized pustular psoriasis demonstrating marked erythema studded with numerous pustules (courtesy of William James, MD).

psoriasis of the palms and soles (Fig. 1B). It is unclear whether pustular eruptions of the palms and soles represent a form of localized psoriasis or a different disease called pustular bacterid.

Variants of **generalized pustular psoriasis** include generalized pustular psoriasis of von Zumbusch, exanthematic generalized pustular psoriasis, and impetigo herpetiformis. The von Zumbusch variant presents as generalized pustules in patients with preexisting plaque-type psoriasis or erythrodermic psoriasis. Exanthematic generalized pustular psoriasis arises suddenly without preceding psoriasis (Fig. 1C). Impetigo herpetiformis is associated with pregnancy. Hypocalcemia is also frequently present.

5. Do any factors precipitate generalized pustular psoriasis?

The most important inciting factor is the administration of systemic corticosteroids. In a study of 104 patients, they were implicated as the precipitating factor in 37 patients (36%). This association is one of the primary reasons that psoriasis is not treated with systemic corticosteroids. Less common precipitating factors included infection (13%), hypocalcemia (9%), and pregnancy (3%).

6. Is pustular psoriasis treated differently than classic plaque-type psoriasis?

Most treatments that are used on classic plaque-type psoriasis can also be used for the management of pustular psoriasis. The retinoids, especially acitretin, are particularly effective in pustular psoriasis and are the treatment of choice for generalized pustular psoriasis.

7. What is pustular bacterid?

Pustular bacterid (of Andrews) is a controversial clinical eruption. Many dermatologists consider it to be a form of pustular psoriasis localized to the palms and soles. As originally defined by Andrews, pustular bacterid is a pustular eruption of the palms and soles in which the patient has no history or other clinical signs of psoriasis. The lesions are induced by low-grade bacterial infection in occult or evident foci, such as the teeth, tonsils, or gallbladder. The pustular eruption totally resolves with eradication of the infection. A later study has noted that injected Candida antigen aggravated up to 37% of patients with this disorder, suggesting that this phenomenon may not be restricted to bacterial infections. The recent recognition of bacterial "superantigens" provides a possible immunologic mechanism for induction of this disorder.

8. Why do some consider pustular bacterid a form of localized pustular psoriasis of the palms and soles?

The argument is based on the observation that some patients with pustular eruptions of the palms and soles also have typical psoriasis elsewhere. The clinical appearance and histologic findings of the palmar lesions are identical to those of pustular bacterid. Some dermatologists prefer the term palmar and plantar pustulosis as a noncommittal name for this entity.

9. What is subcorneal pustular dermatosis (Sneddon-Wilkinson disease)?

Subcorneal pustular dermatosis is a rare, benign, chronic, relapsing dermatosis that was described by Sneddon and Wilkinson in 1956. It most commonly affects middle-aged women, although any age group including children may be affected. The lesions typically occur in the flexural and intertriginous areas, where they present as superficial vesiculopustules or pustules that often assume annular or gyrate patterns. The lesions may demonstrate peripheral extension and resolve with variable crusting and scaling. Typically, patients are otherwise healthy, but there are isolated case reports of an associated seronegative rheumatoid-like arthritis.

10. Discuss the pathogenesis of subcorneal pustular dermatosis.

The pathogenesis of subcorneal pustular dermatosis is unknown; even the nosology is controversial. While most authors accept this condition as a distinct entity, a few consider it to be synonymous with, or a variant of, pustular psoriasis. Histologically, both entities demonstrate a subcorneal vesicle filled with neutrophils. The strongest points against the relationship of subcorneal pustular dermatosis and psoriasis are that it has a distinct clinical presentation, patients do not have preceding plaque-type psoriasis, and they are not likely to develop classic psoriasis during the course of their disease. It has been recently demonstrated that some cases of subcorneal pustular dermatosis may demonstrate intraepidermal IgA between the keratinocytes. It is not known whether this is related to the pathogenesis or it is an epiphenomenon. Some drugs such as lithium carbonate may exacerbate subcorneal pustular dermatosis by increasing neutrophil migration into lesions.

11. How is subcorneal pustular dermatosis treated?

Subcorneal pustular dermatosis cannot be cured, but it can be managed. The disease is uncommon enough that good therapeutic studies comparing different treatment modalities are not available. Anecdotal reports have described excellent therapeutic results with dapsone and acitretin. Less frequently used therapies include oral prednisone, topical corticosteroids, sulfapyridine, vitamin E, and ultraviolet B therapy.

12. What is superficial IgA pemphigus?

Recently it has been demonstrated that some cases of what where formerly classified as subcorneal pustular dermatosis may demonstrate intraepidermal IgA between the keratinocytes. Most authorities feel that cases with intraepidermal IgA on direct immunofluorescence should be reclassified as superficial IgA pemphigus (Fig. 2). It has been demonstrated that the IgA autoantibodies are directed against desmocollin 1 and possibly desmocollin 2, which are two molecules that are important for normal adhesion between keratinocytes.

13. What are the cutaneous findings in Reiter's disease?

The classic triad of Reiter's disease consists of nongonococcal urethritis, conjunctivitis, and arthritis. However, this triad is present in only 40% of the cases at the time of presentation, and the mucocutaneous findings are helpful in establishing the diagnosis. The mucocutaneous find-

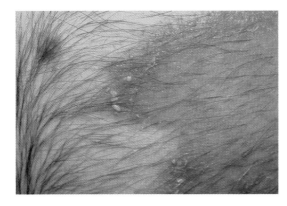

FIGURE 2. Isolated pustule and annular lesions demonstrating scale-crust and superficial pustules in a patient with IgA pemphigus. In the past this would have been considered to be subcorneal pustular dermatosis.

ings include a nonspecific stomatitis, nail changes (subungual hyperkeratosis and onycholysis), circinate balanitis, and keratoderm blennorrhagicum. Keratoderma blennorrhagicum is present in about one-third of cases and presents as pinpoint erythematous papules that progress to pustules and hyperkeratotic papules and plaques. These are most commonly seen on the bottom of the feet but may also occur on the scalp, elbows, knees, buttocks, and genitalia. Histologically, the findings are identical to the pustules seen in pustular psoriasis.

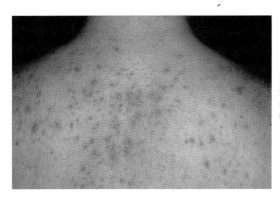

FIGURE 3. Corticosteroids-induced acne manifesting as the explosive onset of numerous follicular based papules and pustules.

14. Which drugs are commonly associated with pustular drug eruptions?

Drugs may produce different patterns of pustular drug eruptions, including aggravation of preexisting pustular eruptions such as psoriasis or subcorneal pustular dermatosis. Primary pustular drug eruptions can be classified as acneiform, halogenodermas, and toxic erythema with pustules.

- *Acneiform drug eruptions:* systemic corticosteroids (steroid acne), phenytoin, lithium, iodides, bromides, isoniazid (Fig. 3)
- *Halogenodermas:* iodides, bromides; may produce both acneiform drug eruptions and nonfollicular pustules (Fig. 4)
- *Drug-induced toxic erythema with pustules* (acute generalized exanthematous pustulosis): an uncommon drug eruption that presents as fever, malaise, and diffuse erythema studded with small pustules; caused by numerous medications including co-trimoxazole, erythromycin, hydroxychloroquine, streptomycin, terbinafine, and cephalosporins

15. What is acne necrotica miliaris?

This chronic folliculitis of the scalp, which primarily affects middle-aged men, presents as follicular-based pustules that quickly develop into perifollicular crusts and scale. The eruption may be asymptomatic or pruritic. If the lesions are pruritic, secondary excoriations may predominate. Acne necrotica miliaris does not result in permanent scarring or hair loss. Most patients respond to low-dose tetracycline, which may need to be continued for years.

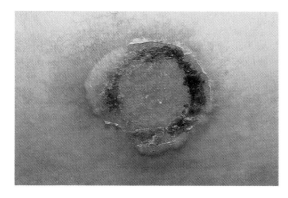

FIGURE 4. Annular pustular eruption of the back secondary to oral potassium iodide (iododerma).

16. What is folliculitis decalvans?

Folliculitis decalvans (Quinquaud's disease) is a rare, scarring alopecia of unknown etiology. Clinically, it presents as follicular-based pustules that may assume annular or circinate configurations. The pustules rapidly form crusts; in many patients, the crusts may predominate. The hairs are permanently lost, leaving patches of atrophic hairless skin.

Treatment is generally unsatisfactory; topical corticosteroids and oral antibiotics are typically used. Anecdotal reports have described isolated success with oral rifampin or oral zinc sulfate.

17. Discuss the pathogenesis of miliaria pustulosa.

All forms of miliaria result from the retention of sweat secondary to **occlusion of the sweat ducts.** The pathogenesis of miliaria pustulosa is not entirely understood, but it is believed that heat and occlusion result in the proliferation of surface bacteria which produce toxins that damage the acrosyringium (intraepidermal portion of the eccrine sweat duct).

Depending on the level of occlusion, different patterns of disease are produced. If significant numbers of neutrophils are attracted to the acrosyringium, a flaccid pustule develops, producing **miliaria pustulosa**. If the disease is less severe or the inflammatory response muted, then only an erythematous papule is present, producing the clinical lesion called **miliaria rubra** (heat bumps, prickly heat). If the damage to the acrosyringium is entirely mechanical, such as occurs following a sunburn, the inflammatory response is minimal and small superficial vesicles are formed at the acrosyringium, producing the variant referred to as **miliaria crystallina.**

18. How is miliaria pustulosa treated?

Once miliaria pustulosa has developed, there is no satisfactory treatment except removing the patient from the hot and humid environment. Occlusive wear that may have aggravated the condition should also be eliminated. Anecdotally, some dermatologists have tried weak solutions of salicylic acid to produce exfoliation or tape stripping of the stratum corneum to remove the obstruction to sweating, but there are no studies to document the efficacy of these treatments. Some patients may require weeks or even months to establish normal sweating after severe attacks.

19. What is the differential diagnosis of a pustular eruption in a neonate?

Erythema toxicum neonatorum	Staphylococcal infection
Transient neonatal pustular melanosis	Herpes simplex (more commonly vesicular)
Incontinentia pigmenti (more	Candidiasis
commonly vesicular)	Congenital syphilis

20. How do erythema toxicum neonatorum and transient neonatal pustular melanosis differ?

Erythema toxicum neonatorum (ETN) and transient neonatal pustular melanosis (TNPT) are both benign vesiculopustular disorders of unknown etiology that present during the first few days of life. ETN does not demonstrate a racial predilection and is very common, with up to 20% of neonates being affected. Clinically, it usually presents as macular erythema that usually affects the face initially; approximately 10–20% of cases develop pustules within the center of the areas of macular erythema. Biopsies of the pustules demonstrate an acute superficial folliculitis composed primarily of eosinophils. Peripheral eosinophilia may be present in 20% of cases. The lesions resolve without permanent sequelae in 7–10 days.

Epidemiologically, TNPT differs from ETN in that it occurs in about 5% of black neonates but < 1% of white neonates. Clinically, it presents as vesiculopustules that are not associated with surrounding erythema. The vesiculopustules resolve within 48 hours and are followed by hyperpigmented macules that may take 3 months to resolve. In contrast to ETN, biopsies demonstrate subcorneal pustules that are not follicular-based, and the primary inflammatory cells are neutrophils. Peripheral eosinophilia is absent.

Both conditions are benign and self-limited. Treatment is not recommended.

21. What is infantile acropustulosis?

Infantile acropustulosis, also referred to as acropustulosis of infancy, is an inflammatory disease first described in 1979. Most case reports have been in black infants from the southern United States, but it has also been reported from other racial groups and countries including Scandinavia. Clinically, the condition is characterized by recurrent crops of 1–2-mm intensely pruritic vesiculopustules on the extremities (Fig. 5). Histologically, there are well-circumscribed intraepidermal pustules filled with neutrophils. Most cases spontaneously resolve by 2 years of age.

22. What causes infantile acropustulosis?

The etiology and pathogenesis are unknown. It has been postulated that this condition represents a nonspecific host response to arthropod bites. In support of this, some infants with scabies demonstrate similar acral vesiculopustules.

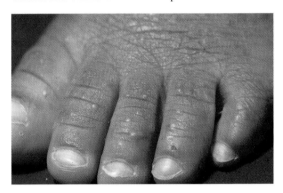

FIGURE 5. Infantile acropustulosis demonstrating typical, pruritic acral pustules in a black child.

23. What is the best treatment of infantile acropustulosis?

None. The disease is self-limited; it usually disappears spontaneously by age 2 years. Patients with severe pruritus can be treated with high doses of antihistamines. Rare patients may require treatment with oral dapsone.

BIBLIOGRAPHY

1. Baker H, Ryan TJ: Generalized pustular psoriasis: A clinical and epidemiologic study of 104 cases. Br J Dermatol 80:771–793, 1968.
2. Barr RJ, Globerman LM, Werber FA: Transient neonatal pustular melanosis. Int J Dermatol 18:636–638, 1979.
3. Harris J, Schick B: Erythema neonatorum. Am J Dis Child 92:27, 1956.
4. Jarratt M, Ramsdell W: Infantile acropustolosis. Arch Dermatol 115:834–836, 1979.
5. Kempinaire A, De Raeve L, Merckx M, et al: Terbinafine-induced acute generalized exanthematous pustulosis confirmed by a positive patch-test result. J Am Acad Dermatol 37:653–655, 1997.
6. Lyons JH: Generalized pustular psoriasis. Int J Dermatol 26:409–428, 1987.
7. Stevens DM, Ackerman AB: On the concept of bacterids (pustular bacterid, Andrews). Am J Dermatopathol 6:281–286, 1984.
8. Ündar L, Göze F, Hah MM: Subcorneal pustular dermatosis with seronegative arthritis. Cutis 42:229, 1988.

12. LICHENOID SKIN ERUPTIONS

Martin L. Johnson, M.D., LTC, MC, USAF

1. How does a lichenoid eruption differ from other papulosquamous conditions?

The lichenoid skin eruptions are part of the papulosquamous category of skin eruptions; i.e., they demonstrate primary lesions that are scaling papules. They differ from many papulosquamous diseases, however, in that their scale is often subtle and the papules tend to remain small and discrete, although at times plaques may form.

2. What does "lichenoid" mean?

The term *lichenoid* has at least three generally accepted applications:

1. Originally, the term referred to the clinical resemblance of the eruption to lichens.

2. Because lichen planus (LP) is the prototypical lichenoid eruption, eruptions sharing clinical features with LP are often described as lichenoid.

3. Lichenoid refers to the histologic tissue reaction of a band-like lymphocytic infiltrate hugging the dermal-epidermal junction, which is typical of LP.

3. Name the most common lichenoid skin disease.

Lichen planus. While not frequent, LP is a relatively common disorder in medical practice, accounting for about 1% of dermatology patient visits. The disease most commonly affects middle-aged adults and shows no consistent gender predilection.

4. Where does LP most frequently present?

The skin and oral mucosa are the most common sites of involvement, and involvement in one should prompt examination of the other. The relative frequency of involvement of these areas is somewhat controversial; patients with oral disease often demonstate no skin lesions, but approximately 50% of patients with cutaneous disease have oral lesions.

5. Describe the characteristic primary cutaneous lesions of LP.

LP is a disease characterized by "*P*" words:

Plentiful	Polished	Papular
Pruritic	Purple	Planar
Polygonal		

The primary lesions on the skin are 1–5-mm, flat-topped, violaceous shiny papules (Fig. 1). While the papules often are clustered, individual lesions tend to be discrete with angulated borders. **Wickham's striae,** a lacy white network on the surface of the papules, is typical and of great diagnostic value.

6. What are the characteristic oral findings in LP?

The mucosal lesions of LP differ from cutaneous lesions by demonstrating Wickham's striae in the absence of a papular component. The usual finding is a white netlike or reticulated, patterned discoloration of the buccal mucosa or other oral mucosal surfaces (Fig. 2).

7. Where do cutaneous lesions of LP usually present?

The flexor aspects of the wrist and forearm. However, LP can involve any cutaneous site, with additional preferred sites including the lateral surfaces of the neck, buttock, sacrum, anogenital region, penis, and ankle.

8. Describe the isomorphic response in LP.

The isomorphic response (**Koebner's phenomenon**) refers to the development of new lesions in response to external trauma. This phenomenon is characteristic of psoriasis and LP. The

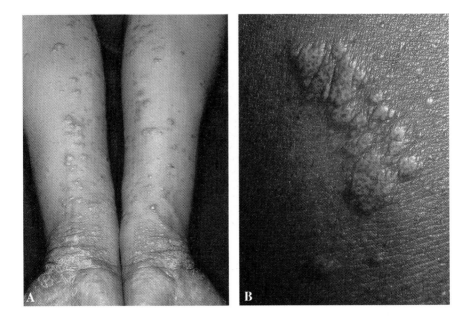

FIGURE 1. Lichen planus. *A*, Typical violaceous flat-topped, polygonal papules. The location on the volar wrist is characteristic. *B*, Note the Wickham's striae. (Courtesy James E. Fitzpatrick, MD.)

isomorphic response may be induced by scratching, physical trauma, or other cutaneous injury. In LP, linear aggregates of typical papules may be caused by scratching or rubbing.

9. What causes LP?

LP remains an idiopathic condition. Etiologic hypotheses include hypersensitivity, viral infection (particularly hepatitis C), autoimmune reaction, and psychogenic origin. In support of these hypotheses are case reports linking LP to viral hepatitis, neurologic disease, and severe psychic trauma. Furthermore, identical lichenoid eruptions may be seen in certain drug eruptions and after allogeneic bone marrow transplantation as a manifestation of graft-versus-host disease. Oral and, to a lesser degree, cutaneous LP have been associated with hypersensitivity to dental amalgams. Most cases of LP occur in otherwise healthy people, and no cause is identified.

10. What are the less common presentations of LP?

Nail changes occur in 10% of patients and include onychodystrophy (including "20-nail dystrophy") as well as the less severe manifestations of longitudinal ridging, irregular pitting, nailplate splitting, nail loss, and pterygium formation (Fig. 2). Desquamative vaginitis may occur. Hypertrophic, ulcerative, vesiculobullous, follicular, and actinic LP are specific variants.

11. How is 20-nail dystrophy related to LP?

The etiology of 20-nail dystrophy is controversial. This nail disorder affects mostly children and is not associated with cutaneous LP. It involves all 20 nails, showing excessive longitudinal ridging with thin, brittle, opalescent nails. Although some consider LP as a possible etiology, nail biopsy studies have shown a spongiotic inflammation and not a lichenoid process.

12. Is LP associated with systemic diseases?

LP has been associated with numerous disorders, but the relationships are weak and perhaps fortuitous. Associated conditions include viral hepatitis, chronic active hepatitis, primary biliary cirrhosis, diabetes mellitus, internal malignancy, and autoimmune or connective tissue diseases.

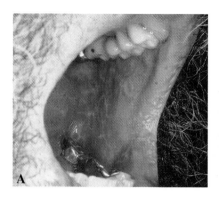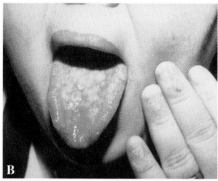

FIGURE 2. *A*, Lichen planus, showing reticulated leukoplakia of the buccal mucosa (courtesy James E. Fitzpatrick, MD). *B*, Patient with ulceration of the oral mucosa and dystrophic nails (courtesy William James, MD).

13. What is the prognosis of LP?

The duration of LP is related to the involved sites. Particularly, oral involvement portends a chronic course, perhaps lasting decades. Cutaneous involvement alone usually clears within 1 year. Patients with both mucosal and cutaneous involvement have an intermediate prognosis. Certain clinical subtypes, such as ulcerative, palmoplantar, and actinic LP, are more recalcitrant. Twenty percent of patients may have a relapse after initial clearing.

14. What is the primary symptom of LP?

Pruritus is typically intense in LP. Most patients report severe itching, although it is rarely absent. The pruritus is of a special quality in that it usually induces rubbing, rather than scratching, for relief. The rubbing may account for the polished appearance of the papules. If excoriation does occur, new lesions are likely to develop in the wounds.

15. LP has a distinctive histopathologic appearance. Describe the key features.

- The statum corneum is thickened (hyperkeratotic) with no retained keratinocytic nuclei (no parakeratosis).
- The granular layer is accentuated.
- The Malpighian layer is irregularly thickened, demonstrating "sawtooth" acanthosis and occasional necrotic keratinocytes.
- The basal layer is disrupted and appears lost or flattened.
- The dermal-epidermal junction is vacuolated and obscured by a band-like **lymphocytic infiltrate** which fills the upper dermis. The lymphocytic infiltrate is so typical of LP that any similar pattern is referred to as a "lichenoid infiltrate."

16. What is the primary differential diagnostic possibility of an LP-like eruption?

LP-like drug eruptions are common and may be indistinguishable from classic LP. Essentially, any exogenous chemical may be causative, but common etiologic agents are listed below. Clinical clues suggesting LP-like drug eruptions include atypical distribution and lack of mucosal involvement; histopathogic clues are parakeratosis and eosinophils in the infiltrate.

Common Etiologic Drug Classes in LP-like Drug Eruptions

Antihypertensives	Antimalarials
Beta-blockers	Chloroquine
Angiotensin-converting enzyme inhibitors	Quinacrine
Thiazides	Anticonvulsants
Furosemide	Carbamazepine

Table continued on next page.

Common Etiologic Drug Classes in LP-like Drug Eruptions (Cont.)

Methyldopa	Phenytoin
Antibiotics	Neurologic
Acyclovir	Benzodiazepines
Isoniazid	Phenothiazines
Tetracyclines	Photodevelopers
Anti-inflammatory agents	Sulfonylureas
Nonsteroidal anti-inflammatory drugs	Chlorpropamide
Gold salts	Miscellaneous
Sulfones	Allopurinol
	Penicillamine

17. Are LP and sytemic lupus erythematosus related?

Systemic lupus erythematous (SLE) has occasionally been diagnosed in patients with LP, and there may be an "LP-LE overlap" syndrome. Acrally located papulosquamous lesions of SLE may resemble LP. In such cases, typical features of SLE are also present.

18. Why is graft-versus-host disease a consideration in lichen planus?

Graft-versus-host disease (GVHD) is a common complication of allogeneic bone marrow transplantation. In GVHD, the foreign bone marrow reacts against antigens in its new host. A lichenoid eruption that may be clincially and histopathologically indistinguishable from classic LP is a common presentation of chronic GVHD. However, lichenoid GVHD is usually more generalized than classic LP.

19. Describe the primary lesion of lichen nitidus.

Lichen nitidus (LN) manifests numerous, 1–2 mm, round or polygonal, flat-topped, shiny, flesh-colored papules typically occurring in a circumscribed area on the extremities, abdomen, or penis (Fig. 3). Rarely are mucosal or nail changes present.

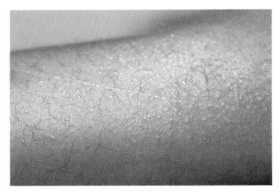

FIGURE 3. Lichen nitidus, with numerous 1–2-mm, shiny, flat-topped papules. Note the linear lesions secondary to the isomorphic phenomenon.

20. What are the other clinical features of lichen nitidus?

LN is relatively uncommon relative to LP and has no gender, age, or race predilection. The eruption is idiopathic, chronic, and, fortunately, asymptomatic. It may demonstrate the isomorphic response. The disease is often self-limited, resolving spontaneously over months or years. There are no recognized systemic disease associations. Response to treatment, generally limited to mild topical corticosteroids, is often poor. Reassurance is frequently the best therapy.

21. Does lichen nitidus demonstrate a lichenoid infiltrate?

No. LN is clinically lichenoid, but histopathologically it is granulomatous. Typically, the epidermis is atrophic centrally, but peripherally, clawlike ridges extend into the papillary dermis around a loosely nested collection of lymphocytes and histiocytes.

22. What is lichen striatus?

Lichen striatus is an uncommon idiopathic dermatosis presenting as a linear plaque, most commonly on the extemities or neck of a child. The primary lesions appear abruptly as a small group of flesh- to rose-colored lichenoid papules. The papules coalesce and may extend to form a linear band several centimeters wide coursing the entire length of the extremity.

23. Discuss the natural history and prognosis of lichen striatus.

Lichen striatus develops rapidly over a period of weeks. Pruritus is common but often minimal. Spontaneous resolution within several months, rarely more than a year, is characteristic. Minimally symptomatic patients require only reassurance; recalcitrant or intensely pruritic cases may respond to topical corticosteroids.

24. What is lichen simplex chronicus?

Lichen simplex chronicus (LSC) is not a disease but a reaction pattern of the skin to chronic friction from rubbing or scratching. LSC can be superimposed on normal skin but is commonly a secondary change seen on chronically inflamed skin. The clinical appearance, termed **lichenification,** is characteristic regardless of the underlying etiology. Lichenification is an inflammatory thickening of the skin with accentuation of the normal skin lines. Closely set lichenoid papules may be discerned peripherally. Frequently, the lichenified plaque has a dusky violaceous hue.

25. How is lichen simplex chronicus treated?

LSC is a self-perpetuating dermatosis; it may persist indefinitely after the initiating stimulus is eliminated. Therefore, cessation of the itch-scratch cycle is imperative to the resolution of LSC. Persistent dermatitis is usually treated with a short course of medium- or high-potency topical corticosterioids. Covering the plaque is very important, as this acts as a physical barrier to continued frictional trauma and as an occlusive adjunct to the topical preparation. Patients must know the cause of their condition and be motivated to stop scratching.

BIBLIOGRAPHY

1. Boyd AS, Nelder KH. Lichen planus. J Am Acad Dermatol 25:593–619,1991.
2. Boyd AS: Update on the diagnosis of lichenoid dermatitis. Adv Dermatol 11:287–315, 1996.
3. Braun-Falco O, Plewig G, Wolff HH, Winkelmann RK. Dermatology. New York, Springer-Verlag, 1991.
4. Bricker SL. Oral lichen planus: A review. Semin Dermatol 13:87–90, 1994.
5. Cribier B, Frances C, Chosidow O: Treatment of lichen planus. An evidence-based medicine analysis of efficacy. Arch Dermatol 134:1521–1530, 1998.
6. Ellgehausen P, Elsner P, Burg G: Drug-induced lichen planus. Clin Dermatol 16:325–332, 1998.
7. Fitzpatrick TB, Eisen AZ, Wolff K, et al (eds): Dermatology in General Medicine, 4th ed. New York, McGraw-Hill, 1993.
8. Halevy S, Shai A: Lichenoid drug eruptions. J Am Acad Dermatol 29:249–255, 1993.
9. Jerastus S, Suvanprakorn P, Kitchawengkul O: Twenty-nail dystrophy. Arch Dermatol 126:1068–1070, 1990.
10. Johnson ML, Farmer ER: Graft-versus-host reactions in dermatology. J Am Acad Dermatol 38:369–392, 1998.
11. Kennedy D, Rogers M: Lichen striatus. Pediatr Dermatol 13:95–99, 1996.
12. Ostman PO, Anneroth G, Skoglund A: Amalgam-associated oral lichenoid reactions. Clinical and histologic changes after removal of amalgam fillings. Oral Surg Oral Med Oral Pathol Oral Radiol Endod 81:459–465, 1996.
13. Rebora A: Lichen planus and the liver. Int J Dermatol 31:392–395, 1992.
14. Sanchez-Perez J, De Castro M, Buezo GF, et al: Lichen planus and hepatitis C virus: Prevalence and clinical presentation of patients with lichen planus and hepatitis C virus infection. Br J Dermatol 134:715–719, 1996.
15. Shai A, Halevy S: Lichen planus and lichen planus-like eruptions: Pathogenesis and associated diseases. Int J Dermatol 31:379–384, 1992.

13. GRANULOMATOUS DISEASES OF THE SKIN

Troy Richey, M.D., and James E. Fitzpatrick, M.D.

1. What is meant by "granulomatous diseases of the skin?"

Quite simply, the granulomatous disorders of the skin comprise a broad category of diseases that are characterized histologically by the presence of granulomas.

2. What are granulomas?

A granuloma (or granulomatous infiltrate) is a focal infiltrate composed primarily of macrophages and their variants, which include epithelioid macrophages and multinucleated giant cells. Macrophages develop from bone marrow–derived monocytes that leave the circulation and enter the skin. Lymphocytes and varying numbers of eosinophils, neutrophils, plasma cells, and fibroblasts also may be present in a granulomatous infiltrate.

3. Explain the role of histiocytes in granulomas.

Many textbooks use the confusing term *histiocyte* when discussing granulomas. *Histiocyte* may be used interchangeably with macrophage or monocyte, but the term is not specific and may be applied also to transformed lymphocytes (e.g., histiocytic lymphoma), fibroblasts that demonstrate phagocytosis (e.g., fibrous histiocytoma, reticulohistiocytoma), and antigen-presenting cells (e.g., histiocytosis X).

4. What causes granulomas?

Granuloma formation is the local tissue response to a poorly soluble substance. The mechanism by which this occurs is not completely understood, but it appears to be via the cell-mediated arm of the immune system. The persistent presence of a poorly soluble substance in the skin causes the activation of T cells, which secrete cytokines causing the ingress, activation, and proliferation of macrophages in the area. The activated macrophages try to phagocytize and destroy the inciting agent or at least to wall it off to keep it from harming the host. In general, granulomas are produced either by infectious agents, foreign bodies, or alterations in the host immune system.

5. List some common granulomatous diseases that affect the skin.

Agents and Diseases that Can Produce Granulomas

Infectious Agents

Fungi	*Bacteria*	*Miscellaneous*
Blastomycosis	Actinomycosis	Leishmaniasis
Candidiasis	Cat scratch fever	Protothecosis (algae infection)
Chromomycosis	Granuloma inguinale (donovanosis)	
Coccidioidomycosis	Mycobacterial infections	
Cryptococcosis	Nocardiosis	
Histoplasmosis	Syphilis	
Sporotrichosis	Tularemia	
	Lymphogranuloma venereum	

Foreign Body Agents		**Miscellaneous Diseases**
Exogenous	Talc	Actinic granuloma
Aluminum	Tattoo pigment	Crohn's disease
Beryllium	Thorns	Granuloma annulare
Hair	Zirconium	Necrobiosis lipoidica
Insect parts	*Endogenous*	Rheumatoid nodules
Paraffin	Bone	Rosacea
Sea urchin spines	Calcium	Sarcoidosis
Silica	Cholesterol	
Silicone	Keratin	
Splinters	Sebum	
Starch	Urate	
Sutures		

6. Can granulomas be recognized clinically?

Sometimes. Granulomas usually present as dermal nodules, although epidermal changes can be present. Foreign body granulomas may demonstrate a central erosion or ulceration secondary to an attempt by the body to extrude the foreign material through an elimination tract. Granulomas often present as nonspecific erythematous nodules. However, they also may present as dermal nodules with an apple-jelly hue that is highly suggestive of an underlying granulomatous process. This apple-jelly hue can frequently be better appreciated by using **diascopy** (applying pressure to the lesion with a glass slide).

7. How do endogenous "foreign" bodies cause granulomas?

Endogenous substances produce a granulomatous reaction when they are exposed to tissues that normally surround them. For example, one of the most common foreign body reactions occurs when an epidermoid cyst wall ruptures and its keratin contents come in contact with the dermis. Normally, the keratin within the cyst is protected from the dermis by the cyst's epithelial lining. However, when a cyst ruptures, the keratin is exposed to the dermis, and being a poorly soluble substance, it produces a granulomatous response.

A second mechanism occurs when endogenous substances that are normally soluble crystallize into large aggregates, which then provoke a granulomatous foreign body reaction (e.g., uric acid crystals in gouty tophi and calcium in calcinosis cutis).

8. What are the sources of the exogenous foreign body agents?

Sources of Foreign Bodies

AGENT	SOURCE
Silicone	Breast implants, joint prostheses, soft tissue injections, hemodialysis tubing
Silica	Soil and rock (very abundant), glass
Paraffin (oils)	Cosmetic injection (historically), factitial injection, grease gun injury
Starch	Surgical gloves contaminating wounds
Graphite	Pencil lead (Fig. 1A)
Thorns	Roses, cactus, yucca (Fig. 1B)
Hair	Barbers, dog groomers, sheep shearers
Talc	IV drug use, wound contamination
Aluminum	Adjuvant in DPT immunizations
Zirconium	Deodorant sticks
Beryllium	Metal, ceramic, and electronic industries; fluorescent lamp workers (historically, as this ceased in 1951)

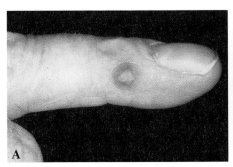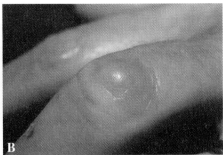

FIGURE 1. *A*, Typical graphite granuloma due to pencil lead injury. *B*, Skin-colored nodule due to yucca thorn embedded in skin for several years.

9. Can the cause of a foreign body reaction be diagnosed histologically?

Sometimes. Often, a tattoo granuloma may retain some color or pigment that can help with the diagnosis. Silicone, paraffin, and other oils are often accompanied by fibrosis and a characteristic

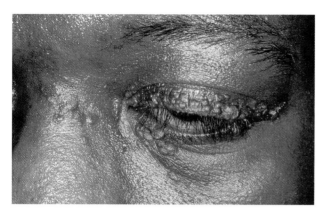

FIGURE 2. Typical numerous periocular papules in a patient with sarcoidosis.

"Swiss cheese" appearance. The Swiss cheese–like holes are actually cavities formerly filled with the oily material that is lost during tissue processing. Also, some foreign bodies are birefringent under polarized light—e.g., talc, starch, silica, and some types of sutures.

10. What is sarcoidosis?

The Seventh International Conference on Sarcoidosis gave the following definition:

"Sarcoidosis is a multisystem granulomatous disorder of unknown etiology. It most commonly affects young adults and presents most frequently with bilateral hilar lymphadenopathy, pulmonary infiltration, [and] skin or eye lesions. The course and prognosis may correlate with the mode of onset. An acute onset with erythema nodosum heralds a self-limiting course and spontaneous resolution, whereas an insidious onset may be followed by relentless, progressive fibrosis."

11. How often is the skin involved in sarcoidosis?

The skin is involved in 20–35% of patients. These findings may be divided into specific and nonspecific lesions. Specific lesions demonstrate sarcoid granulomas on histology, while nonspecific lesions demonstrate some other reactive change.

12. Describe the specific cutaneous findings in sarcoidosis.

The most common cutaneous findings are small papules that may be skin-colored, red, violaceous, yellow-brown, brown, or hypopigmented. The surface is typically smooth but variable scale or umbilication may be present. They are most commonly found around eyelids, nasal alae and nasolabial folds, and malar and neck regions (Fig. 2).

The second most common specific skin lesions are plaques that may assume an annular configuration. Like the papules, the plaques may be skin-colored, red, violaceous, yellow-brown,

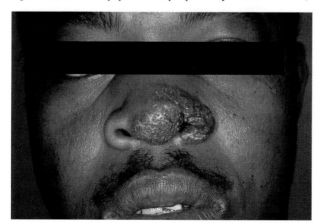

FIGURE 3. Indurated plaque on the nose of a patient with lupus pernio.

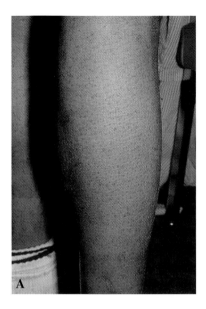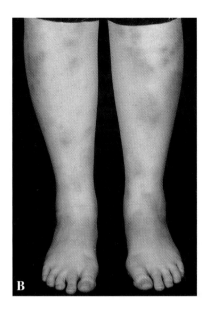

FIGURE 4. *A*, Acquired ichthyosis in a patient with sarcoidosis. *B*, Patient with Löfgren's syndrome demonstrating tender red subcutaneous lesions characteristic of erythema nodosum.

brown, or hypopigmented and the surface may be smooth or demonstrate variable scale. Plaques are usually more recalcitrant to therapy. Plaques with marked overlying vascular dilatation are termed **angiolupoid sarcoidal plaques**.

Uncommon types of specific cutaneous lesions include subcutaneous nodules, involvement of scars and tattoos, erythroderma, ulcerations, verrucous lesions, dystrophic nails, scarring alopecia, and pustular lesions.

13. What is lupus pernio?

This distinct form of cutaneous sarcoidosis presents as purplish plaques around the nose, ears, lips, face, and fingers (Fig. 3). It is usually an insidious process with slow progression that results in scarring, fibrosis, and deformity. It rarely involutes spontaneously and is associated with bony involvement specifically and systemic disease in general.

14. Describe the nonspecific cutaneous lesions of sarcoidosis.

The most common nonspecific cutaneous lesion is erythema nodosum, which may be present in up to 17% of patients. Clinically and histologically it is identical to erythema nodosum associated with other conditions. Less common nonspecific cutaneous lesions include acquired ichthyosis (Fig. 4A), calcinosis cutis, erythema multiforme, and nail clubbing.

15. Does sarcoidosis ever present in the skin without extracutaneous involvement?

Yes. Even though sarcoidosis is defined as a multisystem disorder, some patients present with lesions that are clinically and histologically identical to sarcoidosis without any evidence of involvement of other organ systems. It is possible that some of these patients have involvement of other organ systems but it is minimal and asymptomatic.

16. What is Löfgren's syndrome?

This is the classic acute presentation of sarcoidosis. It consists of bilateral hilar adenopathy, fever, arthralgias, erythema nodosum, and uveitis (Fig. 4B). Sarcoidosis that presents in this manner has an approximately 80% chance of resolving within 2 years.

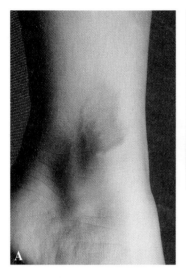
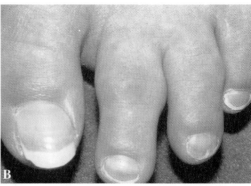

FIGURE 5. *A,* Typical lesion of granuloma annulare demonstrating raised annular lesions without scale. *B,* Subcutaneous granuloma annulare of proximal second toe.

17. What is Heerfordt's syndrome?

Heerfordt's syndrome or uveoparotid fever is a variant of sarcoidosis presenting as uveitis, facial nerve palsy, fever, and parotid gland swelling. Central nervous system involvement is also more common in this presentation.

18. How should cutaneous sarcoidosis be treated?

Treatment of cutaneous sarcoidosis should always be tempered by the fact that 60–80% of cases resolve without treatment in 1–2 years, especially those patients who present with Löfgren's syndrome. For patients with mild cutaneous disease, potent topical corticosteroid (e.g., clobetasol) or intralesional corticosteroid is the treatment of choice. For patients with extensive cutaneous involvement or systemic disease, prednisone is the treatment of choice. Antimalarials have also been shown to be effective in the chronic plaque form of cutaneous sarcoidosis, and these can be a useful alternative to prednisone. Miscellaneous treatments reported to be of benefit in select patients include azathioprine, chlorambucil, cyclosporine, levamisole, and methotrexate.

19. What is the typical presentation of granuloma annulare?

Granuloma annulare (GA) typically presents with violaceous or flesh-colored dermal papules arranged in an annular or semiannular configuration (Fig. 5A). The lesions may be solitary or multiple. Most commonly it affects the dorsum of the hands or feet, but it can also occur on the forearms, arms, legs, or thighs. It tends to affect children or young adults with a 2:1 female preponderance. Several less common variants of granuloma annulare include the macular and erythematous forms, subcutaneous nodules (Fig. 5B), actinically induced lesions, perforating type, and disseminated form. Biopsies of GA demonstrate a characteristic palisaded granuloma associated with collagen destruction (necrobiotic granuloma) and increased dermal mucin.

20. Do any systemic associations occur with granuloma annulare?

Patients who present with localized lesions that are few in number have no systemic associations, and no work-up needs to be done. However, several studies have suggested an association between the disseminated form of GA and diabetes mellitus. Therefore, an appropriate work-up should be done in these patients.

21. What is the typical course of granuloma annulare?

In the classic localized form of GA, the tendency is for spontaneous resolution. Recurrences are fairly common, but the recurrences tend to resolve more quickly than the original lesions. Most studies note that at 2 years post-onset of GA, 50–80% of patients will be lesion-free. However, patients who present with disseminated lesions tend to have a much more protracted course and are frequently less responsive to therapy.

22. How is granuloma annulare treated?

Since GA may spontaneously resolve, expectant observation is certainly a good treatment option. Numerous therapies have been anecdotally reported to be successful, including radiotherapy, cryotherapy, laser, PUVA, niacinamide, isotretinoin, salicylates, potassium iodide, dapsone, antimalarials, and chlorambucil. None has met with overwhelming success. The treatment of choice at this time is strong topical corticosteroids with or without occlusion or intralesional corticosteroids. Corticosteroid therapy usually makes the lesions resolve, but potent preparations are necessary to get a good response and may produce secondary thinning of the skin.

23. What is actinic granuloma?

Actinic granuloma, also called annular elastolytic giant cell granuloma, is a granulomatous process that tends to occur in older patients on sun-exposed skin of the face, arms, and neck. Clinically the lesions are annular and resemble GA, although some cases demonstrate subtle atrophy in the center of the lesion (Fig. 6). Histologically it is also similar to GA in that it demonstrates necrobiotic granulomas but it differs in that it is usually more superficial, demonstrates more foreign body giant cells and prominent elastophagocytosis (macrophages engulfing and breaking down elastic fibers), and mucin is not increased. Some authorities consider it to be a variant of GA but the majority favors it being a disease sui generis. The treatment is the same as for GA but should also include sun protection.

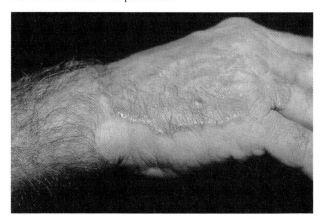

FIGURE 6. Actinic granuloma demonstrating large annular lesion on sun-exposed skin

24. Are rheumatoid nodules really a granulomatous disorder?

Yes, rheumatoid nodules demonstrate sharply demarcated, palisading granulomas with macrophages surrounding areas of fibrinoid degeneration of collagen deep in the dermis or subcutis. A similar histologic picture can be seen in granuloma annulare, necrobiosis lipoidica, and rheumatic fever nodules.

The differentiation of rheumatoid nodule from deep granuloma annulare is difficult but possible in most cases. GA demonstrates increased dermal mucin, while rheumatoid nodules demonstrate marked fibrinoid change that is very eosinophilic. Some cases of deep granuloma annulare cannot be differentiated histologically and require clinical correlation.

25. Where do rheumatoid nodules typically occur?

These are typically present as asymptomatic, firm, fixed, or mobile subcutaneous nodules adjacent to bony structures. The most common site is the elbow (Fig. 7). Other common locations include the extensor aspects of the fingers, flexor sheath tendons in the palms, Achilles tendons, ischial tuberosities, and sacrum. Rheumatoid nodules occur in approximately 25% of patients with rheumatoid arthritis.

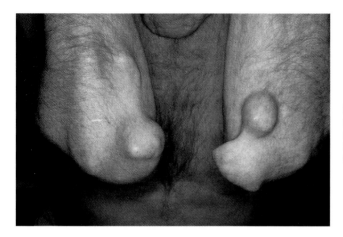

FIGURE 7. Unusually large dermal and subcutaneous rheumatoid nodules in a patient with severe rheumatoid arthritis.

26. What causes rheumatoid nodules?

Most investigators believe that the initial insult is an immune-mediated small vessel vasculitis. Immune complexes and rheumatoid factor have been found within the nodules. This vascular inflammation produces tissue necrosis distal to the damaged vessels. The palisaded macrophages that collect at the periphery of the necrotic area are probably part of a normal healing process. A 65-kDa heat shock protein has also been detected in rheumatoid nodules and it also has been hypothesized that this protein may stimulate T-cells that may play a role in the production of lesions.

27. Are rheumatoid nodules specific for rheumatoid arthritis?

No. They are not pathognomonic for rheumatoid arthritis. They are seen in 5–7% of patients with systemic lupus erythematosus and in a rare condition in children called benign pseudorheumatoid nodules, in which the nodules grow rapidly and then spontaneously involute. These children are usually rheumatoid factor–negative and some authorities feel that many of these cases represent deep GA. Another rare presentation is rheumatoid nodulosis, in which patients present with multiple rheumatoid nodules about the hands. They are rheumatoid factor-positive but have a remarkably benign course.

BIBLIOGRAPHY

1. Dabski K, Winkelmann RK: Generalized granuloma annulare: Clinical and laboratory findings in 100 patients. J Am Acad Dermatol 20:39–47,1989.
2. Felner EI, Steinberg JB, Weinberg AG: Subcutaneous granuloma annulare: A review of 47 cases. Pediatrics 100:965–967, 1997.
3. Johns CJ, Scott PP, Schonfeld SA: Sarcoidosis. Annu Rev Med 40:353–371, 1989.
4. McGrae JD Jr: Actinic granuloma: A clinical, histopathologic, and immunocytochemical study. Arch Dermatol 122:43–47, 1986.
5. McGrath MH, Fleischer A: The subcutaneous rheumatoid nodule. Hand Clin 5:127–135, 1989.
6. Mowry RG, Sams WM, Caulfield JB: Cutaneous silica granuloma. Arch Dermatol 127:692–694, 1991.
7. Peñas PF, Jones-Caballero M, Fraga J, et al: Perforating granuloma annulare. Int J Dermatol 36:340–348, 1997.
8. Travis WD, Balogh K, Abraham JL: Silicone granulomas: Report of 3 cases and review of the literature. Hum Pathol 16:19–27, 1985.
9. Williams WJ: Beryllium disease. Postgrad Med J 64:511–516, 1988.
10. Zax RH, Callen JP: Sarcoidosis. Dermatol Clin 7:505–515, 1989.

14. DRUG ERUPTIONS

Alexandra Theriault, M.D.

1. How do adverse drug reactions differ from drug intolerances and drug allergies?
Drug intolerances and drug allergies are types of adverse reactions. An adverse reaction to a drug is an undesirable and usually unanticipated response independent of the intended therapeutic purpose of the medication. An adverse drug reaction may be either immunologic (i.e., drug allergy) or nonimmunologic (i.e., drug intolerance). Drug allergies are estimated to account for < 10% of all adverse drug reactions, with drug intolerance accounting for the other 90%.

2. Name some nonimmunologic drug reactions.
- Nonimmunologic activation of effector pathways, such as direct release of histamine from mast cells and basophils by opiates, polymyxin B, D-tubocurarine, and radiocontrast media
- Overdosage
- Cumulative toxicity, such as the accumulation of drugs or metabolites in the skin
- Normal pharmacologic effects of the drug that are not the primary therapeutic objective (e.g., alopecia following chemotherapy)
- Drug interactions (e.g., administration of ketoconazole may lead to higher levels of cyclosporine and increased toxicity)
- Metabolic changes, such as warfarin producing a hypercoagulable state that results in warfarin necrosis
- Exacerbation of preexisting dermatologic diseases (e.g., lithium can exacerbate acne, psoriasis, and subcorneal pustular dermatosis)
- Ecological changes, such as antibiotics that reduce the bacteriologic flora, predisposing the patient to candidal infections
- Inherited enzyme or protein deficiencies (e.g., the phenytoin hypersensitivity syndrome occurs in patients deficient in epoxide hydrolase, an enzyme required for metabolism of a toxic epoxide derived from phenytoin)

3. What is the safest method of administering a drug to avoid sensitization?
Oral administration of a drug is the route least likely to produce sensitization. Intramuscular is the most likely parenteral way of eliciting drug sensitization, whereas intravenous is less likely.

4. What is the most common manifestation of an adverse drug reaction?
Cutaneous reactions are the most common adverse drug reaction and produce a wide range of manifestations: pruritus, maculopapular eruptions, urticaria, angioedema, phototoxic and photoallergic reactions, fixed drug reactions, erythema multiforme, vesiculobullous reactions, and exfoliative dermatitis. Drug-attributed skin reactions are seen in 2.2% of inpatients and 1–3% of outpatients.

5. How does a cutaneous drug eruption typically present?

Exanthema (maculopapular or morbilliform)	46%
Urticaria and angioedema	26%
Fixed drug eruptions	10%
Erythema multiforme	5%
Stevens-Johnson syndrome	4%
Exfoliative dermatitis	4%
Photosensitivity reactions	3%
Anaphylaxis	1.5%
Toxic epidermal necrolysis	1.3%

6. How should a suspected drug reaction be evaluated?

Six variables should be evaluated:

- Previous experience or relative reaction rates of a given drug
- Rule out alternative etiologies, such as exacerbation of a previous dermatosis or a new skin disease unrelated to the drug
- Timing of events (most drug reactions occur within 1–2 weeks of initiation of therapy)
- Drug levels
- Reaction to dechallenge (most drug reactions clear within 2 weeks of discontinuing drug)
- Response to rechallenge—most definitive

7. Which commonly used drugs are most likely to produce a cutaneous reaction?

DRUG	REACTIONS PER 1,000 PATIENTS
Amoxicillin	51.4
Trimethoprim-sulfamethoxazole	47
Ampicillin	42
Ipodate sodium	27.8
Whole blood	28
Cephalosporins	13
Allopurinol	
Carbamazepine	

8. Can preexisting diseases enhance the chance of getting a maculopapular skin eruption when using amoxicillin or ampicillin?

Amoxicillin or ampicillin produces a maculopapular eruption in about 5% of patients taking these drugs (Fig. 1). In patients with infectious mononucleosis, the risk of developing a maculopapular eruption increases to 69–100%. In chronic lymphocytic leukemia, the incidence is 60–70%. Some studies report that maculopapular eruptions are more common in patients who are also taking allopurinol, but this is not accepted by all authorities. The pathogenesis for this phenomenon is unknown.

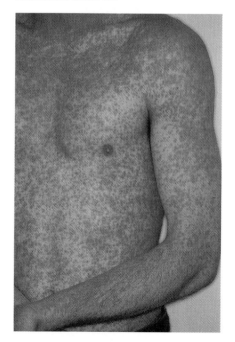

FIGURE 1. Amoxicillin-induced maculopapular (morbilliform) drug eruption in a patient with infectious mononucleosis. In most studies, morbilliform drug eruptions are the most common cutaneous side effect. (Courtesy Scott D. Bennion, MD.)

9. What infectious disease increases the chance of a cutaneous adverse reaction to trimethoprim-sulfamethoxazole?

AIDS. The normal incidence of cutaneous reactions to trimethoprim-sulfamethoxazole is 3%, but this increases to 29–70% in patients with the acquired immunodeficiency syndrome. Incidence of morbilliform drug reactions is tenfold higher in HIV-infected persons.

10. Which feared drug eruption results in sloughing of the entire skin surface and mucous membranes?

Toxic epidermal necrolysis (TEN) is one of the most severe cutaneous drug eruptions. The skin is initially erythematous and tender but quickly sloughs off in large sheets like "wet wallpaper" (Fig. 2). Up to 20–100% of the total cutaneous surface may be involved. The condition can progress very rapidly, with 1 of 7 patients losing their entire epidermis in 24 hours. Without an epidermis, the body has difficulty keeping fluids in and bacteria out. Despite aggressive supportive care, the mortality rate ranges from 11 to 35%. The oral mucosa also may be involved, making oral intake of nourishment very painful, which may further aggravate the fluid and electrolyte imbalances produced by loss of the skin. Ocular conjunctiva is involved in about 85% of patients, and ophthalmologists should be consulted in most cases. The diagnosis can be confirmed by a skin biopsy that demonstrates necrosis of the basal cell layer or entire epidermis with a minimal infiltrate.

The nosology and pathogenesis of toxic epidermal necrolysis are controversial. Some authorities consider it to be a severe form of erythema multiforme, which is an immunologically mediated disease. Other authorities believe it to be an idiosyncratic toxic effect of certain drugs or their metabolites on epithelial cells.

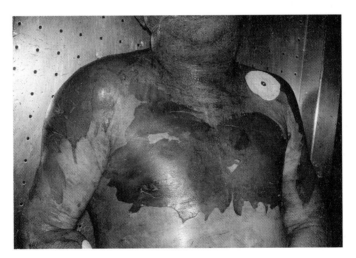

FIGURE 2. Fatal case of toxic epidermal necrolysis secondary to captopril. The skin characteristically sloughs off in large sheets. (Courtesy James E. Fitzpatrick, MD.)

11. Which drugs are most likely to produce toxic epidermal necrolysis?

The etiology of all cases of TEN cannot be proved, but drugs are most commonly implicated. In one series, 77% of cases were clearly established as drug-induced. Since the average patient with TEN is on 4.4 drugs, identifying the offending drug can be problematic. Frequent offenders include allopurinol, ampicillin, amoxicillin, carbamazepine, NSAIDs, phenobarbital, phenytoin, sulfonamides, and lamictal.

12. How soon after starting a drug does TEN develop?

Most cases of TEN start 1–3 weeks after starting the drug. Phenytoin is an exception, requiring 2–8 weeks. If the patient had a similar eruption in the past, the time interval drops to < 48 hours.

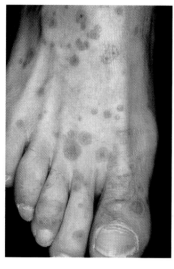

FIGURE 3. Classic lesions of erythema multiforme secondary to co-trimoxazole demonstrating targetoid appearance. (Courtesy James E. Fitzpatrick, MD.)

13. How often is TEN fatal?

The mortality rate is 25–70% depending on the series quoted, with secondary infection being the most common cause of death. Surviving patients heal in 3–4 weeks, but up to 50% have residual, potentially disabling ocular lesions.

The best therapy is to discontinue all likely drugs if possible, make sure the patient is well-hydrated, and continually assess the patient for signs of secondary infection. Corticosteroids are contraindicated. Severe cases are best handled in burn units.

14. What drugs are typically associated with Stevens-Johnson syndrome (erythema multiforme major)?

Commonly implicated drugs include allopurinol, amoxicillin, ampicillin, barbiturates, carbamazepine, gold, NSAIDs, phenobarbital, phenytoin, and sulfonamides. *Mycoplasma pneumoniae* and other infections are also well documented to produce Stevens-Johnson syndrome (Fig. 3).

15. Which type of drug reaction can result in a quick death?

Systemic anaphylaxis, which is IgE-mediated, may present with variable findings, including mild pruritus, erythema, urticaria, asthma, circulatory collapse, laryngeal edema, and death. When a patient gives a history of reaction to a drug, the health care provider *must* ask for details about the previous reaction, particularly seeking a history of urticaria, breathing problems, collapse, and hospitalization.

16. What class of drugs are the most common cause of anaphylaxis?

Beta-lactam antibiotics. Anaphylactic reactions occur in 1–5 per 10,000 administrations of penicillin. Most allergic reactions to beta-lactam antibiotics produce urticaria and angioedema, but 10% may result in life-threatening hypotension, bronchospasm, or laryngeal edema. Approximately 1% of all anaphylactic reactions are fatal. Fatal reactions may occur within minutes of parenteral administration of these drugs.

17. Name the commonly used drug that can exacerbate a preexisting urticaria.

Aspirin may both induce urticaria and aggravate urticaria from other causes. If possible, stop this drug in all patients with urticaria.

18. Name the drugs most likely to induce urticaria.

ACE inhibitors, gamma-globulin, NSAIDs, penicillins, and sulfonamides. Urticaria produced by drugs is clinically indistinguishable from urticaria produced by other allergens.

19. How is drug-induced urticaria mediated?

Urticaria may be produced by both nonimmunologic and immunologic mechanisms. Drugs such as codeine, morphine, amphetamine, hydralazine, quinine, vancomycin, and x-ray contrast media produce urticaria by the nonimmunologic release of histamine by mast cells. Allergic urticaria may be due to a type I (Coombs and Gell) reaction mediated by IgE, causing the release of histamine. This usually develops within minutes to hours (usually within 1 hour) after giving the offending drug, and may precede or be associated with anaphylaxis. Urticaria may also be produced by a type III reaction mediated by antigen–antibody complexes. In contrast to type I reactions which occur within hours, type III urticaria usually develops 1–3 weeks after beginning the drug.

20. A 45-year-old white man comes to the emergency room with large areas of nonpitting edema over the face, eyelids, neck, tongue, and mucous membranes which developed 6 hours ago. Ten days earlier, he started a new drug for hypertension. What is the most likely cause of his reaction?

The clinical description is that of a patient who has **angioedema.** An **angiotensin-converting enzyme** (ACE) inhibitor, such as captopril, enalapril, or lisinopril, is the most likely antihypertensive drug to produce this reaction. A recent study reported that 35% of 17 patients seen for angioedema during a 5-year period were on ACE inhibitors. In another study, 77% of patients experienced the reaction within 3 weeks of starting treatment.

21. A patient is evaluated for a several-day history of fever, malaise, urticaria, arthralgias, lymphadenopathy, and a peculiar erythema along the sides of his palms and soles. He has been started on several new medications in the last few weeks. What is the most likely diagnosis?

The patient most likely has a **serum sickness-like drug eruption** caused by immune complexes and complement activation. The diagnostic cutaneous finding is the characteristic erythema on the sides of the palms and soles; a finding seen in 75% of cases of serum sickness-like drug eruptions. Other typical findings include fever and malaise (100%), urticaria (90%), arthralgias (50–67%), and lymphadenopathy (13%). Glomerulonephritis is common in serum sickness reactions in animals but uncommon in humans. Reactions occur 7–21 days after the drug is given but may occur with the first administration of the drug. Commonly implicated drugs include beta-lactam antibiotics, sulfonamides, thiouracil, cholecystographic dyes, and hydantoin.

22. A man complains of a recurrent burning eruption on his penis. He develops a single blister over the glans penis that heals over 1–2 weeks with hyperpigmentation. This same pattern has happened on three occasions in the last 2 years. What does he have?

The history is characteristic of a **fixed drug eruption.** Fixed drug eruptions are cutaneous reactions that recur at the same site with each administration of the drug. Characteristically, it occurs on the face or genitalia but may occur anywhere (Fig. 4). It is a well-demarcated erythematous lesion that often blisters and heals with hyperpigmentation. Drugs commonly associated include phenolphthalein in laxatives, sulfonamides, beta-lactam antibiotics, tetracycline, barbiturates, gold, oral contraceptives, and aspirin. Foods have also been implicated in fixed drug reactions.

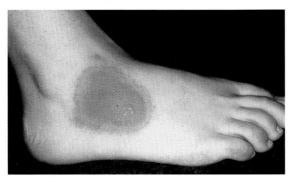

FIGURE 4. Sulfonamide-induced fixed drug eruption of the ankle manifesting an erythematous plaque and focal blisters. (Courtesy James E. Fitzpatrick, MD.)

23. How does drug-induced lupus erythematosus (LE) differ from idiopathic systemic lupus erythematosus (SLE)?

Drug-induced LE is generally milder than idiopathic SLE. Drug-induced LE usually manifests as fever, malaise, pleuritis, pneumonitis, and arthralgias. Skin, mucous membrane, and central nervous system findings, and renal disease are more commonly seen in idiopathic SLE. The antinuclear antibodies in drug-induced LE are usually antihistone and single-stranded DNA antibodies, whereas idiopathic SLE is associated with double-stranded DNA and Sm antibodies. Drug-induced LE usually resolves simply by stopping the drug. Drug-induced LE constitutes 5–10% of all cases of SLE.

24. What drugs are usually associated with drug-induced LE?

Of patients treated continuously with procainamide, 90% develop antinuclear antibodies after 2 years, and 10–20% develop symptoms of LE. Other commonly implicated drugs include hydralazine, isoniazid, chlorpromazine, procainamide, hydantoin, D-penicillamine, methyldopa, and quinidine.

25. Which drug is usually associated with erythema nodosum?

Erythema nodosum, which is a form of panniculitis that characteristically presents as tender erythematous nodules over the shins, is most commonly associated with **oral contraceptives.** Sulfonamides, bromides, iodides, tetracycline, penicillin, and 13-cis retinoic acid have also been associated with erythema nodosum.

26. What drugs are associated with lichenoid skin eruptions?

Lichenoid drug eruptions clinically and histologically resemble lichen planus. The lesions are usually multiple, purple, discrete, flat-topped polygonal papules and plaques. This differs from other drug reactions in that it may take weeks to years following administration of the drug to develop the lesions. Sulfonamides (especially thiazide diuretics), gold, captopril, propranolol, and antimalarials are the most common drugs that produce these reactions. It may take months for the rash to resolve following discontinuation of the drug.

27. Name the drugs most likely to produce cutaneous hyperpigmentation and discoloration.

Drugs produce cutaneous hyperpigmentation and discoloration by different mechanisms. The two main mechanisms of hyperpigmentation and discoloration are **drug deposition** (e.g., heavy metals) and **stimulation of melanocytic** activity.

Drugs Producing Changes in Skin Pigmentation

COLOR	DRUG
Slate gray	Chloroquine
	Hydroxychloroquine (Fig. 5A)
	Minocycline
	Phenothiazines
Slate blue	Amiodarone
Blue-gray	Gold (chrysoderma)
Yellow	Beta-carotene
	Quinacrine
Red	Clofazimine
Brown (hyperpigmentation)	ACTH
	Bleomycin
	Oral contraceptives
	Zidovudine

28. What drugs can produce subepidermal bullae and erosions on the dorsum of the hands?

The description is characteristic of the eruption seen in porphyria cutanea tarda and, less commonly, variegate porphyria and hereditary coproporphyria. This reaction is called **pseudoporphyria** since the porphyrin levels are normal (Fig. 5B). Tetracycline, nalidixic acid, furosemide and other sulfonamides, dapsone, naproxen, and pyridoxine are most likely to induce pseudoporphyria.

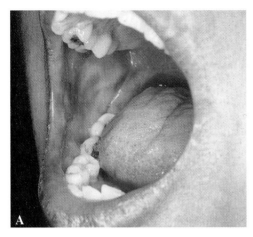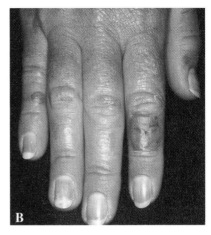

FIGURE 5. *A*, Hydroxychloroquine-induced slate gray pigmentation of the buccal mucosa. *B*, Tetracycline-induced pseudoporphyria demonstrating hemorrhagic blisters and erosions over the back of the hand. (Courtesy James E. Fitzpatrick, MD.)

29. Name two drugs that commonly exacerbate porphyria cutanea tarda.
Ethanol and estrogens.

30. A 30-year-old white woman is evaluated with a new case of "acne." Over the last few days, she has suddenly developed erythematous follicular papules and pustules over her upper trunk. She was admitted 3 weeks earlier with an acute exacerbation of SLE that is now improving. What is the most likely diagnosis?
Steroid acne is the most likely diagnosis. Her history indicates a high probability that she was started on corticosteroids during the admission. Steroid acne typically presents with inflammatory papules and pustules, but comedones and cysts are typically absent. In contrast to acne vulgaris, steroid acne preferentially involves the trunk and demonstrates lesions in the same stage of development. Other drugs associated with similar eruptions include lithium, isoniazid, bromides, and iodides.

31. What is the "red neck" or "red man" syndrome? What drug causes it?
The red man syndrome is a histamine-like reaction associated with intravenous **vancomycin.** It is characterized by pruritus, erythema over the upper body, and angioedema. Usually, it is a mild reaction, but rarely cardiovascular shock may occur. The total dose of drug and the rate of intravenous infusion of vancomycin influence the release of histamine and the development of the signs and symptoms of this syndrome. Antihistamines are effective in preventing it.

32. Describe a typical presentation of warfarin necrosis.
The patient is typically a woman who has been given a loading dose of warfarin (Coumadin). Three to 5 days after starting the drug, the patient develops one or more lesions over the thighs, buttocks, or breasts. Initially painful and red, it rapidly becomes necrotic with hemorrhagic bullae and an erythematous edge (Fig. 6). A necrotic eschar rapidly develops.
Rapid recognition of the characteristic lesions in the typical situation is the key to reducing tissue destruction. Therapy includes discontinuing warfarin, administering vitamin K to reverse the effect of warfarin, giving heparin as an anticoagulant, and administering monoclonal antibody-purified protein C concentrate. Therapy may also include debridement, grafting, and even amputation. Warfarin necrosis has frequently been associated with low levels of protein C.

33. Is it always necessary to discontinue warfarin in these patients?
Although most references state that warfarin should be discontinued, this is controversial. There are numerous examples in the literature of patients who have continued to receive this drug

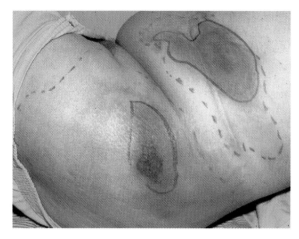

FIGURE 6. Characteristic lesions of warfarin necrosis, demonstrating early necrosis and hemorrhagic bullae surrounded by a ring of eythema.

who did not develop new skin lesions or exacerbate established lesions. One reason for discontinuing warfarin appears to be medicolegal—to prevent malpractice suits.

34. Where are photoinduced drug eruptions usually seen?
- The face (eyelids are spared), neck (submental area is spared), and V-area of the chest
- Outer aspects of the forearms and dorsal hands
- Delineation is seen at the level of short-sleeved shirts on the upper arm
- The left arm is usually involved more often than the right if the patient drives frequently
- The area covered by the watchband is usually spared
- The dorsal feet and lower legs are often involved in women

35. Name and describe the two types of photo-induced drug eruptions.
Phototoxic drug reactions and photoallergic drug reactions. Phototoxic reactions occur within minutes to hours after exposure to both the drug and light and occur in all individuals given the specific drug and UV exposure. The rash clinically resembles a sunburn and stinging is a prominent feature. Photoallergic drug reactions are mediated by type IV delayed hypersensitivity and occur 24–48 hours after UV exposure. Clinically the lesions are on sun-exposed sites, but are not as well demarcated as phototoxic reactions. They are also eczematous and pruritic.

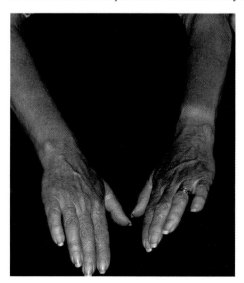

FIGURE 7. Demeclocycline-induced phototoxic reaction on the dorsum. (Courtesy James E. Fitzpatrick, MD.)

36. What drugs commonly cause phototoxic drug reactions?

Amiodarone, chlorpromazine, demeclocycline (Fig. 7), doxycycline, psoralens, and tetracycline.

37. What drugs commonly cause photoallergic drug reactions?

Griseofulvin, quinine, quinolones, sulfonamides, phenothiazines, quinidine, hydrochlorothiazides, piroxicam, and pyridoxine.

BIBLIOGRAPHY

1. Anderson JA: Allergic reactions to drugs and biological agents. JAMA 268:2845–2857, 1992.
2. Avakian R, Flowers FP, Araujo OE, Ramos-Caro FA: Toxic epidermal necrolysis: A review. J Am Acad Dermatol 25:69–79, 1991.
3. Blacker KL, Stern RS, Wintroub BU: Cutaneous reactions to drugs. In Fitzpatrick TB, Eisen AZ, Wolff K, et al (eds): Dermatology in General Medicine, 4th ed. New York, McGraw-Hill, 1993, pp 1783–1795.
4. Breathnach SM: Drug reactions. In Champion RH, Burton JL, Ebling FJG (eds): Textbook of Dermatology, 5th ed. Oxford, Blackwell Scientific Publications, 1992, pp 2961- 3035.
5. Fritsch PO, Elias PM: Erythema multiforme and toxic epidermal necrolysis. In Fitzpatrick TB, Eisen AZ, Wolff K, et al (eds): Dermatology in General Medicine, 4th ed. New York, McGraw-Hill, 1993, pp 585–600.
6. Guillaume J-C, Roujeau J-C, Revus J, et al: The culprit drugs of toxic epidermal necrolysis (Lyell's syndrome). Arch Dermatol 123:1166–1170, 1987.
7. Hedner T, Samuelsson O, Lunde H, et al: Angio-edema in relation to treatment with angiotensin converting enzyme inhibitors. BMJ 304:941–946, 1992.
8. Megerian CA, Arnold JE, Berger M: Angioedema: 5 years' experience, with a review of the disorder's presentation and treatment. Laryngoscope 102:256–260, 1992.
9. Millikan LE: Drug eruptions (dermatitis medicamentosa). In Moschella SL, Hurley HJ (eds): Dermatology, 3rd ed. Philadelphia, W.B. Saunders, 1992, pp 535–573.
10. Poh-Fitzpatrick M: Porphyria, pseudoporphyria, and pseudopseudoporphyria. Arch Dermatol 122:403–404, 1986.
11. Ramsay CA: Drug induced pseudoporphyria. J Rheumatol 18:799–800, 1991.
12. Roujeau J-C, Chosidow O, Saiag P, Guillaume J-C: Toxic epidermal necrolysis (Lyell's syndrome). J Am Acad Dermatol 23:1039–1058, 1990.
13. Roujeau JC, Stern RS: Severe cutaneous reactions to drugs. N Engl J Med 331:1272–1285, 1994.
14. Wallace MR, Mascola JR, Oldfield III EC: Red man syndrome: Incidence, etiology, and prophylaxis. J Infect Dis 164:1180–1185, 1991.

15. VASCULITIS

Curt P. Samlaska, M.D.

1. How are vasculitic disorders defined and classified?
A vasculitis is simply defined as **inflammation of blood vessels.** However, vascular syndromes are multisystemic disorders which frequently involve organ systems with the richest vascular supply, such as the skin.

Classification is enigmatic due to the lack of standardization and definition. The most accepted classification scheme is based on the size of the involved blood vessels, as shown in the table below. Subclassification of the various vasculitic syndromes is based on clinical and histologic criteria that have been determined to be suggestive of a specific disorder. The American College of Rheumatology Subcommittee on Classification of Vasculitis has determined classification criteria for many of these disorders. These criteria are analogous to the diagnostic criteria established for systemic lupus erythematosus.

Classification of Systemic Vasculitis—Adopted by the Chapel Hill Consensus Conference on the Nomenclature of Systemic Vasculitis, 1994

VESSEL SIZE	VASCULAR SYNDROME
Large-vessel vasculitis	Giant cell (temporal) arteritis
	Takayasu arteritis
Medium-sized–vessel vasculitis	Polyarteritis nodosa (classic PAN)
	Kawasaki disease
Small-vessel vasculitis	Wegener's granulomatosis
	Churg-Strauss syndrome
	Microscopic polyangiitis (polyarteritis)
	Henoch-Schönlein purpura
	Essential cryoglobulinemic vasculitis
	Cutaneous leukocytoclastic vasculitis

Adapted from Jennette JC, Falk RJ, Andrassy K, et al: Nomenclature of systemic vasculitides: Proposal of an International Consensus Conference. Arthritis Rheum 37:187–192, 1994.

2. Are there specific serologic markers for any of these vasculitic disorders?
Yes. Anti-myeloperoxidase antibodies directed against cytoplasmic components of neutrophils have been used to help identify patients with segmental necrotizing glomerulonephritis and systemic vasculitis. Antibodies directed against cytoplasmic anti-neutrophil cytoplasmic antibodies (c-ANCA) have been detected in 66–90% of patients with active Wegener's granulomatosis. Patients with pulmonary-renal syndrome who have antibody staining showing a peripheral anti-neutrophil cytoplasmic pattern (p-ANCA) are most likely to have microscopic polyangiitis.

3. What is a leukocytoclastic vasculitis?
Patients with leukocytoclastic vasculitis, also referred to as leukocytoclastic angiitis and allergic or necrotizing vasculitis, present with characteristic purpuric papules, most frequently involving the extremities, known as **palpable purpura** (Fig. 1). The histopathology of the lesions is also important, showing a perivascular infiltrate comprised of intact and fragmented neutrophils (nuclear dust). The vessel walls also demonstrate fibrinoid changes or necrosis.

4. Name the systemic disorders known to be associated with leukocytoclastic vasculitis.

Wegener's granulomatosis	Macroglobulinemia
Microscopic polyangiitis	Systemic lupus erythematosus
Churg-Strauss syndrome	Rheumatoid arthritis
Henoch-Schönlein purpura	Dermatopolymyositis
Cryoglobulinemic vasculitis	Ulcerative colitis
Multiple myeloma	Inherited deficiencies of complement components

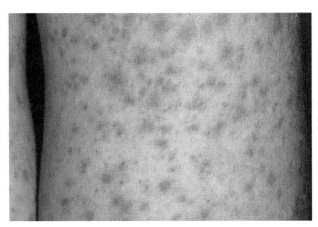

FIGURE 1. Leukoclastic vasculitis secondary to ampicillin. Typical lesions of palpable purpura are seen.

5. What other conditions can cause a leukocytoclastic vasculitis?

Infections—bacterial (streptococcal infections, bacterial endocarditis), viral (parvovirus B19, HIV, hepatitis A–C), mycobacterial (Hansen's disease, tuberculosis), fungal (*Candida albicans*), protozoan (*Plasmodium malariae*), helminthic (*Schistosoma haematobium, S. mansoni, Onchocerca volvulus*)

Drugs—aspirin, sulfonamides, penicillins, barbiturates, amphetamines, propylthiouracil

Malignancy—lymphomas, colonic carcinoma, hairy cell leukemia, multiple myeloma, lung cancer, renal cell carcinoma, prostate cancer, breast cancer, head and neck cancer

6. What is the difference between giant-cell (temporal) arteritis and Takayasu arteritis?

Both disorders affect large vessels. **Takayasu's arteritis** manifests with a progressive granulomatous inflammation of the aorta and its major branches and most frequently afflicts patients aged < 50 years. **Giant-cell arteritis** usually affects patients > 50 years old with a granulomatous vasculitis that also can involve the aorta and its major branches. However, giant cell arteritis shows a predilection for the extracranial branches of the carotid artery, particularly the temporal artery, which can progress to visual loss and blindness if not treated with systemic steroids.

7. What are the major organs involved in classic polyarteritis nodosa (PAN)?

Kidneys, heart, liver, GI tract, and peripheral nerves. PAN, in its classic form, is a multisystem, segmented necrotizing inflammation of small and medium-sized muscular arteries (Fig. 2). Signs and symptoms are nonspecific and constitutional, reflecting the organ involvement. Pulmonary arteries are typically not involved. The mean age of onset is 48 years, with a male:female ratio of about 4:1. Diagnosis is by demonstrating vasculitic changes on biopsy of involved organs or by demonstrating typical aneurysms of medium-sized vessels on angiography.

8. How is classic polyarteritis nodosa different from Kawasaki disease?

Both disorders affect medium-sized vessels. **PAN** produces a necrotizing inflammation of medium-sized and/or small arteries without producing glomerulonephritis or vasculitis in arterioles, capillaries, or venules. Patients with **Kawasaki disease** are most often children with mucocutaneous lymph node syndrome (adenopathy, glossitis, cheilitis, conjunctivitis, etc.) with arteritis involving large (often resulting in coronary arteritis, coronary artery aneurysms, and myocardial infarctions), medium-sized, and small arteries.

9. What is the primary difference between microscopic polyangiitis and PAN?

The distinguishing feature for these two systemic disorders is a vasculitis involving arterioles, venules, or capillaries. Patients with microscopic polyangiitis have involvement of minute vessels, whereas individuals with classic PAN have involvement of medium-sized arteries. Some authors consider microscopic polyarteritis a subset of PAN, while others consider it a distinct form of vasculitis.

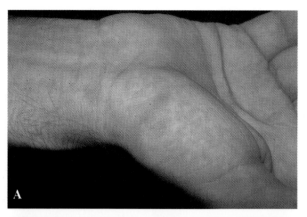

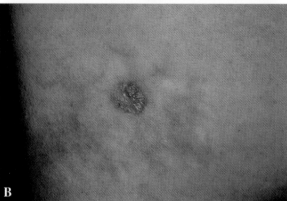

FIGURE 2. Cutaneous polyarteritis nodosa. *A*, Characteristic linear erythematous lesion. Note the Y-shaped bifurcation. *B*, Reticulated hyperpigmented lesion with an associated ulceration. (Courtesy of James E. Fitzpatrick, MD.)

10. What are the main features of Churg-Strauss syndrome?

Clinical Features of Churg-Strauss Syndrome

FINDING	SENSITIVITY
Asthma	100%
Blood eosinophilia > 10%	95%
Paranasal sinus abnormalities	86%
Mono- or polyneuropathy	75%
Pulmonary infiltrates	40%
Extravascular (perivascular) eosinophils	14%
History of seasonal allergies	—

Pulmonary involvement helps discriminate Churg-Strauss syndrome (also known as allergic angiitis and granulomatosis) from PAN. Although palpable purpura involving the extremities has been observed in up to 45% of patients and is considered by many physicians to be a major feature of Churg-Strauss syndrome, it is not considered to be discriminating in comparison to other vasculitic syndromes. Nevertheless, cutaneous involvement should be considered an important feature when present, and biopsies frequently demonstrate perivascular eosinophilia, which is one of the diagnostic criteria.

11. What were those features again?

To recall the diagnostic criteria for Churg-Strauss syndrome, remember the mnemonic **BEAN SAP: B**lood **E**osinophilia, **A**sthma, **N**europathy, **S**inus abnormalities, **A**llergies, and **P**erivascular eosinophils. The American College of Rheumatology has recently established these six criteria for the diagnosis of Churg-Strauss syndrome, with the presence of four of these six criteria yielding a diagnostic sensitivity of 85% and a specificity of 99.7%.

12. List the main features of Wegener's granulomatosis.
There are four criteria for establishing the diagnosis of Wegener's granulomatosis:
1. Abnormal urinary sediment (red cell casts or > 5 red blood cells/high-power field)
2. Abnormal findings of chest radiographs (nodules, cavities, or fixed infiltrates)
3. Oral ulcers or nasal discharge
4. Granulomatous inflammation on biopsy

The presence of two or more of the four criteria gives a diagnostic sensitivity of 88% and a specificity of 92%.

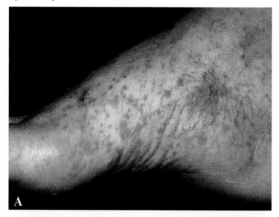

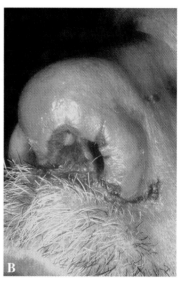

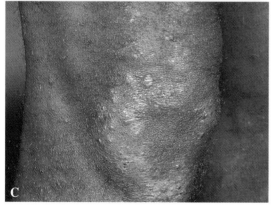

FIGURE 3. Wegener's granulomatosis. *A,* Fatal case demonstrating purpuric lesions. This patient was c-ANCA–positive. *B,* Nasal erosions and ulcerations. *C,* Nonspecific papules on the knee in a patient with limited Wegener's granulomatosis involving the sinuses and the skin (courtesy of James E. Fitzpatrick, MD).

13. Is there an easy way to remember these diagnostic criteria?
Simply remember the mnemonic **ROUGH:**
- **R** = Chest **R**adiograph
- **O** = **O**ral ulcers
- **U** = **U**rinary sediment
- **G** = **G**ranulomas
- **H** = **H**emoptysis

Hemoptysis during illness has been added as a fifth criteria.

14. List the cutaneous findings in Wegener's granulomatosis.
Leukocytoclastic vasculitis   Urticaria
Papules   Erythema

Petechiae   Purpura
Ulcerative lesions   Pyoderma gangrenosum
None of these cutaneous findings is specific for Wegener's granulomatosis.

15. Wegener's granulomatosis and Churg-Strauss syndrome seem very similar. How do you distinguish between them?

It is often difficult to distinguish between Wegener's granulomatosis and Churg-Strauss syndrome, due to the presence of nasal, sinus, and pulmonary involvement in both diseases and due to the fact that all the classic features are rarely found in a single patient. There are many situations in which the features of systemic vasculitides overlap, and these are referred to as overlap vasculitis syndromes, similar to the overlap syndromes reported for other rheumatologic conditions.

The use of cytoplasmic anti-neutrophil cytoplasmic antibodies (c-ANCA) for differentiating between these two disorders is helpful (c-ANCA is usually present in high titers in Wegener's but not in Churg-Strauss), but is not included in the current diagnostic criteria for either syndrome. The presence or absence of other features should confirm the diagnosis in most cases.

	Wegener's Granulomatosis	Churg-Strauss Syndrome
Asthma	−	+
Blood eosinophilia	−	+
Perivascular eosinophils on biopsy	−	+
Hemoptysis	+	−
Microhematuria	+	−

16. What forms of treatment are available for Wegener's granulomatosis and Churg-Strauss syndrome?

Systemic corticosteroids are the mainstay for treatment of most forms of systemic vasculitis. Cyclophosphamide is very effective in the treatment of Wegener's granulomatosis and is one of the most important reasons for distinguishing between these two disorders.

17. Describe the clinical features of Henoch-Schönlein purpura (HSP).

The mnemonic **PAPAH** (pä′ pä) can be used to remember the clinical features of HSP: **P**urpura, **A**bdominal **P**ain, **A**rthralgias, **H**ematuria.

Also known as anaphylactoid purpura, HSP is characterized by intermittent purpura that typically involves the extremities and buttocks. Skin biopsies frequently demonstrate detectable IgA antibodies on immunofluorescence studies. Although HSP may occur at any age, it usually afflicts children between 3–10 years of age. Treatment is supportive.

18. What are cryoglobulins?

Cryoglobulins are abnormal circulating IgG and IgM immunoglobulins that precipitate at low temperatures and redissolve at 37°C. Precipitation within the microvasculature can result in a variety of cutaneous findings, including purpura (leukocytoclastic vasculitis on biopsy), blisters, ulcerations, Raynaud's phenomenon, and distal extremity cyanosis. Because the extremities experience lower temperatures, there is a propensity for extremity involvement. Cryoglobulins are frequently found in patients with paraproteinemias, such as multiple myeloma and macroglobulinemia. Mixed cryoglobulinemia, with more than one antibody class involved, has been reported in systemic lupus erythematosus, rheumatoid arthritis, Sjögren's syndrome, and hepatitis B and C infection.

19. Are there any obscure disorders known to dermatologists, but little known to other subspecialties, that could be classified as systemic vasculitis?

Erythema elevatum diutinum. Described in 1894, this chronic disorder is characterized by persistent, elevated, erythematous plaques and/or nodules, with a predilection for overlying joint spaces, such as the fingers, wrists, elbows, knees, ankles, and toes. The lesions are usually painful. Vasculitis, particularly of the leukocytoclastic type, is demonstrated on biopsy. It is considered a chronic fibrosing leukocytoclastic vasculitis. There may be an associated IgA or IgG monoclonal gammopathy. Some patients have shown a dramatic response to dapsone.

BIBLIOGRAPHY

1. Callen JP: Cutaneous vasculitis. Arch Dermatol 134:355–357, 1998.
2. Callen JP: Vasculitis. In Callen JP, Jorizzo JL, Greer KE, et al (eds): Dermatologic Signs of Internal Disease, 2nd ed. Philadelphia, W.B. Saunders, 1995, pp 31–39.
3. Daoud MS, Gibson LE, Specks U: Cutaneous leukocytoclastic vasculitis with positive anti-neutrophil cytoplasmic antibodies. Acta Derm Venereol 79:328–329, 1999.
4. de Groot K, Gross WL: Wegener's granulomatosis. Lupus 7:285–291, 1998.
5. Dillon MJ: Childhood vasculitis. Lupus 7:259–265, 1998.
6. Evans J, Hunder GG: The implications of recognizing large-vessel involvement in elderly patients with giant cell arteritis. Curr Opin Rheumatol 9:37–40, 1997.
7. Irvine AD, Bruce IN, Walsh MY, Bingham EA: Microscopic polyangiitis: Delineation of a cutaneous-limited variant associated with antimyeloperoxidase autoantibody. Arch Dermatol 133:474–477, 1997.
8. Jennette JC, Falk RJ, Andrassy K, et al: Nomenclature of systemic vasculitides: Proposal of an International Censensus Conference. Arthritis Rheum 37:187–192, 1994.
9. Koldingsnes W, Gran JT, Omdal R, Husby G: Wegener's granulomatosis: Long-term follow-up of patients treated with pulse cyclophosphamide. Br J Rheumatol 37:659–664, 1998.
10. Langford CA, Sneller MC: New developments in the treatment of Wegener's granulomatosis, polyarteritis nodosa, microscopic polyangiitis, and Churg-Strauss syndrome. Curr Opin Rheumatol 9:26–30, 1997.
11. Leavitt RY, Fauci AS, Bloch DA, et al: The American College of Rheumatology 1990 criteria for the classification of Wegener's granulomatosis. Arthritis Rheum 33:1101–1107, 1990.
12. Lotti T, Ghersetich I, et al: Cutaneous small-vessel vasculitis. J Am Acad Dermatol 39:667, 1998.
13, Nakajima H, Ikeda M, Yamamoto Y, Kodama H: Erythema elevatum diutinum complicated by rheumatoid arthritis. J Dermatol 26:452–456, 1999.
14. Noguchi M, Tatezawa T, Nakajima S, Ishikawa O: Giant cell (temporal) arteritis involving both external and internal carotid arteries. J Dermatol 26:469–473, 1999.
15. Pak H, Montemarano AD, Berger T: Purpuric nodules and macules on the extremities of a young woman: Cutaneous polyarteritis nodosa. Arch Dermatol 134:231–232, 1998.
16. Papi M, De Pita O, Frezzolini A, Didona B: Prognostic factors in leukocytoclastic vasculitis: What is the role of antineutrophil cytoplasmic antibody? Arch Dermatol 135:714–715, 1999.
17. Penas PF, Porras JI, Fraga J, et al: Microscopic polyangiitis: A systemic vasculitis with a positive P-ANCA. Br J Dermatol 134:542–547, 1996.
18. Sais G, Vidaller A, Jucgla A, et al: Prognostic factors in leukocytoclastic vasculitis: A clinicopathologic study of 160 patients. Arch Dermatol 134:309–315, 1998.
19. Saulsbury FT: Henoch-Schoenlein purpura in children. Medicine (Baltimore) 78:395–409, 1999.
20. Soni BP, Williford PM, White WL: Erythematous nodules in a patient infected with the human immunodeficiency virus: Erythema elevatum diutinum (EED). Arch Dermatol 134:232–233, 1998.
21. Stein SL, Miller LC, Konnikov N: Wegener's granulomatosis. Pediatr Dermatol 15:352–356, 1998.
22. Tatsis E, Schnabel A, Gross WL: Interferon-alpha treatment of four patients with the Churg-Strauss syndrome. Ann Intern Med 129:370–374, 1998.
23. Veraldi S, Mancuso R, Rizzitelli G, et al: Henoch-Schoenlein syndrome associated with human parvovirus B19 primary infection. Eur J Dermatol 9:232–233, 1999.

16. DEPOSITION DISORDERS

Lori Lowe, M.D.

1. How are the deposition disorders defined?

Deposition disorders comprise a diverse group of conditions or diseases in which there is accumulation, deposition, or production of substances in the skin. Typically, these substances are products of abnormal metabolism or degenerative phenomena occurring locally or systemically. The major cutaneous deposits may be subdivided into the hyalinoses, mucinoses, and mineral salts.

2. What is amyloid?

Amyloid is a protein with distinct tinctorial and ultrastructural properties found as extracellular deposits. It is composed of a nonfibrillary protein known as the amyloid P component and a fibrillary component that is derived from various sources. The amyloid fibril has an antiparallel, β-pleated sheet configuration. Electron microscopy reveals amyloid to be composed of rigid, nonbranching, nonanastomosing fibrils measuring 6–10 nm in diameter.

3. How is amyloid identified?

With light microscopy, amyloid appears as amorphous, hyalinelike, eosinophilic deposits. Amyloid typically demonstrates green birefringence with the alkaline Congo red stain, reddish metachromasia with crystal violet, and yellow-green fluorescence with thioflavine-T stain. These stains are not absolutely specific for amyloid, as false-positive results may occur with the other hyalinelike deposition disorders.

4. Name the various types of amyloidosis.

Classification of Amyloidosis

CLINICAL DISORDER	AMYLOID PROTEIN PRECURSOR	AMYLOID PROTEIN
Primary systemic amyloidosis	Immunoglobulin light chain	AL
Myeloma-associated amyloidosis	Immunoglobulin light chain	AL
Secondary systemic amyloidosis	Serum amyloid A lipoprotein	AA
Primary localized cutaneous amyloidosis		
Macular amyloidosis	Keratinocyte tonofilaments	—
Lichen amyloidosis	Keratinocyte tonofilaments	—
Nodular amyloidosis	Immunoglobulin light chain (produced locally by plasma cells)	AL

Amyloidosis may be classified according to clinical presentation and type of amyloid fibril protein deposition. The amyloid in the macular and lichenoid variants is derived from degenerated tonofilaments of keratinocytes. Nodular amyloidosis is formed from light chain-derived AL protein produced locally by plasma cells. It cannot be distinguished from primary systemic amyloidosis, and therefore, systemic disease should be excluded in all patients with nodular amyloidosis.

5. What are the cutaneous manifestations of primary or myeloma-associated systemic amyloidosis? How often do they occur?

Cutaneous lesions are seen in about 30% of cases of primary or myeloma-related systemic amyloidosis. The most common skin lesions are petechiae or ecchymoses due to amyloid deposition within blood vessel walls with subsequent fragility and dermal hemorrhage. These are often seen at sites predisposed to trauma, such as the hands or intertriginous areas. Pinching the skin gives characteristic purpuric lesions known as "pinch purpura." Purpura around the eyes may occur spontaneously but also frequently is seen following proctoscopy or vomiting ("post-proctoscopic purpura") (Fig. 1). Waxy papules, nodules, or plaques may be seen. Less common cutaneous lesions include sclerodermoid plaques and bullae. Alopecia and nail dystrophy also may develop.

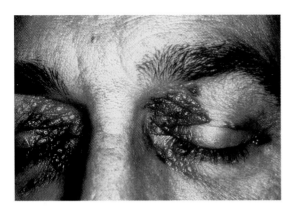

FIGURE 1. Primary systemic amyloidosis. Characteristic periorbital purpuric plaques.

6. Name the other organ systems that may be involved in primary or myeloma-associated amyloidosis.

Mucous membrane involvement with macroglossia occurs in 20% of cases. Hepatomegaly is found in about 50% of cases. Cardiac involvement may manifest as a restrictive cardiomyopathy or constrictive pericarditis. Peripheral nerve involvement results in paresthesias, peripheral neuropathy, and median nerve entrapment (carpal tunnel syndrome). Renal failure usually develops late in the disease course but may be a cause of death.

7. Compare lichen amyloidosis and macular amyloidosis.

Lichen amyloidosis, also known as papular amyloidosis, is the most common form of localized cutaneous amyloidosis. Lesions are pruritic, flesh-colored to brown papules, often with overlying scale (Fig. 2A). Papules may coalesce into verrucous plaques. The shins are the most common site of involvement.

In **macular amyloidosis,** pruritic macular hyperpigmentation occurs most commonly in the interscapular area. The chest or extremities are less commonly involved. The lesions may have a characteristic reticulate or rippled appearance.

Both of these variants of primary localized cutaneous amyloidosis occur more frequently in patients from the Middle East, Asia, and Central and South America.

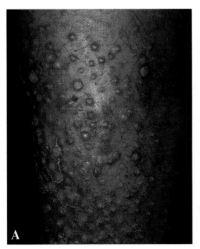

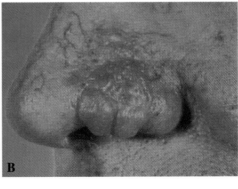

FIGURE 2. *A*, Lichen amyloidosis. Numerous, pruritic scaly papules on the anterior shin. *B*, Nodular amyloidosis demonstrating large waxy nodule on the nose.

8. How does nodular amyloidosis present? What is it associated with?

Nodular amyloidosis typically presents as solitary or multiple waxy nodules (Fig. 2B). Common sites of involvement include the face, scalp, lower extremities, and genitalia. It may be associated with the subsequent development of systemic amyloidosis in 15% of cases.

9. In what setting is secondary systemic amyloidosis seen?

Secondary systemic amyloidosis is associated with chronic systemic disease, such as infection, collagen vascular disease, or neoplasm. Examples of disease associations include tuberculosis, leprosy, osteomyelitis, rheumatoid arthritis, scleroderma, pustular psoriasis, leukemia, and lymphoma.

10. What are the systemic manifestations of secondary systemic amyloidosis?

Organs commonly involved in secondary systemic amyloidosis include the liver, spleen, and kidneys, resulting in hepatosplenomegaly and nephrotic syndrome, respectively. The skin appears clinically uninvolved except for exceptional cases that may show purpura. Although skin lesions are generally lacking, biopsy of subcutaneous abdominal fat may demonstrate amyloid deposition.

11. What is lipoid proteinosis?

Lipoid proteinosis, also known as hyalinosis cutis et mucosae, is a rare autosomal recessive genodermatosis in which skin and mucous membranes are infiltrated with a hyaline scleroprotein. The presenting symptom, hoarseness, develops in infancy due to involvement of the vocal cords with the hyaline deposits. Bullae, pustules, and crusts, followed by acneiform scars, are seen on the face and extremities. Waxy papules develop on the face and eyelids, producing a characteristic "string of beads" appearance. Later, verrucous plaques may develop on the elbows and knees.

12. Which histologic feature or "deposit" is common to all porphyrias?

The porphyrias are a group of diseases resulting from defects in the enzymes that regulate heme biosynthesis. The biochemical and clinical features are different for each type of porphyria, yet all demonstrate similar cutaneous histology with **deposits of eosinophilic, hyaline material around blood vessels.** This material stains positively with the periodic acid–Schiff stain and represents reduplicated basal lamina or type IV collagen.

13. Which porphyria classically demonstrates the largest deposits? What are its cutaneous features?

Erythropoietic protoporphyria, also termed protoporphyria, has the largest eosinophilic deposits in the cutaneous lesions. This autosomal dominant disorder of porphyrin metabolism is caused by a deficiency of the enzyme ferrochelatase (heme synthetase). Symptoms include photosensitivity, pruritus, burning, erythema, and edema, and often begin in early childhood. Chronic changes include a waxy, "cobblestone" thickening of the skin and shallow scars or pits. Increased protoporphyrin may be identified in the feces and blood, although urinary porphyrins are normal.

14. Name some of the cutaneous mucinoses.

The mucinoses are a heterogeneous group of disorders characterized by **dermal mucin deposition.** This mucin is largely hyaluronic acid, an acid mucopolysaccharide, with smaller amounts of chondroitin sulfate and heparin.

Disorders resulting in diffuse mucin deposition include generalized myxedema, pretibial myxedema, lichen myxedematosus, scleredema, reticular erythematous mucinosis, and the mucopolysaccharidoses (storage diseases). Mucin deposition may also be focal or localized, as with follicular mucinosis, cutaneous focal mucinosis, and digital mucous cyst.

15. Describe the clinical lesions seen in pretibial myxedema and its disease associations.

Patients with pretibial myxedema develop nodules or diffuse plaques typically located on the anterior lower legs, although involvement of other sites has been rarely reported (Fig. 3A). The lesions result from large amounts of dermal mucin deposition. Pretibial myxedema is seen in 1–4% of patients with Graves' disease and, less commonly, in patients with autoimmune thyroiditis.

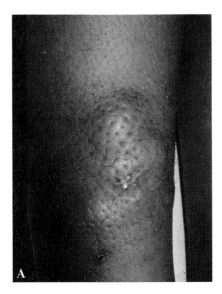 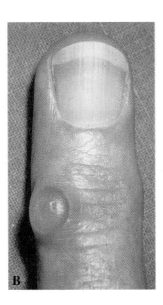

FIGURE 3. *A*, Pretibial myxedema. Thick plaques on anterior lower legs with peau d'orange change secondary to dermal mucin. *B*, Digital mucous cyst. Dome-shaped cystic nodule overlying the DIP joint.

16. Describe the clinical lesions seen in lichen myxedematosus.

In lichen myxedematosus, also known as papular mucinosis, numerous flesh-colored to erythematous, densely grouped lichenoid papules are found primarily on the face and arms. Lesions may be generalized. There is coalescence of papules into indurated plaques in the scleromyxedema variant. Lesions result from an increase in dermal mucin and an increase in fibroblasts.

17. What serum abnormality has been associated with lichen myxedematosus?

Serum paraproteinemia, usually IgG with lambda light chains. Rare cases with kappa light chains have been reported. Waldenstrom's macroglobulinemia or multiple myeloma may be rarely associated.

18. What is a digital mucous cyst?

A digital mucous cyst is a solitary, asymptomatic, semitranslucent, dome-shaped nodule typically present on the dorsal finger near the proximal nailfold or distal interphalangeal joint (Fig. 3B). It may distort the nail matrix, resulting in a groove in the nail plate. Clear, gelatinous mucoid material can be expressed from the cyst. It may rarely communicate with the underlying joint space. The digital mucous cyst arises spontaneously and may represent focal myxoid degeneration of collagen.

19. What substance is elevated in gout?

Gout is a heterogeneous group of disorders of purine metabolism resulting in elevated levels of **uric acid** (monosodium urate). Patients have either increased uric acid production or decreased renal excretion. The former may be seen with myeloproliferative disorders, and the latter, with renal disease and/or diuretic therapy.

20. Where is the uric acid deposited in gout? What are the resulting clinical manifestations?

Uric acid crystals in gout are most commonly deposited in the synovium, kidneys, soft tissues, and skin. The most common site is the synovium of joints, producing **acute gouty arthritis.** The metatarsophalangeal joint of the great toe is classically involved. Uric acid crystal deposition in the kidneys may result in **gouty nephropathy** with progressive renal failure and secondary hypertension. Uric acid urolithiasis or uric acid renal stones may also occur.

Uric acid deposition in the skin and soft tissues results in **gouty tophi,** which are seen in 20–50% of patients. Common sites of involvement include the helix of the ear, elbows, and digits (Fig. 4). These gouty tophi may ulcerate and discharge monosodium urate crystals that appear as a thick chalky material. Under light microscopy, these crystals are needle-shaped and birefringent.

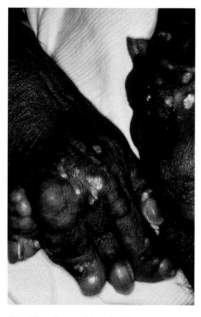

FIGURE 4. Gouty tophi. Tophaceous deposits of gout overlying digits.

21. How is gout treated?
Acute attacks of gout may be treated with a variety of agents, including colchicine, phenylbutazone, nonsteroidal anti-inflammatory agents, or systemic corticosteroids. Long-term therapy may include colchicine, allopurinol, probenecid, or urine alkalinization (to increase uric acid solubility).

22. How many types of calcinosis cutis are there?
1. **Dystrophic calcinosis cutis** occurs when there is deposition of calcium salts within inflamed or damaged tissue. Calcium and phosphorus metabolism is normal. It may be localized, such as within acne scars or epidermoid cysts, or widespread. Widespread dystrophic calcinosis cutis most often occurs in association with connective tissue disease, such as dermatomyositis or scleroderma.

2. **Metastatic calcinosis cutis** is seen with aberrations in calcium or phosphorus metabolism. It occurs when the serum calcium-phosphorus product exceeds 60.

3. The term **idiopathic calcinosis cutis** is used when no obvious underlying cause can be identified for tissue calcification. As with dystrophic calcification, this variant may be widespread, such as in calcinosis universalis, or localized, as in tumoral calcinosis or scrotal calcinosis.

23. What underlying medical conditions have been associated with metastatic calcinosis cutis?

Hyperparathyroidism	Sarcoidosis
Pseudohypoparathyroidism	Destructive bone disease
Vitamin D toxicity	Malignancies
Milk-alkali syndrome	Chronic renal failure

24. Where does metastatic calcinosis occur?
In metastatic calcinosis, calcium deposits are found in the skin, subcutaneous tissues, blood vessels, tendon, muscle, and internal organs.

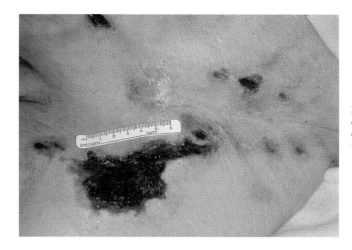

FIGURE 5. Metastatic calcinosis cutis. Necrosis of overlying skin in a patient with chronic renal failure.

25. Describe the cutaneous lesions in metastatic calcinosis.

In metastatic calcinosis cutis, yellowish-white to bluish-white rock-hard nodules or plaques are seen. There is a predilection for these deposits to occur over large joints, in the flexural areas, and in fingertips. Lesions may ulcerate, draining a white chalky material. If calcium deposition occurs within vessels, there may be infarction of the overlying skin and extensive tissue necrosis (Fig. 5). The term **calciphylaxis** is used for the development of extensive systemic and cutaneous calcification, usually with tissue necrosis, seen in patients with chronic renal failure and hyperparathyroidism.

BIBLIOGRAPHY

1. Armijo M: Mucoid cysts of the fingers. J Dermatol Surg Oncol 7:317–322, 1989.
2. Breathnach SM: Amyloid and amyloidosis. J Am Acad Dermatol 18:1–16, 1988.
3. Dinneen AM, Dicken CH: Scleromyxedema. J Am Acad Dermatol 33:37–43, 1995.
4. Elder GH: The cutaneous porphyrias. Semin Dermatol 9:63–69, 1990.
5. Ivker RA, Woosley J, Briggaman RA: Calciphylaxis in three patients with end-stage renal disease. Arch Dermatol 131:63–68, 1995.
6. Jambrosic J, From L, Hanna W: Lichen amyloidosis: Ultrastructure and pathogenesis. Am J Dermatopathol 6:151–158, 1984.
7. Konstantinov K, Kabakchiev P, Karchev T, et al: Lipoid proteinosis. J Am Acad Dermatol 27:293–297, 1992.
8. Mascaro JM: Porphyrias in children.Pediatr Dermatol. 9:371–372, 1992.
9. Palmer DG, Highton J, Hessian PA: Development of the gout tophus: An hypothesis. Am J Clin Pathol 91:190–195, 1989.
10. Rogioletti F, Rebora A: The new cutaneous mucinoses: A review with an up-to-date classification of cutaneous mucinoses. J Am Acad Dermatol 24:265–270, 1991.
11. Somach SC, Helm TN, Lawlor KB, et al: Pretibial mucin: Histologic patterns and clinical correlation. Arch Dermatol 129:1152–1156, 1993.
12. Tan SY, Pepys MB: Amyloidosis. Histopathology 25:403–414, 1994.
13. Truhan AP, Roenigk HH: The cutaneous mucinoses. J Am Acad Dermatol 14:1–18, 1986.
14. Venencie PY, Powell FC, Su WPD, et al: Scleredema: A review of 33 cases. J Am Acad Dermatol 11:128–134, 1984.
15. Walsh JS, Fairley JA: Calcifying disorders of the skin. J Am Acad Dermatol 33:693–706, 1995.

17. PHOTOSENSITIVE DERMATITIS

Kathleen M. David-Bajar, M.D., COL, MC

1. What is the definition of photosensitivity?

Although there is not a uniform definition accepted by all, most dermatologists define photosensitivity as the development or exacerbation of a skin eruption and/or symptoms (including pruritus or pain) following exposure to sunlight. In some instances, a patient may not specifically relate the eruption to sun exposure, usually due to a delay in the onset of signs or symptoms following sun exposure. Thus, if a skin eruption is photodistributed, even without a definite history of exacerbation following sun exposure, many dermatologists classify it as a photosensitive dermatosis. Some photosensitivity reactions (e.g., phototoxic drug reactions) are very similar to sunburn but occur with less intense sun exposure than would normally be required to induce sunburn in that individual.

2. How are photosensitive dermatoses classified?

Classification of Photodermatoses

ACUTE	CHRONIC
Sunburn	Polymorphous light eruption
Phototoxic drug eruptions	Porphyria cutanea tarda
Photocontact dermatitis	Subacute cutaneous lupus erythematosus
Solar urticaria	Discoid lupus erythematosus
Erythropoietic protoporphyria (becomes chronic)	Hydroa aestivale and vacciniforme
Acute cutaneous lupus erythematosus	Pellagra
Persistent light reactivity	
Actinic reticuloid	

It is useful to think of photosensitivity in terms of acute versus chronic dermatoses. There is some overlap, as some acute photoeruptions may become chronic when unrecognized and untreated. Chronic photodermatoses, such as polymorphous light eruption, may present acutely each spring. **Acute** photodermatoses usually develop within minutes to hours of light exposure. A sunburn is a classic example. **Chronic** photodermatoses develop less acutely and may be very persistent. Chronic cutaneous lupus erythematosus (discoid lupus erythematosus) is a classic example of a photosensitive dermatosis that may be induced by light but persist for a long time. Many forms of skin cancer are also due to chronic sun exposure (see Chapters 47 and 48).

3. Are any other dermatoses photoreactive?

In addition to the classic photosensitive dermatoses, a number of other skin eruptions may occasionally, but not always, be triggered or exacerbated by sun exposure: some viral diseases (e.g., herpes simplex labialis), erythema multiforme, granuloma annulare, disseminated superficial actinic porokeratosis, and pemphigus erythematosus.

4. What are the important questions to ask a patient with suspected photosensitivity?

1. How long does it take for the skin reaction to develop following light exposure? Some reactions (e.g., solar urticaria) occur within minutes following sun exposure, while others (e.g., chronic cutaneous lupus erythematosus) may take weeks to develop.

2. Have you ever had a similar skin reaction to light? Some reactions (e.g., polymorphous light reaction) tend to be recurrent or seasonal, while others may be one-time events (e.g., photosensitive drug reaction).

3. Is there a family history of similar skin reactions to light? Some photosensitive disorders are familial (e.g., erythropoietic protoporphyria) or occur more frequently in certain racial groups (e.g., polymorphous light reaction in North American Indians).

4. What do you put on your skin? Numerous products (soaps, perfumes, sunscreens) may produce photoallergic contact dermatitis in some individuals.

5. What medications do you take by mouth? Numerous drugs, both prescription and non-prescription, can occasionally produce photosensitive reactions.

6. Are there any associated cutaneous symptoms? Pruritus is a typical complaint associated with certain diseases (such as photoallergic contact dermatitis), while pain or burning is associated with other diseases (erythropoietic protoporphyria).

7. Do you have any other symptoms? Some photosensitive dermatoses are confined to the skin, while others (e.g., systemic lupus erythematosus) are associated with internal involvement.

5. What is the key physical finding in a patient with a photodermatosis?

The distribution of skin lesions. Lesions typically occur on sites most exposed to direct sunlight, such as the face, neck, upper or "V" area of chest, and the dorsal hands and arms. Areas more protected from sunlight, such as the scalp, upper eyelids, infranasal and submental areas, as well as fully-clothed areas, are typically spared. In photocontact dermatitis, the affected areas are those areas with exposure to both sunlight and the causative topical agent.

6. What are the most common causes of photosensitive dermatoses?

Medications, both systemic and topical, are frequent causes of photosensitivity. Polymorphous light eruption is the most common cause of chronic photodermatitis. Other causes of photosensitivity include the porphyrias, lupus erythematosus (see also Chapter 22), and dermatomyositis.

7. Discuss drug-induced photodermatitis.

Comparison of Phototoxic and Photoallergic Drug Eruptions

	PHOTOTOXIC	PHOTOALLERGIC
Frequency	Common	Rare
Morphology	Often resembles sunburn	Variable, may resemble contact dermatitis
Onset following first exposure	May occur	Usually not
Specific immune reaction involved	No	Yes

Phototoxic reactions are more common, often resemble sunburn (Fig. 1), and can occur on first exposure to a drug, without an incubation period. **Photoallergic** drug reactions are much less common and are believed to be mediated through specific immune reactions. They do not occur on first exposure to the drug without an incubation period. Passive transfer of photoallergic drug reactions has been described in animals.

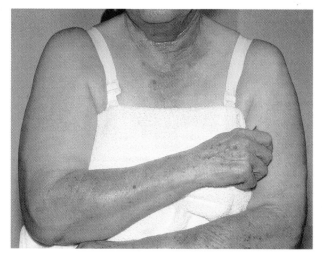

FIGURE 1. Phototoxic drug eruption. Sunburn-like erythema on the cheeks, neck, "V" area of the chest, and dorsal forearms.

8. What drugs are commonly associated with photodermatitis?

Phototoxic Reactions	*Photoallergic Reactions*
Tetracyclines	Halogenated salicylanilides (antimicrobials)
Furosemide	Phenothiazines
Benoxaprofen	Sulfanilamides
Thiazides	Para-aminobenzoic acid (PABA) esters
Piroxicam	Fragrances (musk ambrette, 6-methylcoumarin)
Naproxen	Benzophenone
Amiodarone	Avobenzone
Phenothiazines	

Some agents, such as phenothiazines, can produce either a phototoxic or photoallergic reaction. Because the list of potentially photosensitizing drugs is continually expanding, each drug used by a patient presenting with a photosensitive eruption should be considered as a possible etiologic agent. References such as Bruinsma's *The Guide to Drug Eruptions* may be used to determine if photoreactions have been reported with each drug in question.

9. Which topical agents are most likely to produce photocontact dermatitis?
Coal tar derivatives, psoralens, halogenated salicylanilides, sunscreen agents such as PABA (Fig. 2A) and benzophenones, and fragrances such as musk ambrette and 6-methylcoumarin. In addition, various plants that contain furocoumarins have been associated with photocontact dermatitis, termed phytophotodermatitis. Plants associated with phytophotodermatitis include figs, celery, parsnip, meadow grass, fennel, ferns, clover, lime, and lemon. Furocoumarins are found in the skin of the limes, so please take precautions when preparing gin and tonics at your next pool party (Fig. 2B).

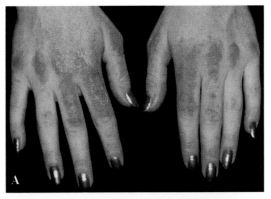

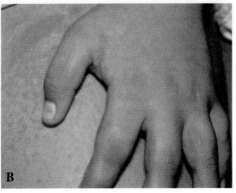

FIGURE 2. Photocontact dermatitis. *A,* Erythema of the dorsal hands and fingers, due to a sunscreen containing PABA. *B,* This patient was squeezing limes at a family picnic the day before this pruritic eruption occurred. Linear erythema is present on the lateral fingers and upper thigh, where lime juice contacted her skin in the presence of sunlight.

10. What is persistent light reactivity?

In persistent light reactivity, photodermatitis believed to be triggered by topical or systemic drugs persists long after the presumed causative agent has been discontinued. These unfortunate patients may be sensitive to a broad range of light, even visible light, and be totally incapacitated by this disease. Actinic reticuloid is a related disease involving persistent and severe photodermatitis and occurs primarily in older men.

11. What is polymorphous light eruption (PMLE)?

PMLE is a common, chronic photoeruption that typically begins in the first three decades of life. There may be a positive family history of sunlight sensitivity. Patients characteristically report the onset of skin disease beginning with sun exposure in spring or early summer. Patients sometimes demonstrate gradual improvement with continuing sun exposure, a phenomenon termed "hardening."

The specific skin lesions of PMLE may be of numerous (polymorphous) types, but one or two morphologic types usually predominate in individual patients. These include erythematous macules, patches, papules, plaques (Fig. 3), and vesicles and bullae. Lesions are photodistributed, often on the face and neck, chest, and dorsal arms and hands. The lips may also be involved.

PMLE is not infrequent among Native Americans from both North and South America (in whom the term **actinic prurigo** is often used). In this population, the family history is usually positive. The etiology of PMLE is unknown, and most patients with PMLE do not have anti-nuclear antibodies. Patients with PMLE have been reported to be sensitive to ultraviolet B, ultraviolet A, or both.

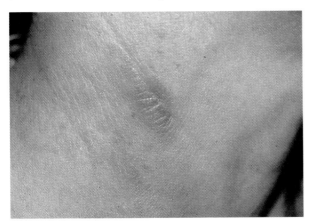

FIGURE 3. Polymorphous light eruption. Erythematous, scaly plaque on the lateral neck, which tended to recur each spring.

12. How is a polymorphous light eruption diagnosed?

PMLE is a clinical diagnosis, based on the history of a recurrent photoeruption, usually occurring each spring or early summer, with a consistent skin biopsy. There is no individual clinical, histologic, or laboratory finding that can establish a diagnosis of PMLE. Thus, it is important to exclude other causes of photosensitive dermatoses, such as lupus erythematosus and photodrug eruptions. Generally, the skin biopsy is helpful in this regard. In addition to routine histology, other negative tests include direct immunofluorescence testing of lesional skin (to exclude cutaneous lupus erythematosus), testing for anti-nuclear antibodies (including anti-Ro/SS-A antibodies), and a porphyrin screen (to rule out erythropoietic protoporphyria). Light testing may demonstrate a lowered minimal erythema dose (MED)—i.e., the dose of ultraviolet light required to produce erythema is less than one would predict on the basis of skin type.

13. How is polymorphous light eruption treated?

Sunscreens and other sun-protective measures are helpful, but a number of patients are not controlled with such measures. Topical steroids, beta-carotene, antimalarials, and psoralens with ultraviolet A light (PUVA; see Chapter 54) are alternatives that may be successful.

14. What is solar urticaria?

Urticaria, or hives, may be triggered by ultraviolet or even visible light. The urticarial papules or plaques usually develop on exposed areas within minutes of sun exposure and are accompanied by pain or pruritus. Rarely, systemic reactions leading to anaphylactic shock can occur.

15. Discuss the differential diagnosis of photodermatoses in infants or young children.

In the neonatal period, photodermatoses are uncommon, probably due in part to the minimal degree of exposure to sunlight. However, cutaneous lesions of **neonatal lupus erythematosus** typically occur very early in life and are often photoexacerbated. These patients develop erythematous, often annular plaques, usually distributed on the face and scalp. Cardiac conduction defects may also be seen. Nearly all of these infants, and their mothers, have circulating anti-Ro/SS-A antibodies, and possibly anti-La/SS-B antibodies.

The differential diagnosis also includes several genodermatoses that may present as photosensitivity early in life. Other childhood photodermatoses include polymorphous light eruption, photo-drug eruptions, photocontact dermatitis, hydroa aestivale, hydroa vacciniforme, erythropoietic protoporphyria, and cutaneous lupus erythematosus.

Genodermatoses Associated with Photosensitivity

DISEASE	SKIN FINDINGS	INHERITANCE	OTHER
Cockayne's syndrome	Scaly facial photodermatitis	Autosomal recessive	Dwarfism, bird-like facies, deafness, retardation
Bloom syndrome	Erythema, telangiectasia of cheeks	Autosomal recessive	Small at birth, severe growth retardation, respiratory infections, malignancy
Rothmund-Thomson syndrome	Facial erythema, edema followed by atrophy and telangiectasia	Autosomal recessive	Cataracts, usually normal intelligence
Hartnup disease	Pellagra-like eruption	Autosomal recessive	Cerebellar ataxia

16. How do hydroa aestivale and hydroa vacciniforme differ?

These rare, vesiculopapular photoeruptions of unknown etiology occur in childhood. Lesions occur primarily on the face, especially the ears, nose, and cheeks, and on the chest and dorsal hands. **Hydroa aestivale** occurs more commonly in females and is not associated with scarring. **Hydroa vacciniforme** is more common in males and heals with shallow, vacciniform scars.

17. Which porphyrias are associated with photodermatoses?

The most common porphyria with prominent cutaneous findings is **porphyria cutanea tarda** (PCT). There is a delay in the onset of lesions following sun exposure; thus, many PCT patients do not specifically complain of photosensitivity. The cutaneous changes seen in PCT may also be seen in other porphyrias, including variegate porphyria, hereditary coproporphyria; in pseudoporphyrias associated with hemodialysis; and with certain medications, such as furosemide, nalidixic acid, tetracycline, and naproxen.

More acute photosensitivity is seen in erythropoietic protoporphyria, congenital erythropoietic porphyria, and erythropoietic coproporphyria.

18. Describe the cutaneous changes in porphyria cutanea tarda.

Skin fragility with minor trauma is a common complaint, particularly over the dorsal fingers and hands. Skin lesions are usually found on the dorsal hands, fingers, and feet, and sometimes on the face and upper trunk. Tense vesicles and bullae develop in these sites, and heal with erosions, scarring, atrophy, milia, and pigmentary changes (Fig. 4). Hypertrichosis and thickened, sclerotic plaques may develop on the face and chest. Patients may not relate the skin changes to sun exposure, but on questioning, they often have a history of worsening in the summer months or following other periods of intense sun exposure.

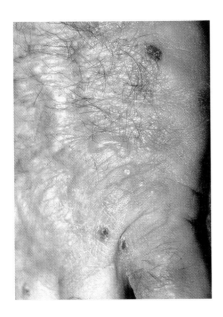

FIGURE 4. Porphyria cutanea tarda. Vesicles, crusts, and milia on the hand of a patient with alcohol-triggered PCT.

19. What causes porphyria cutanea tarda?

The porphyrias are due to specific enzyme deficiencies that lead to accumulation of porphyrins. Porphyrins absorb light in the 400–405-nm (Soret band) range, in the lower range of visible light. This absorbed light energy is then transferred to cellular structures or to molecular oxygen, causing damage to tissues.

PCT is due to a deficiency of the enzyme **uroporphyrinogen decarboxylase.** There are two main categories of PCT patients, acquired and hereditary. Patients with acquired PCT have the enzyme deficiency in the liver only and often have attacks triggered by agents such as alcohol, estrogen, hexachlorobenzene, and iron. PCT may also develop in patients with chronic liver disease, e.g., hepatitis C infection. In hereditary PCT, uroporphyrinogen decarboxylase is deficient in most tissues, not just the liver. Both heterozygous and homozygous inheritance of enzyme deficiencies have been described.

20. How is porphyria cutanea tarda diagnosed?

Fluorescent spectrophotometric analysis of plasma is a rapid screen for porphyria. Plasma is exposed to an excitation wavelength of 400–410 nm, and the emission peaks are measured. A sharp emission peak at 619 nm confirms a porphyrin disorder. To differentiate the specific porphyrins further, a 24-hour urine specimen is submitted for porphyrin studies. In PCT, the major porphyrins elevated in urine are uroporphyrin I and 7-carboxylporphyrin III. In addition, stool porphyrins should be tested; PCT patients have normal levels of protoporphyrins but increased isocoproporphyrins in the stool.

21. How is variegate porphyria distinguished from porphyria cutanea tarda?

Variegate porphyria (VP) may produce cutaneous lesions that are indistinguishable from those seen in PCT, but patients with VP have increased levels of protoporphyrins in their stool and only moderately increased urine porphyrins. Unlike PCT patients, VP patients often have acute attacks of porphyria similar to those seen in patients with acute intermittent porphyria, and thus it is important to distinguish VP from PCT.

22. What treatments are used in porphyria cutanea tarda?

1. Eliminate any agents that may trigger PCT, such as alcohol.
2. Protect from both ultraviolet and visible light.

3. Phlebotomy is most often the treatment of choice. Phlebotomy is believed to work by decreasing excessive iron stores. Removal of about 500 ml of whole blood is done at periodic intervals as tolerated, until the hemoglobin level is about 10–11 gm/dl or until side effects are experienced.

4. Low-dose chloroquine therapy is an alternate treatment that requires very close monitoring for hepatotoxicity.

23. What are the cutaneous findings in erythropoietic protoporphyria?

Patients with erythropoietic protoporphyria usually have complaints beginning in childhood, though cases presenting in adult life are well documented. Photosensitivity may be severe, with almost immediate burning and stinging of the exposed skin following sun exposure. Erythema, edema, hive-like lesions, vesicles, and purpura may then develop, particularly on the nose, cheeks, and dorsal hands. With time, these areas develop atrophic, waxy scars. The skin over the knuckles may become thickened, wrinkled, and shiny, giving the appearance of very aged hands.

24. How is a diagnosis of erythropoietic protoporphyria made?

Erythropoietic protoporphyria is believed to be due to a deficiency of the enzyme ferrochelatase. Red blood cells (RBCs) and feces show increased levels of protoporphyrins. In addition, if fresh RBCs are examined with a fluorescence microscope, 5–30% of RBCs will fluoresce a coral red color. This fluorescence is transient and light-sensitive; thus, RBCs should be collected and examined in a dark room.

25. What treatments are used in erythropoietic protoporphyria?

Therapy is primarily preventative, aimed at protecting the skin from ultraviolet and visible radiation. Beta-carotene capsules given orally may be helpful.

26. Do any other medical problems occur in patients with erythropoietic protoporphyria?

About 11% of patients with erythropoietic protoporphyria have a mild anemia of unknown etiology. Cholelithiasis is seen and may occur at a very early age. Liver disease is common but only rarely leads to fatal hepatic failure.

BIBLIOGRAPHY

1. Addo HA, Frain-Bell W: Actinic prurigo—A specific photodermatosis? Photodermatology 1:119–128, 1994.
2. Bickers DR, Pathak MA, Lim HW: The porphyrias. In Freedberg IM, et al (eds): Fitzpatrick's Dermatology in General Medicine, 5th ed. New York, McGraw-Hill, 1999.
3. Bowers AG: Phytophotodermatitis. Am J Contact Dermat 10:89–93, 1999.
4. Bruinsma W: A Guide to Drug Eruptions, 5th ed. Oosthuizen, The Netherlands, The File of Medicines, 1990.
5. Hawk JLM, Norris PG: Abnormal responses to ultraviolet radiation: Idiopathic. In Freedberg IM, et al (eds): Fitzpatrick's Dermatology in General Medicine, 5th ed. New York, McGraw-Hill, 1999.
6. Ryckaert S, Roelandts R: Solar urticaria: A report of 25 cases and difficulties in phototesting. Arch Dermatol 134:71–74, 1998.
7. Vassileva SG, Mateev G, Parish LC: Antimicrobial photosensitive reactions. Arch Intern Med 158:1993–2000, 1998.
8. Walsh DS, Beard JS, James WD: Fluorescent spectrophotometric analysis in the evaluation of porphyria. JAMA 272:1580–1581, 1994.

18. DISORDERS OF PIGMENTATION

Joseph Yohn, M.D.

1. What are the four components of normal skin pigmentation?

What we view as normal skin pigmentation is the combination of four pigments in the epidermis and dermis:

1. Oxygenated hemoglobin (red) in the arterioles and capillaries
2. Deoxygenated hemoglobin (blue) in the venules
3. Any ingested carotenoids or incompletely metabolized bile (yellow)
4. Epidermal melanin (brown)

Of all the pigments, melanin, which is synthesized by epidermal melanocytes, is the most important pigment in determining skin color.

2. How are racial differences in pigmentation determined?

Racial differences in pigmentation are determined by the type of melanin synthesized and the amount distributed to the surrounding keratinocytes. Fair-skinned individuals make a light brown form of melanin, pheomelanin, and distribute only small amounts to surrounding keratinocytes. On the other hand, melanocytes of darkly pigmented individuals make a dark brown form of melanin, eumelanin, and distribute large amounts of it to neighboring keratinocytes. All of the skin colors in between are due to a mixture of light brown pheomelanin and dark brown eumelanin.

3. How frequently do pigmentation disorders occur?

Most patients, over a lifetime, will suffer from a pigmentation disorder. Fortunately, the most common pigmentation disorders are benign, self-limited, and reversible. For example, one of the most common develops following a cutaneous inflammatory reaction, when the skin is either more darkly pigmented (postinflammatory hyperpigmentation) or less pigmented (postinflammatory hypopigmentation) than surrounding normal skin. Postinflammatory changes in pigmentation slowly revert to normal over several months.

4. Name the two major types of cutaneous dyspigmentation.

Leukoderma and melanoderma. Patients with **leukoderma** present with areas of skin that appear lighter than surrounding normal skin, whereas patients with **melanoderma** have skin that appears darker than normal. The major forms of cutaneous dyspigmentation can be broken down further into subtypes depending on whether there is alteration in melanocyte number or pigment content of the skin (see table on next page.)

5. Are some disorders of pigmentation markers for systemic disease?

Pigmentation Pattern	Associated Disease
Ash-leaf hypopigmented macules	Tuberous sclerosis
Generalized hypopigmentation	Albinism
Axillary and inguinal freckles	Neurofibromatosis
Generalized hyperpigmentation	Addison's disease

6. How do you diagnose a pigmentation disorder?

Clinical history: The history is the most important aspect of the investigation of a pigmentation disorder. It should focus on the time of onset (such as at birth, during childhood, or later in life) and a family history. Other facts to be determined include any associated illness or symptoms, drug ingestion, chemical exposure, occupation, and exposure to sunlight, artificial ultraviolet light, or ionizing radiation. Finally, a careful **review of systems** should be performed.

Skin examination: The entire skin surface should be evaluated with attention to the lesion(s) color, shape, and distribution. Lesion **color** helps to place the disorder into a specific category to

Classification of Epidermal Disorders of Pigmentation

	LEUKODERMA (DECREASED PIGMENTATION)		MELANODERMA (INCREASED PIGMENTATION)	
	Decreased Melanocyte Number	*Decrease or Absence of Melanin*	*Increased Melanocyte Number*	*Increased Melanin*
Genetic	Vitiligo (some forms) Piebaldism Waardenburg's syndrome Woolf's syndrome Ziprowski-Margolis syndrome	Albinism Phenylketonuria Homocystinuria Histidinemia Tuberous sclerosis	Lentigines Moynihan's syndrome Peutz-Jegher syndrome	Café au lait macule, neurofibromatosis Café au lait macule, Albright's syndrome Becker's melanosis Nevus spilus Ephiledes (freckles)
Chemical or drug	Monobenzyl ether of hydroquinone *para*-Substituted phenols	Hydroquinone Chloroquine and hydroxychloroquine Arsenicals Mercaptoethyl amines Corticosteroids (topical and intradermal)	Stem cell factor Melanocyte-stimulating hormone (MSH)	Arsenicals Busulfan Psoralens 5-Fluorouracil Cyclophosphamide Topical nitrogen mustard Bleomycin
Endocrine or metabolic	Vitamin B$_{12}$ deficiency	Kwashiorkor Nephrotic syndrome Intestinal malabsorption Hypopituitarism Addison's disease Hyperthyroidism	—	Addison's disease ACTH- and MSH-producing tumors ACTH or estrogen therapy Pregnancy Melasma Porphyria cutanea tarda Kwashiorkor Pellagra Intestinal malabsorption
Physical	Burns (thermal, ionizing radiation, etc) Trauma	Trauma	UVR (tanning) Solar lentigo PUVA-induced lentigo	UVR (tanning) Thermal radiation (infrared) Ionizing radiation Trauma
Inflammation and infection	Vitiligo (some forms) Pinta Yaws Onchocerciasis Cutaneous T-cell lymphoma Scleroderma	Sarcoidosis Secondary syphilis Leprosy Tinea versicolor Pityriasis alba Eczema Psoriasis Discoid lupus	—	Postinflammatory hyperpigmentation Lichen planus Discoid lupus erythematosus Lichen simplex chronicus Atopic dermatitis Psoriasis Tinea versicolor Scleroderma

aid in narrowing the diagnostic possibilities. (A clinical pearl: anesthetic leukoderma is highly suggestive of leprosy.) The **shape** of a lesion is sometimes diagnostic. Linear areas of depigmentation, often in areas of trauma, are suggestive for vitiligo, whereas ash-leaf-shaped hypopigmented macules suggest tuberous sclerosis. **Distribution** of pigmentary changes also helps in diagnosis. Symmetrical depigmentation on the arms, legs, and/or torso suggests vitiligo. Increased pigmentation of the oral mucosa, axillae, and palmar creases is associated with Addison's disease.

Other diagnostic tests: Wood's lamp examination is sometimes helpful. Skin biopsy, with or without special stains for melanin (silver nitrate or the Fontana-Masson stain), determines epidermal melanocyte number and the extent and location of epidermal and dermal pigmentation.

7. What is a Wood's lamp?

A hand-held black light. Wood's lamp emits light in a narrow spectrum of long-wave ultraviolet to short-wave visible light. Hypopigmented areas appear lighter, and depigmented areas appear pure white. Furthermore, epidermal hyperpigmentation is enhanced (appears darker), whereas dermal hyperpigmentation is not enhanced.

LEUKODERMA

8. Name some heritable forms of leukoderma.

- **Ziprowski-Margolis syndrome** is a rare X-linked recessive disorder characterized by deaf-mutism, heterochromic irides, and hypomelanosis of the skin.
- **Waardenburg's syndrome** is an autosomal dominant disorder associated with congenital deafness, heterochromic irides, hypomelanotic skin macules, white forelock, laterally displaced medial canthi, and widening of the nasal root.
- **Woolf's syndrome (piebaldism)** is a rare autosomal dominant depigmentation disorder that is characterized by a white scalp forelock, hyperpigmented macules within areas of skin depigmentation, and associated deafness.
- **Vitiligo** is a much more common disorder affecting approximately 1:100 people worldwide, and although the culprit gene(s) have not been identified, some patients with vitiligo have a genetic tendency for this disorder.

9. Name the skin disorder that manifests with complete loss of skin pigmentation.

Vitiligo is a depigmenting disorder due to loss of epidermal melanocytes. There are both familial and nonfamilial forms, and the overall incidence is 1%. Vitiligo has been reported to be associated with autoimmune disorders, including thyroid disease and diabetes mellitus. Many patients have circulating anti-melanocyte antibodies that may play a role in melanocyte destruction. However, the cause of vitiligo is unknown. Vitiligo affects all races and affects both sexes equally.

Typically, lesions of vitiligo are stark white with a well-demarcated border and no other skin changes. Sometimes, the border is hyperpigmented and rarely erythematous. Areas commonly affected are the periorbital, perioral, and anogenital areas, as well as the elbows, knees, axillae, inguinal folds, and forearms. Frequently, lesions of vitiligo develop symmetrically on the trunk and extremities (Fig. 1). Vitiligo also causes depigmentation of hair (leukotrichia).

10. When does vitiligo have its onset?

The peak incidence occurs in the third decade of life, but 50% of cases occur before age 20. Vitiligo has been reported in all age groups with onset as early as birth and as late as 81 years.

11. Do any factors influence the onset of vitiligo?

The patient presenting with vitiligo usually describes asymptomatic areas of skin that have rapidly lost all pigment. Rarely does the patient recall an associated illness, but skin trauma is commonly reported to cause vitiligo lesions. One caveat—vitiligo only occurs in patients predisposed to the condition. Thus, skin trauma will not induce vitiligo in nonpredisposed individuals.

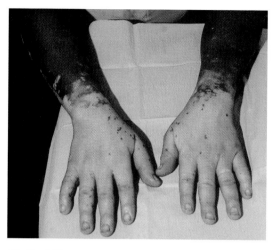

FIGURE 1. African-American man with vitiligo. Note the complete loss of skin pigmentation of the hands and wrists.

12. Is vitiligo treatable?

Yes. The most effective treatment is psoralen plus ultraviolet A radiation (PUVA).

Vitiligo repigments in small part from the border and mostly from the hair follicle. Therefore, the more deeply penetrating UVA is necessary to stimulate the hair follicle melanocytes. The use of psoralen allows for lower doses of UVA per treatment. For most cases, psoralen is administered systemically in the form of pills.

Fifty to 75% of patients will repigment following PUVA given twice weekly. Most patients require 15–25 treatments to initiate repigmentation and 100–300 treatments for maximal repigmentation. Following repigmentation, the patient is slowly weaned off PUVA. Fully repigmented skin has an 85% chance of remaining pigmented.

For patients who decline PUVA treatment, topical steroids are helpful. All patients with vitiligo should use sunscreens to protect depigmented skin from sun damage.

13. What is piebaldism?

Piebaldism is an uncommon autosomal dominant depigmentation disorder that is characterized by a white scalp forelock and hyperpigmented macules within areas of skin depigmentation. Piebaldism is due to decreased melanocyte expression of stem cell factor receptor, which is required for normal melanocyte migration to the skin. Melanocytes migrate during embryologic development in a dorsal-to-ventral direction, and melanocytes with decreased stem cell factor receptor expression are unable to migrate to ventral skin surfaces, such as the forehead, abdomen, and volar arms and legs. For this reason, depigmented areas in piebaldism predominate on ventral skin surfaces. Patients are otherwise healthy. There is no treatment available for piebaldism. Piebaldism with deafness is called Woolf's syndrome.

14. What is albinism?

Albinism is a group of inherited disorders of the melanin pigment system. All forms are autosomal recessive, except dominant albinoidism and X-linked ocular albinism. In albinism, there is either a defect in the enzyme tyrosinase with a decrease in melanin synthesis or a defect in packaging of melanin in melanosomes. Generally, albinism presents as depigmented or hypopigmented skin and hair, nystagmus, photophobia, and decreased visual acuity (Fig. 2). There are 10 different forms of albinism. Some forms affect the skin, hair, and eyes (oculocutaneous albinism); other forms primarily affect the eyes (ocular albinism). There is no treatment available for albinism.

15. How does albinism differ from the other inherited leukodermas?

The common feature of vitiligo, piebaldism, and the rarer leukoderma syndromes is a decrease or total absence of epidermal melanocytes. By comparison, patients with albinism have normal epidermal melanocyte number, but the melanocytes synthesize inadequate amounts of melanin.

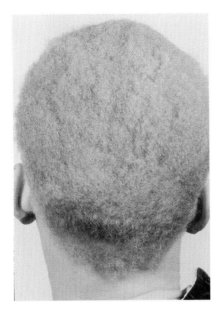

FIGURE 2. Albino African-American boy with generalized hypopigmentation.

16. Can disorders of amino acid metabolism cause leukoderma?

Inherited Disorders of Amino Acid Metabolism with Related Leukoderma

DISORDER	AFFECTED AMINO ACID	INCIDENCE	INHERITANCE	MANIFESTATIONS
Phenylketonuria	Phenylalanine	1:11,000	AR	Hypopigmentation of hair, eyes, and skin; mental retardation if not treated early
Histidinemia	Histidine	1:10,000	AR	Hypopigmentation, mental retardation
Homocystinuria	Methionine	1:45,000	AR	Hypopigmentation of skin, hair, and eyes; CNS abnormalities, skeletal abnormalities (Marfan's-like), thromboembolic disease

AR, autosomal recessive.

17. How do chemicals cause skin depigmentation or skin hypopigmentation?

Monobenzyl ether of hydroquinone (MBEH) and *para*-substituted phenols (PSP) cause skin depigmentation by destroying melanocytes. It is believed that both MBEH and PSP are taken up by melanocytes and metabolized into toxic products that kill the melanocytes.

Hydroquinone, a commonly used skin-lightening agent, causes decreased melanin synthesis by competing with tyrosine and dihydroxyphenylalanine for the enzyme tyrosinase. With hydroquinone bound to its active site, tyrosinase is unable to synthesize melanin. Other chemicals, such as arsenic, mercaptoethyl amines, chloroquine, hydroxychloroquine, and corticosteroids, all act to metabolically suppress melanocytes, resulting in decreased melanin synthesis and skin lightening. In most cases, the effects of these chemicals are reversible.

18. Can patients with nutritional disorders suffer from leukoderma?

Yes. Patients suffering from protein loss or deficiency diseases, including kwashiorkor, intestinal malabsorption, and nephrotic syndrome, often manifest with facial, truncal, and extremity hypopigmentation. The hypopigmentation is believed to be due to dysregulation of normal melanogenesis secondary to lack of amino acid precursors for melanin synthesis and for normal melanin polymer formation. Normal pigmentation returns following treatment of the nutritional disorder.

19. What disorders should the clinician consider in a patient with hypopigmented macules and patches?

Tuberous sclerosis, sarcoidosis, discoid lupus erythematosus, eczema, psoriasis, secondary syphilis, leprosy, and tinea versicolor.

20. What is tuberous sclerosis?

Tuberous sclerosis (TS), an autosomal dominant disorder with an incidence of 1/6,000 births, is a multifaceted disorder that causes tumors in nearly every organ in the body (see also chapter 5). The most common presenting symptom is seizures, although many patients are asymptomatic. The hypopigmented macules of TS classically are referred to as ash-leaf spots. Less commonly, they are smaller and clustered and are called confetti spots. Hypopigmented macules are not diagnostic of TS, but they are suggestive of the disease; and because many people are asymptomatic, the presence of hypopigmented macules requires further investigation. They are present at birth, before the various tumors develop, and are important markers of TS.

21. What pigmentation abnormalities are associated with sarcoidosis, discoid lupus, cutaneous T-cell lymphoma, scleroderma, eczema, and psoriasis?

Hypopigmented lesions. Inflammatory mediators commonly elevated in these disorders have been shown to inhibit human melanocyte melanization.

22. What infectious disorders can have associated leukoderma?

Secondary syphilis, pinta, yaws, onchocerciasis, and leprosy. The inflammatory reaction associated with these diseases alters melanocyte homeostasis, with resultant decreased melanin synthesis and transfer to keratinocytes.

23. Describe the pigmentation changes seen with the treponematoses.

Secondary syphilis: Hypopigmented macules can be found on the neck, shoulders, upper chest, and axillae in patients with secondary syphilis (due to *Treponema pallidum*). The hypopigmented neck lesions have been termed the "necklace of Venus."

Pinta: Pinta is a chronic nonvenereal disease caused by *T. carateum* that is endemic in Central and South America. The primary lesion, at the site of inoculation, is a **hypopigmented patch or plaque** on the arm, leg, or torso. Secondary pinta lesions (pintides) are at first erythematous and then become hyper- and hypopigmented. Later in the disease, pinta lesions become more uniformly hypopigmented.

Yaws: Yaws is a nonvenereal disease caused by *T. pallidum* ssp. *pertenue* that is common in children in impoverished areas of Central America. The primary lesion heals as an **atrophic hypopigmented scar.** Secondary yaws often heals without dyspigmentation, but the gummatous tertiary yaws lesions localized to the lower extremities, volar wrists, and dorsal hands are depigmented.

24. What cutaneous lesions are seen with Hansen's disease?

Hansen's disease, or leprosy, is a chronic infectious disease caused by *Mycobacterium leprae*. *M. leprae* infects the skin and peripheral nerves and manifests with anesthetic, hypopigmented patches, plaques, or nodules. Patients with indeterminate and tuberculoid leprosy have one or few lesions, whereas patients with lepromatous leprosy have many lesions. Lesions may repigment following antibiotic cure.

25. Why is lesional skin of tinea versicolor frequently hypopigmented?

Tinea versicolor is caused by overgrowth of the skin normal flora yeast, *Pityrosporum orbiculare. Pityrosporum,* in its pathogenic hyphal form, secretes an enzyme that breaks down epidermal unsaturated fatty acids to azelaic acid, which inhibits melanocyte tyrosinase. Tinea versicolor is common in tropical and temperate climates and is found in all races and age groups. The typical lesion is a scaly, slightly erythematous macule or patch located on the proximal anterior and posterior torso (Fig. 3). Tinea versicolor may be either hypopigmented or hyperpigmented.

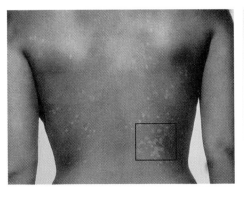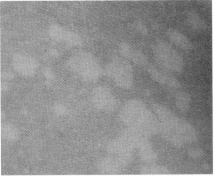

FIGURE 3. Multiple hypopigmented macules and patches on the torso of a woman with tinea versicolor.

MELANODERMA

26. What are lentigines? What heritable disorders manifest these?

Lentigines are brown to dark-brown, 1–5 mm macules that may occur on any cutaneous surface. They resemble freckles, but on biopsy, these lesions have increased numbers of melanocytes and increased melanocyte and basal keratinocyte pigmentation.

A benign condition characterized by the rapid development of hundreds of lentigines widespread over the skin surface in adolescents or young adults has been described. The presence of multiple lentigines at a young age is suggestive of autosomal dominant disorders, especially Moynahan's syndrome or Peutz-Jeghers syndrome (Fig. 4).

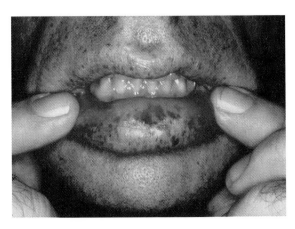

FIGURE 4. A 45-year-old man with numerous hyperpigmented macules of Peutz-Jeghers syndrome.

27. Describe the clinical manifestations of Moynahan's syndrome.

Patients with Moynahan's syndrome have hundreds of lentigines on the face, trunk, and extremities. The mnemonic LEOPARD has been applied to the clinical symptoms associated with this syndrome:

    L = **L**entigines
    E = **E**lectrocardiographic conduction defects
    O = **O**cular hypertelorism
    P = **P**ulmonic stenosis
    A = **A**bnormal genitalia
    R = Growth **R**etardation
    D = **D**eafness

28. Why is Peutz-Jeghers syndrome associated with carcinoma?

Patients with Peutz-Jeghers syndrome have widespread cutaneous lentigines that also involve the lips, buccal mucosa, palate, tongue, and eyelids.

In addition, they suffer from gastrointestinal polyps, usually in the small bowel, which by the second decade of life can become symptomatic with diarrhea, hemorrhage, obstruction, or intus-susception. Malignant degeneration of GI polyps has been reported, with carcinomas developing most commonly in the large intestine but also in the small intestine and stomach.

29. Are there pigmentation disorders associated with neurofibromatosis?

Yes. Common pigmented lesions of neurofibromatosis 1 (NF1, von Recklinghausen's disease) are café au lait macules (CALM) and inguinal and axillary freckling. CALM are, as the name would imply, flat, tan to light-brown lesions located anywhere on the body; these range from a few millimeters to several centimeters in diameter. Greater than 90% of CALM of NF1 are present at birth or within the first year of life. NF1 is a relatively common autosomal dominant disorder that occurs in 1:3,000 live births.

30. Do any other disorders manifest with CALM?

Yes. In 1937, Albright reported a syndrome consisting of osteitis fibrosa disseminata, endocrine dysfunction with precocious puberty in females, and CALM. The CALM of **Albright's syndrome** differ from those of NF1 by occurring predominantly on the forehead, posterior neck, sacrum, and buttocks. CALM of Albright's syndrome tend to be unilateral and do not cross the midline, whereas CALM of NF1 exist in a random, generalized pattern. CALM of Albright's syndrome appear at or soon after birth.

31. What is Becker's melanosis?

Becker's melanosis (also known as Becker's pigmented hairy hamartoma and Becker's nevus) is a benign pigmented lesion that develops in the second or third decade of life with a male:female ratio of 5:1. There is no predominance of race, and one large study reported a prevalence of 0.52% in males between ages 17–26 years. Greater than 80% of lesions occur on the trunk, appearing as a tan to dark-brown patch with an irregular border ranging in size from 100–500 cm^2 (Fig. 5). Excess hair growth has been reported in 56% of cases. With onset in the teen years and young adulthood, Becker's melanosis is easily differentiated from a congenital nevus and CALM of Albright's syndrome, which are present at birth. Once fully developed, Becker's melanosis remains stable for the life of the patient.

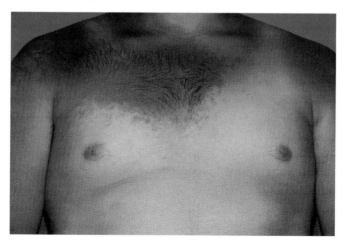

FIGURE 5. Becker's melanosis demonstrating increased hair on the shoulder and upper chest. (Courtesy of James E. Fitzpatrick, MD.)

32. What is a nevus spilus?

Nevus spilus is a CALM that contains darkly pigmented, 1–3-mm-diameter macules or papules. The lesion is present at birth and can involve any cutaneous surface. The darkly pigmented macules and papules of nevus spilus are junctional or compound nevi, respectively (see also Chapter 43.)

33. Do any natural factors stimulate human epidermal pigmentation?

Melanocyte-stimulating hormone	Insulin-like growth factor
Stem cell factor	Endothelin-1
Basic fibroblast growth factor	Leukotriene C4 and B4

34. What drugs are usually used to stimulate skin pigmentation? How do they work?

The psoralens or furocoumarins, potent photosensitizing drugs, have been used for thousands of years to stimulate skin pigmentation. The most commonly used agent in dermatology for skin photosensitization is **8-methoxypsoralen** (8-MOP). The exact mechanism of skin photosensitization is not known, but 8-MOP is preferentially taken up by epidermal cells, where it binds to cell membranes and is concentrated within cell nuclei. Upon photoactivation, 8-MOP causes alteration in cell membrane signaling and forms covalent bonds with DNA that leads to the formation of psoralen–DNA adducts. Together, the altered cell membrane signaling and psoralen–DNA adducts incite a cascade of events that stimulate melanocyte melanin synthesis and melanin transfer to keratinocytes, resulting in increased skin pigmentation.

35. Can other drugs cause increased skin pigmentation?

Yes. Arsenicals, busulfan, 5-fluorouracil, cyclophosphamide, topical nitrogen mustard (mechlorethamine), and bleomycin most commonly cause increased skin pigmentation. The mechanisms by which these drugs cause hyperpigmentation are unknown, but it is possible that the drug or a metabolite either directly stimulates epidermal melanocytes to increase melanin synthesis or indirectly stimulates metabolic pathways that cause increased epidermal melanization.

36. How does sun tanning occur? What are the other effects of sunlight on human skin pigmentation?

Sunlight stimulates human epidermal melanocytes to increase melanin synthesis and stimulates increased melanocyte transfer of melanosomes to keratinocytes. This melanocyte response to sunlight is called **tanning.** The action spectrum of sunlight that causes tanning is the ultraviolet spectrum (wavelengths 290–400 nm). Excess sunlight exposure causes abnormal melanocyte function, resulting in areas of melanocyte overproduction of melanin and increased melanocyte proliferation. Overproduction of melanin in a localized area causes the development of brown macules called **freckles.** Skin lesions that are made up of increased numbers of melanocytes and increased melanin synthesis are called **solar lentigines.**

37. Can endocrine and metabolic disorders cause altered skin pigmentation?

Yes. **Addison's disease** is the prototype disorder with diffuse hypermelanosis associated with pigment accentuation in mucous membranes, skinfolds, palmar creases, and pressure points (elbows, knees, knuckles, and coccyx). Adrenocorticotropic hormone (ACTH) or melanocyte-stimulating hormone (MSH)-producing **tumors** can cause increased skin pigmentation. Similarly, systemic administration of ACTH and MSH may cause skin hyperpigmentation. **Pregnancy** and **estrogen therapy** can cause hyperpigmentation, usually of the nipples and anogenital skin. Additionally, a mask-like hyperpigmentation, called melasma, can develop on the forehead, temples, cheeks, nose, and upper lip in pregnant women and women receiving estrogen therapy.

Patients with **porphyria cutania tarda** can have profound hyperpigmentation of sun-exposed skin associated with facial hirsutism. Nutritional disorders, such a **kwashiorkor, pellagra,** and **intestinal malabsorption,** can cause skin hyperpigmentation along with areas of hypopigmentation.

38. Can forms of radiation other than ultraviolet radiation cause increased skin pigmentation?

Yes. Thermal (infrared) and ionizing radiation skin injury can result in hyperpigmentation, probably due to melanocyte-stimulating inflammatory mediators and immune cytokines released in response to injury from these different forms of radiation.

BLUE-GRAY DYSPIGMENTATION

39. Are there other types of dyspigmentation besides leukoderma and melanoderma?

Yes. **Blue-gray skin discoloration** can develop from melanin in dermal melanocytes, dermal melanin deposition, or nonmelanin dermal dyspigmentation.

Classification of Dermal Hyperpigmentation

	MELANODERMA (INCREASED PIGMENTATION)		NON-MELANIN PIGMENTS
	Increased Melanocyte Number	*Increased Melanin*	
Genetic	Mongolian spot Nevus of Ota Nevus of Ito	—	—
Chemical or drug	—	Fixed drug eruption	Silver Mercury Bismuth Gold Antimalarials Phenothiazines Minocycline Amiodarone
Endocrine or metabolic	—	Chronic nutritional deficiency	Ochronosis
Physical	—	Erythema ab igne	—
Inflammation and infection	—	Macular amyloidosis Erythema dyschromium perstans Postinflammatory hyperpigmentation	—

40. Name the different types of hyperpigmentation due to excess numbers of dermal melanocytes.

Mongolian spot, nevus of Ota, and nevus of Ito.

41. Differentiate a nevus of Ota from a nevus of Ito.

Nevus of Ota (oculodermal melanocytosis) is an acquired disorder of dermal melanocytosis with an age of onset in early childhood or young adulthood. Less than 1% of Asiatic individuals are affected, and nonAsiatic races are affected even less frequently. Females are affected five times more frequently than males, with color hues ranging from dark brown, to purplish-brown, to blue-black. In its most common form, it involves the periorbital skin of one eye, although bilateral forms can occur, and pigmentation can extend to involve the temple, forehead, periorbital cheek, nose areas, and ocular structures.

A variant of nevus of Ota, called **nevus of Ito,** can occur over the shoulder and neck region and has the same natural history as nevus of Ota.

42. What types of hyperpigmentation are due to dermal melanin deposition?

- Macular amyloidosis   Brownish-gray macules
- Fixed drug eruption   Reddish-brown to blue-gray macule, with erythema, edema, scale, and sometimes blisters

- Erythema ab igne

  Blue-gray patches, sometimes with erythema and scale

- Erythema dyschromium perstans

  Erythematous, ash-gray macules and patches

- Postinflammatory hyperpigmentation

  Brown to gray macules and patches (Fig. 6)

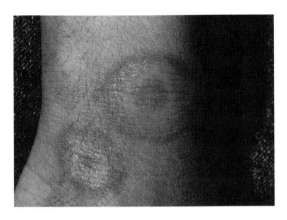

FIGURE 6. Two target-shaped patches of postinflammatory hyperpigmentation on the dorsal wrist of a woman following resolution of erythema multiforme.

43. Describe the presentation of fixed drug eruption.

Fixed drug eruption is a localized form of cutaneous drug reaction that commonly presents as a reddish-brown to blue-gray macule. Usually, a fixed drug eruption develops in the same location with each exposure to a particular drug. Initially, the skin area is erythematous, slightly edematous, and scaly, sometimes with blister formation. Inflammation resolves with sharply marginated skin hyperpigmentation. Any skin surface can be involved, including the face, digits, and oral and genital mucosa. Tetracyclines, barbiturates, salicylates, and phenolphthalein are frequently implicated, and eliminating the offending agent results in disappearance of the eruption.

44. How does erythema ab igne occur?

Erythema ab igne is a skin reaction to thermal injury. Chronic heating pad use is a common cause of this disorder. Usually, the affected area has a net-like pattern of blue-gray discoloration, sometimes with associated erythema and scale. Patients often complain that the affected area burns, stings, or itches. Treatment requires discontinuing heating pad use. Skin dyspigmentation slowly resolves over several months to a year, although permanent dermal scarring and hyperpigmentation can result.

45. Are there any metabolic disorders associated with nonmelanin skin dyspigmentation?

Yes. Ochronosis (alkaptonuria) is a rare autosomal recessive inherited deficiency of homogentisic acid oxidase that results in accumulation of homogentisic acid in connective tissue, where it causes a dark brown to bluish-gray dyspigmentation. Commonly affected skin areas include the pinna, tip of the nose, sclera, extensor tendons of the hands, fingernails, and tympanic membranes. Less commonly, blue macules develop on the central face, axillae, and genitalia.

Homogentisic acid also deposits in the bones and articular cartilage, causing **ochronotic arthropathy** that results in premature degenerative arthritis. Overall, the course of ochronosis is progressive dyspigmentation and articular degeneration with no successful treatment available.

46. What pigmentation disorders are associated with heavy metal deposition in the dermis?

Silver, mercury, bismuth, arsenic, and gold can cause brown to blue-gray discoloration due to metal deposition in the dermis. Silver, mercury, and bismuth toxicity result in blue-gray discoloration of the skin, nails and mucosa. Silver toxicity (argyria) is most prominent in sun-exposed areas. Chrysoderma is an uncommon brown skin pigmentation that develops following parenteral gold administration and is most prominent in sun-exposed areas.

47. What drugs can deposit in the dermis and cause pigmentary changes?

Amiodarone, bleomycin, busulfan, chloroquine, chlorpromazine, clofazimine, minocycline, trifluoperazine, thioridazine, and zidovudine cause blue-gray pigmentation of the skin and mucosa.

BIBLIOGRAPHY

1. Crowson AN, Magro CM: Recent advances in the pathology of cutaneous drug eruptions. Dermatol Clin 17:537–560, 1999.
2. Franz DN: Diagnosis and management of tuberous sclerosis complex. Semin Pediatr Neurol 5:253–268, 1998.
3. Hearing VJ: Biochemical control of melanogenesis and melanosomal organization. J Invest Dermatol Symp Proc 4:24–28, 1999.
4. Hemminki A: The molecular basis and clinical aspects of Peutz-Jeghers syndrome. Cell Mol Life Sci 55:735–750, 1999.
5. Jozwiak S, Schwartz RA, Janniger CK: LEOPARD syndrome (cardiocutaneous lentiginosis syndrome). Cutis 57:208–214, 1996.
6. Kovacs SO: Vitiligo. J Am Acad Dermatol 38:647–666, 1998.
7. Mosher DB, Fitzpatrick TB, Ortonne JP, Hori Y: Normal skin color and general considerations of pigmentary disorders. In Freedberg IM, Eisen AZ, et al (eds): Fitzpatrick's Dermatology in General Medicine, 5th ed. New York, McGraw-Hill, 1998, pp 936–1017.
8. Orlow SJ: Albinism: An update. Semin Cutan Med Surg 16:24–29, 1997.
9. Rosenmann E, Rosenmann A, Ne'eman Z, et al: Prenatal diagnosis of oculocutaneous albinism type I: Review and personal experience. Pediatr Dev Pathol 2:404–414, 1999.
10. Ruggieri M: The different forms of neurofibromatosis. Childs Nerv Syst 15:295–308, 1999.
11. Scholzen TE, Brzoska T, Kalden DH, et al: Effect of ultraviolet light on the release of neuropeptides and neuroendocrine hormones in the skin: Mediators of photodermatitis and cutaneous inflammation. J Investig Dermatol Symp Proc 4:55–60, 1999.
12. Spritz RA: Piebaldism, Waardenburg syndrome, and related disorders of melanocyte development. Semin Cutan Med Surg 16:15–23, 1997.
13. Spritz RA, Hearing VJ Jr: Genetic disorders of pigmentation. Adv Hum Genet 22:1–45, 1994.
14. Vassileva SG, Mateev G, Parish LC: Antimicrobial photosensitive reactions. Arch Intern Med 158:1993–2000, 1998.
15. Verghese S, Newlin A, Miller M, Burton BK: Mosaic trisomy 7 in a patient with pigmentary abnormalities. Am J Med Genet Dec 87:371–374, 1999.
16. Wolverton SE: Update on cutaneous drug reactions. Adv Dermatol 13:65–84, 1997.

19. PANNICULITIS

James W. Patterson, M.D.

1. What is panniculitis?

Panniculitis represents infiltration of subcutaneous tissue by inflammatory and/or neoplastic cells. This condition presents clinically as an apparent deep induration or swelling of the skin. Associated signs and symptoms may include erythema, ulceration, drainage, warmth, and pain or tenderness. Under certain circumstances, induration or nodularity may be present without significant inflammation, or they may persist after inflammation has largely subsided.

2. Name the various types of panniculitis. How are they classified?

Major Forms of Panniculitis

Septal panniculitis	Metabolic derangements
Erythema nodosum	Altered melting/solidification points of fat
Subacute nodular migratory panniculitis	Sclerema neonatorum
(Scleroderma panniculitis)	Subcutaneous fat necrosis of the newborn
Lobular and mixed panniculitis	Pancreatic (enzymic) fat necrosis
Vasculitis and connective tissue disease	Alpha-1 antitrypsin deficiency panniculitis
Nodular vasculitis (erythema induratum)	Traumatic panniculitis
Lupus panniculitis	Infectious panniculitis
Other types of connective tissue panniculitis	Malignancy and panniculitis
	Lipodystrophy

Although no single classification seems to be totally satisfactory, disorders tend to be grouped by a combination of histopathologic features and etiologies. **Septal panniculitis** refers to a predominance of inflammation involving the connective tissue septa between fat lobules, whereas **lobular panniculitis** indicates predominant involvement of the fat lobules themselves. **Lipodystrophy** may be an end-stage change of the fat brought about by several different phenomena, including inflammation, trauma, or metabolic or hormonal alterations.

3. What is erythema nodosum?

Erythema nodosum consists of an eruption of erythematous, tender nodules, typically over the pretibial areas (Fig. 1A) but occasionally elsewhere, that is regarded as a hypersensitivity response to some antigenic challenge. It is typically an acute process, but a more chronic variety also occurs. Some experts consider the condition termed **subacute nodular migratory panniculitis** (Villanova's disease) to be a chronic variant of erythema nodosum.

4. What causes erythema nodosum?

Erythema nodosum is usually considered to represent a delayed hypersensitivity response that reflects a common reaction pattern to a wide variety of eliciting factors. This interpretation is supported by recent work that demonstrates a role for T-lymphocytes in the disorder. Reactive oxygen intermediates may be involved in the tissue damage and inflammation that accompany erythema nodosum.

5. List some of the common underlying conditions associated with erythema nodosum.

Streptococcal infection (e.g., streptococcal pharyngitis) and drugs (especially oral contraceptives, possibly halogens) are among the most common. Others include tuberculosis, deep fungal infections (such as coccidioidomycosis and blastomycosis), *Yersinia* infection, sarcoidosis, ulcerative colitis, regional enteritis, and leukemia.

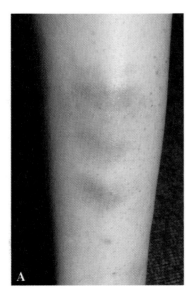 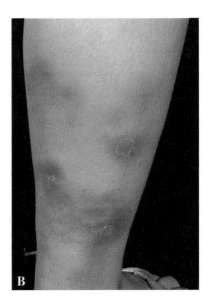

FIGURE 1. *A*, Typical lesion of erythema nodosum on the leg. *B*, Erythema induratum demonstrating characteristic indurated subcutaneous nodules. Spontaneous ulceration is common. (Courtesy of James E. Fitzpatrick, MD.)

6. How should a biopsy of erythema nodosum be obtained?

Biopsy should be obtained from the most fully developed (central) portion of the lesion. It is absolutely critical that the biopsy be deep enough to incorporate subcutaneous fat. Incisional biopsies that include a generous horizontal expanse of subcutis are preferred to small punch biopsies.

7. What are the characteristic microscopic features of erythema nodosum?

The typical histologic features include a predominantly septal panniculitis, with a light spillover of inflammatory cells into the fat lobules in a "lacelike" configuration. Cell types may include lymphocytes, neutrophils, and/or eosinophils. Perivascular infiltrates are common, but true vasculitis is not observed. In chronic forms of the disease, small microgranulomas are sometimes observed within connective tissue septa.

8. How is erythema nodosum treated?

Treatment of the underlying disorder, if known, is of primary importance. Salicylates or nonsteroidal anti-inflammatory drugs, bedrest, and potassium iodide (particularly in chronic forms of the disease) are also helpful. One study has shown that 77% of infection-associated cases heal within 7 weeks of onset, while 30% of idiopathic cases may persist for 6 months or more.

9. What is nodular vasculitis?

This form of panniculitis commonly occurs over the posterior lower legs (Fig. 1B), although other sites include the feet, thighs, buttocks, and forearms. Ulceration and drainage sometimes occur. It was originally considered a tuberculid and termed *erythema induratum*. Recent studies confirm that many cases are associated with *Mycobacterium tuberculosis* infection. However, a similar eruption has been recognized that is idiopathic or associated with other forms of infection.

10. What is the pathogenesis of nodular vasculitis?

Nodular vasculitis is considered to be an immune complex vasculitis that is triggered by a variety of antigenic stimuli. Mycobacterial infection is one such stimulus, and a number of investigators have identified mycobacterial DNA in these lesions using the polymerase chain reaction.

11. Describe the microscopic features of nodular vasculitis.

Nodular vasculitis presents as a lobular panniculitis with a mixed infiltrate that may be granulomatous. Vasculitis of a medium-sized artery or vein is present but often obscured by dense inflammation, and additional sectioning may be necessary to demonstrate it. Caseous necrosis is present in up to 50% of cases. Although necrosis can occur in cases not associated with tuberculosis, one recent study suggests that the incidence of necrosis may be slightly higher among those patients whose lesions are positive for *Mycobacterium tuberculosis*-complex DNA.

12. What is the differential diagnosis of nodular vasculitis?

Clinical clues to an association with tuberculosis include constitutional symptoms, elevated erythrocyte sedimentation rate, an abnormal chest x-ray, or a positive tuberculin skin test. Both polyarteritis nodosa and superficial thrombophlebitis show vasculitis involving medium-sized vessels in the subcutis. In both conditions, the inflammation is more specifically directed toward the vessel, and extensive lobular inflammation obscuring the vessel changes is uncommon. The clinical findings are also quite different in these two disorders (e.g., hypertension, renal and CNS disease in systemic polyarteritis, association with internal malignancy in superficial migratory thrombophlebitis). In my experience, true examples of nodular vasculitis are seldom seen, but this might change with the recent rise in numbers of cases of tuberculosis.

13. How should nodular vasculitis be treated?

Treatment should be directed toward any underlying infection, especially tuberculosis. Studies have demonstrated the responsiveness of mycobacteria-associated lesions to combination antituberculous therapy. Symptomatic care includes bedrest, bandages, anti-inflammatory agents, and avoidance of potential aggravating factors such as smoking. A recent report documented a favorable response to oral gold therapy in one patient.

14. What are the clinical features of lupus panniculitis?

Lupus panniculitis, also termed lupus profundus, consists of erythematous or flesh-colored subcutaneous nodules (Fig. 2). Unlike some other forms of panniculitis, these lesions do not predominate on the lower legs but frequently occur in unusual locations, such as the face, upper outer arms, shoulders and trunk, including the breast. They sometimes show overlying follicular plugging or epidermal atrophy, changes associated with cutaneous (discoid) lupus erythematosus.

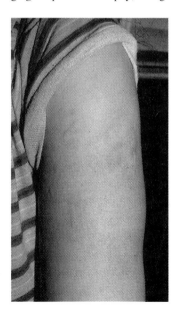

FIGURE 2. Lupus panniculitis presenting as atrophic indurated areas over the upper arms. (Courtesy of James E. Fitzpatrick, MD.)

15. Describe the microscopic features of lupus panniculitis.

There is typically a mixed septal-lobular panniculitis with a predominance of lymphocytes in a patchy or diffuse and perivascular distribution. Nodular aggregates of lymphocytes surrounded by plasma cells, or lymphoid follicles, may be present, and mucin deposition or hyalinization sometimes occur. Overlying epidermal changes associated with cutaneous lupus erythematosus may be seen in close to one-half of cases.

16. Is a diagnosis of lupus panniculitis significant?

Panniculitis may be a presenting finding of either cutaneous or systemic lupus erythematosus. A small percentage of patients presenting with lupus panniculitis fulfill criteria for systemic lupus erythematosus, and other complications have been reported, such as the development of antiphospholipid antibody syndrome. Antinuclear antibodies are common, and occasionally other circulating antibodies are detected, such as anti-neutrophil cytoplasmic antibodies. Because of the unusual clinical features of lupus panniculitis, the true diagnosis may not be suspected for months or years. Early biopsy and direct immunofluorescence study of these lesions may provide the first clue to the diagnosis of lupus erythematosus and may allow for early institution of appropriate therapy. Treatments for the panniculitis include intralesional corticosteroids, systemic antimalarials, or dapsone.

17. Aren't sclerema neonatorum and subcutaneous fat necrosis of the newborn the same thing?

No. In these conditions, there are varying degrees of sclerosis of the subcutaneous fat of newborns. **Sclerema neonatorum** arises in premature infants and is characterized by diffusely cold, rigid, board-like skin; early death is common. In **subcutaneous fat necrosis of the newborn**, relatively discrete, firm subcutaneous nodules develop several weeks after birth (Fig. 3). Hypercalcemia may be present. The prognosis for survival and resolution of the lesions is excellent.

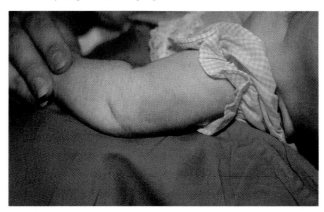

FIGURE 3. Subcutaneous fat necrosis of the left upper arm in an otherwise healthy infant. (Courtesy of James E. Fitzpatrick, MD.)

18. How similar are the microscopic features of sclerema neonatorum and subcutaneous fat necrosis of the newborn?

Both conditions show needle-shaped clefts within lipocytes, presumably representing triglyceride crystals that have been dissolved out during tissue processing. Sclerema tends to show thickened fibrous septa and little inflammation, while subcutaneous fat necrosis shows a substantial lobular panniculitis.

19. What causes these disorders?

Neonatal fat has an increased ratio of saturated to unsaturated fatty acids, which results in higher melting and solidification points for stored fat. This plus other possible metabolic defects lead to crystal formation, fat necrosis, and inflammation when the fat is subject to such stresses as vascular compromise or trauma.

20. What is pancreatic fat necrosis?

This consists of subcutaneous nodules (Fig. 4), on the legs or elsewhere, associated with acute pancreatitis, pancreatic carcinoma, pancreatic pseudocysts, or traumatic pancreatitis. Visceral fat may also be involved. Although immune mechanisms may play a role in producing this form of fat necrosis, the weight of evidence favors the effects of circulating amylase and/or lipase on subcutaneous fat. Treatment is directed toward the underlying pancreatic disease.

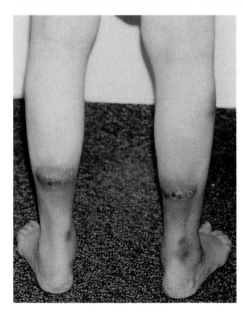

FIGURE 4. Pancreatic fat necrosis (panniculitis) involving the lower legs.

21. Are there any characteristic histopathologic features of pancreatic fat necrosis?

Pancreatic fat necrosis may begin as a septal panniculitis, but later changes are rather unique, and include formation of lipocyte remnants with thick, shadowy walls ("ghost cells") and pools of basophilic material that represent saponification of fat by calcium salts.

22. What is the role of alpha-1 antitrypsin (proteinase inhibitor) deficiency in the development of panniculitis?

Since the mid-1970s, it has become apparent that patients with this proteinase inhibitor deficiency, especially those most severely affected and having the PiZZ phenotype, are prone to develop painful subcutaneous nodules that ulcerate and drain. It is believed that in such individuals, a variety of triggering factors, such as trauma, may initiate a sequence of events that includes unchecked complement activation, inflammation, endothelial cell damage, and tissue injury. Microscopic clues to the diagnosis include diffuse neutrophilic infiltration of the reticular dermis and liquefactive necrosis of the dermis and fibrous septa, with resultant separation of fat lobules. Current treatments, which include dapsone and systemic corticosteroids, will soon be joined by the parenteral administration of proteinase inhibitor, which has been successful in experimental studies.

23. What types of trauma can produce panniculitis?

Numerous forms of trauma, either accidental or purposeful, can produce painful subcutaneous nodules or plaques. These include cold injury, injection of foreign substances such as oils or medications, or blunt trauma. There are some unique microscopic clues for each of these types of injury, so biopsy is particularly helpful when traumatic panniculitis is suspected. Polarization microscopy is one simple test for detecting the presence of refractile foreign material in tissue sections. The therapeutic challenge lies mainly in finding and removing the source of the injury that has produced the panniculitis.

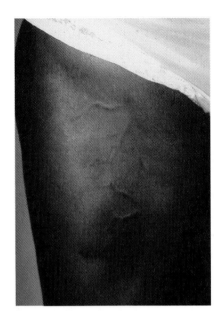

FIGURE 5. Severe lipoatrophy secondary to panniculitis associated with an ill-defined collagen vascular disease. (Courtesy of James E. Fitzpatrick, MD.)

24. How does infection produce panniculitis?

Panniculitis can result from localized or generalized infection caused by gram-positive and gram-negative bacteria, mycobacteria, *Nocardia*, *Candida*, and *Fusarium* species. Other organisms that have been associated with panniculitis include streptococci, *Toxocara*, *Trypanosoma*, and *Borrelia burgdorferi*, the latter being the etiologic agent of Lyme disease. Immunosuppressed patients appear to be particularly at risk for infectious panniculitis. Microscopic features vary and can occasionally mimic other forms of panniculitis. However, findings that should suggest the possibility of infection include mixed septal-lobular involvement, neutrophilic infiltration, vascular proliferation and hemorrhage, and sweat gland necrosis. Special stains and culture studies are keys to making the correct diagnosis and instituting appropriate antimicrobial therapy.

25. What is the role of malignancy in producing panniculitis?

Malignant infiltrates can sometimes produce subcutaneous nodules that mimic other forms of panniculitis. Complicating the issue is the realization that forms of more traditional inflammatory panniculitis can also accompany malignancy, including erythema nodosum, migratory thrombophlebitis, and pancreatic fat necrosis. Therefore, diagnosis again is heavily dependent on biopsy. Microscopic clues to the recognition of malignant infiltrates include a monotonous cell population and/or cytologic atypia, "lining up" of atypical cells between collagen bundles, and minimal alteration of connective tissue in the face of dense cellular infiltration. Malignancies that are capable of producing panniculitis-like lesions include poorly differentiated carcinomas, lymphomas, multiple myeloma, and leukemias.

26. What is lipodystrophy?

Lipodystrophy presents as either depression or, less commonly, induration of the skin due to changes in subcutaneous tissue. **Lipoatrophy** (Fig. 5) occurs in a bewildering array of forms, some of which are idiopathic, while others may be associated with syndromes of insulin-resistant diabetes mellitus, complement abnormalities, or administration of injectable insulin and corticosteroids. There have been numerous recent reports of lipoatrophy with administration of HIV-1 protease inhibitors. In some of these cases, there has also been a redistribution of subcutaneous fat, with accumulation of fat in abdominal and cervical areas. Experimental evidence suggests that these protease inhibitors inhibit adipogenesis in a dose-responsive manner. Probably the most common form of lipoatrophy is postinflammatory in nature and can occur following several types of panniculitis.

Lipohypertrophy, which manifests as induration of involved skin, occurs in some individuals due to repeated injections of insulin. This effect is apparently independent of the source of insulin, and can even occur with human recombinant insulin. Growth hormone injections have also resulted in lipohypertrophy. Microscopically, lipoatrophy features "collapse" of fat lobules, with formation of variably sized lipocytes and development of numerous capillaries in a mucinous background stroma. In lipohypertrophy, lipocytes are enlarged and appear to encroach upon the midportion of the dermis. A variety of plastic surgical procedures has been used to improve or correct lipoatrophy. Rotation of insulin injection sites is a key to management of lipohypertrophy, both to prevent or minimize the hypertrophic changes and to assure adequate insulin absorption.

27. Why hasn't Weber-Christian disease been discussed up to this point? What is its relationship to other forms of panniculitis?

Weber-Christian disease, or relapsing, febrile, nonsuppurative panniculitis, was originally described in 1925 and 1928, and to this day, many cases of panniculitis seen on hospital wards receive this arbitrary classification. However, recent medical advances have allowed more precise definition of many forms of panniculitis, and as a result, few cases remain that are ill-defined enough to be placed into this nonspecific category. Conditions that at one time might have been termed "Weber-Christian disease" include factitial panniculitis, pancreatic fat necrosis, lupus panniculitis, or alpha-1 antitrypsin deficiency panniculitis.

28. Dicuss the approach to use when attempting to diagnose an "unknown" case of panniculitis.

1. Careful history and physical examination are of greatest importance, with an emphasis on the location of the eruption as well as its timing in relation to any possible drug ingestion, infection, or trauma.

2. Laboratory studies should be guided by the clinical history but might include cultures (e.g., for possible streptococcal pharyngitis in erythema nodosum), anti-nuclear antibody determination (to rule out lupus panniculitis), or measurement of alpha-1 antitrypsin levels (for evaluation of proteinase inhibitor deficiency panniculitis).

3. Skin biopsy can be of tremendous benefit, and recognition of established microscopic patterns of disease can be complemented by special stains and polarization microscopy.

4. Immunohistochemistry can be useful in selected cases where malignancy is a possibility, and x-ray microanalysis is a specialized test that can be used to determine the identity of foreign material in cases of traumatic panniculitis.

BIBLIOGRAPHY

1. Adame J, Cohen PR: Eosinophilic panniculitis: Diagnostic considerations and evaluation. J Am Acad Dermatol 34:229–234, 1996.
2. Ball NJ, Adams SP, Marx LH, Enta T: Possible origin of pancreatic fat necrosis as a septal panniculitis. J Am Acad Dermatol 34:362–364, 1996.
3. Baselga E, Margall N, Barnadas MA, et al: Detection of *Mycobacterium tuberculosis* DNA in lobular granulomatous panniculitis (erythema induratum-nodular vasculitis). Arch Dermatol 133:457–462, 1997.
4. Bohm I, Bruns A, Schupp G, Bauer R: ANCA-positive lupus erythematodes profundus: Successful therapy with low-dosage dapsone. Hautarzt 49:403–407, 1998.
5. Bohn S, Buchner S, Itin P: Erythema nodosum: 112 cases. Epidemiology, clinical aspects and histopathology (see comments). Schweiz Med Wochenschr 127:1168–1176, 1997.
6. Boonchai W, Suthipinittharm P, Mahaisavariya P: Panniculitis in tuberculosis: A clinicopathologic study of nodular panniculitis associated with tuberculosis. Int J Dermatol 37:361–363, 1998.
7. Burden AD, Krafchik BR: Subcutaneous fat necrosis of the newborn: A review of 11 cases. Pediatr Dermatol 16:384–387, 1999.
8. Cho KH, Lee DY, Kim CW: Erythema induratum of Bazin. Int J Dermatol 35:802–808, 1996.
9. Chung HS, Hann SK: Lupus panniculitis treated by a combination therapy of hydroxychloroquine and quinacrine. J Dermatol 24:569–572, 1997.

10. Durden FM, Variyam E, Chren MM: Fat necrosis with features of erythema nodosum in a patient with metastatic pancreatic carcinoma. Int J Dermatol 35:39–41, 1996.

11. Geller JD, Su WPD: A subtle clue to the histopathologic diagnosis of early alpha-1 antitrypsin deficiency panniculitis. J Am Acad Dermatol 31:241–245, 1994.

12. Granter SR, Barnhill RL, Duray PH: Borrelial fasciitis: Diffuse fasciitis and peripheral eosinophilia associated with Borrelia infection. Am J Dermatopathol 18:465–473, 1996.

13. Hauner H, Stockamp B, Haastert B: Prevalence of lipohypertrophy in insulin-treated diabetic patients and predisposing factors. Exp Clin Endocrinol Diabetes 104:106–110, 1996.

14. Hendrick SJ, Silverman AK, Solomon AR, et al: Alpha-1 antitrypsin deficiency associated with panniculitis. J Am Acad Dermatol 18:684–692, 1988.

15. Holland NW, McKnight K, Challa VR, Agudelo CA: Lupus panniculitis (profundus) involving the breast: Report of 2 cases and review of the literature. J Rheumatol 22:344–346, 1995.

16. Kano Y, Shiohara T, Yagita A, Nagashima M: Erythema nodosum, lichen planus and lichen nitidus in Crohn's disease: Report of a case and analysis of T-cell receptor V gene expression in the cutaneous and intestinal lesions. Dermatology 190:59–63, 1995.

17. Kunz M, Beutel S, Brocker E: Leukocyte activation in erythema nodosum. Clin Exp Dermatol 24:396–401, 1999.

18. Loche F, Tremeau-Martinage C, Laplanche G, et al: Panniculitis revealing qualitative alpha-1 antitrypsin deficiency (MS variant). Eur J Dermatol 9:565–567, 1999.

19. Martens PB, Moder KG, Ahmed I: Lupus panniculitis: Clinical perspectives from a case series. J Rheumatol 26:68–72, 1999.

20. Nousari HC, Kimyai-Asadi A, Santana HM, et al: Generalized lupus panniculitis and antiphospholipid syndrome in a patient without complement deficiency. Pediatr Dermatol 16:273–276, 1999.

21. O'Riordan K, Blei A, Rao MS, Abecassis M: Alpha-1 antitrypsin deficiency–associated panniculitis: Resolution with intravenous alpha 1-antitrypsin administration and liver transplantation. Transplantation 63:480–482, 1997.

22. Ollert MW, Thomas P, Korting HC, et al: Erythema induratum of Bazin: Evidence of T-lymphocyte hyperresponsiveness to purified protein derivative of tuberculin: Report of two cases and treatment. Arch Dermatol 129:469–473, 1993.

23. Patterson JW, Brown PC, Broecker AH: Infection-induced panniculitis. J Cutan Pathol 16:183–193, 1989.

24. Riarte A, Luna C, Sabatiello R, et al: Chagas' disease in patients with kidney transplants: Seven years of experience 1989-1996. Clin Infect Dis 29:561–567, 1999.

25. Roper NA, Bilous RW: Resolution of lipohypertrophy following change of short-acting insulin to insulin lispro (Humalog). Diabet Med 15:1063–1064, 1998.

26. Ruvalcaba RH, Kletter GB: Abdominal lipohypertrophy caused by injections of growth hormone: A case report. Pediatrics 102:408–410, 1998.

27. Shaffer N, Kerdel FA: Nodular vasculitis (erythema induratum): Treatment with auranofin. J Am Acad Dermatol 25:426–429, 1991.

28. Zhang B, MacNaul K, Szalkowski D, et al: Inhibition of adipocyte differentiation by HIV protease inhibitors. J Clin Endocrinol Metab 84:4274–4277, 1999.

20. ALOPECIA

Leonard C. Sperling, M.D., COL, MC

1. How is alopecia classified?

Alopecia (hair loss) can be divided into (1) disorders of the hair shaft and (2) all other forms of hair loss. Abnormalities of the hair shaft can produce alopecia because the shafts are fragile and "break off." The other forms of alopecia can be divided into scarring and nonscarring alopecia. In scarring alopecia, hair is lost permanently. Both scarring and nonscarring alopecia can be divided into diffuse and patterned hair loss. In the diffuse pattern, hair is lost evenly from all parts of the scalp, and discrete "bald spots" do not occur. In patterned hair loss, certain areas of the scalp are affected more than others.

2. What are some common types of patterned hair loss?

Patchy—**multiple** scattered lesions; **moth-eaten**—myriad, diffusely distributed, small lesions; **ophiasis**—hair loss around periphery of scalp; **male-pattern baldness**—symmetrical hair loss predominantly affecting the vertex and crown of the scalp

3. Can scarring and nonscarring alopecia be differentiated clinically?

In the setting of alopecia, scarring means that there has been permanent destruction of hair follicles, with their replacement by fibrous tissue. Usually, an obvious scar such as that seen after wounding is not evident, but there is a loss of follicular openings that gives the scalp a smooth and shiny appearance (Fig. 1). The texture of the scalp may remain soft and supple, although sometimes induration or firmness is palpable.

4. What causes common balding?

People who are bald have hair follicles that are genetically programmed to miniaturize under the influence of post-pubertal androgens. Probably several genes (inherited from both mother and father) influence the severity of balding. Until very late in the balding process, the number of hairs does not decrease, but the hairs become progressively smaller until they are no longer visible to the naked eye. Except in very marked and long-standing balding, very fine, short hairs can be seen exiting from follicular orifices if a magnifying lens is used.

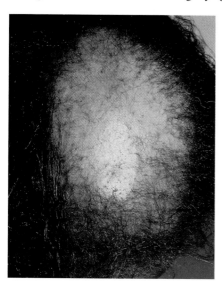

FIGURE 1. Follicular degeneration syndrome, a form of scarring alopecia. The smooth skin, devoid of most follicular openings, reflects light like a mirror.

5. How effective are medical treatments for common balding?

About one-third of balding patients who use topical minoxidil solution experience significant (cosmetically obvious) hair regrowth. Any regrowth that occurs is only maintained while the drug is used. If therapy is stopped, hair density reverts to its pretreatment state. Oral finasteride may be somewhat more effective, and can be used in combination with topical minoxidil.

6. How do you treat balding due to hyperandrogenism?

Women whose balding is a manifestation of hyperandrogenism (excessive production of circulating androgens) may benefit from therapy directed at the cause of hyperandrogenism. Polycystic ovarian disease, late-onset congenital adrenal hyperplasia, Cushing's syndrome, and adrenal and ovarian neoplasms are potential causes of hyperandrogenism. In the absence of elevated circulating androgens, nonspecific therapy directed at suppressing ovarian androgen production or blocking the peripheral effect of androgens is sometimes tried. Oral contraceptive agents and spironolactone are most often used for this purpose.

7. What are the surgical options for treatment of balding?

Men, and occasionally women, can achieve permanent cosmetic improvement by undergoing a **hair transplantation** procedure. Hair follicles from the occipital area (donor site) are moved to the balding area (recipient site). The procedure is tedious and expensive, but the cosmetic results can be satisfactory. Various other surgical procedures, including scalp reductions (which involve removing the bald areas) and scalp flaps, are also used sometimes in selected patients.

8. Discuss the common causes of circular bald spots.

Although many forms of alopecia can result in a circular bald patch, the most common causes are tinea capitis and alopecia areata. **Tinea capitis** is a superficial fungal infection with a predilection for children, especially black children. The surface of the skin is scaly and sometimes inflamed, and small dark stubs of hair ("black dots") may be scattered within the affected area. In this condition, the hair shaft is invaded and replaced by myriad circular fungal spores. In the United States, *Trichophyton tonsurans* is usually the culprit. A circular, scaly or crusted bald spot on the scalp of a black child should be considered to be tinea capitis until proved otherwise (Fig. 2A).

Alopecia areata also commonly affects children, but adults more often develop the condition. In alopecia areata, the affected areas may be totally hairless, but the scalp surface looks otherwise normal, without scaling and minimal, if any, erythema. A few short hairs may be present in the bald spot; these "exclamation mark" hairs taper and lose pigment as they approach the scalp and may appear to float on the scalp surface (Fig. 2B).

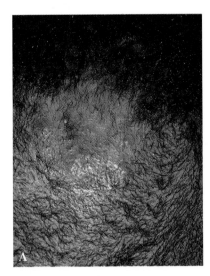

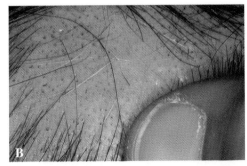

FIGURE 2. *A*, Tinea capitis. A large bald patch studded with small inflammatory papules surrounded by smaller, similar lesions. Close examination may reveal "black dots" scattered within the bald area. *B*, A patch of alopecia areata showing several "exclamation mark hairs."

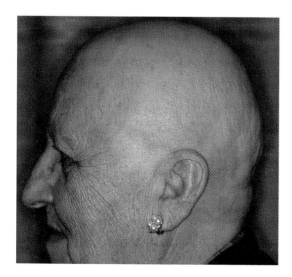

FIGURE 3. Alopecia totalis demonstrating total loss of scalp hair and most of eyebrows. (Courtesy of James E. Fitzpatrick, MD.)

9. What is alopecia totalis?

Alopecia areata may cause one or many bald spots. If it affects the entire scalp, it is called **alopecia totalis** (Fig. 3). If the entire body is affected, it is referred to as **alopecia universalis.**

10. How is alopecia areata treated?

When a solitary lesion of alopecia areata is **small** (<5 cm in diameter), no treatment may be needed. The prognosis for such a lesion is excellent, and spontaneous regrowth often occurs. Intralesional corticosteroids, and sometimes potent topical corticosteroids, may hasten regrowth.

The **larger** or more **numerous** lesions carry a more guarded prognosis. Intralesional corticosteroid injections are usually started. For extensive hair loss involving 30–100% of the scalp surface, a short (e.g., 3-month) course of systemic corticosteroids (usually prednisone) may be required. If hair regrowth does not resume or if hair loss recurs once corticosteroids are stopped, the prognosis is poor. The use of systemic corticosteroids to treat extensive alopecia areata is controversial. Appropriate risk-versus-benefit considerations must be carefully analyzed.

Although spontaneous regrowth may occur even in alopecia totalis, no therapy has been found to be consistently safe and effective for **severe** disease. Topical immunotherapy with chemicals causing allergic contact dermatitis (e.g., diphencyprone) seems to offer the most hope.

11. How do you treat tinea capitis?

Although topical antifungal agents work well for tinea corporis, they are of little value in tinea capitis. Systemic antifungal agents are required to eradicate the spores that invade affected hair shafts. A course of treatment generally takes 1–3 months. **Griseofulvin** is the treatment of choice because it is safe and effective, rarely causing significant side effects. Ultramicrosized formulations of griseofulvin can be given in half the dose required with microsized forms of the drug. Fungal resistance to griseofulvin is rare. For the few patients whose tinea capitis is resistant to griseofulvin or who cannot tolerate griseofulvin because of side effects (such as headache or gastrointestinal upset), ketoconazole, terbinafine, and itraconazole are acceptable alternatives.

12. What is trichotillomania?

Compulsive hair pulling.

13. Who is most likely to be affected by trichotillomania?

The typical patient is an adolescent girl, although the condition can affect children of both sexes as well as adults. In trichotillomania, hairs are forcibly plucked out of the scalp by the patient, usually as a mechanism for relieving tension or stress. Less often, trichotillomania is a manifestation of psychosis or an obsessive-compulsive neurosis. Although the patient may deny

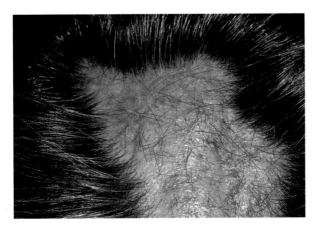

FIGURE   4. Trichotillomania. The highly irregular shape, sharp circumscription, and presence of "broken-off" hairs of various lengths are typical of this condition.

plucking, the often bizarre shape of the bald area, combined with the presence of short hairs of various lengths within the area of thinning, suggests the diagnosis (Fig. 4). The diagnosis may be confirmed by a scalp biopsy that may demonstrate diagnostic features or by creating a "hair growth window." This test is performed by weekly shaving of an involved area to prevent plucking; the hair will recover and regain normal density within the shaved area.

14. Why do cancer patients lose their hair?

Cancer patients are susceptible to two forms of diffuse hair loss. **Anagen effluvium** is a direct effect of anticancer treatment. Patients receiving radiation therapy to the scalp or systemic chemotherapy can shed all or most of their hair within a few weeks of starting treatment. This hair loss is a direct effect of the chemotherapy or radiotherapy on the hair follicle, whose rapidly dividing cells are very susceptible to injury. When the hair matrix (the epithelial root that produces the hair shaft) is exposed to radiation or chemical toxins, it can produce only a thinned hair shaft that eventually tapers to a point (Fig. 5A). This marked tapering makes the shaft extremely fragile, and the hair shaft can literally be combed away or broken off by minor trauma. Unless the dose of radiation or chemotherapy is very high, regrowth of hair occurs once therapy is stopped.

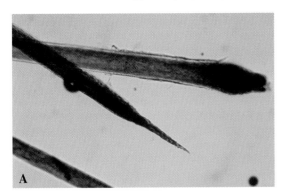

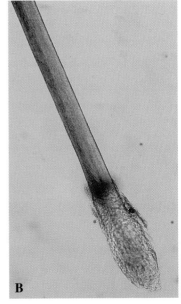

FIGURE 5. Hair loss in cancer therapy. *A,* Anagen effluvium. The shaft tapers to a pencil-like point and easily separates from the follicle. *B,* Normal telogen hair. About 50–100 telogen hairs such as these are normally shed during the course of the day. Much higher numbers are shed during a telogen effluvium.

In **telogen effluvium,** the metabolic and emotional "stress" of severe, debilitating illness causes many of the actively growing (anagen) hairs to enter the shedding (telogen) phase of hair growth prematurely. The hairs remain in telogen for about 3 months before they are finally shed (Fig. 5B), so there is a "lag" time between the onset of severe disease and actual hair loss. Seldom is more than 50% of the hair shed in telogen effluvium, so patients develop thin hair but do not become completely bald. If the patient recovers and is no longer debilitated, hairs re-enter the actively growing phase and the hair regrows.

15. In what other clinical settings can a telogen effluvium occur?

Normally, about 10% of scalp hairs are in the telogen (preshedding) phase at any given time. Whenever an abnormally large number of otherwise normal telogen hairs are present, a telogen effluvium occurs.

1. There are several clinical situations in which a telogen effluvium is found, including severe illness such as metastatic cancer, but any serious illness or major surgical procedure can also result result in a telogen effluvium.

2. The most common form of telogen effluvium occurs in women about 3 months after giving birth.

3. Virtually all newborn infants develop a telogen effluvium during the first 6 months of life, which is why many babies have more hair at birth than at 3 or 4 months of life.

Causes of Telogen Effluvium

Physiologic effluvium of the newborn	Postsurgical (major procedure or major trauma)
Postpartum	Hypothyroidism and other endocrinopathies
Postfebrile (e.g., malaria)	Crash or liquid protein diets; starvation
Severe infection	Drugs (retinoids, anticoagulants, anticonvulsants,
Debilitating chronic illness	antithyroid, heavy metals)

16. To which forms of hair loss are black patients susceptible?

1. Black children are particularly prone to acquiring tinea capitis.

2. Hair-shaft fragility disorders are common among African-American women because of certain hair grooming techniques using chemical hair "relaxers." These products are effective in straightening kinky or curly hair but are harsh, and with continued use, the hair shaft becomes frayed. The foci of fraying have a special appearance termed **trichorrhexis nodosa,** which looks like the bristles of two paint brushes that have been pushed together (Fig. 6). The hair shafts easily fracture at the points of trichorrhexis nodosa, leaving abnormally short hair shafts behind. Patients have scalp hair of very uneven length and may complain that their hair "falls out" with combing or "won't grow." In fact, their hair is growing but breaking off.

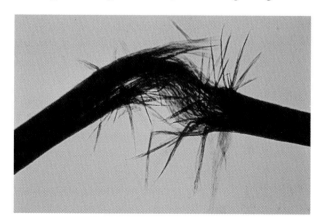

FIGURE 6. Trichorrhexis nodosa fracture in a woman using chemical hair straighteners.

17. Discuss the mechanism of follicular degeneration syndrome.

The most common form of scarring alopecia in black patients has been called the **follicular degeneration syndrome,** or "hot-comb alopecia." The condition more often affects adult women than men and typically causes hair loss that is most severe on the central crown of the scalp and slowly progresses centrifugally (see Fig. 1). When the bald patches are carefully examined, a few normal hairs may be found, but most follicular openings have been completely obliterated, suggesting a scarring process. Scattered inflammatory, perifollicular papules may be found in the peripheral zone where hair thinning has just begun. Scalp biopsy confirms that hair follicles are completely destroyed and replaced with fibrous tissue. "Hot combs" are rarely used nowadays for straightening hair, so hot comb alopecia is a misnomer. It is doubtful that hair care products are primarily responsible for hair loss in these patients, but chemical relaxers and other cosmetics may exacerbate the condition.

18. Name some medications that cause hair loss.

Anticancer medications, colchicine, thallium (rat poisons and insecticides), antiepileptic drugs (phenytoin, valproic acid, carbamazepine), anticlotting drugs (heparin, coumarin), and retinoids (etretinate).

19. What is alopecia mucinosa?

The term actually refers to two entirely different causes of hair loss. The conditions have in common a similar histologic finding—**follicular mucinosis,** the accumulation of mucin (acid mucopolysaccharides) within the follicular epithelium, resulting in hair damage and hair loss.

The first form of alopecia mucinosa is a benign condition found in young and otherwise healthy individuals. One or more oval or circular hairless patches or plaques are present, which can be hypopigmented or erythematous and may be scaly, eczematous, or studded with minute papules. The condition usually involves the head, neck, upper arms, or upper torso. Spontaneous resolution usually occurs in months to years.

The second form of alopecia mucinosa occurs in patients with mycosis fungoides, a form of cutaneous T-cell lymphoma. Patients are usually elderly, and numerous and often large, hairless, erythematous, and indurated plaques are found. Histologically, follicular mucinosis is present, but an atypical lymphocytic infiltrate that often invades the epidermis and follicles is also seen. This

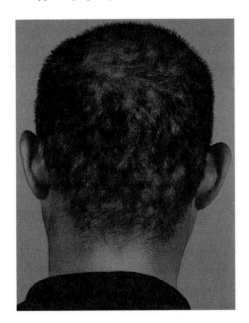

FIGURE 7. Moth-eaten alopecia.

atypical cellular infiltrate allows for the diagnosis of mycosis fungoides. The hairless lesions and histologic follicular mucinosis are merely manifestations of the underlying lymphoma.

20. What is meant by the term moth-eaten alopecia?

"Moth-eaten alopecia" is a form of nonscarring, patterned hair loss in which there are myriad small foci of alopecia scattered over the scalp (Fig. 7). This pattern of alopecia is described as the classic form of alopecia seen in patients with secondary syphilis. However, other etiologies, such as alopecia areata and systemic lupus erythematosus, can result in the same pattern of hair loss. Furthermore, hair loss in syphilis can be diffuse as well as moth-eaten.

BIBLIOGRAPHY

1. Brodin M: Drug-related alopecia. Dermatol Clin 5:571–579, 1987.
2. Hebert AA: Tinea capitis: Current concepts. Arch Dermatol 124:1554–1557, 1988.
3. Hordinsy M: Alopecia areata. In Olsen E (ed): Disorders of Hair Growth. New York, McGraw-Hill, 1994, pp 195–222.
4. Kaufman KD, Olsen EA, Whiting D, et al: Finasteride in the treatment of men with androgenetic alopecia: Finasteride Male Pattern Hair Loss Study Group. J Am Acad Dermatol 39:578–589, 1998.
5. Kligman AM: Pathologic dynamics of human hair loss: I. Telogen effluvium. Arch Dermatol 83:175–198, 1961.
6. Krafchik B, Pelletier J: An open study of tinea capitis in 50 children treated with a 2-week course of oral terbinafine. J Am Acad Dermatol 41:60–63, 1999.
7. Leyden J, Dunlap F, Miller B, et al: Finasteride in the treatment of men with frontal male pattern hair loss. J Am Acad Dermatol 40:930–937, 1999.
8. Muller SA: Trichotillomania. Dermatol Clin 5:595–601, 1987.
9. Nickoloff BJ, et al: Benign idiopathic vs. mycosis fungoides-associated follicular mucinosis. Pediatr Dermatol 2:201, 1985.
10. Orfanos CE: Androgenetic alopecia: Clinical aspects and treatment options. In Orfanos CE, Happle R (eds): Hair and Hair Diseases. Berlin, Springer-Verlag, 1990, pp 485–527.
11. Rudolph AH: Diagnosis and treatment of tinea capitis due to *Trichophyton tonsurans*. Int J Dermatol 24:426–431, 1985.
12. Sperling LC, Mezebish DS: Hair diseases. Med Clin North Am 82:1155–1169, 1998.
13. Sperling LC, Sau P: The follicular degeneration syndrome in black patients: "Hot comb alopecia" revisited and revised. Arch Dermatol 128:68–74, 1992.
14. Sperling LC, Skelton HG 3rd, Smith KJ, et al: Follicular degeneration syndrome in men. Arch Dermatol 130:763–769, 1994.

21. ACNE AND ACNEIFORM ERUPTIONS

John L. Aeling, M.D.

1. How common is acne?

One hundred percent of boys and 90% of girls will have some acne lesions during puberty. So, the question is not how often but how severe. Acne can affect all age groups, from neonates to senior citizens. Nearly 85% of persons aged 12–25 will have some acne lesions. In 1990, 4.5 million visits were made to dermatologists for acne-related skin problems. A recent study of clinical acne that examined 749 individuals reported a 3% prevalence in men and 12% in women ages 25 and older and the incidence did not substantially decrease until after age 44.

2. Name the acne subtypes.

Acne presents in many forms and variations. The most common form is acne vulgaris, which is classified according to the predominant lesion type as comodonal, papular, pustular, or cystic. It can be graded as mild, moderate, or severe (Fig. 1).

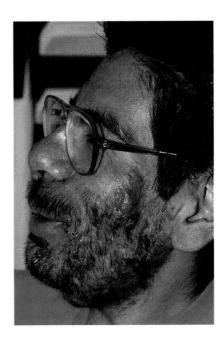

FIGURE 1. Severe inflammatory cystic acne vulgaris.

Clinical Subtypes of Acneiform Skin Lesions

Acne vulgaris	Drug-induced acne
Acne conglobata	Hidradenitis suppurativa
Neonatal acne	Scalp dissecting cellulitis
Infantile acne	Keloidal acne (Fig. 2A)
Acne rosacea	Pyoderma faciale
Gram-negative acne	Acne venenata (contact acne)
Perioral dermatitis	Acne excoriée
Acne mechanica	Acne fulminans
Nevoid acne	Favre-Racouchot syndrome (Fig. 2B)

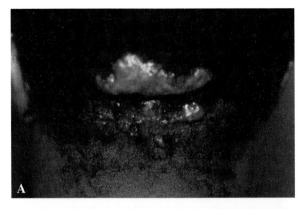

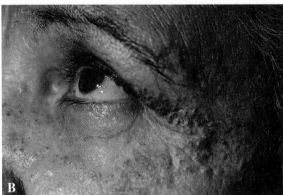

FIGURE 2. Clinical subtypes of acneiform skin lesions. *A*, A male patient with keloidal acne on the posterior neck. *B*, An elderly patient with Favre-Racouchot syndrome. Solar elastosis and comedones associated with chronic sun exposure.

3. Discuss the psychosocial impact of acne.

The psychological effect of acne vulgaris is the major factor that brings patients to physicians for treatment. Acne patients frequently have feelings of inferiority, low self-esteem, anger, depression, frustration, and embarrassment. Recent studies have shown poor academic performance in students with severe acne. Another study has shown a significant difference in unemployment in patients with severe acne compared to age-and sex-matched controls; in a study of 625 patients, there was 16.2% unemployment in men with acne as compared to 9.2% in controls and 14.3% in women compared to 8.7% in controls.

4. How much is known about the pathogenesis of acne?

Many factors play a role in the pathogenesis of acne, including a hereditary predisposition, androgenic hormones, and many other external and internal factors. The four primary pathogenic factors include increased sebum production, the presence of *Proprionibacterium acnes* (an anaerobic diphtheroid bacterium), abnormal follicular keratinization, and inflammation. The primary lesion in the development of acne is abnormal keratinization within the follicular infundibulum (that portion of the follicle between the sebaceous gland and surface epidermis). Patients with acne have a lower concentration of linoleic acid in their lipids than controls without acne, which may play an important role in the development of follicular retention hyperkeratosis and subsequent comedo formation.

5. How does the composition of sebum differ between the sebaceous gland and the skin surface?

The major constituent of **sebaceous lipid** is triglyceride, which makes up over 50% of the lipid; wax esters account for 25%, squalene 15%, and there are small amounts of cholesterol esters and free cholesterol. The **surface lipid** contains 15% free fatty acids, while sebaceous gland lipid contains none. This is due to hydrolysis of triglycerides on the skin surface.

6. Is there a difference between neonatal acne and infantile acne?

Yes. **Neonatal acne** occurs in up to 20% of newborns and may be present at birth or develop during the first few months of life. It is more common in males, is relatively mild, and regresses spontaneously in most infants by age 6 months. It is not associated with significant scarring or an increased incidence of acne in later life.

Infantile acne usually begins between the third and sixth month of life and may persist to age 5 and rarely longer. It is rare and is also more common in males. It can be severe, with nodules, cysts, and significant residual scarring. Some cases are associated with virilizing tumors. Some studies show an increased incidence of severe acne in later life.

7. What are some common myths regarding the etiology of acne?

- **Chocolate and fatty foods cause acne.** Much folklore exists regarding diet and acne. Acne is less common in some countries where diets are markedly different from those in the United States, but this difference may be due to genetic factors. There is very little scientific information to implicate diet in playing a significant role in the pathogenesis of acne.
- **Sunlight exposure improves acne.** There are no studies that show ultraviolet light improves acne. A tan may mask erythema and provide some cosmetic improvement. PUVA (psoralen and UVA) exposure has been reported to cause acne.
- **Poor hygiene causes acne.** If acne was caused by a deficiency of soap and water, it would occur between the toes. In fact, too much scrubbing and friction aggravate acne (acne mechanica).
- **Acne is a disease primarily affecting teenagers.** Many adults have acne or acne variants. Acne rosacea is primarily a disease of adults aged 20–50.
- **Masturbation causes acne.** The *People's Common Sense Medical Adviser* by R. V. Pierce, M.D., published in 1895, attributes everything from blindness, dyspepsia, deafness, and terrible skin eruptions to this "unspeakable affliction." In fact, the author devotes a whole chapter to the afflictions caused by "spermatorrhea."

8. How much does 1 year of topical acne therapy cost?

Clindamycin, 60 ml, bid application = $114.24
Tretinoin, 45-gm tube, qd application = $94.56
Benzoyl peroxide erythromycin, bid application = $94.04
Erythromycin, 60 ml, bid application = $26.76
Benzoyl peroxide, 42.5 gm, bid application = $21.58

9. Who is at risk for gram-negative acne?

Gram-negative acne occurs in 2–5% of young patients, mostly males, who have been on long-term antibiotic therapy for acne vulgaris. It presents with inflammatory follicular pustules and nodules about the nose in patients who previously have been in good control with standard acne therapy. When this condition is suspected, bacterial cultures should be taken. These will reveal one or more gram-negative organisms, including *Klebsiella, Escherichia coli, Proteus,* and/or *Pseudomonas* species. Standard broad-spectrum antibiotics should be discontinued, and appropriate gram-negative antibiotic treatment instituted. Isotretinoin can be used for resistant cases.

10. How much does it cost to treat acne with systemic antibiotics for 1 year?

Tetracycline, 500 mg, bid	$45.04
Erythromycin, 500 mg, bid	$174.00
Minocycline, 100 mg, bid	$1,445.50
Doxycycline (generic), 100 mg, bid	$280.28

11. How much does it cost to treat acne with systemic isotretinoin for 20 weeks?

Isotretinoin, 70 mg, qd	$1,326.75
Office consultation and five follow-up visits	$315.00
Lab studies, including complete blood count, liver function tests, lipid profile, and urine pregnancy test	$568.80
Total cost	$2,210.55

12. What is pyoderma faciale?

This is an acute, ferocious skin disease of women aged 15–40. It strikes like a hurricane, often in patients with no previous history of acne. It most commonly involves the central face but may affect the upper trunk. It is characterized by severe pustules, nodules, cysts, and draining sinus tracts (Fig. 3). Many of the patients have a history of flushing, and some authors regard it as a severe variant of acne rosacea. It has been reported in some patients during pregnancy or immediately postpartum.

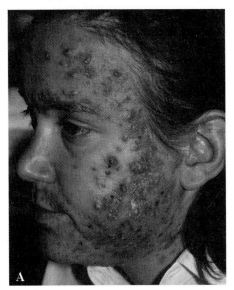 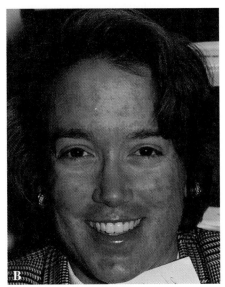

FIGURE 3. Pyoderma faciale. *A*, This fulminant eruption developed when the patient was tapered off systemic corticosteroids. *B*, Same patient post-treatment with a tapered course of prednisone and accutane. The eruption did not recur.

13. How do you treat pyoderma faciale?

This is one of the few times that oral steroids should be used to treat acne. Prednisone in a dose of 40–60 mg daily tapered over 3–4 weeks is indicated. Isotretinoin should be started in a dose of 1 mg/kg /day in conjunction with the prednisone and continued for 4–6 months. Once the disease has been brought under control, it rarely, if ever, recurs.

14. What is acne fulminans?

This rare systemic disease is seen predominately in young men. Its clinical features include fever, polyarthritis, leukocytosis, malaise, weight loss, anorexia, and severe acute cystic and often ulcerative acne lesions. It occurs primarily on the upper trunk, but lesions may also be seen on the buttocks, proximal extremities, neck, and face (Fig. 4). The etiology is unknown, but it is thought to be immunologically mediated. It has been described in young men, particularly soldiers, who are introduced into a tropical environment where they are exposed to high humidity, temperature, and the friction of wearing a backpack. Like pyoderma faciale, it usually responds well to treatment with isotretinoin and oral prednisone.

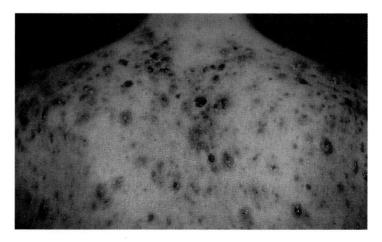

FIGURE 4. A male patient with acne fulminans. Note the ulcerative lesions on the upper back.

15. What is perioral dermatitis?

This common distinctive acneiform skin eruption occurs almost exclusively in women aged 20–40. It rarely occurs in men, children, or teenagers. Perioral dermatitis is characterized by erythema, scaling, and follicular papules that occur around the mouth, nose, and, less frequently, on the eyelids. The etiology is unknown, but many patients have used mid- or high-potency topical steroids inappropriately. Many patients with perioral dermatitis are heavy users of cleansers, moisturizers, and makeup. It responds well to treatment with oral tetracycline. A 6–8-week course of therapy is recommended.

16. What is chloracne?

Chloracne is a subtype of contact acne (acne venenata) that is induced by exposure to halogenated hydrocarbons. Although usually due to contact, rarely it can be caused by systemic exposure through inhalation or ingestion. Many chemicals have been implicated, including insecticides, herbicides, preservatives, and flame retardants. Many of these compounds are also potent hepatic toxins. There have been many industrial accidents related to these chemicals, resulting in major legal battles.

17. Describe the clinical presentation and course of chloracne.

Numerous comedones are the hallmark of chloracne. Frequently, noninflammatory cysts may be present, with inflammation occurring as a secondary event. The main areas of involvement are the face, neck, axilla, penis, and scrotum. The entire hair-bearing skin surface can be affected in extreme cases. The disease is often chronic, lasting years or even decades.

18. Do any drugs cause or aggravate acne?

A wide range of drugs have been reported to cause or aggravate acne, although many of these associations are isolated case reports.

Drugs That Cause or Aggravate Acne

Steroid Hormones	Halogens
Topical corticosteroids	Iodides
Systemic corticosteroids	Bromides
Anabolic steroids	Halogenated hydrocarbons
Some progestins	Antituberculous drugs
Testosterone	Isoniazid
Antidepressants	Miscellaneous drugs
Lithium	Thiourea
Aminoptine	Thiouracil
Antiepileptic drugs	PUVA
Phenytoin	
Trimethadione	

19. How does steroid acne differ from acne vulgaris?

Steroid acne has a sudden onset, the lesions are monomorphic (all lesions at the same stage of development), and comedones are absent. It occurs primarily on the upper trunk, less frequently on the face, and clears when the drug is withdrawn.

20. A patient asks you if her oral contraceptive is aggravating her acne. What do you tell her?

The answer is yes, no, and maybe, because it depends on the pill. Oral contraceptive pills (OCPs) that are estrogen-dominant tend to improve acne. If the OCP contains a progestin which has significant androgenic activity, it may aggravate acne. There are eight progestins presently used in OCPs, and they all have varying degrees of androgenic activity. The progestins with the highest androgenic activity are norethindrone acetate, norgestrel, and levonorgestrel. Norplant, the long-acting subdermal implant, uses norgestrel as the active ingredient, and the most common skin complaint is acne. It should be mentioned that the flaring or production of acne with these products is idiosyncratic and unpredictable. Ortho Tri-Cyclen is FDA-approved to treat moderate acne in females age 15 or older who have no contraindications to oral contraceptives.

21. Does tetracycline increase the risk of ovulation in women who are taking oral contraceptives?

Maybe. There are no well-controlled studies proving that broad-spectrum antibiotics increase the risk of ovulation in women taking OCPs, but there is certainly a theoretic risk. The best documentation of this phenomenon is with rifampin. Other implicated antibiotics include tetracyline, griseofulvin, penicillins, ampicillin, and sulfonamides. The use of progesterone-only contraceptives as an alternative for women using OCPs and taking long-term antibiotics has been recommended by some authors. Any physician who is prescribing these medications should warn patients of this theoretic risk.

22. What is hidradenitis suppurativa?

Hidradenitis is a chronic, suppurative, recurring inflammatory disease that affects apocrine gland follicles. It is more common in females and begins after puberty. It is characterized by inflammatory nodules, abscess formation, scarring, and sinus tract formation. The disease presents in skin that contains apocrine glands. The axilla and groin are most frequently involved, but the disease is also seen on the perineum, buttocks, neck, and scalp (Fig. 5).

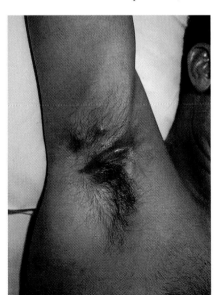

FIGURE 5. Hidradenitis suppurativa of the axilla with cysts and draining sinus tracts.

23. How do you treat hidradenitis suppurativa?

- This frustrating chronic disease is treated by measures that reduce friction and moisture. Weight reduction, loose undergarments, topical antiseptic soaps, and topical aluminum chloride are helpful in some patients.
- Acute exacerbations can be treated with systemic antibiotics. Problem cases should have bacterial cultures and sensitivities taken, although not all cultures grow pathogenic bacteria. The chronic use of topical clindamycin proves beneficial in some patients.
- Chronic inflammatory nodules can be treated with intralesional steroids. Systemic retinoids may help some patients but are not as effective as when used to treat severe acne vulgaris, and relapses are quite common.
- Severe refractory hidradenitis is best treated by complete surgical excision of the involved area. Incision and drainage should be minimized because it often leads to chronic sinus tract formation.

24. Discuss acne rosacea.

Acne rosacea is a chronic skin disease that most commonly occurs in the third to fourth decade of life, although it can be seen in adolescents and elderly patients. It is characterized by flushing, telangiectasia, follicular papules, and pustules, and in severe late-stage disease, patients may develop chronic facial lymphedema and rhinophyma. It is usually symmetrical and is most commonly seen on the convex areas of the face, including the nose, cheeks, forehead, and chin (Fig. 6). Blepharitis, conjunctivitis, and keratitis are common associations.

The etiology of rosacea is unknown. Genetic factors seem to play a role in that the disease is more common in persons of Celtic ancestry and is less common in blacks. Factors that stimulate flushing, such as hot beverages, alcohol, ultraviolet light exposure, and emotional factors, frequently exacerbate the disease.

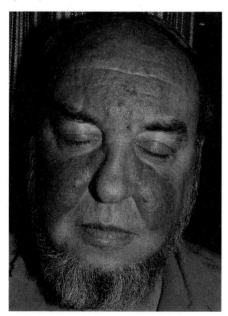

FIGURE 6. Acne rosacea involving the convex surfaces of the face.

25. How is acne rosacea treated?

Trigger factors that produce flushing should be avoided. These triggers vary greatly from patient to patient.

Tetracycline is very effective in suppressing inflammatory lesions. A starting dose of 1 g daily in divided doses is recommended for 3–4 weeks. The dose is then tapered to maintenance depending on the patient's response. Often, a maintenance dose of 250 mg daily or on alternate days will provide excellent control. Erythromycin, doxycycline and minocycline are also effective. They can be taken with food but are more expensive. Both oral and topical metronidazole are effective if an alternate treatment is needed.

Oral isotretinoin is helpful for severe resistant cases, but the drug is not as effective as when used for severe cystic acne, and relapses are more common. Oral antibiotics have little effect on flushing, telangiectasia, lymphedema, or rhinophyma. Isotretinoin may provide some benefit for early rhinophyma, but severe rhinophyma is best treated by surgical paring or electrosurgery. Persistent telangiectasia can be treated by tunable dye vascular laser with good cosmetic results.

26. When should a patient be started on isotretinoin therapy?

Isotretinoin is indicated for severe nodular and/or cystic acne vulgaris that is unresponsive to conventional therapy, including an adequate course of systemic antibiotics. It should be used as a first-line drug in patients with acne fulminans and pyoderma faciale in combination with a short 3–4-week tapered course of systemic prednisone. The recommended dose is 0.5–2 mg/kg given for 16–20 weeks.

Isotretinoin is also beneficial for patients with severe hidradenitis suppurativa, acne rosacea, and gram-negative acne who are unresponsive to conventional therapy. However, it is not as effective in these diseases as it is in severe acne vulgaris, and relapses are more frequent. Isotretinoin is also used in several diseases of keratinization, including Darier's disease, pityriasis rubra pilaris, and some types of psoriasis. It is often used in combination with PUVA (psoralen and UVA phototherapy) to treat severe inflammatory or pustular psoriasis.

27. What is the most serious side effect associated with isotretinoin therapy?

This drug is a major teratogen. Of the pregnancies that have occurred in patients taking isotretinoin, one-third have resulted in spontaneous abortion, one-third ended in therapeutic abortion, and the one-third that continued to term showed a major fetal malformation in 20%, including the brain, heart, and ears. Unfortunately, many of the reported patients who had a pregnancy while taking isotretinoin were pregnant when the drug was started. When treating women of childbearing years, the drug should be started on the second day of the next menstrual period, after a negative pregnancy test, and only if the patient is using adequate contraception.

28. Discuss the topical therapy of acne vulgaris.

The single most important topical medication used to treat acne are retinoids. We now have numerous topical preparations to choose from that are less irritating and decrease the most common complaints associated with other medications. These include adapalene (Differin), tazarotene (Tazorac), and tretinoin (Avita, Retin-A). The patient should be instructed that it may take 12–16 weeks of use for maximum benefit. These are the only drugs that normalize keratinization within the follicular infundibulum and prevent comodone formation.

Other topical treatmens include benzoyl peroxide, topical antibiotics (erythromycin, clindamycin, and sodium sulfacetamide), alpha-hydroxy acids, salicylic acid, and azelaic acid. Antibiotic resistance of *Propionibacterium acnes*, the anaerobic bacterium associated with acne pathogenesis, has become more common. More than half of patients undergoing therapy with a topical antibiotic will develop resistance. No bacterial resistance has been reported with topical benzoyl peroxide.

29. Can shaving cause acne vulgaris?

No. Shaving can cause pseudofolliculitis barbae (PFB) in genetically predisposed individuals. PFB occurs most frequently on the neck of black men, but it can occur in all races. It also can develop from shaving facial, pubic, and leg hair (Fig. 7). The problem starts with close shaving of curly hair that grows flat to the skin, resulting in ingrown hair that produce an inflammatory reaction. The treatment of choice is to stop shaving, allow the inflammation to subside, and then recommend an alternative method of hair removal such as clippers, depilatories, or laser hair removal.

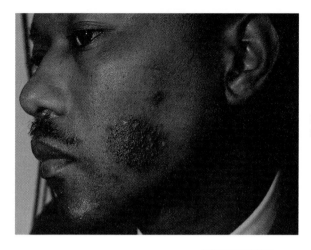

FIGURE 7. A male patient with pseudofolliculitis barbae.

BIBLIOGRAPHY

1. Bergfeld WF, Odom RB: New perspectives on acne. Clinician 12:1–32, 1994.
2. Champion RH, Burton JL, Ebling FJG: Textbook of Dermatology, 5th ed. Oxford, Blackwell Science, 1993.
3. Cunliffe WJ: Acne and unemployment. Br J Dermatol 115:379–383, 1986.
4. Downing DT, Stewart ME, Wertz PW, et al: Essential fatty acids and acne. J Am Acad Dermatol 14:221–225, 1986.
5. Espersen F: Resistance to antibiotics used in dermatological practice. Br J Dermatol 139:4–8, 1998.
6. Farrell LN, Strauss JS, Stranieri AM: The treatment of severe cystic acne with 13-cis retinoic acid: Evaluation of sebum production and the clinical response in a multiple dose trial. J Am Acad Dermatol 3:602–611, 1980.
7. Fitzpatrick TB, Eisen AZ, Wolff K, et al: Dermatology in General Medicine. New York, McGraw-Hill, 1993.
8. Goulden V, Stables GI, Cunliffe WJ: Prevalence of facial acne in adults. J Am Acad Dermatol 41:577–580, 1999.
9. Guidelines of care for acne vulgaris. J Am Acad Dermatol 22:676–680, 1990.
10. Kligman AM: Postadolescent acne in women. Cutis 48:75–77, 1992.
11. Krowchuk DP, Stancin T, Keskinen R, et al: The psychological effects of acne on adolescents. Pediatr Dermatol 8:332–338, 1991.
12. Lucky AW, Biro FM, Huster GA, et al: Acne vulgaris in premenarchal girls. Arch Dermatol 130:308–314, 1994.
13. Motley RJ, Finlay AY: How much disability is caused by acne? Clin Exp Dermatol 14:194–198, 1989.
14. Plewig G, Jansen T, Kligman AM: Pyoderma faciale. Arch Dermatol 128:1611–1617, 1992.
15. Plewig G, Kligman AM: Acne and Rosacea, 2nd ed. Berlin, Springer Verlag, 1993.
16. Reed BR: The pill. Fitzpatrick's J Clin Dermatol 2:41–44, 1994.

22. COLLAGEN VASCULAR DISEASES

Kathleen M. David-Bajar, M.D., COL, MC

1. Discuss the skin changes of lupus erythematosus.

Skin changes occur very frequently in lupus erythematosus (LE) and are second in frequency only to musculoskeletal complaints in this condition, occurring in about 85% of patients. It is useful to classify the eruptions seen in LE as to their possible diagnostic and prognostic significance.

Skin lesions that are diagnostic of LE have been called **lupus-specific eruptions.** Skin biopsies of these lesions show characteristic histopathologic changes of cutaneous LE. Further classification of the lupus-specific eruptions into subtypes of cutaneous LE is also useful, as some lesions of cutaneous LE are more strongly associated with systemic lupus erythematosus.

Lupus patients also develop many skin changes that are not specific for LE, termed **lupus-nonspecific eruptions.** These eruptions do not help to establish a diagnosis of LE, but they may still be very important to note, as specific systemic findings may be associated with them. For example, cutaneous lesions of palpable purpura in a patient with LE are not lupus-specific—i.e., such lesions may be seen in patients who do not have LE. However, they may be associated with vasculitic lesions of the kidney or CNS, and thus they have significance in the evaluation and treatment of lupus.

Classification of Cutaneous Disease in Lupus Erythematosus

Lupus-specific eruptions	Lupus-nonspecific eruptions
Acute cutaneous lupus erythematosus (ACLE)	Nonscarring alopecia
Subacute cutaneous lupus erythematosus (SCLE)	Telangiectasia
Annular	Livedo reticularis
Papulosquamous	Palpable purpura
Psoriasiform	Periungual erythema
Pityriasiform	
Chronic cutaneous lupus erythematosus	
Discoid lupus erythematosus (DLE)	
Hypertrophic DLE	
Lupus panniculitis	
Bullous eruption of systemic lupus erythematosus (SLE)	
Neonatal lupus erythematosus (NLE)	

2. What is acute cutaneous lupus erythematosus (ACLE)?

ACLE presents as an acute malar or more generalized photodistributed eruption. The malar erythema has been described as a "butterfly rash," since the pattern across the cheeks resembles the wings of a butterfly (Fig. 1). Nearly all patients presenting with ACLE will have systemic lupus erythematosus (SLE), often in an acute flare. ACLE is usually transient, improving when the SLE improves, and generally does not result in scarring of the skin.

3. Are there any common skin eruptions that may be confused with acute cutaneous lupus erythematosus?

Many patients have complaints of erythema of the face due to a wide variety of conditions, but not all of them are photoinduced. The differential diagnosis of photosensitive eruptions of the face is not as broad and includes polymorphous light eruption, photoreactions to systemic medications and topical products, and certain types of porphyria (see chapter 17). In addition, certain facial eruptions, such as rosacea, occasionally may be triggered or worsened by sun exposure. ACLE is an important cutaneous finding since it is strongly associated with SLE. Thus, patients with ACLE will have additional systemic complaints relating to SLE and will nearly always have a positive anti-nuclear antibody (ANA) test.

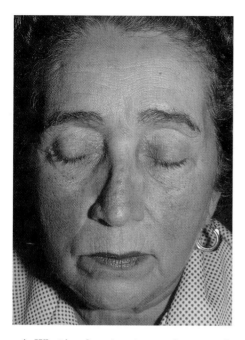

FIGURE 1. Acute cutaneous lupus erythematosus. Note the classic malar erythema ("butterfly rash").

4. What is subacute cutaneous lupus erythematosus (SCLE)?

This type of cutaneous LE was first described and characterized in the late 1970s. These patients have an eruption that is more persistent than that of ACLE, lasting weeks to months or longer. The lesions of SCLE consist of scaly, superficial, inflammatory macules, patches, papules, and plaques that are photodistributed, particularly on the upper chest and back, lateral neck, and dorsal arms and forearms. Several different morphologic types of SCLE have been described: annular lesions, and two types of papulosquamous lesions, psoriasiform and pityriasiform (Fig. 2). Some patients have more than one morphologic type of lesion.

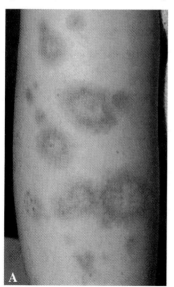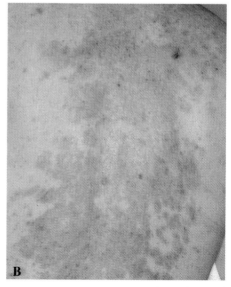

FIGURE 2. Subacute cutaneous lupus erythematosus. *A*, Annular lesions on the upper arms. *B*, Erythematous papules and plaques on the back.

5. Do patients with SCLE have SLE?

About one-half of patients with SCLE will have four or more criteria for the classification of SLE, though most SCLE patients do not have serious renal or CNS lupus erythematosus. Typically, they have skin disease, photosensitivity, and musculoskeletal complaints. Dry eyes and dry mouth are also common. Some patients with SCLE experience severe manifestations of SLE, and thus all SCLE patients should be monitored for systemic disease.

6. How do you make a diagnosis of SCLE?

SCLE is a clinical diagnosis based on the presence of a typical photodistributed eruption and a skin biopsy consistent with cutaneous LE. Direct immunofluorescence testing may also be helpful. In addition to granular deposition of immunoreactants at the dermal-epidermal junction, particulate deposition of IgG within the epidermis has been described in SCLE. Most patients with SCLE have circulating antibodies to Ro/SS-A (Sjögren's syndrome A) and, less commonly, to La/SS-B (Sjögren's syndrome B). These antibodies are not demonstrable in all patients with SCLE, thus their absence does not exclude this diagnosis.

7. What is the initial work-up of SCLE?

Once a diagnosis of SCLE is made, it is important to evaluate for the presence of SLE:

1. History and physical examination to identify manifestations of SLE in other organ systems.

2. Laboratory testing should be directed by findings on the history and physical exam but will generally include a complete blood count with differential, urinalysis, serum chemistries including renal function tests, and an ANA panel to include anti-Ro/SS-A, anti-La/SS-B, and anti-native DNA antibodies. Complement determinations may be ordered as some SCLE patients have partial or complete complement deficiencies.

3. A medication history is very important as SCLE may be triggered or worsened by a number of medications, especially thiazide diuretics. Some physicians recommend avoiding estrogens and sulfonamides in any patient with LE.

Medications Associated with Subacute Cutaneous Lupus Erythematosus

Hydrochlorothiazide	Gold	Diltiazem	Interferon β
Piroxicam	Procainamide	Naproxen	Captopril
Penicillamine	Sulfonylureas	Oxyprenolol	Griseofulvin
Glyburide	Verapamil	Cinnarizine	Cilazapril
Aldactone	Nifedipine	Terbinafine	Ranitidine

8. How is SCLE managed?

Cutaneous complaints are often of most concern to these patients, and thus dermatologists are generally the physicians managing this disease. Broad-spectrum sunscreens and sun-protective measures, including lifestyle changes and clothing, are perhaps the most important initial measures. Some patients respond to topical steroids, although potent topical steroids are usually required. Oral antimalarial therapy is also beneficial in many patients. Less commonly used treatments include dapsone, gold, immunosuppressive drugs, retinoids, and systemic steroids.

9. What is chronic cutaneous lupus erythematosus?

There are several types of cutaneous LE that are very persistent, termed chronic cutaneous lupus erythematosus. Discoid lupus erythematosus (DLE) is the most common of these chronic forms of cutaneous LE. An unusual variant of DLE with thick keratotic scale is referred to as hypertrophic DLE. Lupus panniculitis is another form of chronic cutaneous LE.

10. Describe the skin changes of discoid lupus erythematosus.

DLE is a chronic inflammatory disease consisting of fixed, indurated, erythematous papules and plaques that are often distributed on the head and neck (Fig. 3A). Without intervention, DLE lesions may last for many years and are associated with extensive scarring, a feature that helps distinguish DLE from SCLE. When DLE occurs on the scalp, permanent scarring alopecia may result.

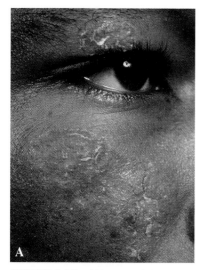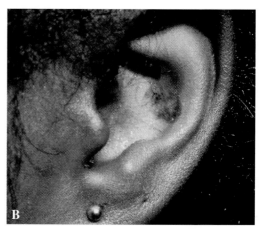

FIGURE 3. Discoid lupus erythematosus. *A,* Fixed, erythematous, indurated, scaly plaques of DLE on the cheek and upper eyelid. *B,* DLE lesion in the concha of the external ear. Hypopigmented and hyperpigmented areas, erythema, and scarring are present.

Pigmentary changes, both hyperpigmentation and hypopigmentation, are also frequently associated with lesions of DLE. Epidermal changes, including scale, keratotic plugging of the hair follicles, and sometimes crusting, are also generally present. The external ears are often involved in DLE (Fig. 3B); thus, this area should be carefully examined in patients with suspected DLE.

11. Do patients with DLE develop systemic lupus erythematosus?
   If the initial work-up of a patient with localized lesions of DLE does not reveal evidence of SLE, the risk of developing SLE is about 5%. If lesions are generalized, the risk is slightly higher. However, DLE lesions are not uncommon in patients with an established diagnosis of SLE. About 25% of SLE patients will develop lesions of DLE at some time in the course of their disease.

Comparison of Lupus-Specific Eruptions

DISEASE	DURATION	% OF PATIENTS WITH SLE	PHOTOSENSITIVE
ACLE	Hours–weeks	99%	Yes
SCLE	Weeks–months	50%	Yes
DLE	Months–years	5%	+/−

12. How is discoid lupus erythematosus treated?
   As with other types of cutaneous LE, sunscreens and sun-protective measures are the foundation of therapy. Potent topical steroids and intralesional corticosteroids are often helpful. Antimalarial drugs are also used. Less often, therapy with gold, immunosuppressive medications, or systemic corticosteroids is offered.

13. What is minocycline-induced lupus?
   This condition has been reported in patients taking minocycline for acne. Most patients are young females who have taken minocycline chronically. The most common symptom is symmetric polyarthralgia, but other findings such as fatigue, fever, elevated liver enzymes, pneumonitis, and anemia have also been reported. Lupus-specific skin eruptions, such as acute cutaneous LE or discoid LE, have not been reported. Nearly all patients will have a positive screening ANA test, Once minocycline is discontinued, most patients have resolution of symptoms.

14. What is lupus panniculitis?

In lupus panniculitis, inflammation involves the subcutaneous tissue, resulting in inflamed nodules that often resolve with depressed scars. There may be overlying lesions of DLE. When lupus panniculitis occurs with an overlying DLE lesion, it may be called **lupus profundus.** About one-half of patients with lupus panniculitis have four or more criteria for the classification of SLE.

The diagnosis is confirmed by an adequate excisional biopsy. Small punch biopsies are not adequate to rule out other causes of panniculitis. Direct immunofluorescence examination may be helpful in establishing the diagnosis. The treatment of choice is antimalarial drugs.

15. Describe the bullous eruption of SLE.

This rare blistering eruption has been described primarily in patients with established SLE. The histopathologic findings are quite different from those of other forms of cutaneous LE. Biopsies demonstrate a separation of the epidermis from the dermis and a neutrophil-rich inflammatory cell infiltrate. Antibodies to type VII collagen, a component of anchoring fibrils (see chapter 1), have been described in some patients with the bullous eruption of SLE. It has been proposed, but not proven, that these antibodies are involved in the pathogenesis of this disease.

16. How is the bullous eruption of systemic lupus erythematosus treated?

These patients typically respond to therapy with **oral dapsone.** Systemic corticosteroids have also been used.

17. What is neonatal lupus erythematosus (NLE)?

In NLE, infants develop skin disease (50%), heart disease (50%), or both (10%). The skin lesions occur most commonly on the face and head, morphologically resemble SCLE lesions, and are transient, resolving within a few months. The heart disease usually manifests as isolated complete heart block, although lesser degrees of heart block have been reported. The heart block is generally permanent and may require a pacemaker. About 10% of infants with NLE and heart disease die from cardiac complications. A few infants with NLE also have thrombocytopenia and/or liver disease.

Nearly all infants with NLE have anti-Ro/SS-A and sometimes anti-La/SS-B antibodies, as will their mothers. A few NLE patients have been reported to have anti-U1RNP antibodies in the absence of anti-Ro or anti-La antibodies. These antibodies are transient and are not detectable after a few months of life. They are of maternal origin, transferred via the placenta.

18. Which tests should be done in an infant with suspected NLE?

Serum from both the infant and mother should be assayed for ANA, and specifically for anti-Ro/SS-A, anti-La/SS-B, and anti-U1RNP antibodies. A skin biopsy for routine histology and direct immunofluorescence is also recommended. The biopsy will show histopathologic and direct immunofluorescence changes similar to those seen in SCLE.

Antibody Associations with Selected Collagen Vascular Diseases

DISEASE	ASSOCIATED ANTIBODY
Systemic lupus erythematosus	Anti-nuclear, anti-nDNA, anti-Sm antibodies
Subacute cutaneous lupus erythematosus	Anti-Ro/SS-A, anti-La/SS-B
Neonatal lupus erythematosus	Anti-Ro/SS-A, La/SS-B, U1RNP
CREST syndrome	Anti-centromere antibodies
Dermatomyositis	Anti-Jo-1

19. Once a diagnosis of NLE is made, what work-up should be done?

A physical examination should be performed, including cardiac examination and electrocardiogram. Because of reports of involvement of the liver and platelets, liver function tests and a platelet count should also be done. Additional tests or procedures may be done as indicated by physical findings. Mothers of infants with NLE should also be examined, as some will have or develop SCLE, SLE, or symptoms of Sjögren's syndrome.

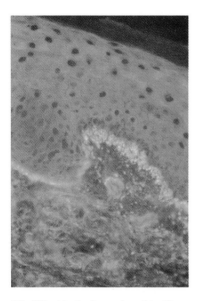

FIGURE 4. Lupus band test. Band-like deposition of IgM is seen at the junction between the epidermis and dermis in a skin biopsy specimen taken from a lesion of DLE. (Courtesy of James E. Fitzpatrick, MD.)

20. What is the lupus band test?

This direct immunofluorescence test is performed either on lesional skin or on normal, non-lesional skin. Granular deposits of immunoglobulins and complement are detected in a band-like pattern at the dermal-epidermal junction (Fig. 4). When this pattern is seen in lesional skin, it supports a diagnosis of cutaneous LE. When found in nonlesional skin, it is suggestive of SLE.

21. What is scleroderma?

Scleroderma is a chronic disease that involves the microvasculature and connective tissue and results in fibrosis. It may be localized, as in **morphea,** or more generalized and involving visceral organs, as in **progressive systemic sclerosis.** In morphea, sclerotic, indurated plaques develop that may be solitary, multiple, linear, or generalized. The surface is usually smooth, with the center of the lesion a whitish or ivory color, whereas the border of active lesions is often violaceous. Morphea usually involves the skin and subcutaneous tissues but may involve deeper structures, even bone. Patients with morphea generally do not develop systemic sclerosis.

22. What is the CREST syndrome?

C = **C**alcinosis cutis
R = **R**aynaud's phenomenon
E = **E**sophageal dysfunction
S = **S**clerodactyly
T = **T**elangiectasia

CREST syndrome, or Thibierge-Weissenbach syndrome, is generally considered a type of limited systemic scleroderma. In addition to the cutaneous changes of calcinosis cutis, Raynaud's phenomenon, sclerodactyly, and telangiectasia, these patients often develop hyperpigmentation, particularly in sun-exposed areas (Fig. 5). Most patients with the CREST syndrome have circulating antibodies to centromeres, called anti-centromere antibodies.

23. Describe the early cutaneous findings in progressive systemic sclerosis (PSS).

The earliest cutaneous complaints of PSS are often swelling of the hands and feet or symptoms associated with Raynaud's phenomenon. Telangiectasia may also develop early in the course of disease. The proximal nailfolds show changes in the capillaries, including avascular areas (dropout) and marked dilatation. Over time, the skin of the digits becomes thickened and sclerotic (Fig. 6). Sclerotic changes are often progressive, involving the face and extremities, and may eventually involve large areas of the body. Other late changes include digital ulcers and even loss of the digits.

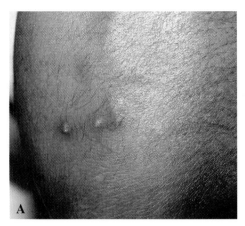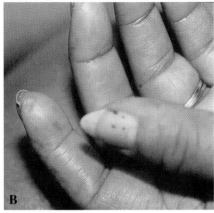

FIGURE 5. CREST syndrome. *A,* Firm, tender, whitish papules of calcinosis cutis on the elbow. *B,* Sclerodactyly and telangiectasia on the fingers.

24. What is dermatomyositis?

Dermatomyositis is a chronic inflammatory disease involving the skin and skeletal muscles. Its etiology is unknown. **Polymyositis** is the term used for involvement of the skeletal muscles without cutaneous involvement. The muscle involvement usually presents as proximal muscle weakness, sometimes with pain, and later with muscle atrophy. Muscle involvement may precede, follow, or occur simultaneously with skin disease and, in some instances, may not be detectable, a condition called **amyopathic dermatomyositis.** A number of cutaneous changes are present, including blotchy erythema, erythematous to violaceous papules and plaques particularly on extensor surfaces, poikilodermatous changes, and calcinosis cutis.

25. Are there skin changes diagnostic of dermatomyositis?

Two cutaneous findings have been described as pathognomonic of dermatomyositis: Gottron's papules and Gottron's sign. **Gottron's papules** are erythematous to purplish flat papules on the extensor surfaces of the interphalangeal joints. **Gottron's sign** consists of symmetric violaceous erythema, sometimes with edema, over the dorsal knuckles of the hands, elbows, knees, and medial ankles (Fig. 7A). Other skin findings that are characteristic of dermatomyositis are

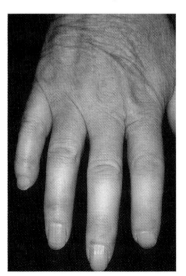

FIGURE 6. Progressive systemic sclerosis. Characteristic sclerodactyly manifesting as tight, shiny, thickened skin. (Courtesy of James E. Fitzpatrick, MD.)

periorbital edema with a lilac-colored erythema (heliotrope, Fig. 7B), periungual telangiectasia with cuticle dystrophy, and a photodistributed violaceous erythema of the forehead, sun-exposed areas of the neck, upper chest, shoulders, dorsal arms, forearms, and hands.

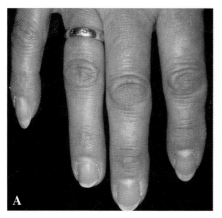 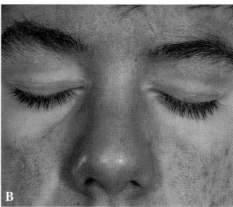

FIGURE 7. Dermatomyositis. *A*, Characteristic violaceous erythema over dorsal knuckles in a patient with associated breast cancer. *B*, Characteristic photodistributed erythema associated with heliotrope of upper eyelids. (Courtesy of James E. Fitzpatrick, MD.)

26. How do you diagnose dermatomyositis?

1. Skin biopsy may be helpful, although the histopathologic changes are consistent with, rather than diagnostic of, dermatomyositis.

2. Serum levels of muscle enzymes are typically elevated, with the creatine phosphokinase (CPK) level the most reliable indicator of disease activity.

3. An electromyogram of an affected muscle will generally be abnormal.

4. Biopsy of an affected muscle may be diagnostic, but nonspecific changes are also seen. The use of magnetic resonance imaging has been reported recently to be helpful in identifying muscle groups that would most likely yield significant findings on muscle biopsy.

5. Although many patients with dermatomyositis have a positive screening ANA, only a small percentage will have specific ANAs detected, such as anti-Jo-1.

27. Are any diseases associated with dermatomyositis?

Adults with dermatomyositis have been reported to have a variety of malignancies that sometimes follow a clinical course of exacerbation and remission in concert with the dermatomyositis. Screening with a careful history and physical examination is recommended in adult patients with dermatomyositis. Female patients should be carefully screened for ovarian cancer.

BIBLIOGRAPHY

1. Callen JP: Collagen vascular diseases. Med Clin North Am 82:1217–1237, 1998.
2. Dunn CL, James WD: The role of magnetic resonance imaging in the diagnostic evaluation of dermatomyositis. Arch Dermatol 129:1104–1106, 1993.
3. Euwer RL, Sontheimer RD: Amyopathic dermatomyositis (dermatomyositis siné myositis): Presentation of six new cases and review of the literature. J Am Acad Dermatol 24:959–966, 1991.
4. Gilliam JN: The cutaneous signs of lupus erythematosus. Contin Educ Fam Physician 6:34–70, 1977.
5. Lee LA: Neonatal lupus erythematosus. J Invest Dermatol 100:9S–13S, 1993.
6. Lee LA, David KM: Cutaneous lupus erythematosus. Curr Prob Dermatol 1:161–210, 1989.
7. Sontheimer RD: Subacute cutaneous lupus erythematosus: A decade's perspective. Med Clin North Am 73:1073–1091, 1989.
8. Sontheimer RD, Provost TT (eds): Cutaneous Manifestations of Rheumatic Diseases. Baltimore, Williams & Wilkins, 1996.
9. Sontheimer RD: SCLE: Experience gained from two decades of observation. Yale University/Glaxo Dermatology Lectureship Series in Dermatology. Beechwood Associates, 1993.

23. URTICARIA AND ANGIOEDEMA

Harold S. Nelson, M.D.

1. What percentage of the population experiences acute urticaria during their lifetime?

An estimated 10–20% of the population will experience at least one episode of urticaria during their lifetime (Fig. 1).

2. Is chronic urticaria primarily of allergic etiology?

No. In a large series of patients with chronic urticaria, a personal or family history of allergy was no more common than in the general population, suggesting that there is no connection between chronic urticaria and allergy. On the other hand, patients with atopic disorders (eczema, hayfever, asthma) had acute urticaria lasting 1–3 days more often than the normal population. In this atopic group, the acute urticaria frequently occurred on an obvious allergic basis, in many cases due to foods.

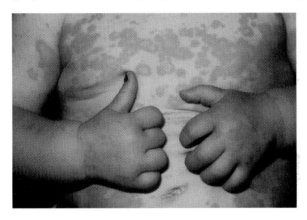

FIGURE 1. Urticaria in a child. Note that some lesions demonstrate an annular appearance. (Courtesy of James E. Fitzpatrick, MD.)

3. What is the "cause" of most chronic urticaria?

In most patients seen in referral centers, chronic urticaria remains unexplained despite extensive work-up. Excluding patients with physical urticarias, perhaps 95% remain "idiopathic."

4. How common are the physical urticarias?

Of 554 patients with urticaria seen in a university clinic in England, physical urticarias constituted 17.5% of the total, most of the remainder being idiopathic. The most frequent of the physical urticarias were dermographism (8.5%) (Fig. 2), cholinergic (5.1%), and acquired cold (2.5%).

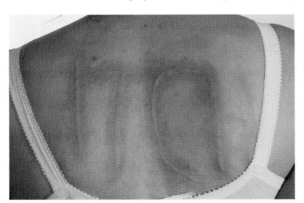

FIGURE 2. Dermographism: Whealing immediately following pressure.

5. What association has been described between autoantibodies and chronic urticaria?

Anti-thyroid microsomal antibodies have been reported in 13–14% of patients with chronic idiopathic urticaria, more than twice as frequent as in normal controls. A number of patients with chronic urticaria react to intradermal injection of their own serum by developing a wheal and flare that persists up to 8 hours. Many of these patients have IgG antibodies in their serum that react with the alpha subunit of the high-affinity IgE receptor on mast cells and basophils. In other patients, the IgG antibody appears to react with IgE itself. The frequency of these IgG autoantibodies in patients with chronic urticaria is not yet established but has been reported to be as high as 60% and 10%, respectively, in a referral clinic.

6. Name the components of the "triple response."
1. Vasodilatation (erythema)
2. Increased vascular permeability (wheal)
3. Axon reflex (flare)

The triple response is classically produced by injection of histamine into the skin.

7. What is the mechanism of the axon reflex?

The axon reflex is produced by stimulation of cutaneous sensory nerve endings, with antidromic conduction of the impulse and release of the neurokinin substance P. Substance P causes vasodilatation directly and also causes the release of histamine and other mediators from cutaneous mast cells.

8. List five mediators that are capable of directly causing vasodilatation and increased vascular permeability in the skin.

Histamine	Platelet-activating factor (PAF)
Prostaglandin D_2 (PGD$_2$)	Bradykinin
Leukotriene C_4 and D_4	

9. Name three mediators that may cause vasodilatation and increased vascular permeability indirectly through action on the mast cell.

Substance P; the anaphylatoxins C3a, C4a, and C5a; and histamine-releasing factors all cause release of mast cell mediators. Only substance P also has direct action on blood vessels.

10. Which cells synthesize histamine-releasing factors?

Thus far, substances that release histamine and other mediators from basophils and/or mast cells have been reported to be released by neutrophils, platelets, alveolar macrophages, T lymphocytes, B lymphocytes, and monocytes.

11. Certain physical urticarias can be passively transferred with the patient's serum. Which physical urticarias can be so transferred?

IgE-mediated transfer has been described for acquired cold urticaria, some solar urticarias, and for dermatographism. The susceptibility of this activity to inactivation by heat as well as adsorption studies have established an IgE-mediated basis for this transfer.

12. In what form of physical urticaria are subjects at risk of drowning?

Patients with acquired cold urticaria may have massive mediator release if immersed in cold water. Such release has resulted in drowning, presumably because the patient went into shock from the massive mediator release.

13. How quickly after the application of cold does whealing develop in acquired cold urticaria?

Whealing in cold urticaria does not develop during the exposure to the cold stimulus, but rather upon rewarming (Fig. 3). The delay is probably due to the decrease in cutaneous blood flow during exposure to the cold.

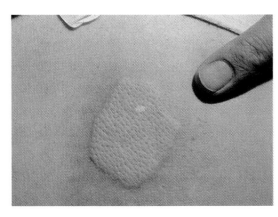

FIGURE 3. Positive ice cube test in a patient with acquired cold urticaria. (Courtesy of James E. Fitzpatrick, MD.)

14. Only one form of urticaria has whealing that is sufficiently characteristic to suggest a specific diagnosis. Which one?

The wheals in **cholinergic urticaria** are quite different from those in other forms of urticaria. They are small, punctuate (often referred to as pencil-eraser-sized) with a prominent erythematous flare. They may become confluent, however, and form larger areas of whealing.

15. Where does cholinergic urticaria usually develop?

On the upper thorax and neck. It may progress to involve the extremities.

16. What are the precipitating events for cholinergic urticaria? By what mechanism do they produce the whealing?

Exercise, warm baths and showers, and emotions are the classic triggers of cholinergic urticaria. There is an elevation of the core body temperature, which is perceived centrally, resulting in efferent cholinergic output to the skin and leading to mast cell degranulation.

17. How are the solar urticarias classified?

Solar urticarias are classified according to the inciting wavelength.

Type I	280–320 nm	Type IV	400–500 nm
Type II	320–400 nm	Type V	280–500 nm
Type III	400–500 nm	Type VI	400 nm (protoporphyrin IX)

18. What is Darier's sign?

Darier's sign is a finding in urticaria pigmentosa. Urticaria pigmentosa is a frequent manifestation of mastocytosis in which yellow-tan to red-brown macules containing increased numbers of mast cells are scattered over the body. Stroking the skin over the pigmented macules causes an urticarial wheal to form that is limited to the area of the pigmented lesion (Fig. 4).

19. How often does aspirin cause or exacerbate urticaria?

Aspirin is rarely a cause of urticaria in an otherwise asymptomatic patient, but many patients with chronic urticaria will have increased whealing if they take aspirin or nonsteroidal anti-inflammatory drugs when their disease is active. These same patients are usually able to take aspirin with impunity when their urticaria is inactive, indicating that aspirin is not the cause but a nonspecific exacerbating factor, presumably acting on a pharmacologic basis. Prospective and retrospective data suggest that aspirin administration will cause a flare in 20–40% of patients with active urticaria.

20. What is the prognosis of chronic urticaria?

Champion followed 554 patients with urticaria seen at a hospital clinic in England. After 6 months, 50% still had active disease. Of these patients, 40% continued to have at least intermittent symptoms 10 years later. The prognosis was somewhat worse in patients with only angioedema and even poorer if both urticaria and angioedema were present.

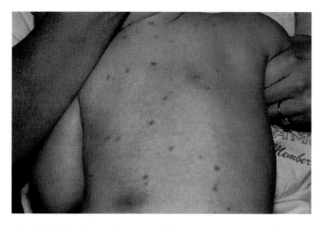

FIGURE 4. Child with urticaria pigmentosa demonstrating multiple tan papules and a positive Darier's sign in two lesions that have been stroked. (Courtesy of James E. Fitzpatrick, MD.)

21. Much has been discovered in recent years regarding the histopathology of chronic idiopathic urticaria. What three major types of cells may be encountered in increased numbers in these biopsies?

The characteristic histopathologic finding of nonvasculitic chronic urticaria is a perivascular infiltrate. There are increased numbers of **lymphocytes. Mast cells** are increased some 10-fold, and there is increased histamine on biopsy of the skin. Although **eosinophils** are often not prominent, increased deposition of the major basic protein of the eosinophil is present in the tissue in 50% of patients, indicating eosinophil involvement in the inflammatory process.

22. In contrast to chronic idiopathic urticaria, what are the typical histologic features of urticarial vasculitis?

Biopsy specimens from patients with urticarial vasculitis typically reveal necrotizing vasculitis of the small venules with deposition of immunoglobulin and complement. In those with low serum complement (hypocomplementemic urticarial vasculitis), polymorphonuclear leukocytes commonly predominate, while in those with normal serum complement, a lymphocytic infiltrate is more typical.

23. Can clinical findings suggest the presence of urticarial vasculitis?

The individual lesions of vasculitis may resemble those of idiopathic urticaria; however, they may feel firmer, tend to persist for > 24 hours, and on clearing they tend to leave an ecchymotic area due to leakage of red blood cells into the perivascular tissue (Fig. 5). Associated systemic symptoms, such as arthralgias and myalgias, are also common. The erythrocyte sedimentation rate is often increased, autoantibodies may be present, and there may be evidence of renal disease.

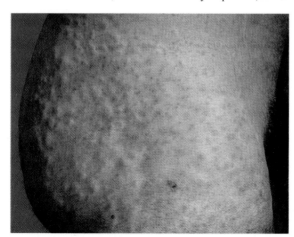

FIGURE 5. Lesions of urticarial vasculitis demonstrating characteristic pinpoint hemorrhages. (Courtesy of James E. Fitzpatrick, MD.)

24. A number of clues in the patient's history may suggest that a patient with recurrent angioedema has the hereditary form. Name some.

Seventy-five to 85% of patients with hereditary angioedema (HAE) give a positive family history of similar attacks. The attacks of angioedema themselves are characterized by absence of urticaria and pruritus, both common with idiopathic angioedema. In HAE, episodes of angioedema are often triggered by trauma or surgery. Significant upper airway obstruction is seen almost exclusively in HAE, as opposed to ordinary idiopathic angioedema. Attacks of severe abdominal pain are common in HAE, representing edema of the bowel wall. Finally, attacks of HAE typically progress for several days and respond poorly to treatment with antihistamines or epinephrine.

25. Why is C1 esterase deficiency not a part of the differential diagnosis of chronic urticaria?

Hereditary deficiency of C1 esterase inhibitor is the underlying defect in HAE. These individuals have recurring attacks of nonpruritic angioedema but do not have urticaria. Therefore, HAE never is part of the differential diagnosis of urticaria.

26. Name the recommended screening laboratory test for hereditary angioedema.

Serum C4. C2 is usually within normal limits when the patient is between attacks. C1 esterase inhibitor can be normal but without function in 15–20% of patients. The normal immunoassay will not detect these patients; a functional assay is required but is usually not readily available and is more expensive than a determination of C4 level.

27. What is the treatment of choice for HAE? How does it work?

HAE is inherited in an autosomal dominant pattern. Attenuated androgens, such as danazol or stanozolol, induce synthesis of normal C1 esterase inhibitor by the liver in these patients. Patients with the functionally abnormal C1 esterase inhibitor also respond, since they too have one normal gene.

28. How may a patient with HAE be treated prophylactically prior to elective surgery?

Effective prophylactic treatment to prevent attacks of HAE triggered by the trauma of surgery includes epsilon-amino caproic acid, 15 gm/day for 2–3 days, or the administration prior to surgery of 2–3 units of fresh frozen plasma to restore normal levels of C1 esterase inhibitor.

29. A 60-year-old patient presents with a new onset of attacks of nonpruritic angioedema and a depressed C4 level. What is the first diagnosis you consider?

Acquired C1 esterase inhibitor deficiency. This situation is usually encountered in patients with lymphoma who have a circulating low-molecular-weight IgM, depressed C1 esterase inhibitor level, and low levels of the C1–C4. The mechanism of C1 activation is by reaction with immune complexes or by binding of the C1 to anti-idiotypic antibody bound to the immunoglobulin on the surface of the tumor cells. Acquired C1 esterase deficiency has also been reported with connective tissue disorders such as systemic lupus erythematosus, with carcinoma, and with an IgG antibody directed toward C1 esterase inhibitor. In the latter circumstance, the C1 levels are usually normal. Androgen therapy benefits patients with acquired C1 esterase inhibitor deficiency by increasing C1 esterase inhibitor production by the liver.

30. Certain drugs have been identified as being particularly effective for a subset of patients with chronic urticaria or angioedema. What are these drugs, and when is a trial with them indicated?

- Cyproheptadine has been reported to be particularly effective in controlling acquired cold urticaria.
- Corticosteroids and nonsteroidal anti-inflammatory drugs prevent the lesions of delayed pressure urticaria, whereas antihistamines are completely without benefit.
- Hydroxychloroquine has been effective in some cases of hypocomplementemic urticarial vasculitis.
- The attenuated androgens, such as danazol and stanozolol, increase synthesis of C1 esterase inhibitor, thereby preventing attacks of hereditary angioedema.

31. What three mediator antagonists have been reported to be useful in symptomatic control of urticaria?

Competitive antagonists of the H_1 and H_2 histamine receptor and antagonists of leukotriene D_4 receptor have been reported to be useful in treating urticaria. The latter two are usually used in conjunction with an H_1 antagonist. Recent studies suggest that the non-sedating H_1 antagonists are just as effective in treating urticaria as the classic, sedating antagonists.

BIBLIOGRAPHY

1. Bensch GW, Borish L: Leukotriene receptor antagonists in the treatment of chronic idiopathic urticaria (abstract). J Allergy Clin Immunol 103:S154, 1999.
2. Champion RH, Roberts SOB, Carpenter RG, Roger JH: Urticaria and angio-edema: A review of 554 patients. Br J Dermatol 81:588, 1969.
3. Elias J, Boss E, Kaplan AP: Studies of the cellular infiltrate of chronic idiopathic urticaria: Prominence of T-lymphocytes, monocytes, and mast cells. J Allergy Clin Immunol 78:914–918, 1986.
4. Grattan CEH, Francis DM, Hide M, Greaves MW: Detection of circulating histamine releasing autoantibodies with functional properties of anti-IgE in chronic urticaria. Clin Exp Allergy 21:695–704, 1991.
5. Hide M, Francis DM, Grattan CEH, et al: Autoantibodies against the high-affinity IgE receptor as a cause of histamine release in chronic urticaria. N Engl J Med 328:1599–1604, 1993.
6. Kaplan AP: Urticaria and angioedema. In Middleton E Jr, Reed CE, Ellis EF, et al (eds): Allergy: Principles and Practice. St. Louis, Mosby, 1998.
7. Leznoff A, Sussman GL: Syndrome of idiopathic chronic urticaria and angioedema with thyroid autoimmunity: A study of 90 patients. J Allergy Clin Immunol 84:66–71, 1989.
8. Monroe EW, Bernstein DI, Fox RW, et al: Relative efficacy and safety of loratadine, hydroxyzine, and placebo in chronic idiopathic urticaria. Arzneimittelforschung 42:1119–1121, 1992.
9. Moore-Robinson M, Warin RP: Effect of salicylates in urticaria. BMJ 4:262–264, 1967.
10. Ormerod AD: Urticaria: Recognition, causes and treatment. Drugs 48:717–730, 1994.
11. Schocket AL (ed): Clinical Management of Urticaria and Anaphylaxis. New York, Marcel Dekker, 1993.
12. Tong LJ, Balakrishnan G, Kochan JP, et al: Assessment of autoimmunity in patients with chronic urticaria. J Allergy Clin Immunol 99:461–465, 1997.

IV. Infections and Infestations

24. VIRAL EXANTHEMS

William L. Weston, M.D.

1. What is the difference between an exanthem and an enanthem?

Any skin rash associated with a viral infection is called an **exanthem.** If the rash occurs on mucosal surfaces, it is termed an **enanthem.**

2. What viruses cause exanthems?

Of the hundreds of viruses that infect humans, most have been associated with an exanthem. Some viral infections which almost always cause an exanthem include measles, rubella, human herpesviruses including herpes simplex and varicella-zoster virus, and parvovirus B19. The most frequently seen viral exanthems are those caused by enteroviruses, followed by measles, varicella, herpes simplex, and parvovirus B19.

3. How do viruses cause exanthems?

In almost all viral exanthems studied to date, the responsible virus is within the skin lesions. It is presumed that the virus disseminates to the skin through the blood during a viremic phase of the viral illness. It is suspected that the exanthem observed is the result of the local cutaneous host response to the virus.

4. Describe the clinical types of viral exanthems that are seen.

- Widespread macular and papular eruptions are the most frequently seen and are called **morbilliform eruptions** after the appearance of measles (morbilli) (Fig. 1A).
- Acral-located papules are called **papular acrodermatitis.**
- **Blistering** eruptions may be seen as discrete blisters on a red base (dew drops on a rose petal) or as grouped blisters.
- A widespread **lacy red eruption** is characteristic of erythema infectiosum.
- Viruses can also produce widespread **diffuse redness** that mimics scarlet fever or acral-located papulovesicular eruptions.

5. Which viruses cause morbilliform eruptions?

Measles, rubella, human herpesvirus 6 (roseola), infectious mononucleosis (Epstein-Barr virus and cytomegalovirus), and enteroviruses.

6. Which viruses cause blistering eruptions?

Varicella, herpes simplex, herpes zoster (Fig. 1B), and coxsackieviruses (hand, foot and mouth syndrome) (Fig. 1C).

7. Which viruses cause lacy eruptions?

Parvovirus B19 (Fig. 2).

8. What viruses cause scarlet fever-like eruptions?

Enteroviruses, adenoviruses, and hepatitis B and C.

9. Which viruses cause acral-located eruptions?

Areas of skin where the skin surface temperature is low are distally located and called acral. Those included are the fingers, toes, hands, feet, ears, nose, and buttocks. Some viral infections preferentially locate to acral areas, including those that produce the Gianotti-Crosti syndrome or

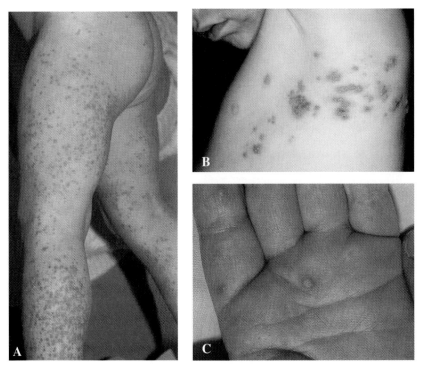

FIGURE 1. Morbilliform eruptons. *A*, Numerous widespread red macules and papules. *B*, Grouped vesicles limited to a dermatome in herpes zoster infection (courtesy of James E. Fitzpatrick, MD). *C*, Discrete palmar vesicle in epidermic hand, foot, and mouth syndrome.

papular acrodermatitis (Fig. 3). These viruses include hepatitis B, cytomegalovirus, Epstein-Barr virus, and coxsackievirus A16.

10. Can viral exanthems be unilateral?

Yes, there is a described laterothoracic periflexural exanthem that involves only one side of the body (Fig. 4). The cause of this eruption is thought to be viral, but it has not been proven.

11. Discuss the differential diagnosis of viral morbilliform eruptions.

Drug eruptions are most commonly confused with viral morbilliform exanthems. Also, bacterial scarlet fever, insect bites, early lesions of guttate psoriasis, and urticaria may mimic morbilliform eruptions.

Differential Diagnosis of Morbilliform Eruptions

Common viruses	Drug eruptions
Measles	Ampicillin
Rubella	Penicillin
Roseola	Nonsteroidal anti-inflammatory drugs
Erythema infectiosum	Salicylic acid
Infectious mononucleosis	Barbiturates
Pityriasis rosea	Phenytoins
Common bacteria	Phenothiazines
Scarlet fever	Thiazide diuretics
Reactive erythemas	Isoniazid
Urticaria	Papulosquamous disorders
Papular urticaria	Guttate psoriasis
Erythema multiforme	Graft-versus-host disease

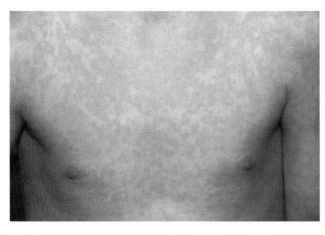

FIGURE 2. Lacy rash of chest in erythema infectiosum.

12. What are the components of the STAR complex?

In some viral exanthems, a monoarthric arthritis may accompany the syndrome, particularly in adolescent girls. It may present as the so-called STAR complex, which includes **S**ore **T**hroat, **A**rthritis, and **R**ash.

13. What causes the STAR complex?

Rubella and human parvovirus B19 are the most likely viruses responsible. Other causes include hepatitis B, adenovirus, echoviruses, coxsackieviruses, and Epstein-Barr virus.

14. How does sunlight exposure influence viral exanthems?

Many viral exanthems will be photoexaggerated, that is, they will have many more skin lesions within the areas of sun exposure and have few lesions in sun-protected areas. This is particularly true of the human herpesviruses, particularly varicella.

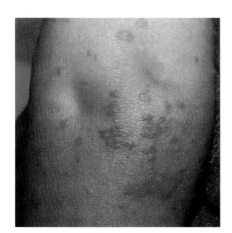

FIGURE 3. Acral-located red papules in Gianotti-Crosti syndrome.

15. What is the traditional numbering of the "original" six exanthematous illnesses?

First disease	Measles
Second disease	Scarlet fever
Third disease	Rubella (German measles)
Fourth disease	Duke's disease (scarlatinella)
Fifth disease	Erythema infectiosum
Sixth disease	Exanthem subitum (roseola)

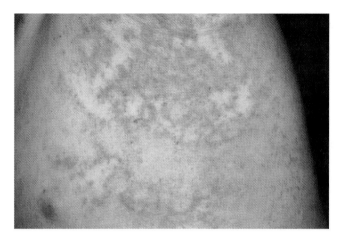

FIGURE 4. Lacy eruption of axilla in periflexural exanthem.

BIBLIOGRAPHY

1. Baldari U, Monti A, Righini MG: An epidemic of infantile papular acrodermatitis [Gianotti-Crosti syndrome] due to Epstein-Barr virus. Dermatology 188:203, 1994.
2. Brown KE, Young NS, Liu JM: Molecular, cellular and clinical aspects of parvovirus B19 infection. Crit Rev Oncol Hematol 16:1, 1994.
3. Drago F, Ranieri E, Malaguti F, et al: Human herpesvirus 7 in pityriasis rosea. Lancet 349:1367–1368, 1997.
4. Hall CB, Long CE, Schnabel KC, et al: Human herpesvirus-6 infection in children. N Engl J Med 331:432, 1994.
5. Hogan PA, Morelli JG, Weston WL: Viral exanthems. Curr Probl Dermatol 4:35, 1992.
6. Jones VF, Badgett JT, Marshall GS: Repeated photoreactivation of herpes simplex virus type 1 in an extrafacial dermatomal distribution. Pediatr Infect Dis J 13:238, 1994.
7. Jundt JW, Creager AH: STAR complexes: Febrile illness associated with sore throat, arthritis and rash. South Med J 86:521, 1993.
8. Lajo A, Borque C, Del Castillo F, et al: Mononucleosis caused by Epstein-Barr virus and cytomegalovirus in children: A comparative study of 124 cases. Pediatr Infect Dis J 13:56, 1994.
9. Mancini AJ: Exanthems in childhood: An update. Pediatr Ann 27:163–170, 1998.
10. Mangi RJ: Viral arthritis—The great masquerader. Bull Rheum Dis 43:5, 1994.
11. McCuaig CC, Russo P, Powell J, et al: Unilateral laterothoracic exanthem: A clinicopathologic study of forty-eight patients. J Am Acad Dermatol 34:979–984, 1996.
12. Norval M, El-Ghorr A, Garssen J, et al: The effects of ultraviolet light irradiation on viral infections. Br J Dermatol 130:693, 1994.
13. Weston WL: Viral exanthems. In Weston WL, Lane AT, Morelli JG (eds): Color Textbook of Pediatric Dermatology, 2nd ed. St. Louis, Mosby, 1995.
14. Weston WL, Morelli JG: Newly recognized infectious exanthems. Dermatol Nurs 10:191–193, 1998.

25. BULLOUS VIRAL ERUPTIONS

Sylvia L. *Brice*, M.D.

1. What are the most likely etiologic agents in bullous viral eruptions?

VIRUS	DISEASE
Herpes simplex virus types 1 and 2 (HSV-1), (HSV-2)	Herpes labialis (oral herpes) Herpes genitalis (genital herpes)
Varicella zoster virus (VZV)	Varicella (chickenpox) Herpes zoster (shingles)

2. To what family of viruses do HSV and VZV belong?

HSV-1 and 2 and VZV are members of the human herpesvirus family. Other members of this family include cytomegalovirus, Epstein-Barr virus, human herpesvirus-6, human herpesvirus-7, and human herpesvirus-8. The human herpesviruses all contain double-stranded DNA, share certain structural features and mechanisms for infection and replication, and have the capacity to establish latent infection in the human host.

HERPES SIMPLEX

3. What happens during primary HSV infection?

Primary infection refers to an individual's first infection with HSV, either type 1 or 2, at any site. These patients are seronegative initially but subsequently develop HSV-specific antibodies.

HSV gains access to the host through the epithelial surface. Following active replication within the skin or mucosa, HSV infects the associated cutaneous neurons and migrates to the sensory root ganglia, where a latent infection is established. Primary HSV infection may be associated with extensive cutaneous lesions, severe pain, and systemic symptoms. However, in many cases, the primary infection is asymptomatic (or unrecognized).

4. What about recurrent infection?

Recurrent HSV infection represents reactivation of the latent virus in the sensory ganglia. "Reactivated" virus particles migrate back along the nerves to the site in the skin where the primary infection occurred, with subsequent viral replication and the development of clinical lesions. The most common sites for recurrent herpes simplex infection are the lips (herpes labialis, "cold sores"), genitalia, and sacral area (Fig. 1). Often, individuals experience a prodrome of tingling or burning in the skin prior to the development of visible lesions. Certain factors, such as fever, stress, menses, and sun exposure may precipitate recurrent infection. The frequency of recurrent infection varies greatly between individuals. In most individuals, clinically evident recurrence becomes less frequent over time.

5. What is the difference between a primary and an initial HSV infection?

When an individual without preexisting antibodies to either HSV-1 or HSV-2 develops an infection with herpes (either type 1 or 2), it is referred to as the **primary infection**. When an individual with preexisting antibodies to one type of HSV then experiences an infection with the other HSV type, it is referred to as the **initial (or initial, non-primary) infection**.

6. Define asymptomatic shedding.

In some cases of recurrent infection, clinical lesions may not be visible, but virus can be recovered if the skin or mucosal site is cultured appropriately and the virus can be transmitted to another person. In these instances, the host immune response is believed to eliminate the focus of virus before a full-fledged recurrence develops.

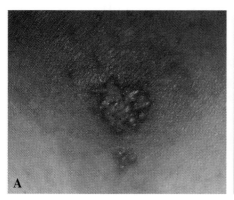 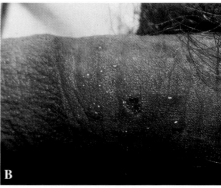

FIGURE 1. *A,* Classic lesion of recurrent herpes simplex with grouped vesicles on an erythematous base. *B,* Recurrent herpes genitalis.

7. How is herpes simplex virus transmitted?

HSV is transmitted by direct contact of the infected cutaneous surface(s) of one indivdual with the mucosa or skin of an uninfected individual. HSV does not survive long outside its normal habitat, and so transmission by contact with fomites is extremely uncommon. It is assumed that HSV-1 is most commonly transmitted during childhood inadvertently from infected family members, whereas infection with HSV-2 may develop later when individuals become sexually active.

8. How long is HSV's incubation period, the time from initial infection to appearance of vesicles?

The time interval between exposure and development of primary disease is estimated to be 3–14 days. However, not all cases of primary disease are symptomatic, and so the first evidence of infection may be a recurrent episode, well after the actual exposure.

9. Can you have "herpes" and not know it?

Yes. Many individuals who give no history of HSV infection are seropositive for HSV-specific antibodies. In addition, if repeated viral cultures of the oral or genital mucosa are performed, HSV can be recovered periodically from such individuals (asymptomatic shedding). This may be one factor contributing to the widespread transmission of this virus. Based on the seroprevalence of herpes-specific antibody, 70–80% of the population is infected with HSV-1 and 25–30% with HSV-2.

10. What controls HSV latency and reactivation?

The mechanisms for latency and recurrence remain poorly understood. The complete viral genome appears to be present in latent virus, although the latent virus within the ganglia is not in an infectious form and no viral proteins have been detected. In this way, the latent virus is shielded from the host's immune system, both by its location within the CNS and because of its lack of viral-specific antigens. Certain HSV-specific mRNAs, known as latency associated transcripts, are present, but their role in latency and/or reactivation is unknown.

11. Do HSV-1 and 2 differ?

HSV types 1 and 2 are very closely related, sharing approximately 50% homology in their genetic composition. As expected, many of their viral proteins are also similar (known as type-common), although each type also produces unique proteins (type-specific). Immunohistologic techniques can be used to identify these type-specific proteins and thus differentiate HSV-1 from HSV-2 in clinical situations. HSV-1 is usually associated with oral herpes and HSV-2 with genital herpes, although each virus can affect both sites.

12. What can you tell a patient with genital herpes about the risk of transmission to his or her partner?

Giving advice is extremely difficult, primarily because of the phenomenon of asymptomatic shedding. Even between episodes of clinically active disease, patients may shed infectious virus from the genital mucosa. Based on results of viral cultures, estimates of asymptomatic shedding range from an incidence of <1% up to 15%. However, use of more sensitive tests (e.g., PCR) has demonstrated that viral shedding can occur an average of 28% of days. Therefore, the safest practice is the routine use of a condom, even between active episodes. At the very least, avoidance of sexual contact during clinically apparent disease (i.e., until lesions are completely dry) is advised. The antiviral agent, acyclovir, decreases but does not eliminate asymptomatic shedding. The potential protective effect of acyclovir, whether taken routinely by the infected partner or prophylactically by the uninfected partner, has not been established.

13. How do you diagnose HSV infection?

1. **Clinical history:** Recurrent blisters or erosions in the same site (especially in an oral or genital distribution) are highly suspicious for HSV infection. A prodrome of tingling or burning is also consistent with this diagnosis.

2. **Physical exam:** The classic lesion is grouped vesicles on an erythematous base, but more often only nonspecific crusted erosions are seen.

3. **Laboratory methods:** The gold standard remains viral culture, although many new rapid and sensitive techniques for detection of viral-specific proteins may be more cost-effective for routine office use. Use of PCR is also becoming more common in viral laboratories. For any method of detection, the age of the lesion sampled is critical. Vesicles provide the highest percentage of positive results, with culture results available in 12–48 hours. Ulcers or erosions, if they are not dry or crusted, can also yield positive results.

14. How is a Tzanck smear performed?

In a Tzanck smear, the base of the suspected herpetic lesion is gently scraped, and the skin or mucosal cells removed are placed on a glass slide. The cells are stained and then examined by light microscopy for evidence of viral-induced cytologic change, including the characteristic **multinucleated giant cells.** Tzanck smears provide an efficient and inexpensive method of diagnosis, although the results are not always definitive. This technique cannot distinguish HSV from VZV.

15. Who gets herpetic whitlow?

Herpetic whitlow (HSV infection of the hand or fingers) was previously considered a disease of health care professionals, which occurred as a result of contact with infected patients. In fact, as few as 10% of individuals with this disorder fall in that category. The remaining cases are seen in children and young adults and result from autoinoculation from another site of infection (Fig. 2A). In children the etiologic agent is generally HSV-1, while in adults it is HSV-2.

16. What is Kaposi's varicelliform eruption?

Eczema herpeticum, or Kaposi's varicelliform eruption, is an extensive, disseminated cutaneous infection with HSV (Fig. 2B). It occurs most commonly as a complication of a localized herpes infection in patients with atopic dermatitis, although it may also be associated with other dermatoses such as Darier's disease, pemphigus, severe seborrheic dermatitis, and psoriasis. Why this widespread viral dissemination develops in these patients is not clear, although immune dysfunction is suspected. Fortunately, antiviral therapy is beneficial in this process.

17. How does a baby get herpes? Is it a serious problem?

Neonatal herpes is one of the most critical problems associated with the increased incidence of genital herpes. Herpes infection in the neonatal period can be, and often is, devastating because of the inadequate immune response seen in neonates. In most cases, transmission of HSV to the neonate occurs by delivery through an infected birth canal. Postpartum acquisition occurs less commonly. Development of primary or initial non-primary genital herpes by the mother at or near

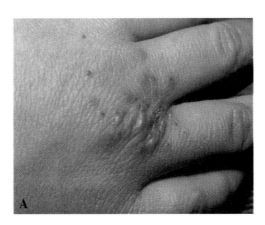
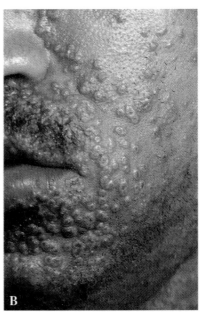

FIGURE 2. *A*, Herpetic whitlow. *B*, Eczema herpeticum (Kaposi's varicelliform eruption) occurring in a patient with atopic dermatitis (courtesy of Scott D. Bennion, MD).

the time of delivery poses a significant risk for the infant. However, most cases of neonatal herpes are the result of asymptomatic shedding in women with no known history of genital herpes. The usual onset of neonatal herpes is 5–21 days following exposure. Approximately 80% of infected neonates have at least some characteristic skin lesions.

18. What are the drugs of choice for treatment of HSV?

There are now three systemic antiviral agents routinely used for the treatment of HSV: acyclovir, valacyclovir, and famciclovir. Valacyclovir is the L-valyl ester of acyclovir with a bioavailability 3–5 times greater than acyclovir. Famciclovir is the diacetyl-6-deoxy analog of penciclovir. It is well absorbed and has a long intracellular half-life. Both valacyclovir and famciclovir offer the advantage of less frequent dosing compared to acyclovir. All three drugs are generally safe and highly effective because of their very specific antiviral activity. The antiviral drug is preferentially taken up by infected cells, where it must be converted to its active form by the viral enzyme thymidine kinase. The active form preferentially inhibits viral DNA synthesis, with little impact on host cell metabolism. For the currently recommended doses of these drugs, see table below.

Recommended Antiviral Therapy for HSV*

Immunocompetent patients	
Primary/initial episode	ACV 200 mg PO 5 times/day or 400 mg tid for 10 days VAL 1 g PO bid for 10 days FAM 250 mg PO tid for 5–10 days
Recurrent episode (best results obtained with early patient-initiated therapy)	ACV 200 mg PO 5 times/day or 400 mg tid for 5–7 days VAL 500 mg PO for 5 days FAM 125 mg PO bid for 5 days For herpes labialis, penciclovir 1% cream applied q 2 hours while awake for 4 days
Suppressive therapy (titrate to lowest required dose)	ACV 200–400 mg PO bid–tid VAL 500–1000 mg PO qd FAM 125–250 mg PO bid

Table continued on next page

Recommended Antiviral Therapy for HSV* (Cont.)

Immunosuppressed patients	
Primary/initial or recurrent	ACV 5–10 mg/kg IV q 8 hours
	If not severe, 400 mg PO 5 times/day for 7–14 days
	VAL 1 g PO tid for 7 days
	FAM 500 mg PO bid for 7 days
Suppressive therapy	ACV 400–800 mg PO tid
	VAL 1 g PO tid
	FAM 500 mg PO bid

*Dose adjustment necessary in renal impairment. ACV, acyclovir; VAL, valacyclovir; FAM, famciclovir.

19. When is chronic suppressive therapy indicated?

Once an episode of recurrent HSV infection (whether oral or genital) has begun, initiation of antiviral therapy often provides only mild symptom improvement. If antiviral therapy is initiated during the prodromal phase, the response may be somewhat better. In patients with frequently recurrent or severe disease, especially with genital herpes, **chronic suppressive therapy** may be considered. After 1 year on therapy, a "drug holiday" may be given to assess the continued need for treatment, since the natural history of recurrent infection is to decrease in frequency with time.

VARICELLA-ZOSTER

20. Describe the natural history of varicella.

Varicella, or chickenpox, is the primary infection with varicella-zoster virus (VZV). It is characterized by the appearance of two to three successive crops of diffuse, pruritic vesicles and papules over several days. These lesions then evolve into pustules and crusted erosions, so that lesions in all stages of development are present together (Fig. 3). Lesions generally persist for up to 1 week.

Varicella most commonly occurs during childhood. It is highly contagious, both via respiratory secretions and contact with the cutaneous lesions. The incubation period ranges from 10–23 days, and the patient is considered contagious from 4 days before the onset of lesions until all lesions have crusted.

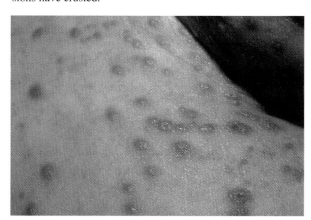

FIGURE 3. Varicella, with skin lesions at all stages of development.

21. What is shingles?

Herpes zoster, or "shingles," is the recurrent form of infection with VZV and represents reactivation of the latent virus in the sensory ganglia. The cutaneous eruption consists of painful and/or pruritic vesicles, which tend to follow a unilateral, dermatomal distribution (Fig. 4). Prodromal pain may often precede the development of visible lesions. The entire course is usually 2–3 weeks in duration. The most common area of involvement for herpes zoster is the trunk (dermatomes innervated by the thoracic nerves), followed by the head (first branch of the trigeminal nerve).

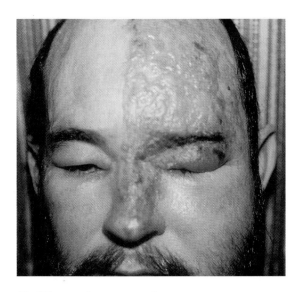

FIGURE 4. Herpes zoster involving a facial dermatome.

22. Who gets herpes zoster?

Anyone who has had varicella may develop herpes zoster. However, it usually develops in persons >50 years of age, and the incidence increases with advancing age. Herpes zoster is also more common in immunocompromised individuals, and the incidence has risen since the advent of AIDS.

23. Can herpes zoster be recurrent?

Approximately 5% of patients with herpes zoster will experience a recurrence, usually in the same dermatome.

24. What is disseminated zoster?

Disseminated zoster is defined as the presence of >20 vesicles outside the primary and adjacent dermatomes. It is uncommon in immunocompetent patients, but up to 40% of immunocompromised patients may develop this complication. In these cases, visceral involvement may also occur.

25. Is a vesicular eruption along a dermatome always herpes zoster?

When a patient presents with a vesicular eruption along a dermatome, a diagnosis of herpes zoster is generally made. However, recurrent herpes simplex may also have a "zosteriform" distribution, indistinguishable from herpes zoster both clinically and on Tzanck smear. Although this presentation is not common, the possibility should be entertained, especially when the dermatomes involved are in the orofacial or genital distribution or the patient presents with recurrent zoster.

26. Is herpes zoster contagious?

Herpes zoster is the result of reactivation of latent VZV in the sensory ganglia. There is no evidence that a person can develop herpes zoster as a result of contact with patients with either varicella or herpes zoster. However, direct contact with the cutaneous lesions may result in transmission of primary varicella to a susceptible host.

27. What is postherpetic neuralgia?

Postherpetic neuralgia is the most common complication of herpes zoster. It is defined as the presence of pain after skin lesions have healed, or pain lasting >4 weeks after the onset of cutaneous lesions. The pain is often severe and debilitating. Overall, it occurs in 10–15% of patients, but the incidence increases dramatically with age so that >50% of patients with herpes zoster who are over age 60 develop postherpetic neuralgia. Other risk factors include prominent prodromal symptoms and moderate or severe pain at presentation. In most cases, postherpetic neuralgia resolves spontaneously within the first 12 months, but it may persist for years.

28. How do you diagnose VZV infection?

For **varicella,** the physical findings of lesions in various stages of development (papules, vesicles, pustules, and erosions), especially with a history of exposure to an individual with varicella (or zoster), is generally enough to make the diagnosis. The diagnosis of **herpes zoster** also is often made on the basis of physical findings. A Tzanck smear may be useful. Additional laboratory testing is generally unnecessary. In atypical cases, a viral culture may be performed, although culturing VZV is more difficult and takes longer than culturing HSV. Immunohistochemical testing (immunofluorescence, immunoperoxidase) to detect viral-specific antigens in infected cells and use of PCR have become more commonly available.

29. What is the treatment for varicella?

Generally, symptomatic therapy, such as calamine lotion and oral antihistamines, is all that is required. Acyclovir is not routinely recommended for otherwise healthy children from a cost-effective standpoint. However, for varicella in an adult or immunocompromised individual, prompt initiation of systemic antiviral therapy is advised (see table below). Routine childhood vaccination to prevent varicella is now recommended for children and adolescents who have not been infected. Vaccination is also recommended for susceptible adults, especially those at high risk for exposure.

Recommended Antiviral Therapy for VZV*

Immunocompetent patients	
Varicella	Start within 24 hours of rash onset
	ACV 20 mg/kg (up to 800 mg) PO bid for 5 days
Herpes zoster	Start within 72 hours of rash onset, especially recommended in patients > 50 years of age or with ophthalmic zoster
	ACV 800 mg PO 5 times/day for 7 days
	VAL 1 g PO tid for 7 days
	FAM 500 mg PO tid for 7 days
Immunosuppressed patients	
Varicella	ACV 10–12 mg/kg IV q 8 hours for 7–10 days
Herpes zoster	If not severe, ACV 800 mg PO 5 times/day for 7 days
	If severe or progressing, ACV 10 mg/kg IV q 8 hours for 7 days

*Dose adjustment necessary in renal impairment. ACV, acyclovir; VAL, valacyclovir; FAM, famciclovir.

30. How about herpes zoster?

Herpes zoster is a self-limited disease and in most young, otherwise healthy persons, symptomatic measures (cool compresses, antihistamines, analgesics) are sufficient. However, for persons who are over 50 years of age, have ophthalmic zoster, or are immunocompromised, systemic antiviral therapy is recommended (see table above). If started within 72 hours of the onset of skin lesions, systemic antiviral therapy reduces the discomfort and duration of the acute infection and may reduce the severity of postherpetic neuralgia.

31. Is there any special concern in treating the patient with ophthalmic zoster?

Ocular disease occurs in 20–70% of patients with ophthalmic zoster, and antiviral therapy is routinely recommended. In addition, patients with involvement in this dermatome should be evaluated by an ophthalmologist.

OTHER VIRAL ERUPTIONS

32. What is hand, foot, and mouth disease?

Hand, foot, and mouth disease, or vesicular stomatitis with exanthem, is usually seen in infants or young children. Following a brief prodrome of fever, malaise, and sore throat, the characteristic enanthem develops. Red macules, vesicles, and ulcers may be seen on the buccal mucosa, tongue, palate, and pharynx (Fig. 5A). Lesions may also occur on the hands and feet (dorsal aspects, as well as the palms and soles) (Fig. 5B). Hand, foot, and mouth disease is caused by one of several enteroviruses, most commonly coxsackievirus A16 or enterovirus 71. It is highly contagious and spreads by direct contact.

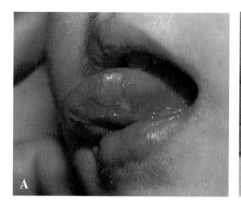
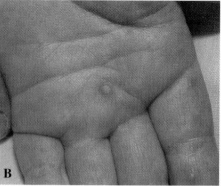

FIGURE 5. Hand, foot, and mouth disease. *A*, Vesicular stomatitis. *B*, Typical lesions on palmar skin. The vesicular lesions are typically gray and often elliptical.

33. What is orf?

Human orf, or ecthyma contagiosum, is caused by a parapoxvirus that is usually contracted by direct exposure to infected sheep or goats. Milkers' nodules are caused by a closely related virus found in cows. Both of these infections may also be contracted by exposure to fomites containing the virus (e.g., fence posts, soil). The lesions of both orf and milker's nodules are identical, consisting of dome-shaped, firm bullae which develop an umbilicated crust (Fig. 6). One to several lesions develop, usually on the hands and forearms, and these generally resolve without therapy in 4–6 weeks.

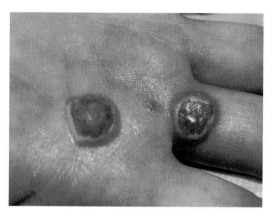

FIGURE 6. Classic lesions of orf demonstrating a central ulceration and a necrotic vesiculobullous edge.

BIBLIOGRAPHY

1. Anonymous: Prevention of varicella: Update recommendations of the Advisory Committee on Immunization Practices (ACIP). MMWR 48(RR-6):1–5, 1999.
2. Balfour HH Jr: Antiviral drugs. N Engl J Med 340:1255–1268, 1999.
3. Bodnar MG, Miller OF 3rd, Tyler WB: Facial orf. J Am Acad Dermatol 40:815–817, 1999.
4. Brown ZA: Genital herpes complicating pregnancy. Dermatol Clin 16:805–810, 1998.
5. Cohen JI, Brunell PA, Straus SE, Krause PR: Recent advances in varicella-zoster virus infection. Ann Intern Med 130:922–932, 1999.
6. Kushner D, Caldwell BD: Hand-foot-and-mouth disease. J Am Podiatr Med Assoc 86:257–259, 1996.
7. McCrary ML, Severson J, Tyring SK: Varicella zoster virus. J Am Acad Dermatol 41:1–14, 1999.
8. Wald A: Herpes: Transmission and viral shedding. Dermatol Clin 16:795–757, 1998.
9. Whitley RJ, Kimberlin DW, Roizman B: Herpes simplex viruses. Clin Infect Dis 26:541–553, 1998.

26. WARTS (HUMAN PAPILLOMAVIRUS INFECTIONS)

Barbara R. Reed, M.D.

Tom Sawyer on Curing Warts
"You got to go all by yourself, to the middle of the woods, where you know there's a spunk-water stump, and just as it's midnight you back up against the stump and jam your hand in and say:
Barley-corn, barley-corn, injun-meal shorts,
Spunk-water, spunk-water, swaller these warts,
and then walk away quick, 11 steps, with your eyes shut, and then turn around three times and walk home without speaking to anybody. Because if you speak the charm's busted."

—Tom Sawyer to Huck Finn
in *The Adventures of Tom Sawyer* by Mark Twain

1. What causes warts?
Warts are caused by a virus, the human papillomavirus (HPV). HPV is a circular, double-stranded DNA virus containing approximately 8,000 base pairs. There are at least 80 types of HPV.

2. Name the common types of warts.

Clinical Presentation of Common Types of Warts

TYPE OF WART	USUAL LOCATION	COMMON PRESENTATION	COMMON HPV TYPES
Common (verruca vulgaris)	Varies	Flesh-colored, rough, hyperkeratotic papules; single or grouped	2, 4, 29
Plantar, palmar	Soles, palms	Thick, hyperkeratotic lesions; may be painful	1, 2, 4, 10
Flat (verruca planae)	Face, hands, knees	Small, 2–5-mm, flat-topped, hyper-pigmented papules; multiple	3, 10
Anogenital (condyloma acuminatum)	Genitalia, anogenital region	Moist, cauliflower-like masses, variably sized; sexually transmitted	6, 11, 42–44

HPV infection is highly specific for epidermis, especially extremities, palms, and soles but also the scalp and mucosal surfaces such as the mouth, larynx, genital areas, and rectal mucosa. Some types of HPV have a predilection for infection in certain locations in the body. For example, flat warts are seen mostly on the face and hands of children and are often caused by HPV types 3 and 10 (Fig. 1A). Common warts occur most often on the fingers and periungual skin and are commonly due to HPV types 2, 4, and 29 (Fig. 1B). Warts in immunosuppressed patients are caused by HPV type 8 and others (Fig. 1C).

3. How frequently are the different cutaneous warts seen?
The three types of cutaneous HPV infections are widespread throughout the general population. Common warts, which represent up to 71% of cutaneous warts, occur frequently among school-aged children, with a prevalence of 4–20%. Plantar warts are most common among adolescents and young adults and represent about 34% of cutaneous warts. Flat warts are least common (4%) and affect mostly children. Other groups at high risk for cutaneous warts are butchers, meat packers, and fish handlers.

4. Can warts cause cancer?
Certain types of HPV infection have been associated with the development of malignancy. Although bowenoid papulosis is not considered a premalignancy, it may be associated with an increased risk of cervical cancer. Carcinomas of the conjunctiva, cornea, nasal cavities, oral cavity, esophagus, and plantar surface of the foot also have been reported in association with various types of HPV.

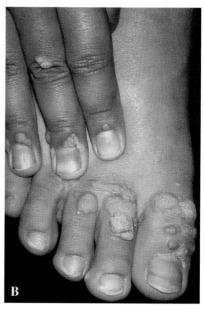

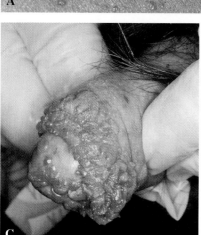

FIGURE 1. Some common types of warts. *A*, Flat warts of the face presenting as multiple 1–2-mm papules. *B*, Multiple common warts of the hands and feet (*A–B* courtesy of James E. Fitzpatrick, MD). *C*, Condyloma accuminatum of the penis presenting as moist cauliflower-like papillomas (courtesy of Scott Norton, MD).

TYPE OF WART	ASSOCIATED CONDITION	HPV TYPES
Bowenoid papulosis	Increased risk of cervical dysplasia and neoplasia in women	16 (majority), 18, 31, 32, 34, 35, 39, 42, 48, 51–54
Buschke-Lowenstein	Verrucous carcinoma in anogenital area	6
Epidermodysplasia verruciformis	Polymorphic: flat warts, pityriasis versicolor–like	5, 8 in 90%; 19–25, 36, 46, 47, 50
Laryngeal tumors	Laryngeal papillomatosis in children	5,11
Squamous intraepithelial neoplasia	Varies	6, 11, 16, 18, 30, 31, 33–35, 39, 40, 42, 45, 51, 52, 56, 58
Invasive anogenital cancers	Varies	16, 18, 31, 33, 35, 45, 51, 52, 56

5. What is epidermodysplasia verruciformis (EV)?

EV is a rare, inherited disorder in which cutaneous HPV infection is generalized and persistent. Most cases are autosomal recessive, but autosomal dominant and X-linked dominant forms are also reported. The lesions are either flat warts or reddish-brown macular plaques, often developing in sun-exposed areas (Fig. 2A). Malignant change occurs in about one-third of cases, but metatasis is uncommon. At least 15 types of HPV are associated with EV, and more than one type of HPV may be found in the same patient.

6. What techniques are used to study warts?

Polymerase chain reaction combined with ELISA, in situ hybridization, or reverse dot-blot hybridization. Nucleotide sequencing may provide further characterization.

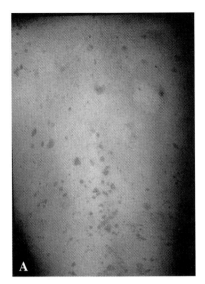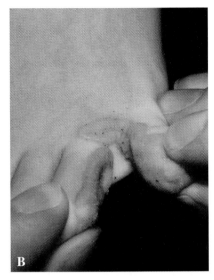

FIGURE 2. *A*, Multiple reddish-brown macules of the back in a patient with epidermodysplasia verruciformis. *B*, "Kissing" warts produced by inoculation of the toe web space. (Courtesy of James E. Fitzpatrick, MD.)

7. How does a person become infected with warts?

HPV infection occurs after exposure to humans or animals with HPV infection. The most common mode of transmission is through **touch** or **contact** from an individual infected with HPV, although HPV may also survive on inanimate objects for unknown amounts of time. Small abrasions or cracks in the skin of exposed persons allow the virus to penetrate. Such infection may commonly occur at a swimming pool, where chlorinated water and rough concrete surfaces may abrade the skin, or at other public places. Genital warts may be transmitted through sexual intercourse. People who work with meat, fish, and poultry also commonly have warts in the hand and forearm area, thought to be promoted through microinjuries sustained during processing of animals or fish as well as from prolonged immersion of the skin in water.

Autoinoculation is another form of transmission. Periungual warts are often found in persons who have a habit of biting their cuticles, for example. Presumably the excoriated areas are more hospitable to virus on contaminated surfaces, but spread of a single common wart is also possible. Flat warts in the beard area or on the legs may be spread by shaving.

8. Do warts spread?

Yes, especially if they are injured. Such injury may happen if the warts are in a location traumatized by shaving or scratching. This reaction is known as the Koebner phenomenon. (The Koebner reaction is also present in skin conditions that have no known viral cause, such as psoriasis and lichen planus.) Close approximation of two surfaces, where one surface is affected and the opposing surface is unaffected, is also associated with an increased likelihood of spreading (e.g., adjacent toe surfaces, Fig. 2B).

9. How long is the incubation period of warts?

Unknown. It is estimated to be several weeks to over 1 year.

10. How can warts be prevented?

No one is certain how to avoid the development of warts.

11. Can HPV live in the human body in a dormant state?

HPV is demonstrable by DNA hybridization and polymerase chain reaction in skin which is clinically normal, indicating the likelihood of a latent or subclinical form of HPV. In addition, it is not uncommon for a wart to recur in the same location many years following apparent resolution.

12. Are plantar warts caused by a special kind of virus? Are they more difficult to treat?

The term *plantar wart* refers to a location rather than to a pattern of behavior. Plantar warts are simply warts on the plantar aspect (sole) of the foot. Warts in this location have a unique appearance from being compressed by the pressure of walking.

Plantar warts are more difficult to eradicate, for reasons which are not entirely clear. Excision by scalpel or laser often results in scarring, and recurrence is common. Repeated liquid nitrogen treatment may be painful, inconvenient, and costly. Home treatments with salicylic acid pads, along with judicious trimming to maintain comfort, seem to be most helpful. Glutaraldehyde, which produces a brown discoloration of treated surfaces, has also been used successfully.

13. What causes the black dots within a wart?

The small black dots, incorrectly referred to as "seeds," are actually thrombosed blood vessels.

14. Can HPV infection have a hereditary basis?

Except in the case of epidermodysplasia verruciformis, warts are not inherited. However, our immune systems are inherited, and some people seem to have inherited an immune system that places them at risk for acquiring HPV infection. For example, women with HPV involving the cervical and/or vaginal areas have given birth to babies with laryngeal warts.

15. Are some people more susceptible to warts than others?

Immunocompromised individuals, such as those with HIV infection or cancer, or transplant patients on immunosuppressive drugs are more susceptible to warts than others. Sexual intercourse at an early age is a known risk factor for acquiring genital warts. Children with atopic dermatitis may have warts that are more extensive and more difficult to eradicate.

16. Should all warts be eradicated?

It is not possible to eradicate certain warts, and it is economically impossible to eradicate all warts in the human population. With nongenital warts, if a wart is large enough to cause discomfort, is disfiguring, or is on a body part that is constantly traumatized, treatment should be considered.

17. How should external genital warts (EGWs) be treated?

Clinical examination is sufficient for evaluation. Treatment goals should be to eliminate symptomatic warts. Sexual partners of patients with EGWs should be evaluated for warts or other sexually transmitted diseases. Women with EGWs should have cervical cytologic screening. HPV detection and EGW typing are not currently required for diagnosis or management. In minors, the presence of EGWs should prompt an evaluation for sexual abuse.

18. What methods are available for the treatment of warts?

Over-the-counter methods for eliminating warts include topical applications of acids such as salicylic or lactic acid. These may be in a liquid form or may be incorporated into plasters.

TREATMENT	WART TYPE	COMMENTS
Destructive methods		
Cryotherapy, electrosurgery	All	Dyschromia, pain
Surgery	Resistant	Scar, recurrence
Laser	Resistant	CO_2 and Nd:YAG lasers
Caustic acids		
Mono-, di-, and trichloracetic acid	Common	Irritation, blisters, scar
Cantharadin	Small, common	Irritation, blisters, hyperpigmentation
Chemotherapeutic agents		
Podophyllotoxin*	External genital	Erythema, erosions, ulcers, pain
Imiquimod*	External genital	Erythema, burning, erosion
Bleomycin (intralesional)*	Common	Pain, nail loss, nail dystrophy, Raynaud's phenomenon
5-Fluorouracil (topical)*	Flat	Irritation

Table continued on next page.

TREATMENT	WART TYPE	COMMENTS
Miscellaneous		
Interferon*	Anogenital	Inject intralesional or intramuscular
Tretinoin (topical)*	Flat	Irritation
Glutaraldehyde	Plantar	Brown discoloration, allergy
Cimetidine (oral)*	Resistant	Best in children
Salicylic acid	Common, plantar	Available over-the-counter
Retinoids*	Immunosuppression	Relapse when drug is discontinued
Formalin*	Plantar	Contact sensitivity

*Avoid during pregnancy.

When choosing a treatment plan for warts, the physician's primary concern should be to *not* make the treatment worse than the warts. For example, a treatment worse than the disease would be to excise and suture a wart on the weight-bearing surface of the foot and then have the wart recur in the middle of a painful scar. Sometimes the best treatment is benign neglect. Resistance and recurrence are common with all treatments.

19. What are common side effects of treatment methods?

Scarring (liquid nitrogen, laser, acids, cantharadin)

Blistering (liquid nitrogen, cantharadin, topical 5-fluorouracil, bleomycin) (Fig. 3A)

Allergy (cantharadin, chemotherapeutic agents, tretinoin, acids, glutaraldehyde)

Persistent hyper- or hypopigmentation (liquid nitrogen)

20. What are "fairy ring" warts?

Satellite warts are not uncommon following any treatment that produces blisters (Fig. 3B).

21. Should any treatments be avoided?

- During pregnancy, chemotherapeutic agents, interferon, and retinoids should be avoided, and careful consideration should be given to use of acids and cantharadin. Liquid nitrogen and laser are safe for use during pregnancy.
- Bleomycin should be avoided around fingernails, as permanent nail dystrophy, Raynaud's phenomenon, and sclerotic changes in the distal finger have been reported.
- X-irradiation is not indicated for treatment of warts. Increased invasiveness of lesions following radiation has been reported.

22. Is there a best way to treat warts?

No single treatment method may be relied upon to eliminate warts permanently. Treatment choice must depend on the location, appearance, and symptoms of the wart.

Facial: These warts are usually flat and can respond to treatment with topical tretinoin cream. Liquid nitrogen may be used cautiously, but persistent hypopigmentation is an undesired side effect.

Weight-bearing (plantar): These warts are treated with combinations of acid plaster or liquid acid preparations and/or liquid nitrogen. Glutaraldehyde, intralesional bleomycin, or laser may be used in refractory cases.

Nails: Periungual warts may be treated with topical acids or cantharadin. Liquid nitrogen, often helpful in the treatment of common warts, should be used cautiously here because of the intense pain it causes, as well as risk of persistent nail deformity.

Genital: Genital warts may be treated with liquid nitrogen, podophyllin or derivatives, topical acids, 5-fluorouracil, imiquimod, or cidofovir. Refractory warts may be treated with interferon. Laser may also be indicated in some cases.

Children: Salicylic acid plasters and liquids, cantharadin, and liquid nitrogen have been used successfully. There are recent reports of success using oral cimetidine in prepubertal children with extensive common warts. Laser may be used in refractory warts.

Many warts regress without treatment. It is speculated that such warts are identified as foreign by the owner's immune system, which then rejects the wart.

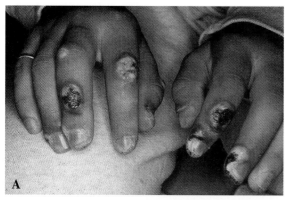

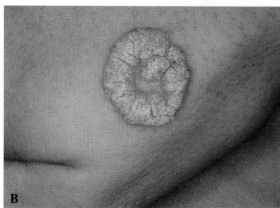

FIGURE 3. Side effects of wart treatment. *A*, Painful blisters produced by cantharadin (courtesy of Brenda Kodomo, MD). *B*, Fairy-ring formation of warts on the wrist, at the periphery of a blister produced by previous liquid nitrogen therapy (courtesy of James E. Fitzpatrick, MD).

23. How can you tell if a wart is gone?
Treatment success is considered the return of normal body skin lines.

24. How can you be sure that warts will never come back?
You can't.

25. Do any warts come from toads?
No. There is no supportive scientific evidence—whether histologic, viral, or other—that the bumps on the skin of a toad are at all related to warts.

BIBLIOGRAPHY

1. Beutner KR, Wiley DJ, et al: Genital warts and their treatment. Clin Infect Dis 28(Suppl 1):S37–S56, 1999.
2. Crum C: Genital papillomaviruses and related neoplasms. Mod Pathol 7:138–145, 1994.
3. Fazel N, Wilczynski S, Lowe L, Su LD: Clinical, histopathologic, and molecular aspects of cutaneous human papillomavirus infections. Dermatol Clin. 17:521–536, 1999
4. Highet AS, Kurtz J: Human papillomavirus (HPV) and warts. In Champion RH, Burton JL, Ebling FJG (eds): Rook/Wilkinson/Ebling Textbook of Dermatology, 5th ed. Oxford, Blackwell Science, 1992.
5. Moscicki AB: Human papillomavirus infection in adolescents. Pediatr Clin North Am 46:783–807, 1999.
6. Orlow SJ, Paller A: Cimetidine therapy for multiple viral warts in children. J Am Acad Dermatol 28:794–796, 1993.
7. Shama SK, Androphy EJ, Galen WK, et al: Guidelines of care for warts: HPV. Dermatol World Aug(suppl): 15–19, 1993.
8. Stern P, Levine N: Controlled localized heat therapy in cutaneous warts. Arch Dermatol 128:945–948, 1992.
9. Syrjanen KJ: Human papillomavirus in genital carcinogenesis. Sex Transm Dis 21(2 Suppl):S86–S89, 1994.

27. BACTERIAL INFECTIONS

James E. Fitzpatrick, M.D.

STAPHYLOCOCCAL INFECTIONS

1. Which bacterium is the most common cause of skin infections?
Staphylococcus aureus.

2. What kinds of skin infections does *S. aureus* produce?

Impetigo (bullous impetigo)	Staphylococcal scalded skin syndrome
Furuncles (boils)	Staphylococcal cellulitis
Carbuncles	Toxic shock syndrome
Superficial folliculitis	Staphylococcal scarlet fever
(impetigo of Bockhart)	Wound infections
Staphylococcal septicemia	Secondary infections of dermatitis

The most common primary infections are impetigo and furuncles.

3. Is *S. aureus* the only bacterium that causes impetigo?
Older textbooks state that the most common cause of impetigo (impetigo contagiosum) is group A β-hemolytic *Streptococcus*. In recent years, most infections in the United States have been due to *S. aureus,* but the prevalence varies geographically. While impetigo may be due to either organism, in many cases both can be cultured. In these cases, it is thought that the streptococci are the primary infection and the staphylococci are secondary invaders after the infection has damaged the skin.

4. What does staphylococcal impetigo look like?
Early lesions of staphylococcal impetigo appear as thin, flaccid blisters that may demonstrate cloudy contents or layering of pus (Fig. 1). The base of the blister may demonstrate variable erythema. Histologically, the blisters are very superficial; the split occurs beneath the stratum corneum. For this reason, the blisters quickly collapse and may demonstrate a shiny lacquered appearance. Older lesions demonstrate a yellowish crust.

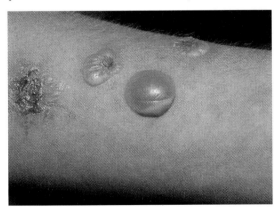

FIGURE 1. Early lesion of bullous staphylococcal impetigo demonstrating fragile bullae with layering of the pus. Collapsed blister with lacquered appearance is also present.

5. Why is staphylococcal impetigo frequently bullous?
Bullous impetigo is caused by staphylococci that produce toxins (exfoliative toxins A and B) capable of causing the split in the epidermis. Group II staphylococci are most commonly implicated.

6. How is bullous impetigo diagnosed?
The **clinical appearance** is usually suggestive but not diagnostic, and other superficial blistering or pustular disorders need to be considered, such as pemphigus, some bullous drug eruptions,

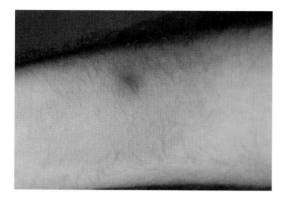

FIGURE 2. Furuncle presenting as a very tender, erythematous follicular-based abscess.

and subcorneal pustular dermatosis. A **Gram stain** of the blister contents should demonstrate abundant gram-positive cocci, but the definitive test is a **culture,** that not only establishes the cause but also provides sensitivities to different antibiotics. The diagnosis can also be established by doing a **biopsy,** which demonstrates a subcorneal blister with neutrophils and cocci in the blister cavity.

7. How is bullous impetigo treated?

Oral dicloxacillin or cephalexin are the antibiotics of choice for severe infections. Oral erythromycin is frequently used in penicillin-allergic patients, although up to 20% or more of all staphylococci are resistant. Topical mupirocin is also effective and can be used if the patient cannot take oral antibiotics.

8. What is the difference between a furuncle and a carbuncle?

A **furuncle** (boil) is a deep follicular abscess, and a **carbuncle** is a more serious subtype in which there is involvement of several adjoining follicles. A furuncle may develop into a carbuncle. Carbuncles are more likely to develop complications, such as cellulitis or septicemia.

9. How do furuncles present?

Furuncles may be solitary or multiple and present as painful, erythematous, deep-seated follicular abscesses (Fig. 2). Patients may demonstrate mild constitutional symptoms in severe cases, or lesions may progress into carbuncles or staphylococcal cellulitis.

10. What is the best way to treat furuncles?

As always, the diagnosis should be confirmed with a culture and antibiotic sensitivities performed at the initial visit, since not all follicular-based abscesses are due to staphylococci. Following culture, the patient should be treated with oral dicloxacillin or oral cephalexin. Oral erythromycin, azithromycin, or clarithromycin can be used if the patient is allergic to penicillin. Oral dicloxacillin is the mainstay of outpatient treatment of staphylococcal infections because 97% of all organisms are sensitive. Nonsuppurative lesions can also be treated with local heat. Fluctuant furuncles should be opened and drained. Smaller lesions may be punctured with a no. 11 blade and the contents drained, while large abscesses may require a larger incision, drainage, and a wick.

11. Why do some patients develop recurrent staphylococcal impetigo or recurrent furunculosis?

Recurrent infections occur when *Staphylococcus aureus* establishes itself as a part of the resident microbial flora. This occurs in up to 20% of individuals. The most common sites of carriage are the anterior nasal vestibule, axilla, groin, and feet. Patients who have virulent strains are prone to the development of recurrent impetigo or furunculosis depending on the strain. A variety of host factors, such as abnormal neutrophil chemotaxis (e.g., hypergammaglobulinemia IgE syndrome), deficient intracellular killing (e.g., chronic granulomatous disease), and immunodeficiency states (e.g., AIDS), are important in a minority of patients. Diabetes mellitus is listed in many references as being associated with recurrent furunculosis, but this is controversial.

12. How is staphylococcal carriage eliminated?

Standard treatment regimens, such as oral dicloxacillin, oral cephalexin, oral erythromycin, or even intravenous vancomycin, eliminate active infection but not staphylococcal carriage. The most commonly used regimen to eliminate staphylococcal carriage is **rifampin** in combination with **dicloxacillin.** Less common regimens utilize oral clindamycin, topical mupirocin ointment, or replacement of the microflora with a less pathogenic strain of *S. aureus* (strain 502A). The success of these regimens varies from 50–70%.

13. What is staphylococcal scalded-skin syndrome?

Staphylococcal scalded-skin syndrome typically occurs in neonates, infants, or immunocompromised adults. Like bullous impetigo, it is due to group II staphylococci that produce an exfoliatoxin; however, it differs in that the infection occurs at a distant site, such as a conjunctivitis or abscess. In neonates and infants, the kidneys are not able to excrete the exfoliatoxin adequately. The high level of exfoliatoxin produces diffuse, tender erythema associated with fever that rapidly progress to flaccid bullae; the bullae wrinkle and exfoliate, leaving an oozing erythematous base (Fig. 3). Mortality in neonates is usually not due to the infection but is secondary to impaired temperature regulation or fluid balance.

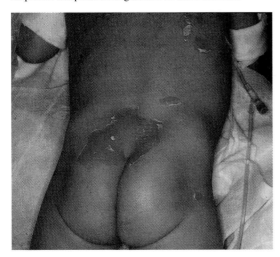

FIGURE 3. Early staphylococcal scalded skin syndrome demonstrating diffuse erythema and early desquamation.

14. Describe the presentation of toxic shock syndrome.

Toxic shock syndrome is an acute febrile illness due to *Staphylococcus aureus* strains that produce pyrogenic exotoxins. These toxin-producing strains have been isolated classically from superabsorbent tampons in menstruating women but are also found in abscesses, wound infections, or the vaginas of nonmenstruating women.

Clinically, the hallmarks are fever, hypotension, and a diffuse erythema that resembles scarlet fever. Other manifestations include pharyngeal erythema, strawberry tongue, conjunctival infection, and gastrointestinal symptoms. Desquamation of the palms and soles occurs 1–2 weeks following resolution of the erythema.

15. Why is *S. aureus* frequently found in secondary infections of dermatitis and wounds?

S. aureus has receptors that allow it to bind to fibrin that is found in abundance on wound surfaces and in dermatitic skin.

STREPTOCOCCAL INFECTIONS

16. What types of cutaneous infections are produced by β-hemolytic streptococci?

β-hemolytic streptococci are responsible for impetigo, blistering distal dactylitis, ecthyma, erysipelas, necrotizing fasciitis, and septicemia.

17. How does streptococcal impetigo present?

Streptococcal impetigo presents as superficial, stuck-on, honey-colored crusts overlying an erosion (Fig. 4). The most common location is the face, but any area may be involved. In contrast to staphylococcal impetigo, blisters are absent.

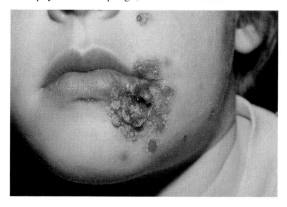

FIGURE 4. Characteristic stuck-on, honey-colored crusts of streptococcal impetigo.

18. What is ecthyma?

Ecthyma is a severe form of streptococcal impetigo in which there is a thick crust overlying a punched-out ulceration of the epidermis (Fig. 5). Typically, it is surrounded by a zone of erythema. In contrast to streptococcal impetigo, which is usually found on the face and does not produce scarring, ecthyma is more commonly located on lower extremities and may heal with scarring.

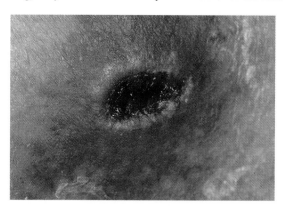

FIGURE 5. Streptococcal ecthyma demonstrating punched-out ulceration surrounded by erythema.

19. What is blistering distal dactylitis?

Blistering distal dactylitis is an uncommon infection typically caused by *Streptococcus pyogenes* but occasionally may be caused by *Staphylococcus aureus*. It typically presents in young children as one or more tender superficial bullae on an erythematous base on the volar fat pad of a finger (Fig. 6). In rare instances toes may be affected.

20. What is erysipelas?

Erysipelas, or St. Anthony's fire, is a form of cellulitis usually caused by β-hemolytic streptococci, rarely by *Staphylococcus aureus*. Patients often have a prodrome of malaise, fever, and headache. Typically, erysipelas presents on the face as an erythematous indurated plaque with a sharply demarcated border and a "cliff-drop" edge (Fig. 7). In severe cases, the epidermis may become bullous, pustular, or necrotic. Untreated erysipelas can be fatal due to vascular thrombosis, bacteremia, or toxin release. **Streptococcal cellulitis** is a more generic term that includes erysipelas but also cellulitis that lacks the characteristic "cliff-drop" border. Known commonly as "blood poisoning," it is most often found on extremities and is associated with lymphangitis (Fig. 8).

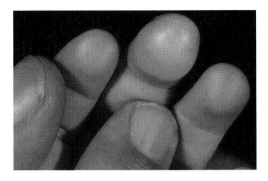

FIGURE 6. Blistering distal dactylitis demonstrating a characteristic tender superficial blister on the volar fat pad.

21. How do you diagnose erysipelas?

The diagnosis usually is made clinically because the organism is difficult to recover in culture. Aspiration of the advancing edge following the injection of nonbacteriostatic saline produces positive cultures in about 20% of cases.

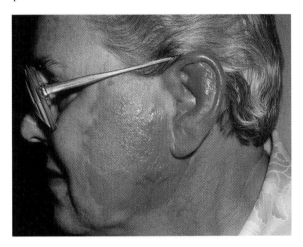

FIGURE 7. Characteristic lesion of erysipelas demonstrating indurated, erythematous plaque with sharply demarcated border.

22. How is erysipelas treated?

Mild or early cases may be treated with an oral penicillin or oral erythromycin. Oral **dicloxacillin** is the best choice since it provides better antistaphylococcal coverage for the rare case of staphylococcal erysipelas. Severe cases or cases with central facial involvement should be hospitalized and treated with intravenous antibiotics, such as vancomycin. Erysipelas usually improves within 48 hours after institution of antibiotic therapy.

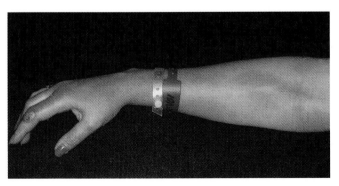

FIGURE 8. Streptococcal cellulitis that started with an injury to the index finger. Note associated lymphangitis extending up the arm.

OTHER BACTERIA

23. Describe the cutaneous manifestations of Lyme disease.

Lyme disease is a multisystem disease caused by *Borrelia burgdorferi* that is transmitted to humans by ticks of the genus *Ixodes*. One to 30 days after the tick bite, patients present with variable constitutional symptoms, including fever, malaise, headache, and arthralgias. Approximately three-fourths of patients develop erythema chronicum migrans that begins as an erythematous papule at the bite site and progresses to an annular erythema that may reach 20 cm or more in size (Fig. 9).

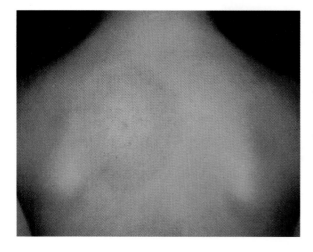

FIGURE 9. Typical lesion of erythema chronicum migrans manifesting as central papule at the tick bite site surrounded by annular erythema.

24. What types of skin infections does *Pseudomonas aeruginosa* produce?

P. aeruginosa is one of the most feared bacterial pathogens in medicine. Cutaneous infections include:

Ecthyma gangrenosum	Wound infections (burn wounds)
Septic vasculitis	Cellulitis
Pseudomonal folliculitis	Necrotizing fasciitis
External otitis media	Onycholysis (green nail syndrome)
Toe web infection	Paronychia

25. How does ecthyma gangrenosum differ from ecthyma?

- Ecthyma is caused by β-hemolytic streptococci, while ecthyma gangrenosum is most commonly caused by *P. aeruginosa*.
- Ecthyma is a localized infection that normally occurs in healthy young adults. Ecthyma gangrenosum usually follows septicemia in a neutropenic patient. Less commonly, it follows primary inoculation into the skin.
- Ecthyma responds rapidly to antibiotics, whereas ecthyma gangrenosum has a high mortality.
- Clinically, ecthyma gangrenosum presents as one or more red macules that become edematous and rapidly progress to hemorrhagic bullae. In the late stages, it may ulcerate or form an eschar surrounded by erythema.

26. Where do you get *Pseudomonas* folliculitis?

In your hot tub. *Pseudomonas* folliculitis is typically associated with hot tub use (hot tub folliculitis). Less commonly, it is associated with whirlpools or swimming pools. It is usually associated with *P. aeruginosa* serotype O:11, although other serotypes have also been reported. *Pseudomonas* folliculitis has also been reported as a complication of depilatories used for the removal of leg hair.

27. How does *Pseudomonas* folliculitis present?

Clinically, it occurs 1–3 days after exposure, presenting as a diffuse truncal eruption. The primary lesion is a follicular-based erythematous papule that frequently demonstrates a follicular pustule. Less commonly, patients may also demonstrate mastitis, abscesses, or lymphangitis. The disease is usually self-limited, although rare patients may continue to develop recurrent folliculitis or abscesses for up to 2 months.

28. What is the best treatment for *Pseudomonas* folliculitis?

Most cases are self-limited and do not require treatment. Severe or recurrent cases can be treated with oral ciprofloxacin. Ultimately, the best treatment is prevention of infection. The most effective measures are frequent drainage of the hot tub or whirlpools to remove the buildup of desquamated skin cells that serve as the prime source of nutrients. Adequate chlorination and bromination are also necessary.

29. How is Wood's light used in diagnosing *Pseudomonas* infections?

P. aeruginosa produces a pigment called pyoverdin that fluoresces yellow-green on Wood's light. The Wood's light is useful in detecting pseudomonads in burn wounds, surgical infections, ulcerated ecthyma gangrenosum, and gram-negative toe web infections.

30. What causes tularemia? Where did the name tularemia come from?

Tularemia is caused by *Francisella* (formerly *Pasteurella*) *tularensis,* a gram-negative coccobacillus. The infection is acquired through handling of infected animals (squirrels and rabbits), tick bites, and deerfly bites. Tularemia gets its name from Tulare County in California, the site where researchers isolated the organism from ground squirrels in 1911. The term was first used by Dr. Francis, who was subsequently honored by having the genus named after him.

31. Describe the skin lesions of tularemia.

Tularemia has six presentations: ulceroglandular, glandular, oculoglandular, oropharyngeal, typhoidal, and pneumonic forms. The ulceroglandular form is the most common presentation and the one that typically demonstrates skin lesions. The primary skin lesion begins as a small papule at the inoculation site, which rapidly necroses. The papule may be surrounded by an area of cellulitis and is characteristically associated with painful regional lymphadenopathy. Systemic symptoms include fever, chills, headache, and malaise.

32. How should tularemia be treated?

The treatment of choice is streptomycin. Alternate therapies include gentamycin, chloramphenicol, and tetracycline.

BIBLIOGRAPHY

1. Berger RS, Seifert MR: Whirlpool folliculitis: A review of its cause, treatment, and prevention. Cutis 45: 97–98, 1990.
2. Cerny Z: Skin manifestations of tularemia. Int J Dermatol 33:468–470, 1994.
3. Chartier C, Grosshans E: Erysipelas. Int J Dermatol 29:459–467, 1990.
4. Chesney PJ: Clinical aspects and spectrum of illness of toxic shock syndrome: Overview. Rev Infect Dis 11(suppl 1): S1–S7, 1989.
5. Demidovich CW, Wittler RR, Ruff ME, et al: Impetigo: Current etiology and comparison of penicillin, erythromycin, and cephalexin therapies. Am J Dis Child 144:1313–1315, 1990.
6. Greene SL, Su WP, Muller SA: Ecthyma gangrenosum: Report of clinical, histopathologic, and bacteriologic aspects of eight cases. J Am Acad Dermatol 11:781–787, 1984.
7. Lina G, Gillet Y, Vandenesch F, et al: Toxin involvement in staphylococcal scalded skin syndrome. Clin Infect Dis 25:1569–1575, 1997.
8. Malane MS, Grant-Kels JM, Feder HM Jr, Luger SW: Diagnosis of Lyme disease based on dermatologic manifestations. Ann Intern Med 114:490–498, 1991.
9. Wheat JL, Kohler RB, Luft FC, White A: Long-term studies of the effect of rifampin on nasal carriage of coagulase-positive staphylococci. Rev Infect Dis 5(Suppl 1): S459–S462, 1981.

28. SYPHILIS

James E. Fitzpatrick, M.D.

"Know syphilis in all of its manifestations and relations, and all other things clinical will be added unto you."

—Sir William Osler, 1897

1. What causes syphilis?

Syphilis is caused by the spirochete *Treponema pallidum,* ssp *pallidum,* which belongs to the order Spirochaetales. *T. pallidum* ssp endemicum is a subspecies that causes bejel, or endemic syphilis. Other pathogenic treponemes for humans include *T. pallidum* ssp *pertenue,* the cause of yaws, and *T. carateum,* the cause of pinta. There are other *Treponema* species that infect other animals or are free-living.

2. Describe the morphologic appearance of *T. pallidum.*

T. pallidum is a delicate spiral bacterium that measures 6–20 μm in length and 0.10–0.18 μm in width (Fig. 1). Because of the narrow width, it is not visible by normal light microscopy and must be visualized by darkfield microscopy or by silver stains (i.e., Warthin-Starry or modified Steiner stains). The spiral coils are regularly spaced at a distance of about 1 μm. The typical spirochete has 6–14 coils. The organism reproduces by transverse fission.

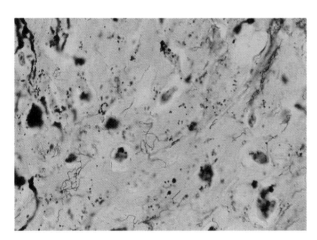

FIGURE 1. Biopsy of secondary syphilis demonstrating numerous spirochetes in the epidermis (Warthin-Starry stain, 1000 ×).

3. Where did syphilis originate?

The origin of syphilis is controversial. An epidemic of syphilis ravaged Europe in the last decade of the 15th century, when it was referred to as the "Great Pox" (as opposed to small pox). Because this epidemic coincided with the return of Columbus from America in 1493, many authorities believe that it was imported from the West Indies. Of interest, Columbus himself is thought to have died from syphilitic aortitis.

The alternative theory is that syphilis was already endemic in the Old World but was spread more rapidly during the wars that occurred shortly after the return of Columbus.

4. How is syphilis transmitted?

Syphilis is most commonly acquired as a sexually transmitted disease but also may be acquired congenitally (see Chapter 56) or, rarely, by blood transfusions. The organism is very fragile and easily killed by heat, cold, drying, soap, and disinfectants. Since the spirochete is so fragile, the possibility that an infection could be acquired from a toilet seat is statistically very remote.

5. What are the chances of getting syphilis from having sexual intercourse with an infected individual?

The definitive study has obviously never been done, but epidemiologic studies show that the chances are about one in three. It is believed that the treponemes cannot penetrate intact epidermis or mucosa and that most infections occur in microscopic or macroscopic breaks in the skin.

6. Following inoculation, how long does it take for the primary chancre to appear?

Experimental study on both rabbits and human volunteers has shown that the appearance of the primary chancre is related to the size of the inoculum. The primary chancre normally appears in 10–90 days, with the average time being about 3 weeks. The organism reaches the regional lymph nodes within hours.

7. Describe the typical Hunterian chancre.

The classic Hunterian chancre develops at the site of inoculation as a painless ulcer with a firm, indurated border (Fig. 2). The size may vary from a few millimeters to several centimeters in diameter. Associated unilateral or bilateral, painless, regional, nonsuppurative lymphadenopathy develops in 50–85% of patients approximately 1 week after the appearance of the primary ulcer. It is important to realize that up to 50% of all chancres are atypical. Painful ulcers, multiple ulcers (Fig. 3) , secondarily infected ulcers, and nonindurated ulcers are variations on the classic chancre.

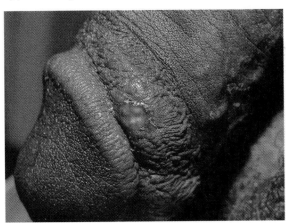

FIGURE 2. Typical Hunterian chancre of syphilis demonstrating characteristic indurated border.

8. Do syphilitic chancres occur on sites other than the genitalia?

Extragenital chancres occur in 5% of all cases of primary syphilis, although the incidence may be as high as 10%. The most common extragenital sites are the lip, which is associated with oral sex, and anus, which is associated with anal intercourse. Anal intercourse may also produce rectal or colonic chancres as high as 20 cm in the bowel. Other reported sites include the tongue, tonsil, finger, eyelid, chin, nipple, umbilicus, axilla, and even the lower limb. A high index of suspicion is required to diagnose extragenital chancres.

9. What is the best way to diagnose primary syphilis?

Diagnosis cannot be based on clinical presentation alone, and unfortunately, *T. pallidum* cannot be cultured. The most specific and rapid method of diagnosing primary syphilis is the demonstration of the spirochete utilizing **darkfield examination** by a trained observer. This test is not readily available to most community physicians and usually requires sending the patient to an STD clinic or medical center. The material for examination can be obtained from either the ulcer or an aspirate from an enlarged lymph node. A single negative darkfield examination does not rule out the possibility of syphilis, and it should not be regarded as negative until there are negative examinations on 3 consecutive days. Primary syphilis can also be diagnosed by **biopsing** the primary ulcer and demonstrating the organism by **special stain.**

In lieu of these procedures, a presumptive diagnosis can be made by serologic tests (see Chapter 3). The **Venereal Disease Research Laboratory** (VDRL) test and **rapid plasma reagin** (RPR) test are negative in early primary syphilis and should be repeated weekly for 1 month to be considered as negative. The diagnosis is more likely if a rising titer can be demonstrated. The **fluorescent treponemal antibody-absorption** (FTA-ABS) test turns positive earlier and is more sensitive.

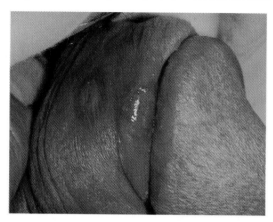

FIGURE 3. Atypical presentation of primary syphilis demonstrating two chancres. (Courtesy of William James, MD.)

10. How is primary syphilis treated?

The recommended treatment for primary syphilis is benzathine penicillin G, 2.4 million units in a single intramuscular dose. Patients who are allergic to penicillin can be treated with either doxycycline (100 mg orally two times per day for 28 days) or tetracycline (500 mg orally four times per day for 28 days), or ceftriaxone (125 mg intramuscularly every day for 10 days, 250 mg intramuscularly every other day, or 1000 mg intramuscularly for 4 doses).

Treatment failures have been reported with all regimens, and patients should have follow-up serologic titers at 3, 6, 12, and 24 months to ensure a fourfold decline in titers. Patients need to be reported to the proper public health agency to ensure tracking of known sexual partners.

11. What is the Jarisch-Herxheimer reaction?

This acute febrile reaction, associated with shaking chills, malaise, sore throat, myalgia, headache, and localized inflammation of infected mucocutaneous sites, usually occurs 6–8 hours following penicillin treatment. Tetracycline, doxycycline, and ceftriaxone are less commonly associated with this reaction. It develops in 50% of patients with primary syphilis, 75% with secondary syphilis, and 30% with neurosyphilis. There is indirect evidence that this reaction is due to the release of a treponemal lipopolysaccharide that acts like a bacterial endotoxin. Similar reactions have been reported with other infectious diseases, including leptospirosis and louse-borne relapsing fever.

12. What is the natural history of the untreated syphilitic chancre?

The untreated syphilitic chancre lasts for about 2–8 weeks and then disappears. The primary chancre may relapse, in which case it is referred to as **chancre redux.**

13. When does secondary syphilis begin?

Secondary syphilis usually begins about 6 weeks after the onset of the primary chancre. In approximately 25% of cases, the primary ulcer will still be present. In one study, 25% of patients with secondary syphilis did not recall a primary chancre.

14. Do patients with secondary syphilis have any symptoms?
The most common reported symptoms include malaise (23–46%), headache (9%–46%), fever (5%–39%), pruritus (42%), and loss of appetite (25%). Less common symptoms include painful eyes, joint or bone pain, meningismus, iritis, and hoarseness. Some textbooks incorrectly state that pruritus is uncommon in secondary syphilis.

15. List the common physical findings in secondary syphilis.

Syphiloderm (rash)	88–100%	Hepatosplenomegaly	23%
Lymphadenopathy	85–89%	Mucous patches	7–12%
Residual primary chancre	25–43%	Alopecia	3–11%
Condylomata lata	9–44%		

16. Describe the syphiloderm of secondary syphilis.
The syphiloderm of secondary syphilis is most commonly a maculopapular dermatitis with variable scale (70%), papular (12%), or macular (10%). Less common morphologic appearances include annular, pustular, and psoriasiform lesions. The rash typically demonstrates a widespread symmetrical distribution, although in some patients, lesions may be localized to a single anatomic region, such as the palms and soles. In a large study done in the United States, the most common sites of involvement, in descending order, were the soles, trunk (Fig. 4A), arms, genitals, palms (Fig. 4B), legs, face (Fig. 4C), neck, and scalp.

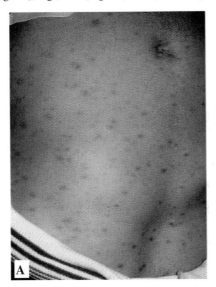
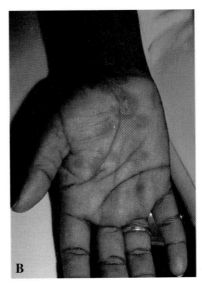
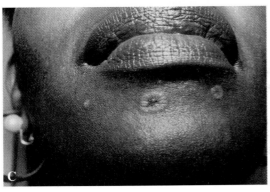

FIGURE 4. Secondary syphilis. *A*, Hyperpigmented macules of secondary syphilis in a patient who was initially treated as chancroid. Note the strong similarity of these lesions to pityriasis rosea. *B*, Characteristic papulosquamous lesions of secondary syphilis on the palm of a nurse. Macular or papulosquamous lesions on the palms are not diagnostic but are suggestive of secondary syphilis. *C*, Annular lesions of secondary syphilis on the face.

17. What are condylomata lata? How do they differ from condylomata accuminata?

Condylomata lata are whitish or grayish, elevated, broad, flat papular lesions of secondary syphilis that primarily occur in moist areas, such as the penis (Fig. 5A), labia, inner thighs, and anal region. These papular lesions may coalesce to form verrucous plaques that are easily confused with **condylomata accuminata,** which are genital warts caused by human papillomavirus. Condylomata lata are more common in women than men.

18. What are mucous patches?

Shallow, usually painless erosions of the mucous membranes (Fig. 5B). Some mucous patches demonstrate linear shapes and have been described as resembling "snail tracks."

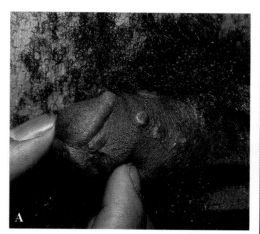
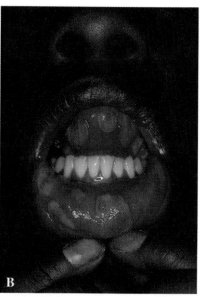

FIGURE 5. *A,* Exophytic condylomata lata of the penis that were referred to the author for treatment of "venereal warts." *B,* Discrete, white, focally eroded mucous patches of secondary syphilis.

19. Is there anything characteristic about the alopecia of secondary syphilis?

The hair loss primarily affects the scalp but may also involve the eyebrows and eyelashes. It presents as a nonscarring, patchy alopecia that is described as a **"moth-eaten" pattern** (see Chapter 20, Fig. 7). This classic pattern appears to be uncommon in the 20th century. The most common pattern of hair loss in secondary syphilis today is a nonspecific diffuse hair loss due to a **telogen effluvium.**

20. How good are physicians at recognizing the signs and symptoms of secondary syphilis?

In a retrospective study of 34 patients with secondary syphilis who had been seen previously by community physicians, only 40% of physicians listed secondary syphilis as the primary diagnosis. Another 14% included secondary syphilis in their differential diagnosis. In sum, almost one-half of physicians did not consider the diagnosis.

21. What is the best way to diagnose secondary syphilis?

The diagnosis of secondary syphilis requires a health care provider with a strong index of suspicion. The cutaneous manifestations of secondary syphilis may mimic other skin diseases, including pityriasis rosea, psoriasis, erythema multiforme, and pityriasis lichenoides et varioliformis acuta, and some drug reactions. It is a good rule of thumb to consider secondary syphilis in any patient having a generalized dermatitis with associated lymphadenopathy.

As with primary syphilis, the most specific tests are the demonstration of the spirochete in either a skin biopsy or on darkfield examination, which can be performed on either the secondary skin lesions or aspirates from lymph nodes. In contrast to primary syphilis, serologic tests are almost invariably positive. The only exception is when there is a false-negative reaction due to a prozone phenomenon which occurs in 1–2% of patients with secondary syphilis. The prozone phenomenon occurs when the titers are very high and can be eliminated by diluting the serum.

22. How should secondary syphilis be treated?
The same as for primary syphilis.

23. What stage follows untreated secondary syphilis?
The mucocutaneous lesions of secondary syphilis usually heal without scarring in 2–10 weeks, although hyperpigmentation or hypopigmentation may persist. Following the resolution of secondary syphilis, patients enter the **latent stage** of infection. During this stage, approximately one-fourth of patients experience relapsing secondary lesions. Most relapses occur in the first year, but these may occur for up to 5 years.

24. How is latent syphilis treated?
For the purpose of treatment, the Centers for Disease Control and Prevention defines infections of <1 year as early latent syphilis and infections of >1 year as late latent. The World Health Organization considers early latent syphilis to extend up to 2 years.

Like primary and secondary syphilis, early latent syphilis is treated with 2.4 million units (mu) of benzathine penicillin G intramuscularly in a single dose. Late latent syphilis or latent syphilis of unknown duration is treated with a total of 7.2 mu of benzathine penicillin G intramuscularly administered as three doses of 2.4 mu intramuscularly at 1-week intervals. Penicillin-allergic patients are treated with doxycycline or tetracycline for 2 weeks in early latent syphilis and for 4 weeks in late latent syphilis.

25. When should lumbar punctures be done in patients with syphilis?
Lumbar punctures to rule out neurosyphilis are recommended for patients with late latent syphilis of more than 1-year duration or unknown duration who demonstrate neurologic symptoms, treatment failure, serum non-treponemal antibody titer equal to or greater than 1:32, other evidence of active syphilis (iritis, aortitis, gumma), non-penicillin treatment, or positive HIV test. Syphilis frequently attacks the central nervous system as demonstrated by the fact that 40% of patients with primary or secondary syphilis demonstrate cerebrospinal fluid pleocytosis and 24% of patients with secondary syphilis demonstrate a reactive VDRL.

26. What happens to patients with untreated latent syphilis?
Approximately one-third of patients with untreated latent syphilis develop tertiary syphilis. The other two-thirds of patients will not develop later effects of the disease.

27. Name the three major presentations of tertiary syphilis.
1. Late benign syphilis
2. Cardiovascular disease
3. Neurosyphilis (general paresis or tabes dorsalis)

28. What are the mucocutaneous features of late benign syphilis?
Late benign syphilis usually occurs 1–46 years after resolution of the secondary skin lesions. Although almost any organ may be involved, the most common organ is the skin (70%) followed by the mucous membranes (10%) and bones (10%). The primary lesion of late benign syphilis is the gumma. A gumma is a granulomatous lesion that contains treponemes only rarely; it probably represents a hypersensitivity reaction.

The skin lesions of late benign syphilis present as nodules and plaques that demonstrate a tendency for central healing and peripheral extension. The central healed areas characteristically demonstrate scarring and atrophy (Fig. 6). The mucosal lesions may involve any mucosal surface but demonstrate a tendency to extend to and destroy the nasal cartilage, producing a "saddle nose" deformity. Involvement of the mucosa over the hard palate may produce a perforation.

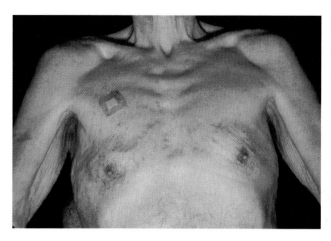

FIGURE 6. Tertiary cutaneous syphilis demonstrating characteristic annular appearance with mild central atrophy. (Courtesy of Richard Gentry, MD.)

BIBLIOGRAPHY

1. Chapel TA: Physician recognition of the signs and symptoms of secondary syphilis. JAMA 246:250–251, 1981.
2. Chapel TA: The signs and symptoms of secondary syphilis. Sex Transm Dis 7:161–164, 1981.
3. Chapel TA, Prasad P, Chapel J, Lekas N: Extragenital syphilitic chancres. J Am Acad Dermatol 13:582–584, 1985.
4. Gourevitch MN, Slewyn P, Davenny K, et al: Effects of HIV infection on the serologic manifestations and response to treatment of syphilis in intravenous drug users. Ann Intern Med 118:350–355, 1993.
5. Hira SK, Patel JS, Bhat SG, et al: Clinical manifestations of secondary syphilis. Int J Dermatol 26:103–107, 1987.
6. Romanowksi B, Sutherland R, Fick GH, et al: Serologic response to treatment of infectious syphilis. Ann Intern Med 114:1005–1009, 1991.
7. Tanabe JL, Huntley AC: Granulomatous tertiary syphilis. J Am Acad Dermatol 15:341–344, 1986.

29. LEPROSY (HANSEN'S DISEASE)

Loren E. Golitz, M.D.

1. Why is leprosy called Hansen's disease?

Leprosy is referred to as Hansen's disease to honor Gerhard Armauer Hansen, a Norwegian physician who discovered the leprosy bacterium in 1873. *Mycobacterium leprae* was the first bacillus to be associated with a human disease.

In addition, as with AIDS, there are considerable social stigmata associated with having leprosy. Therefore, rather than referring to patients as lepers and the disease as leprosy, it is often preferable to use the term Hansen's disease.

2. Was leprosy described in the Bible?

Actually, the condition equated with leprosy in the Bible (Leviticus 13 and 14) has none of the clinical features of leprosy, and most likely it represents another disease or diseases.

3. How is leprosy transmitted?

For years, it was believed that leprosy was transmitted by prolonged skin-to-skin contact, such as between parents and their children. Although the mode of transmission is still uncertain, it seems most likely that *M. leprae* is transmitted via the nasorespiratory route.

4. Are children and adults equally susceptible to acquiring leprosy?

Children and young adults seem to be most susceptible to acquiring leprosy. Only about 5% of adults at risk, such as marriage partners, develop leprosy. As many as 60% of children of a parent with leprosy develop the disease. *M. leprae* may be present in breast milk, and there is some evidence to suggest that the infection can be transmitted via the placenta.

5. Are humans the only host for *M. leprae*?

It was once believed that humans were the only natural reservoir for *M. leprae*. More recently, three other animals have been shown to carry the infection: the nine-banded armadillo, chimpanzee, and sooty mangabey monkey. Up to 10% of wild armadillos in Louisiana and eastern Texas have naturally acquired leprosy.

6. Is leprosy a systemic disease?

Yes. Although the peripheral nerves and skin are most notably affected, leprosy has involved every organ except for the CNS and lung.

7. How common is leprosy?

There are about 5 million persons with leprosy worldwide, about half of whom are receiving antibiotic therapy. Leprosy is endemic in 53 countries, including India, which has an estimated 3 million cases. About 6,000 individuals in the United States have leprosy, many of whom have come from foreign countries.

8. Are there endemic areas for leprosy in the United States?

Southern Texas and Louisiana are considered endemic for leprosy. Southern California and Florida also have many cases. Large cities such as New York and San Francisco have many leprosy cases from other countries.

9. How is leprosy recognized clinically?

The two most useful features are a **skin rash** and areas of **cutaneous anesthesia**. Other features are nerve enlargement, nasal stuffiness, inflammatory eye changes, and loss of eyebrows. A reactional state in lepromatous leprosy causes multiple tender red nodules resembling erythema nodosum (erythema nodosum leprosum).

10. Is there more than one kind of leprosy?

Four major variants of leprosy represent a spectrum of disease: indeterminate leprosy, tuberculoid leprosy, lepromatous leprosy, and dimorphous (or borderline) leprosy (Fig. 1).

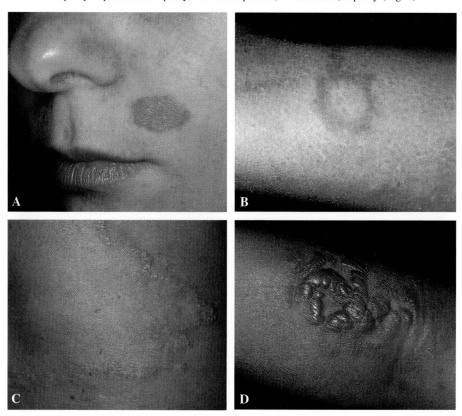

FIGURE 1. Skin lesions in four variants of leprosy. *A,* Indeterminant leprosy. A solitary erythematous macule on the face of a young family member of a patient with lepromatous leprosy. *B,* Tuberculoid leprosy. A solitary well circumscribed, annular anesthetic patch on the leg. *C,* Dimorphous leprosy. A solitary anesthetic annular patch with a scaly border on the trunk. *D,* Lepromatous leprosy. Coalescent brown, firm nodules on an extremity.

11. Are all variants of leprosy equally common?

Although it varies from country to country, about 90% of the leprosy cases in the United States are of the lepromatous type.

12. Does indeterminate leprosy mean that you do not know what type it is?

No. Indeterminate leprosy is believed to be the very first sign of infection with the leprosy bacillus. It usually manifests as a solitary macular skin lesion that is vaguely defined and either erythematous or hypopigmented. Patients with indeterminate leprosy may clear spontaneously or progress to one of the other three types of leprosy.

13. What are the two "polar" forms of leprosy, and how do they differ?

Tuberculoid leprosy and **lepromatous leprosy** are considered the two polar forms, and they tend to remain stable clinically. Patients with tuberculoid leprosy have a high degree of immunity against *M. leprae* and have few skin lesions and few organisms in their skin. Patients with lepromatous leprosy have low immunity against *M. leprae* and have many skin lesions and millions of organisms in their skin.

Clinical Features of Leprosy Skin Lesions

CUTANEOUS LESIONS	TUBERCULOID	DIMORPHOUS	LEPROMATOUS
Number	Few	Numerous	Many
Size	Large	Large and small	Small
Symmetry	Asymmetrical	Symmetrical	Symmetrical
Sensation	Anesthetic	Variable	Variable
Surface	Rough, scaly	Rough, scaly	Smooth
Edge	Sharp	Sharp	Vague

14. Describe dimorphous leprosy.

Dimorphous leprosy, also known as borderline leprosy, shows features intermediate between tuberculoid and lepromatous leprosy. It is a less stable form of leprosy, and its clinical features and immune status may change over time. If dimorphous leprosy develops more features of lepromatous leprosy, it is referred to as dimorphous-lepromatous. If it develops features of tuberculoid leprosy, it is called dimorphous-tuberculoid.

15. What is the unusual feature of the cell-mediated immunity in lepromatous leprosy?

Patients with lepromatous leprosy have a specific energy to *M. leprae*. This is in contrast to diseases such as sarcoidosis and Hodgkin's lymphoma, in which there is loss of immunity to a wide variety of antigens. The clinical spectrum of leprosy appears to depend mainly on an individual's ability to develop effective cell-mediated immunity against *M. leprae*. In endemic areas, most individuals appear to be completely resistant to infection with the leprosy bacillus.

16. How is the diagnosis of leprosy usually made?

The diagnosis of leprosy is usually made by demonstrating cutaneous anesthesia, by finding enlarged superficial nerves, and by demonstrating leprosy bacilli in the skin.

1. **Cutaneous anesthesia** is best diagnosed by using a wisp of cotton to demonstrate loss of light touch. In tuberculoid and dimorphous leprosy, sensation is lost within the center of skin lesions, which are often annular. In lepromatous leprosy, the loss of light touch sensation typically occurs first in fingers and toes, while anesthesia in individual skin lesions may be variable.

2. **Nerve enlargement** in tuberculoid and dimorphous leprosy occurs within or adjacent to specific skin lesions. In lepromatous leprosy, large peripheral nerves can be palpated. The easiest nerves to palpate are the posterior auricular nerve behind the ear and the ulnar nerve at the elbow (Fig. 2).

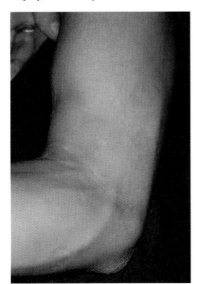

FIGURE 2. Nerve enlargement. Palpable or visually enlarged nerves may be a sign of leprosy.

3. The **demonstration of *M. leprae* in the skin** may be accomplished by a "slit skin smear" by experienced personnel. For those not experienced with the technique, it is easier and more reliable to simply perform a skin biopsy and request a special stain for the leprosy bacillus.

17. What area should be biopsied to detect *M. leprae*?

The raised active margin of tuberculoid and dimorphous skin lesions. For lepromatous leprosy, the biopsy specimen should be taken from a cutaneous papule or nodule.

18. Can the same acid-fast stain used for *Mycobacterium tuberculosis* be used for the leprosy bacillus?

M. leprae is less acid-fast than *M. tuberculosis*, and a modified acid-fast stain known as the Fite stain should be used to demonstrate organisms in tissue (Fig. 3).

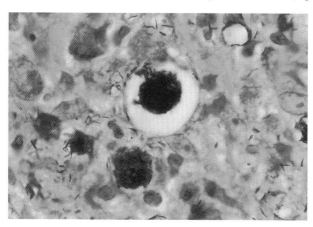

FIGURE 3. Fite stain for *Mycobacterium leprae*. This skin biopsy shows clusters of acid fast leprosy bacilli. The clusters are called glob). (Courtesy of James E. Fitzpatrick, MD.)

19. Is the lepromin skin test helpful in making a diagnosis of leprosy?

No, but it is useful in classifying leprosy into the various subtypes. Lepromin is a crude preparation of killed bacteria from a lepromatous nodule or from infected armadillo liver. An intradermal injection of 0.1 ml of lepromin is read at 48 hours for erythema (Fernandez reaction) or at 3 4 weeks for a papule or nodule (Mitsuda reaction). Patients with tuberculoid leprosy have strongly positive reactions, while dimorphous and lepromatous patients are usually negative. The reaction in indeterminate leprosy is variable.

20. Is the neuropathy in lepromatous leprosy the same as that in diabetic neuropathy?

No. Although the neuropathy is similar in the two diseases, it is a true "stocking-glove" anesthesia in diabetes mellitus. In leprosy, the cooler parts of the skin and nerves are affected, which gives the peripheral neuropathy a spotty and variable expression. For example, the dorsal aspects of the hands may be anesthetic, while the palms are partially spared. This has led some neurologists to misdiagnose leprosy patients as malingerers or neurotics.

21. Describe a patient with advanced lepromatous leprosy.

The skin shows widespread, hyperpigmented papules and nodules with a predilection for cool parts of the body, such as the earlobes, nose, fingers, and toes. There may be loss of the lateral eyebrows (madarosis) (Fig. 4), redness of the conjunctiva, a stuffy nose, flattening of the nasal bridge, and a palpable postauricular nerve. There is marked anesthesia of the extremities with some atrophy of the thenar and hypothenar muscles (Fig. 5A). Contraction of the fourth and fifth fingers may be seen, resulting in difficulty in extending the fingers fully. Ulcers or sores of the hands and feet may be present secondary to minor trauma or burns (Fig. 5B). A plantar ulcer surrounded by hyperkeratotic skin (mal perforans ulcer) may be present over a pressure area (Fig. 5C). The physician should inquire whether the patient is from an endemic area for leprosy.

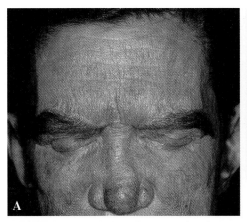
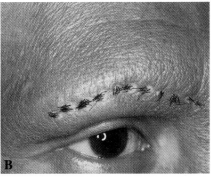

FIGURE 4. Madarosis (loss of eyebrows) is an important sign in leprosy. *A*, This patient has heavy eyebrows due to hair transplants and dark skin color due to the drug clofazamine. *B*, This patient has just received eyebrow transplants.

22. What are the most common complications in leprosy?
1. Traumatic ulcers in anesthetic extremities
2. Reactional states that follow successful drug therapy

23. What are the reactional states of leprosy?
There are two types of reactions that may occur spontaneously but often follow the initiation of antibacterial therapy by months to years. Approximately half of all leprosy patients experience one of these acute inflammatory episodes at some point in their disease course.

Type I reactions, also called **reversal reactions**, complicate unstable dimorphous leprosy and represent alterations in the patient's cell-mediated immunity. The immunity may be either upgraded or downgraded. Typically in type I reactions, existing lesions become acutely inflamed.

Type II reactions, also called **erythema nodosum leprosum** (ENL), occur in lepromatous leprosy (Fig. 6). ENL reactions are believed to represent immune complex precipitation in blood vessels due to released antigens from *M. leprae* organisms that have been damaged by antibiotic therapy. The patients develop red tender nodules mainly on their extremities associated with constitutional symptoms including fever, arthralgias, lymphadenitis, and neuritis.

24. What is chaulmoogra oil?
Chaulmoogra oil is a plant compound that was developed in Burma early in the 1900s. It was found to have weak antileprous properties and was the first effective treatment for leprosy.

25. Is dapsone the treatment of choice for leprosy?
Dapsone was first used to treat leprosy in the early 1940s at the U.S. Leprosarium in Carville, Louisiana. It was the first highly effective agent to treat leprosy and remains an important drug worldwide in the management of the disease. However, during the 1960s and 1970s resistant strains of *M. leprae* developed to monotherapy with dapsone. About half of all new patients have resistant strains, although resistance is believed to be less common in the United States.

26. What drugs are used in multidrug therapy for leprosy?
Because of the resistance to dapsone, multidrug therapy is currently used for leprosy and has resulted in a dramatic improvement in prognosis and a decrease in reported new cases worldwide. Only four drugs are readily available in the United States to treat leprosy: dapsone, rifampin, clofazimine, and ethionamide. Of these agents, only rifampin is bactericidal.

Recommended therapy for **lepromatous leprosy** in the United States is dapsone, 100 mg/day for life, and rifampin, 600 mg/day for 3 years. For **tuberculoid leprosy**, the recommended treatment is dapsone, 100 mg/day for 5 years.

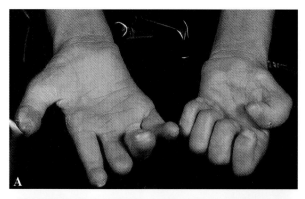

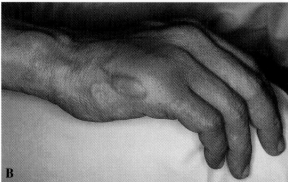

FIGURE 5. Features of advanced lepromatous leprosy. *A*, The hands often show contractures and muscle atrophy of the thenar and hypothenar eminences. *B*, Accidental burn. Because of anesthetic extremities patients with lepromatous leprosy are subject to burns and other minor trauma. *C*, Mal perforans ulcers. Patients with lepromatous leprosy develop foot ulcers surrounded by thick keratin as a result of peripheral anesthesia.

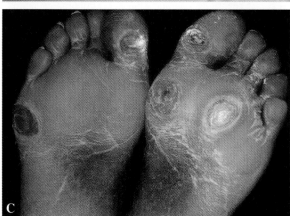

27. Do the recommendations of the World Health Organization differ?

Due to economic and other factors, the WHO treatment recommendations are different from those of the U.S. The WHO recommends three drugs for treatment of **lepromatous leprosy**, due to concern about dapsone resistance, but limits treatment to about 5 years: dapsone, 100 mg/day; rifampin, 600 mg/month (due to the expense of the drug); and clofazamine, 300 mg/day. **Tuberculoid leprosy** is treated with dapsone, 100 mg/day, and rifampin, 600 mg/month for 6 months.

28. Does dapsone have any side effects?

Overall, dapsone is a safe drug and is safe to use during pregnancy. All patients on dapsone experience hemolysis of older red blood cells with a mild drop in hematocrit. Patients who are

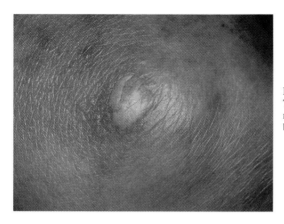

FIGURE 6. Erythema nodosum leprosum. The reactive state in lepromatous leprosy resembles erythema nodosum but may be bullous, as seen in this patient.

glucose-6-phosphatase dehydrogenase deficient may develop severe hemolysis. Methemoglobinemia is also regularly observed but is usually not a significant problem since the level usually does not exceed 12% of the total hemoglobin. Idiosyncratic reactions such as pancytopenia, peripheral neuropathies, acute psychosis, and mononucleosis-like syndrome may also develop.

29. What are the side effects of clofazimine?

The most bothersome side effect of clofazimine is a red to brown to purple discoloration of the skin.

30. How are the reactional states of leprosy treated?

Type I reactions, if severe, require prednisone, 40-80 mg/day. **Mild type II** reactions may be controlled with aspirin, nonsteroidal anti-inflammatory agents, and rest. **More severe type II** reactions may be controlled with thalidomide 400 mg at night. Thalidomide should not be given to women of child-bearing age because of its severe teratogenic effects. If thalidomide is not available, type II reactions can usually be controlled with prednisone, 40-80 mg/day.

31. Should family members of leprosy patients be treated?

Dapsone prophylaxis of all family members is not currently recommended. However, children and spouses should be examined at least once a year by experienced medical personnel.

32. Can leprosy be eliminated as a worldwide disease, like smallpox?

The worldwide prevalence of leprosy has been reduced from 20 million to 5 million, but the disease is far from being eliminated. Leprosy vaccines are being studied.

BIBLIOGRAPHY

1. Bryceson ADM: Leprosy. In Champion RH, Burton JL, Ebling EJG (eds): Rook/Wilkinson/Ebling, Textbook of Dermatology, Oxford, Blackwell Scientific Publications, 1992, pp 1065–1083.
2. Gelber RM: Hansen's disease. West J Med 158:583–590,1993.
3. Goodless DR, Ramos-Caro FA, Flowers FP: Reactional states in Hansen's disease: Practical aspects of emergency management. South Med J 84:237–241,1991.
4. McDougall AC, Ulrich MI: Mycobacterial disease: Leprosy. In Fitzpatrick TB, Eisen AZ, Wolff K, et al (eds): Dermatology in General Medicine. New York, McGraw-Hill, 1993, pp 2395–2409.
5. Meyers WM: Leprosy. Dermatol Clin 10:73–96,1992.
6. Meyers WM, Marty AM: Current concepts in the pathogenesis of leprosy: Clinical, pathological, immunological and chemotherapeutic aspects. Drugs 41:832–856,1991.
7. Okoro AN: Pre-emptive diagnosis of leprosy. Int J Dermatol 30:767–771,1991.
8. Rea TH, Modlin RL: Immunopathology of leprosy skin lesions. Semin Dermatol 10:188–193, 1991.

30. MYCOBACTERIAL INFECTIONS

Syed O. Ali, M.D., CPT, USA, and Karen E. Warschaw, M.D., LTC, USAF

1. What is the classification system of mycobacteria?

Extensive taxonomic work has been done to classify the more than 60 species of organisms belonging to the genus *Mycobacterium*. Runyon, in the 1950s classified the atypical mycobacteria based on their rate of growth, ability to form pigment, and colony characteristics. The classification may also include distinctions among obligate human pathogens requiring direct person-to-person transmission, facultative human pathogens found in the environment rarely responsible for direct person-to-person spread and nonpathogens.

Classification of Pathogenic Mycobacteria

	OBLIGATE HUMAN PATHOGEN	FACULTATIVE HUMAN PATHOGEN
Slow growers		
M. tuberculosis complex		
M. tuberculosis	X	
M. bovis	X	
M. africanum	X	
M. mycoti	X	
Photochromogens (Runyon group 1)		
Form yellow-orange pigment with light		
M. kansasii		X
M. marinum		X
(others include *M. simiae*, *M. intermedium*, and *M. asiaticum*)		
Scotochromogens (Runyon group 2)		
Form orange-red pigment without light		
M. scrofulaceum		X
M. szulgai		X
(others include *M. injectum*, *M. lentiflavum*, and *M. gordonae*)		
Nonchromogens (Runyon group 3)		
Unable to form pigment		
M. avium-intracellulare		X
M. haemophilum		X
M. xenopi		X
M. ulcerans		X
(others include *M. celatum*, *M. genavense*, *M. gastri*, and *M. malmoense*)		
Rapid growers (Runyon group 4)		
Growth within 7 days		
M. fortuitum		X
M. chelonei ssp. *abscessus*		X
M. chelonei ssp. *chelonei*		X
(others include *M. phlei* and *M. smegmatis*)		
Noncultivable		
Unable to cultivate in media		
M. leprae	X	

2. What are the staining characteristics of mycobacteria?

Mycobacteria are aerobic, non–spore-forming, nonmotile bacilli. They do not stain readily, but their most useful staining characteristic is acid fastness. Acid fastness refers to the ability to retain carbol fuchsin dye after washing with acid or alcohol as a result of a high content of cell wall mycolic acids, fatty acids, and other lipids. Other staining methods include the Dieterle, hematoxylin-eosin, auramine-rhodamine, and phenolic acridine orange stains. Acid fastness is also shared by *Nocardia*, *Rhodococcus*, *Legionella micdadei*, *Isospora*, and *Cryptosporidium*.

TUBERCULOSIS

3. How many species of *Mycobacterium* cause infection in human beings?

There are approximately 30 species of *Mycobacterium* that cause disease in humans. The primary culprits include *M. tuberculosis* complex, *M. leprae*, and atypical mycobacteria.

4. Name three mycobacteria in the tuberculosis complex responsible for tuberculosis.

The three species most significant to human disease in the *M. tuberculosis* complex include *M. tuberculosis*, *M. bovis*, and *M. africanum*. Under certain conditions the attenuated strain of *M. bovis*, bacillus Calmette-Guérin (BCG), may also cause disease.

5. What is tuberculosis?

Tuberculosis is a systemic infectious disease that can affect any organ system, including the skin. The lungs, however, are the most commonly involved organ. Cutaneous tuberculosis has a broad clinical spectrum depending on the route of infection, virulence of the organism, and immune status of the host. Lupus vulgaris and scrofuloderma, although rare, are the two most common forms of cutaneous tuberculosis.

Classification of Cutaneous Tuberculosis

	PRIMARY INFECTION (NON-IMMUNE HOST)	SECONDARY INFECTION (IMMUNE HOST)
Exogenous		
Primary inoculation tuberculosis	X	
Tuberculosis verrucosa cutis		X
Endogenous		
Scrofuloderma		X
Orificial tuberculosis		X
Hematogenous/lymphatic		
Lupus vulgaris		X
Acute miliary tuberculosis	X	

6. What is the difference between a primary and secondary infection?

Primary-inoculation tuberculosis occurs in a host not previously infected. A **secondary infection** occurs in a previously infected host either as a reactivation years later from a primary focus, endogenous spread to new areas, or exogenous reinfection.

7. Explain the route of infection in cutaneous tuberculosis.

Cutaneous tuberculosis may be acquired by three possible routes. The first route is **exogenous infection** acquired from an outside source (primary inoculation tuberculosis and tuberculosis verrucosa cutis). The second route of infection is **endogenous spread**. This can occur by contiguous spread (scrofuloderma), or by autoinoculation (orificial tuberculosis) as organisms are passed from internal organ involvement. The final route is through **hematogenous** or **lymphatic dissemination** (lupus vulgaris and miliary tuberculosis).

8. Who is at risk of acquiring tuberculosis?

In the United States the incidence of tuberculosis was decreasing until 1985 when it reached its nadir. Since 1985 the incidence of tuberculosis has been increasing at an alarming rate. Crowded urban environments, immigration, poverty, homelessness, intravenous drug abuse, loss of tuberculosis control programs, and, most importantly, the HIV epidemic account for the rising incidence. High-risk groups include the elderly, urban homeless, alcoholics, intravenous drug abusers, prison inmates, migrant farm workers, minorities and HIV infected individuals.

9. What is the PPD?

PPD stands for the tuberculin **P**urified **P**rotein **D**erivative and is an intracutaneous skin test. Skin testing consists of intradermal injection into the volar surface of the forearm (Mantoux method). A positive reaction is presumptive evidence of prior exposure to mycobacteria. False-positive reactions may be due to nontuberculous mycobacteria including BCG vaccination. A negative PPD does not rule out tuberculosis.

10. Describe the histopathologic hallmark of tuberculosis.
   The tubercle is the histopathologic hallmark of tuberculosis. This consists of giant cells and epithelioid cells and may have varying amounts of caseation necrosis. This pattern can also be seen in other infections and is not pathognomonic.

11. How can one acquire a primary tuberculous chancre?
   Primary-inoculation tuberculosis occurs from direct inoculation of *M. tuberculosis* into the skin and includes the chancre at the site and affected regional lymph nodes. The organism cannot penetrate intact skin and requires a break in the skin, such as a minor cut or abrasion. Unusual reports have implicated "venereal" inoculation during sexual intercourse, transmission during mouth-to-mouth resuscitation and circumcisions performed by tuberculous rabbis.

12. Describe the clinical manifestation of primary-inoculation tuberculosis.
   Primary tuberculosis may occur in any age group, but is most common in children up to 4 years of age and young adults. The face, mucous membranes (conjunctiva and oral mucosa) and lower extremity are the usual sites of infection. A lesion develops 2–4 weeks after inoculation and presents as a small, non-tender, well-demarcated, non-healing ulcer (Fig. 1). Regional, hard, non-painful lymphadenopathy occurs 3–8 weeks after infection. The PPD may initially be negative and diagnosis is confirmed by culture.

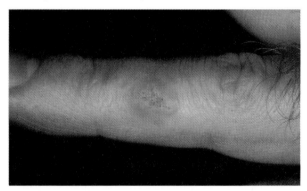

FIGURE 1. Primary-inoculation tuberculosis presenting as an eroded papule. The patient was a microbiologist in a hospital laboratory and this was probably an accidental inoculation. (Courtesy of James E. Fitzpatrick, MD.)

13. What are the different types of cutaneous tuberculosis?
   Tuberculosis of the skin can be divided into two categories; true cutaneous tuberculosis infections and tuberculid reactions. True cutaneous tuberculosis includes lupus vulgaris, tuberculosis verrucosa cutis, cutaneous miliary tuberculosis, cutaneous primary tuberculosis, and tuberculosis cutis orificialis (Fig. 2). A tuberculid refers to a cutaneous or mucosal lesion that represents an immunologic response to a previous infection of tuberculosis at a remote site. Special stains and culture of a tuberculid lesion are negative. Tuberculid reactions include lichen scrofulosorum, papulonecrotic tuberculid, penis tuberculid, erythema induratum.

14. What is the "anatomist's wart"?
   "Anatomist wart" (also known as post mortem wart, prosector's wart, tuberculosis verrucosa cutis, lupus verrucosus, butcher's wart, or warty tuberculosis) is a true cutaneous tuberculosis. It occurs in persons previously exposed to tuberculosis who acquire an exogenous reinfection (secondary infection). Reinfection occurs at sites of abrasions or small cuts, most often on the fingers in Western countries and the lower extremities in tropical regions. Occupations at high risk include medical students, pathologists, and laboratory technicians inoculated during autopsy. Occupations with exposure to cattle such as farmers and butchers may also acquire a similar infection with *M. bovis*.

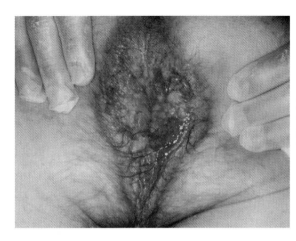

FIGURE 2. Tuberculosis cutic orificialis. Erythematous eroded plaque of perianal area. (Courtesy of James E. Fitzpatrick, MD.)

15. How does the anatomist wart present clinically?

Typically, there is a solitary indurated nodule with a warty surface on the hand or finger. The lesion is asymptomatic and gradually enlarges from a small papule to a hyperkeratotic, irregular red-brown warty plaque that may be confused with a common wart. The regional lymph nodes are generally not involved. The differential diagnosis includes blastomycosis, chromomycosis, and infection due to atypical mycobacteria.

16. Is lupus vulgaris related to lupus erythematosus?

No. Lupus erythematosus is an autoimmune connective tissue disease. Lupus vulgaris is a form of cutaneous tuberculosis. The term lupus is used to depict erosion as if "gnawed by a wolf." Vulgaris means common or ordinary. Both of these terms are used in a variety of unrelated diseases.

17. Describe the clinical manifestations of lupus vulgaris.

Lupus vulgaris is a chronic progressive form of cutaneous tuberculosis that originates from another site and involves the skin or mucous membranes via contiguous, lymphatic, or hematogenous spread. In 40% of patients there is underlying lymphadenitis, and 10–20% have underlying pulmonary involvement. The primary skin lesion is an asymptomatic macule or papule that is brown-red in color and has a soft gelatinous consistency (Fig. 3A). Diascopy, a test where a glass slide is gently pressed against the skin lesion, may be helpful in diagnosing lupus vulgaris. Lupus vulgaris lesions have a characteristic "apple jelly" color with this technique. Squamous cell carcinoma arising in a long-standing lesion is the most serious complication (Fig. 3B).

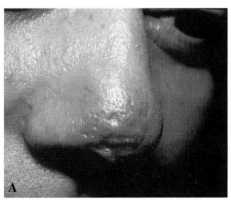
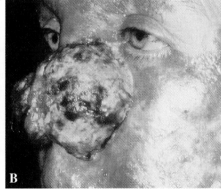

FIGURE 3. Lupus vulgaris. *A*, Red-brown plaque on nasal tip. *B*, Lupus vulgaris with squamous cell carcinoma.

18. Where and when does lupus vulgaris develop?

Lupus vulgaris most often affects patients in their second or third decade of life. The most common site of involvement is the head and neck and in particular, the nose, cheek, and earlobe. There may be extension to involve the oral, nasal or conjunctival mucosa. In the tropics, the buttocks and lower extremities are more often involved.

19. What is scrofuloderma?

Scrofuloderma is a form of cutaneous tuberculosis that originates in tuberculous lymph nodes, bones, joints, or epididymis and spreads directly to the overlying skin. The most common locations include the lateral neck and the parotid, submandibular, and supraclavicular areas. The skin lesion presents as a firm subcutaneous nodule. As the lesion matures there is extensive necrosis leading to a soft, doughy consistency, ulceration with bluish margins, and formation of a sinus tract. Necrotic cheesy material may drain from sinus tracts (Fig. 4).

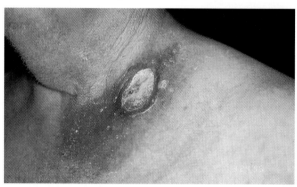

FIGURE 4. Scrofuloderma. Erythematous to violaceous nodule with ulceration. The lesion is an extension from an underlying lymph node.

20. Name the vaccination against tuberculosis. What type of vaccination is it?

Bacillus Calmette-Guérin (BCG) is a live attenuated stain of *Mycobacterium bovis*. It was discovered in 1921, but has not been widely used in the United States with the exception of a very small number of at-risk infants who cannot receive chemoprophylaxis. In third-world countries, the BCG vaccine is widely used. This vaccination is contraindicated in immunosuppressed individuals who are at risk of disseminated *M. bovis* infection.

21. What drugs are used in the treatment of tuberculosis?

Drugs used in the treatment of tuberculosis can be classified into **first-line essential, first-line supplemental**, and **second-line antituberculous drugs**. First-line essential chemotherapeutic agents include isoniazid, rifampin, and rifabutin. First-line supplemental chemotherapeutic agents include pyrazinamide, ethambutol and streptomycin. Isoniazid is the cornerstone of therapy, and rifampin is the second major antituberculous drug. Currently the CDC endorses a number of 6-month and 9-month protocols. The 6-month regimens include an intensive 2-month therapy with three to four agents followed by 4-month therapy with isoniazid and rifampin.

22. What are the major side effects of antituberculous agents?

First-Line Antituberculous Agents and Major Side Effects

DRUG	SIDE EFFECT	SPECIAL COMMENT
Isoniazid	Peripheral neuritis	From pyridoxine deficiency
	Hepatitis	Occurs with 1–2% increased risk with age > 35
Rifampin	Hepatitis	
	Orange stain of secretions	May permanently stain contact lenses
Pyrazinamide	Hyperuricemia	May precipitate gout
Ethambutol	Optic neuritis	Avoid in children under age 13
Streptomycin	Vestibular toxicity	Most common in elderly
	Hearing impairment	

23. What factors have lead to multidrug-resistant tuberculosis?

Multidrug-resistant tuberculosis (MDRTB) is defined as combined resistance to isoniazid and rifampin, and can be either primary or acquired. Primary MDRTB occurs in a person who has not previously been treated, whereas acquired MDRTB is a result of treatment failure. The main factors leading to MDRTB include patient noncompliance in drug therapy, inability or unwillingness to find adequate health care, and inappropriate treatment regimens. Homelessness, intravenous drug use and HIV infection favor the spread of drug resistant tuberculosis. Resistance is prevalent in Asia, South America, and Africa. In the U.S. mini-epidemics of drug resistance are centered in New York City, Miami, and Michigan. Spread to health care workers is a major concern. Treatment cure rates of up to 96% have been published in the medical literature, but this requires aggressive and often very complicated management of the disease.

24. Are there any special treatment considerations for cutaneous tuberculosis?

In general, the treatment of cutaneous tuberculosis is the same as for pulmonary tuberculosis and consists of effective chemotherapeutic agents. Small lesions of lupus vulgaris or tuberculosis verrucosa cutis may be excised, but the treatment must also include standard antituberculous therapy. Surgical drainage of scrofuloderma may shorten the treatment course, and surgical intervention is necessary in any draining lesion.

ATYPICAL MYCOBACTERIA

25. Describe the pathogenesis of the atypical mycobacteria.

Atypical mycobacteria (also known as nontuberculous mycobacteria or NTM) are ubiquitous and are found in soil, water, and domestic and wild animals. As a result of their ubiquitous nature, isolation of these organisms does not necessarily constitute proof of disease. NTMs are generally saprophytes or nonpathogens. In contrast to *M. tuberculosis*, they are not transmitted from person to person. Immunosuppression, organ damage, surgical procedures, or minor cuts and abrasions are a few of the clinical settings in which these organisms can cause disease. Depending on geographic location, atypical mycobacteria may account for 0.5–30% of all mycobacterial infections.

26. What is swimming pool granuloma?

It is an inoculation mycobacteriosis caused by *Mycobacterium marinum*, although very rarely it can be caused by *Mycobacterium gordonae*. *M. marinum* is ubiquitous in aquatic environments, including both fresh and salt water. The organism is inoculated into the skin through small cuts or abrasions while swimming or cleaning aquariums. Following an incubation period of 2–3 weeks (1 week to 2 months in some instances) a small violaceous papule develops at the site of inoculation. The lesion gradually enlarges into a dark red to violaceous plaque. A sporotrichoid pattern may be seen with violaceous nodules along the afferent lymphatics (Fig. 5, *A–B*). The most common sites include hands, feet, elbows, and knees (sites prone to trauma). It is diagnosed through history, biopsy, and culture (Fig. 5C). The lesions typically heal spontaneously, but may disseminate or persist requiring any of a number of different antimicrobial regimens.

27. What is a Buruli ulcer?

Buruli ulcer, caused by *Mycobacterium ulcerans*, is another of the inoculation mycobacteriosis and is the third most common mycobacterial disease in immunocompetent individuals. It occurs in warm tropical climates, most notably Africa, Australia and Mexico. The organism is inoculated into the skin through minor cuts, most commonly on the extensor surface of the extremities. Over a period of 4–6 weeks, a painless subcutaneous swelling develops, which may or may not be pruritic. The swelling then ulcerates and has a necrotic center, undermined borders, and can attain the size of an entire limb. Treatment is primarily surgical.

28. Describe the clinical manifestations of *Mycobacterium avium-intracellulare* complex (MAC) in both non-AIDS and AIDS patients.

Mycobacterium avium complex (MAC) includes both *M. avium* and *M. intracellulare*, although it has recently become clear that *M. avium* is the most common cause. These organisms

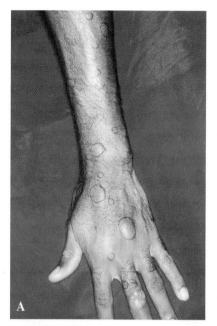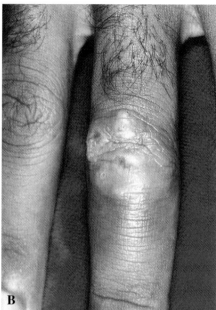

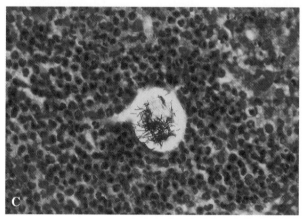

FIGURE 5. Swimming pool granuloma caused by *M. marinum*. *A*, Erythematous nodule on middle finger with sporotrichoid spread along the afferant lymphatics. *B*, Close up of finger nodule. *C*, Ziehl-Nielsen staining demonstrating numerous acid-fast mycobacteria in a patient with swimming pool granuloma (courtesy of James E. Fitzpatrick, MD.)

have gained importance with the epidemic of HIV infection. **HIV-negative persons** most commonly present with pulmonary involvement. Cutaneous disease is rare but may occur as a manifestation of primary intracutaneous inoculation or disseminated disease. The cutaneous lesions are quite variable and include ulcers, abscesses, deep nodules or inflammatory plaques (Fig. 6). **AIDS patients** with MAC generally present with widely disseminated disease (pulmonary, lymph node, gastrointestinal tract, bone). Isolated cutaneous disease is unusual but reported.

29. What is nontuberculous scrofuloderma?
It is a cutaneous manifestation of MAC that usually occurs in young, healthy children. It begins as lymphadenopathy, usually in the cervical region, and slowly enlarges. It may suppurate and rupture, thus forming a chronic draining sinus. It is treated with wide excision of the node.

30. Which atypical mycobacteria are associated with surgical procedures?
The rapidly growing mycobacteria, *M. fortuitum*, *M. chelonei*, and *M. abscessus* (also known as the *M. fortuitum* complex) are ubiquitous and have the ability to survive nutritional depriva-

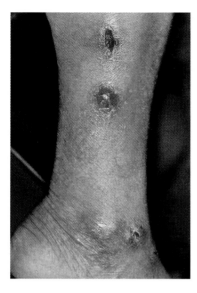

FIGURE 6. *Mycobacterium avium-intracellulare* infection presenting as nodules and ulcerations in an HIV-infected patient. (Courtesy of Margaret Muldrow, MD.)

tion as well as extreme temperatures. These organisms can be found in water, soil, dust, and moist areas in hospitals. Nosocomial infections have included sternal osteomyelitis following open heart surgery, contamination of gentian violet used in preoperative skin markings, hemodialysis, association with various indwelling catheters, and augmentation mammoplasty. Infections also may also be community-acquired through puncture wounds, open fractures, or other trauma (Fig. 7). The incubation period averages 1 month. High-risk patients include those with diabetes. Treatment of the infection consists of debridement of the contaminated area, along with the administration of clarithromycin, clofazimine, and amikacin.

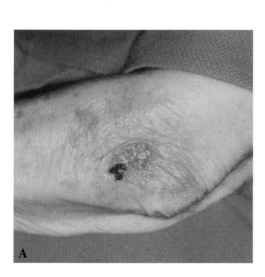

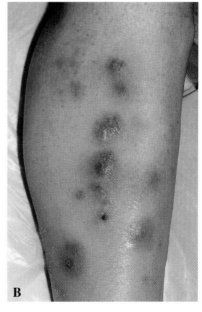

FIGURE 7. Infections with atypical mycobacteria. *A*, Infection caused by *M. fortuitum*. Erythematous plaque with ulceration and necrosis following a puncture wound. *B*, Numerous abscesses and nodules caused by *M. chelonei* infection (courtesy of James E. Fitzpatrick, MD).

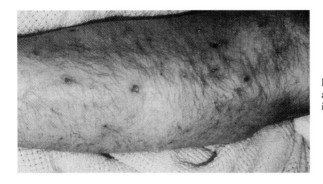

FIGURE 8. Disseminated ulcerated lesions caused by *M. kansasii* in an HIV-infected patient.

31. What are some of the key features of *Mycobacterium kansasii*?

M. kansasii is a photochromogenic acid-fast bacillus. It is found worldwide including the U.S., particularly in the Southwest and the Midwest. The disease is more prevalent in males, elderly, urban, and persons with higher socioeconomic status. It has a predilection for HIV infected individuals (Fig. 8). The usual manifestation of disease in **non–HIV-infected** individuals is pulmonary infection occurring in patients with underlying chronic obstructive pulmonary disease. Cutaneous presentation includes an ulcer with sporotrichoid spread or cellulitis. In **HIV-infected** individuals, almost all colonized patients have disease and require treatment with ethambutol or rifampin.

DISCLAIMER

The opinions or assertions contained herein are the views of the authors and are not to be considered as reflecting the views of the Department of the Air Force, the Department of the Army, or the Department of Defense. This is a work of the U.S. Government and is in the public domain.

BIBLIOGRAPHY

1. Bastian I: Treatment and prevention of multidrug-resistant tuberculosis: Introduction, discussion and summary. Chemotherapy 45(Suppl 2):1–2, 41–45, 1999.
2. Bhattacharya SN: Cutaneous tuberculosis: The evolving scenario. Int J Dermatol 33:97–104, 1994.
3. Connolly B: Scrofuloderma of the lower extremity treated with wide resection: A case report and review of the literature. Am J Orthop 28:417–420, 1999.
4. Edelstein H: Mycobacterium marinum skin infections. Arch Intern Med 154:1359–1364, 1994.
5. Fauci AS (ed): Harrison's Principles of Internal Medicine. New York, McGraw-Hill, 1998.
6. Fitzpatrick TB (ed): Dermatology in General Medicine, 5th ed. New York, McGraw-Hill, 1999.
7. Gart GS: Mycobacterial skin disease: Approaches to therapy. Semin Dermatol 12:352–256, 1993.
8. Kakakhel KU: Cutaneous tuberculosis. Int J Dermatol 28:355–362, 1989.
9. Lao LY: Tuberculin skin testing: Determinants and reaction. Respirology 4:311–317, 1999.
10. Ramesh V: A study of cutaneous tuberculosis in children. Pediatr Dermatol 16:264–269, 1999.
11. Rooney G: Mycobacterium kansasii: Its presentation, treatment and outcome in HIV-infected patients. J Clin Pathol 49:821–823, 1996.
12. Sehgal VN: Cutaneous tuberculosis. Cont Trop Derm 12:645–653, 1994.
13. Van der Werf TS: Mycobacterium ulcerans infection. Lancet 354:1013–1038, 1999.
14. Witzig RS: Clinical manifestations and implications of coinfection with Mycobacterium kansasii and human immunodeficiency virus type 1. Clin Infect Dis 21:77–85, 1995.

31. SUPERFICIAL FUNGAL INFECTIONS

Richard A. Keller, M.D., COL, MC

1. What is a dermatophyte?

A dermatophyte is a fungus that has developed the ability to live on the keratin (hair, nails, or skin scale) of animals. Dermatophytes are classed into three genera: *Microsporum, Trichophyton,* and *Epidermophyton.*

2. How are superficial fungal infections diagnosed?

Superficial fungal infections can usually be suspected clinically, but definitive diagnosis requires the demonstration of fungal pathogens by microscopic examination or culture of skin, nail, or hair scrapings from the suspected lesion. During microscopic examination, hyphae are sought in the material. The material is first placed on a glass slide, and then 1 or 2 drops of 10–20% potassium hydroxide (KOH) are added. A fungal stain such as chlorazol black E may be added to the preparation to aid visualization of the fungal elements. The hyphae of dermatophytes will be septate and typically demonstrate branching. Skin scrapings can also be placed on culture media. Culturing the organism, in addition to being a diagnostic aid, permits speciation of the organism.

3. On a KOH examination, hyphal-like structures arranged in a mosaic pattern are noted. Does this indicate the presence of a dermatophyte?

"Mosaic hyphae" are not really hyphae and do not indicate the presence of a dermatophyte. If you vary the microscope's focus, the pattern can be observed to conform to the cell walls. Mosaic hyphae actually represent thickened stratum corneum cell walls. True hyphae cross the cell walls of keratinocytes and do not conform to the contour of keratinocytes.

4. What are the three most commonly used culture media for the growth of dermatophytes?

Sabouraud's dextrose agar: A nonselective culture medium consisting of peptone, dextrose, agar, and distilled water. It allows the growth of bacteria as well as pathogenic and nonpathogenic yeast and molds.

Mycosel or Mycobiotic Agar: A selective growth medium for dermatophytes. It consists of Sabouraud's agar with cycloheximide (suppresses saprophytic fungi) and chloramphenicol (suppresses bacteria). Dermatophytes and Candida albicans grow readily on this media, while the growth of contaminant bacteria, some yeast, and many opportunistic fungi is inhibited.

Dermatophyte Test Media (DTM): Sabouraud's agar with cycloheximide, gentamicin, and chlortetracycline hydrochloride. It also has a phenol red indicator. If a dermatophyte is present, the color of the media changes from yellow to red. False-positives do occur.

5. Describe some of the presentations of superficial fungal infections caused by dermatophytes.

The superficial dermatophyte infections are classified according to their location on the affected person. This location does not necessarily reveal the identity of the offending organism. The infection will cause the production of scale. The scale may or may not be associated with erythema, vesicles, or annular plaques.

Clinical Presentations of Dermatophyte Infections

Tinea capitis	Scalp
Tinea faciei	Face
Tinea barbae	Beard
Tinea corporis	Trunk, extremities
Tinea cruris	Groin
Tinea manuum (manus)	Hands
Tinea pedis	Feet
Tinea unguium	Nails

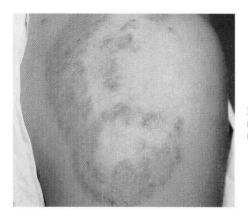

FIGURE 1. Tinea corporis presenting as an erythematous plaque with central clearing. Psoriasis and nummular eczema may look similar to this.

6. Which dermatophyte causes the most fungal infections of skin?
Trichophyton rubrum.

7. What is the most common cause of tinea capitis in the United States?
Until the mid-1950s, *Microsporum audouinii* was the most common cause of endemic tinea capitis in the U.S., but it has since been replaced by *Trichophyton tonsurans*. Several theories have been proposed to explain the almost total disappearance of *M. audouinii* from the U.S., but the most plausible theory is that it was eradicated by the widespread use of griseofulvin. At the same time that *M. audouinii* disappeared, *T. tonsurans,* formerly an uncommon cause of tinea capitis, quickly spread. This species was probably introduced into the U.S. from Central or South America.

8. Name the four clinical patterns of tinea capitis.
1. The **seborrheic** pattern has a dandruff-like scaling of the scalp and should be considered in prepubertal children with suspected seborrheic dermatitis (Fig. 2A).

2. In the **black-dot** pattern, hairs are broken off at the skin line, and black-dots are seen within the areas of alopecia (Fig. 2B). In the United States, this pattern is primarily associated with *T. tonsurans* infections.

3. A **kerion** is an inflammatory fungal infection that may mimic a bacterial folliculitis or an abscess of the scalp (Fig. 2C). The scalp is tender to the touch, and the patient usually has posterior cervical lymphadenopathy.

4. **Favus** is a rare form of inflammatory tinea of the scalp presenting with sites of alopecia that have cup-shaped, honey-colored crusts, which are called *scutula* and are composed of fungal mats.

Tinea capitis is one of the most commonly misdiagnosed skin infections. Any prepubertal child who presents with a scaly scalp dermatitis or carries a diagnosis of seborrheic dermatitis should be presumed to have a dermatophyte infection of the scalp until proven otherwise. Similarly, any child who presents with one or more scalp abscesses most likely has a kerion. Kerions are frequently secondarily infected with *Staphylococcus aureus,* and unsuspecting health care providers often mistakenly treat kerions as bacterial abscesses.

9. What are the types of hair invasion in tinea capitis? What dermatophytes are associated with each type?
Dermatophytes can cause three types of hair invasion:

1. **Endothrix** infections are produced by fungi that invade the inside of the hair shaft and are composed of fungal arthroconidia and hyphae (Fig. 3). A helpful mnemonic to remember the organisms that cause endothrix invasion is: "**TVs** are in houses."—T is *Trichophyton tonsurans*, V is *violaceum*, and S is *soudanense*.

2. **Ectothrix** infections are produced by fungi that primarily invade the outside of the hair shaft. Some agents of small-spore ectothrix cause a fluorescent tinea capitis.

3. **Favus** infections are characterized by invasion of hair by hyphae that do not produce conidia and by the presence of linear air spaces. *T. schoenleinii* is associated with this type of invasion.

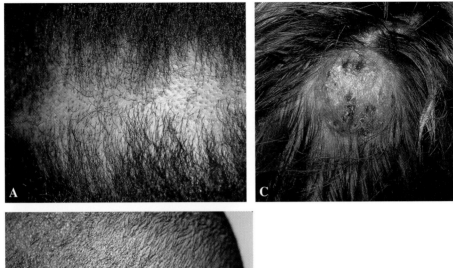

FIGURE 2. Tinea capitis. *A*, Black dot pattern. *B*, Seborrheic pattern. *C*, Kerion presenting as a tender boggy mass in the scalp.

10. What is a Wood's light? What organisms are detected by this exam?

A Wood's light is an ultraviolet light source that emits in the spectrum of 325–400 nm. This light was used extensively for the diagnosis of tinea capitis when *Microsporum audouinii* was the major cause of this disorder. However, it is of limited usefulness today since most cases are now produced by *Trichophyton tonsurans,* which is not fluorescent. The fluorescence is caused by pteridine. The fungi responsible for fluorescent tinea capitis can be remembered by the mnemonic "See Cats And Dogs Fight."

   See—*T. schoenleinii*
   Cats—*M. canis*
   And—*M. audouinii*
   Dogs—*M. distortum*
   Fight—*T. ferrugineum*

Except for *T. schoenleinii,* all of these organisms produce a small spore ectothrix pattern of hair invasion.

11. How is tinea capitis treated?

After the presence of a fungal infection is demonstrated by either culture or a positive KOH smear, treatment with an oral antifungal agent should be instituted. Most patients are placed on griseofulvin. The griseofulvin should be taken with meals to improve absorption. The medication is continued for 4–6 weeks, after which the site is recultured. Using antifungal shampoo may reduce shedding of the organism. Members of the patient's family also should be evaluated for infection or a carrier state and treated if needed. Patients who fail to respond to griseofulvin or are intolerant should be treated with an alternative treatment regimen:

DRUG	DOSE
Fluconazole	6 mg/kg/day for 20 days
Itraconazole	3–5 mg/kg/day for 4–6 weeks
Terbinafine	3–6 mg/kg/day for 4 weeks
	Infections by *M. canis* may require up to 8 weeks of therapy

12. What is meant by a carrier state in tinea capitis?

A carrier is a person who does not have clinical signs of tinea capitis but has a positive fungal culture from the scalp. In families in whom tinea capitis is identified, the carrier rate in adults is around 30%. The presence of these carriers will reduce the cure rate for tinea capitis if they are not treated concomitantly.

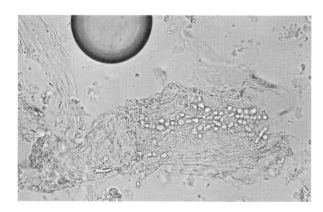

FIGURE 3. Endothrix. The fungal hyphae are seen on the inside of the hair shaft. (Courtesy of Dirk Elston, MD.)

13. Name the three types of tinea pedis. Which dermatophyte is most commonly associated with each?

Interdigital infections, moccasin-type infection, and vesiculobullous or inflammatory infection. **Interdigital** infections present as scaling, maceration, fissuring, or erythema of the webspaces between the toes. This infection is usually associated with *Trichophyton rubrum* or *T. mentagrophytes*. **Moccasin-type** tinea pedis presents as generalized scaling and hyperkeratosis of the plantar surface of the foot. This form of infection is frequently associated with nail involvement. Moccasin-type tinea pedis is typically caused by *T. rubrum*. The **inflammatory** or **vesiculobullous** type will cause a vesicular eruption on the arch or side of the foot and is most often caused by *T. mentagrophytes*.

14. What nondermatophyte mould can cause mycotic infections that mimic moccasin-type tinea pedis?

Scytalidium dimidiatum has been isolated from cases of moccasin-type pedis that are resistant to standard therapy. The organism will not grow on selective dermatophyte media, such as Mycosel, Mycobiotic, or DTM, but it does grow readily on Sabouraud's agar.

15. What is a dermatophytid reaction?

Dermatophytid reactions are inflammatory reactions at sites distant from the site of the associated dermatophyte infection. Types of dermatophytid reactions from tinea pedis include urticaria, hand dermatitis (Fig. 4), or erythema nodosum. The pathogenesis of dermatophytid reactions is not fully understood, but evidence suggests that they are secondary to a strong host immunologic response against fungal antigens.

16. Name and describe the four clinical presentations of onychomycosis.

1. **Distal subungual** onychomycosis presents as onycholysis, subungual debris, and discoloration beginning at the hyponychium that spreads proximally. The most common organism is *Trichophyton rubrum*.

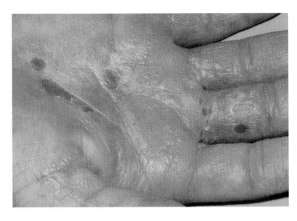

FIGURE 4. Dermatophytid reaction. (Courtesy of Mark Welch, MD.)

2. **Proximal subungual** onychomycosis begins underneath the proximal nailfold and is typically caused by *T. rubrum*. The patient's immune status should be investigated since it is strongly associated with immunosuppressed conditions.

3. **Superficial white** onychomycosis produces a white, crumbly nail surface due to invasion of the top of the nailplate. It is usually caused by *T. mentagrophytes*; however, nondermatophytes such as *Fusarium, Acremonium,* and *Aspergillus* have been associated with this type of infection.

4. **Candidal** onychomycosis is seen in patients with chronic mucocutaneous candidiasis.

17. Can other diseases mimic onychomycosis?

Yes. Psoriasis, Reiter's disease, lichen planus, pachyonychia congenita, Darier's disease, and Norwegian scabies are some of the diseases that can resemble onychomycosis. For this reason, the diagnosis should be established by either a KOH examination or culture before beginning prolonged and often expensive therapies to eradicate the infection.

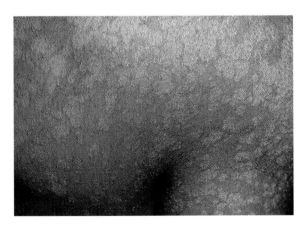

FIGURE 5. Tinea versicolor demonstrating hypopigmented scaly papules.

18. What is tinea versicolor?

Tinea versicolor (pityriasis versicolor) is a hypopigmented, hyperpigmented, or erythematous macular eruption. Macules may coalesce into large patches with an adherent fine scale (Fig. 5). Lesions are located predominantly on the trunk but may extend to the extremities. The proper taxonomic nomenclature of the lipophilic yeast that produces this infection is debatable. Some authorities prefer *Pityrosporum orbiculare,* while others use *Malassezia furfur*. This eruption begins during adolescence, when the sebaceous glands become active. The eruption tends to flare when the temperatures and humidity are high. Immunosuppression, systemic corticosteroids, and sweaty or greasy skin will also cause this disease to flare.

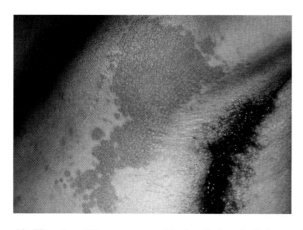

FIGURE 6. Hyperpigmented variant of tinea versicolor. (Courtesy of Dermatology Service, Walter Reed Army Medical Center.)

19. How does *Pityrosporum orbiculare* induce both hyperpigmentation and hypopigmentation in the skin?

P. orbiculare infection induces hypopigmentation because it produces dicarboxylic acid. This compound inhibits the tyrosinase inhibitory activity of melanocytes, which results in diminished melanin production. The dark lesions of tinea versicolor may be due to a variation in the inflammatory response to the infection (Fig. 6).

20. How is tinea versicolor diagnosed? Why is it difficult to culture this organism?

Tinea versicolor is diagnosed by scraping some of the scale from a lesion and looking for the characteristic "meatball and spaghetti" under the microscope. The meatball is the yeast forms, and the spaghetti is the short hyphae. This organism is a lipophilic yeast and will grow only after a source of lipid is added to the culture media. A yellow fluorescence may be seen by Wood's light examination of affected areas.

21. Do *Pityrosporum* yeast cause any other skin disease?

This organism can also produce a folliculitis of the trunk, arms, and neck area. *Pityrosporum* folliculitis presents as pruritic follicular papules and pustules that do not respond to antibiotic therapy. The yeast can be demonstrated by skin biopsies or direct examination of purulent material. The severity of seborrheic dermatitis has been reported to be associated with an increase in the *Pityrosporum* microflora.

22. What is tinea nigra?

A superficial dermatomycosis caused by *Phaeoanellomyces (Exophiala) werneckii*. This is a dematiaceous (pigment-producing) fungus. It causes an asymptomatic tan, brown, or black patch on the palms or soles. The diagnosis is made by demonstrating pigmented hyphae on a KOH examination of the lesion. Tinea nigra has been confused with acral lentiginous melanoma.

23. What is a Majocchi's granuloma?

Majocchi's granuloma is a follicular abscess produced when a dermatophyte infection penetrates the follicular wall into the surrounding dermis. Patients usually present with one or more tender boggy papules or plaques on the legs or, less commonly, arms. Pus may be seen draining from the hair follicle. *Trichophyton rubrum* or *T. mentagrophytes* are the species most commonly isolated from these lesions. Treatment should consist of an oral antifungal agent.

24. What is piedra?

Piedra refers to adherent deposits on the hair shaft caused by superficial fungal infections. **Black piedra,** which is caused by *Piedraia hortae,* presents as firm black nodules on the hair shaft. *Trichosporon beigelii* is the etiologic agent that produces **white piedra,** which results in the formation of less adherent white concretions on the hair shaft.

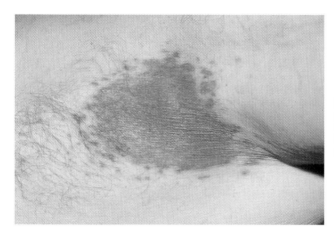

FIGURE 7. Cutaneous candidiasis showing an erythematous plaque with satellite lesion in a body fold area. (Courtesy of Larry Becker, MD.)

25. Name the organism most commonly isolated from cutaneous candidiasis.
Candida albicans is the most common organism isolated from lesions of candidiasis. It is normally part of the microflora of the gastrointestinal tract.

26. How do candidal infections present clinically?
The clinical presentations vary with the sites involved, duration of infection, and immune status of the host. Most sites show erythema, edema, and a thin purulent discharge (Fig. 7).

Clinical Presentations of Cutaneous Candidiasis

DISEASE	CLINICAL DESCRIPTION
Intertrigo	Superficial pustules, erythema, edema, creamy exudates within skin folds
Thrush	White, adherent, cottage cheese-like plaques on oral mucosa
Perlèche	Erythema, fissuring, creamy exudate at the angles of the mouth
Paronychia	Tender, erythematous, indurated proximal nailfold, with or without a purulent discharge
Erosio interdigitalis blastomycetica	Erythema, fissuring, maceration of the webspaces between the fingers

27. What factors predispose to candidiasis?
The factors that predispose to the development of candidiasis are both endogenous and exogenous. Exogenous factors include occlusion, moisture, and warm temperature. Endogenous factors can include immunosuppression, diabetes mellitus, other endocrinopathies, antibiotics, oral contraceptives, Down's syndrome, malnutrition, and pregnancy.

28. Which diseases are associated with adult-onset chronic mucocutaneous candidiasis?
Thymoma, myasthenia gravis, myositis, and aplastic anemia have been associated with the development of chronic mucocutaneous candidiasis after the third decade of life.

29. Name the different classes of oral antifungal agents and their mechanisms of action.

Oral Antifungal Agents

CLASS	EXAMPLES	MECHANISMS OF ACTION
Antibiotic	Griseofulvin	Arrest of cellular division, dysfunction of spindle microtubules
Polyenes	Nyastatin	Binds irreversibly with ergosterol, altering membrane permeability
Azoles	Fluconazole Itraconazole Ketoconazole	Inhibits ergosterol production by inhibiting the cytochrome P–450 lanosterol 14–demethylase
Allyamines	Terbinafine	Blocks ergosterol production by inhibiting squalene epoxidase

30. Which hepatic cytochrome is affected by itraconazole, ketoconazole, and fluconazole?
Cytochrome P-450 3A4.

31. Which drugs should be used with caution when using ketoconazole, itraconazole, or fluconazole? Why? Which drugs are contraindicated and why?
Warfarin, quinidine, digoxin, calcium channel blockers, bulsufan, HIV protease inhibitors, cyclosporine, tacrolimus, oral hypoglycemic agents, hydantoin anticonvulsants, and alcohol. These drugs should be used with caution because the primary effect of azole antifungal drugs on hepatic enzyme metabolism is inhibition. This results in an elevation of the serum level of any drug that requires hepatic metabolism by the cytochrome P-450 3A4 enzyme in order to be removed.

Contraindicated drugs are cisapride, astemizole, terfenadine, lovastatin, midazolam and triazolam. When combined with azole antifungal agents, these drugs can cause severe or life-threatening reactions. Elevated levels of cisapride, astemizole, and terfenadine are associated with cardiac arrhythmias, especially torsades de pointes. The metabolism of lovastatin is markedly reduced and can result in rhabdomyolysis. Simvastatin, atorvastatin, and cerivastatin are metabolized by the same hepatic cytochrome and also should be avoided.

32. Which oral antifungal agents can lower cyclosporine levels?
Griseofulvin and terbinafine.

33. Which drugs can affect antifungal drug levels?
Any drug that raises the gastric pH reduces the absorption of itraconazole and ketoconazole. Rifampin reduces the levels of oral azole and allylamines by induction of hepatic cytochromes. Isoniazid and phenytoin can induce the metabolism of azole antifungal agents. Cimetidine can raise terbinafine levels.

34. Which antifungal drugs have a limited spectrum of activity in the treatment of superficial fungal infections?
Griseofulvin is not effective against tinea versicolor or cutaneous candidiasis. Oral nystatin is not absorbed from the gastrointestinal tract. Topical nystatin and amphotericin are both ineffective against dermatophyte infections. Allylamines have limited effectiveness against tinea versicolor and candidiasis.

BIBLIOGRAPHY

1. Babel D, Baughman S: Evaluation of the adult carrier state in juvenile tinea capitis caused by *Trichophyton tonsurans*. J Am Acad Dermatol 21:1209–1212, 1989.
2. Elewski B: Treatment of tinea capitis: Beyond griseofulvin. J Am Acad Dermatol 40:S27–S30, 1999.
3. Faergemann J: *Pityrosporum* infections. In Elewski B (ed): Cutaneous Fungal Infection, 2nd ed. Malden, MA, Blackwell Science, 1998, pp 73–90.
4. Fitzpatrick JE: Superficial fungal skin diseases. In James WD (ed): Military Dermatology: Textbook of Military Medicine: Part III. Disease and the Environment. Washington, DC, 1994, pp 423–451.
5. Gupta A, Katz I, Shear N: Drug interaction with itraconazole, fluconazole, and terbinafine and their management. J Am Acad Dermatol 41:237–249, 1999.
6. Gupta A, Sauder D, Shear N: Antifungal agents: Part I J Am Acad Dermatol 30:677–698, 1993.
7. Gupta A, Sauder D, Shear N: Antifungal agents: Part II. J Am Acad Dermatol 30:911–933, 1993.
8. Katz HI: Appendix: Oral antifungal adverse drug interactions. In Elewski B (ed): Cutaneous Fungal Infection, 2nd ed. Malden, MA, Blackwell Science, 1998, pp 347–356.
9. Lesher J, Therapeutic agents for dermatologic fungal diseases. In Elewski B (ed): Cutaneous Fungal Infection, 2nd ed. Malden, MA, Blackwell Science, 1998, pp 321–346.
10. Martin A, Kobayashi G: Superficial fungal infection: Dermatophytosis, tinea nigra, piedra. In Freeberg IM, et al (eds): Dermatology in General Medicine, 5th ed. New York, McGraw-Hill, 1999, pp 2337–2357.
11. Martin A, Kobayashi G: Yeast infections: Candidiasis, pityriasis (tinea) versicolor. In Freeberg IM, et al (eds): Dermatology in General Medicine, 5th ed. New York, McGraw-Hill, 1999, pp 2358–2371.
12. Midgley G, Moore M, Cook J, Phan Q: Mycology of nail disorders. J Am Acad Dermatol 31:S68–S73, 1994.
13. Odom R: Common superficial fungal infections in immunosuppressed patients. J Am Acad Dermatol 31:S56–S59, 1994.
14. Wagner D, Sohnle P: Cutaneous defenses against dermatophyte and yeasts. Clin Microbiol Rev 8:317–335, 1995.
15. Wolf F, Jones E, Nathan H: Fluorescent pigment of *Microsporum*. Nature 182:475–476, 1958.

32. DEEP FUNGAL INFECTIONS

Syed O. Ali, M.D., CPT, USA, and Karen E. Warschaw, M.D., LTC, USAF

1. What is a deep fungal infection?

In contrast to the superficial dermatophytes, which are confined to dead keratinous tissue, certain mycotic infections have the capacity for deep invasion of the skin or produce skin lesions secondary to systemic visceral infection. They are typically acquired through direct inoculation, ingestion and/or inhalation of spores from soil or matter. In this chapter, the deep fungal diseases are organized into three categories based on their clinical presentation.

The Deep Fungal Infections

Subcutaneous fungal infections	Sporotrichosis
	Chromomycosis (chromoblastomycosis)
	Mycetoma (Madura Foot)
Systemic or respiratory fungal infections	Blastomycosis
	Histoplasmosis
	Coccidioidomycosis
	Paracoccidioidomycosis
Opportunistic fungal infections	Cryptococcosis
	Aspergillosis
	Mucormycosis
	Penicilliosis

SUBCUTANEOUS FUNGAL INFECTIONS

2. Discuss the characteristics of subcutaneous mycotic infections.

Subcutaneous mycotic infections may be caused by many fungi and are infections of implantation (inoculated directly into the skin through local trauma). The three most important infections are sporotrichosis, chromomycosis, and mycetoma. Lobomycosis, phaeohyphomycosis, rhinosporidiosis, and zygomycosis are significantly less common. As a group these infections primarily involve the skin and subcutaneous tissues and rarely disseminate to produce systemic disease. These organisms are ubiquitous in soil, plants, and trees.

3. What is a dimorphic fungus?

Dimorphic fungi are capable of growing in both the mold and yeast form. Examples of diseases caused by dimorphic fungi include sporotrichosis, histoplasmosis, blastomycosis, paracoccidioidomycosis, and penicilliosis.

4. What occupations are at increased risk of sporotrichosis?

Sporotrichosis is caused by a dimorphic fungus, *Sporothrix schenckii*. This organism is found worldwide except in polar regions and is most common in subtropical and tropical climates. In the U.S. infection is most common in the Midwest. The normal habitat includes soil, thorned plants (especially roses), hay, sphagnum moss, and animals. Cats may carry *Sporothrix* on their paws and can cause infection by scratching their owners or animal handlers. Occupations at risk of cutaneous inoculation include farmers, gardeners, florists, and animal handlers.

5. Describe the clinical manifestations of sporotrichosis.

Cutaneous sporotrichosis is more common than systemic sporotrichosis. Cutaneous sporotrichosis can be further divided into two forms: lymphangitic or lymphocutaneous disease and fixed infection. The lymphocutaneous form accounts for approximately 80% of the cases. This classic form of sporotrichosis begins at the site of inoculation (most commonly upper extremity) as a painless pink papule, pustule or dermal nodule, which rapidly enlarges and ulcerates (Fig. 1A).

Without treatment the infection ascends along the lymphatics, producing secondary nodules and regional lymphadenopathy that may ulcerate (Fig. 1B). The fixed cutaneous variant (20%) is confined to the site of inoculation. The organism may rarely disseminate hematogenously to the joints, bone, meninges or eye. Disseminated disease is most common in immunosuppressed patients. Pulmonary disease is usually due to inhalation and generally occurs in alcoholics or debilitated patients. Diagnosis is made by biopsy and culture. Cutaneous sporotrichosis may be treated with a saturated solution of potassium iodide (SSKI) or itraconazole and extracutaneous disease with amphotericin B, terbenafine, or itraconazole.

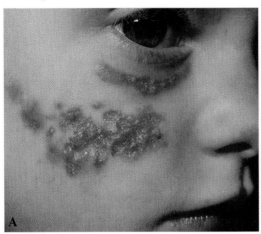
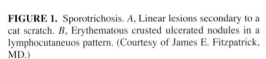
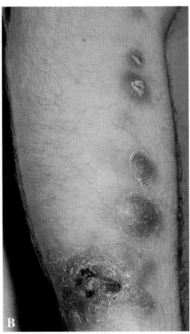

FIGURE 1. Sporotrichosis. *A,* Linear lesions secondary to a cat scratch. *B,* Erythematous crusted ulcerated nodules in a lymphocutaneuos pattern. (Courtesy of James E. Fitzpatrick, MD.)

6. What other organisms may present with lymphocutaneous disease?

Several other diseases may present with a distal ulcer, proximal secondary nodules along the lymphatics and regional lymphadenopathy. The most important organisms include *Mycobacterium marinum, Mycobacterium kansasii, Mycobacterium chelonei,* and *Nocardia.* This pattern of disease is also called sporotrichoid.

7. What are dematiaceous fungi?

Dematiaceous fungi are black pigmented fungi. They are slow growing and can be found in the soil, decaying vegetation, rotting wood and the forest carpet. Subcutaneous-cutaneous disease is caused by traumatic inoculation into the skin. There are three broad categories of dematiaceous fungal infections including chromomycosis, phaeohyphomycosis and some cases of mycetoma (Madura foot).

8. Which organisms may cause chromoblastomycosis?

Five fungal species account for most infections. The most frequent organism worldwide is *Fonsecaea pedrosoi.* Others organisms include *Phialophora verrucosa, Fonsecaea compactum, Wangiella dermatitidis,* and *Cladosporium carrionii.*

9. How does chromomycosis present?

Chromomycosis is a chronic cutaneous and subcutaneous infection that is usually present for years with minimal discomfort. The inciting injury is often times not remembered. The infection is most common on the lower extremity and 95% of cases occur in males. The typical patient is a barefoot, rural agricultural worker in the tropics. At the site of inoculation, red papules develop that eventually coalesce into a plaque. The plaque slowly enlarges and acquires a verrucous or warty surface. Satellite lesions can develop from extension of the infection through scratching. There may also be secondary bacterial infections of the lesion. If the lesion is not treated, it can evolve into a cauliflower-like mass, leading to lymphatic obstruction and elephantiasis-like edema of the lower extremity (Fig. 2). Diagnosis is made through KOH mounts from scrapings, biopsies of the lesions showing the organism and suppurative and granulomatous inflammation, and culture. Rare reports of hematogenous dissemination to the brain have been described. Medical therapy is disappointing; itraconazole, terbenafine, and amphotericin B have been used and shown to be helpful. Surgery may spread the lesions and should only be used after drug therapy.

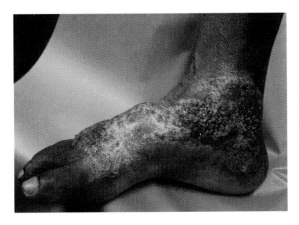

FIGURE 2. Chromomycosis. Cauliflower-like nodules and tumors on the foot and ankle with edema. (Courtesy of James E. Fitzpatrick, MD.)

10. What is cystic chromomycosis?

Cystic chromomycosis (also known as phaeohyphomycosis) is a rare infection caused by some 101 species of dematiaceous fungi, the most common of which are *Exophiala jeanselmei* and *Wangiella dermatitidis*. Clinically, the disease is characterized by inflammatory cysts in the subcutaneous tissue. Treatment is surgical excision of the cysts.

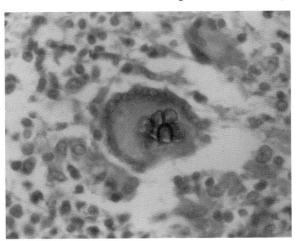

FIGURE 3. Chromomycosis. Diagnostic golden-brown yeast within a multinucleated foreign body giant cell. (Courtesy of James E. Fitzpatrick, MD.)

11. What are Medlar bodies?

Medlar bodies, also called copper pennies or sclerotic bodies, refer to the characteristic brown yeast seen in the biopsies of chromomycosis and are considered to be diagnostic (Fig. 3).

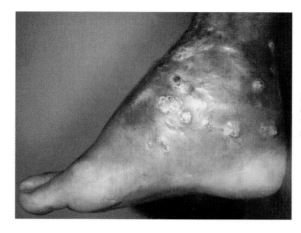

FIGURE 4. Madura foot. Swelling and deformity of the foot and ankle with purulent drainage and fistula formation.

12. What is Madura foot?

Madura foot, a type of mycetoma, is a localized, destructive infection of the skin and subcutaneous tissue that eventually involves deeper structures, such as muscle and bone. It is caused by several different species of fungi or filamentous bacteria.

13. Name some organisms that can cause Madura foot.

Madura foot may be caused by both filamentous bacteria and aerobic actinomycetes (actinomycetomas) and true fungi (eumycetoma). The table below lists the most common organisms by country and category. Although Madura foot may occur throughout the world, it is most common in dry, tropical, rural settings.

Most Frequent Causes of Madura Foot by Country and Classification

COUNTRY	ORGANISM	ACTINOMYCETOMA	EUMYCETOMA
United States	*Pseudallescheria boydii*		X
Canada	*Pseudallescheria boydii*		X
Africa	*Madurella mycetomatis*		X
Latin America	*Nocardia brasiliensis*	X	
Japan	*Nocardia asteroides*	X	
Middle East	*Streptomyces somaliensis*	X	

14. What are the cardinal features of Madura foot?

Madura foot is an indolent localized painless infection with three characteristic features. The first is the formation of nodules in the skin at the site of inoculation, usually a penetrating injury. The second feature is purulent drainage and fistula formation. The third and most characteristic feature is the presence of grains or granules that are visible in the purulent drainage. Seventy percent of cases involve the lower extremity, the foot in particular. Other sites of infection include the hand, head, back and chest. Madura foot is a progressive infection leading to marked swelling and deformity in its latter stages (Fig. 4). Additionally, the lesions have a tendency to become painful in its latter stages when bone involvement and deformity ravage the site. Actinomycetomas generally respond to treatment with combination antibiotic regimens such as dapsone and streptomycin. Treatment is generally unsatisfactory in eumycetomas, and amputation may need to be considered in advanced cases.

15. Where does lobomycosis occur?

Lobomycosis occurs in Central and South America, although it is an extremely rare infection altogether. The typical lesion is that of a keloid-like skin lesion on any part of the body, and is spread by autoinoculation. The mainstay of treatment is surgical removal.

16. How many varieties of subcutaneous zygomycosis are there?

There are two main types of subcutaneous zygomycosis, both occurring in tropical areas. The first type is caused by *Basidiobolus ranarum* and occurs mostly in children. It presents with a firm woody cellulitis in the limb girdle sites. The second type is caused by *Conidiobolus coronatus* and occurs mainly in adults. It begins in the nasal turbinates before spreading to the face with marked deformity and hard, painless swelling. Treatment is with potassium iodide.

SYSTEMIC FUNGAL INFECTIONS

17. Discuss the pathogenesis of the systemic respiratory deep fungi.

The systemic respiratory endemic fungal infections include blastomycosis, histoplasmosis, coccidioidomycosis, paracoccidioidomycosis, and the more recently recognized penicilliosis. These infections are all due to species that show dimorphism. As a group, they cause disease in both healthy immunocompetent individuals as well as the immunosuppressed. These diseases are similar in pathophysiology, but each has distinct clinical characteristics. The causative organisms are found in the soil, and infection occurs with inhalation of the organism into the lung. The primary infection is pulmonary. Dissemination occurs via the lymphohematogenous route, and each fungus has a predilection for particular organ systems.

18. Where is blastomycosis endemic?

Blastomycosis, caused by the soil saprophyte *Blastomyces dermatitidis*, is endemic in North America, especially the southeastern and south central states bordering the Mississippi, Ohio, and St. Lawrence rivers (Kentucky, Arkansas, Mississippi, North Carolina, Tennessee, Louisiana, Illinois, and Wisconsin) and the Great Lakes region. Sporadic cases have occurred in Africa, the Middle East, and India. The typical patient is a middle-aged male with occupational or recreational exposure to the soil.

19. What is the clinical manifestation of blastomycosis?

There can be a subclinical form of infection consisting of a primary chancre (ulcer) with associated lymphadenopathy that develops 1–2 weeks after direct cutaneous inoculation. Acute pulmonary infection occurs following a 30–45-day incubation period. Half of the patients are asymptomatic, and half present with flu-like symptoms (low-grade fever, cough, pleurisy). Progression to chronic pneumonia may ensue. Disseminated disease to the skin is reported in 40–80% of patients. Other distant organ sites include bone in 25–50%, genitourinary tract in 10–30% and central nervous system in 5%.

20. Describe the cutaneous findings in disseminated blastomycosis.

The most characteristic cutaneous presentation is a single (or multiple) crusted, verrucous plaque on exposed skin (face, hands, arms) with color variation from gray to violet (Fig. 5).

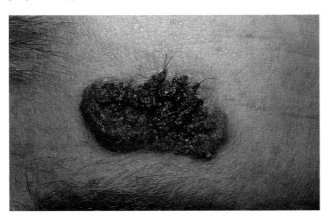

FIGURE 5. Blastomycosis. Classic verrucous plaque. (Courtesy of James E. Fitzpatrick, MD.)

Microabscesses can form, and pus exudes when the crust is lifted off. As the plaque progresses there is central clearing. Ulcerative lesions are a less common cutaneous presentation, and 25% of patients may have nasal or mucosal lesions.

21. Are immunosuppressed patients at increased risk of disseminated disease with blastomycosis?

Blastomycosis, unlike other deep fungal infections (cryptococcosis, histoplasmosis, coccidioidomycosis, mucormycosis, penicilliosis and aspergillosis) infrequently behaves as an opportunistic infection in the immunosuppressed host. There are, however, several reports of disseminated blastomycosis in AIDS patients, organ transplant recipients, and patients receiving glucocorticosteroids and chemotherapy. Central nervous system involvement occurs in 40% of this group, and mortality rates of 30–50% have been reported.

22. What is the treatment of blastomycosis?

The azoles, ketoconazole and intraconazole, are effective in the immunocompetent patient without CNS disease. Minimum treatment time is 6 months. Amphotericin B is the drug of choice in the immunosuppressed and any patient with CNS involvement.

23. Where is histoplasmosis endemic?

Histoplasmosis is caused by *Histoplasma capsulatum*, an environmental saprophyte. It is endemic in the midwestern and south central U.S., where 80% of the population is skin test–positive. It does occur in other parts of the world, but it is not found in Europe. Soil infected with excreta from chickens, pigeons, blackbirds, and bats is inhaled, leading to a pulmonary infection. Rarely, primary cutaneous disease is contracted from traumatic inoculation.

24. What factors are necessary for production of the disease histoplasmosis?

The two most important factors are the number of organisms inhaled and immune status of the host. Cellular immunity is particularly important to host defense, as indicated by severe disseminated disease in HIV-infected patients.

25. Discuss the clinical manifestations of histoplasmosis.

As already mentioned, the clinical manifestations depend on the quantity of organisms inhaled and immune status of the host. Only 1% of patients exposed to a small inoculum develop symptomatic disease; in contrast, 50–100% of persons exposed to a heavy inoculum develop symptoms. The majority of patients with symptoms develop a flu-like acute pulmonary illness characterized by fever, chills, headache, myalgias, chest pain and nonproductive cough. Progressive disseminated histoplasmosis occurs in 1 of 2,000 acute infections. High-risk groups for disseminated disease include patients with impaired cellular immunity such as HIV infection, lymphoma, leukemia and also infants and the elderly. Rarely, there is a primary cutaneous form following direct inoculation into the skin.

26. How common are mucocutaneous findings in disseminated histoplasmosis?

Three different patterns of disseminated histoplasmosis are described: acute, subacute and chronic. The acute syndrome generally occurs in immunosuppressed patients and is characterized by fever, hepatosplenomegaly and pancytopenia, with 18% developing mucocutaneous ulcers. Chronic disseminated histoplasmosis is characterized by involvement of the bone marrow, gastrointestinal tract, spleen, adrenals, and CNS; 67% have painful ulcerations on the tongue, buccal mucosa, gingiva, or larynx (Fig. 6). Although mucous membrane lesions are common, cutaneous lesions are rare in disseminated disease occurring in only 4–6% of immunosuppressed patients, particularly renal transplant patients.

27. Are there any other cutaneous manifestations of histoplasmosis?

Erythema nodosum and less commonly erythema multiforme may be seen in histoplasmosis, coccidioidomycosis, and, rarely, blastomycosis. These cutaneous hypersensitivity reactions are generally associated with a good prognosis.

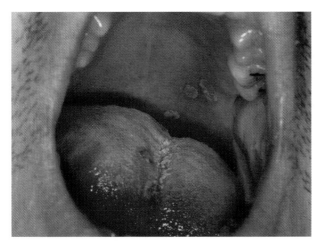

FIGURE   6. Histoplasmosis. Oral ulcerations in an HIV-infected patient. Histoplasmosis more commonly affects the oral mucosa than the skin. (Courtesy of James E. Fitzpatrick, MD.)

28. Where is coccidioidomycosis endemic?

Coccidioidomycosis, also called San Joaquin Valley fever, is caused by *Coccidioides immitis*. It is a dimorphic fungus found in the soil. This organism is endemic in southern California, Arizona, New Mexico, southwestern Texas, northern Mexico, and Central and South America. Over 100,000 people in the U.S. are infected annually, and the number of reported cases has been increasing by as much as 144% throughout the 1990s.

29. What are the clinical manifestations of coccidioidomycosis?

Primary pulmonary infection is asymptomatic in 50% of patients. In 40%, patients present with a mild flu-like illness or pneumonia. Erythema nodosum is present in 5% of patients with acute coccidioidomycosis. Hematogenous dissemination occurs in 0.5% of patients, and the skin is the most common site. Risk factors for dissemination and fatal disease include male sex, pregnancy, immunocompromised status, and race (in order of decreasing risk by race: Filipino, black, and white). Among immunosuppressed patients, lymphocytopenia correlates closely with dissemination. In endemic areas in the U.S. approximately 10% of HIV-positive persons develop acute infection annually. Cutaneous lesions of disseminated coccidioidomycosis are protean. Warty papules, plaques, or nodules are the most characteristic (Fig. 7). Cellulitis, abscesses, and draining sinus tracts also may occur. Other sites of dissemination include bone, joints, and meninges.

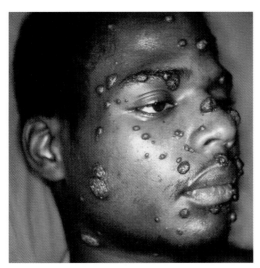

FIGURE 7. Disseminated coccidioidomycosis. Discrete verrucous papules, plaques, and nodules. (Courtesy of James E. Fitzpatrick, MD.)

30. Where is paracoccidioidomycosis endemic?

Paracoccidioidomycosis (South American blastomycosis) previously has been thought to be restricted to Latin America, especially Brazil. Recently there have been reports of cases outside this area. The disease is confined to humid tropical and subtropical forests. *Paracoccidioides brasiliensis* is the causative dimorphic fungus.

31. Why is paracoccidioidomycosis more common in men?

Paracoccidioidomycosis is most common in adult men between the ages of 30–60 years. Skin testing indicates that the rate of infection is equal among the sexes. However, clinical disease is more common in men, with a male:female ratio of 15:1. It has been shown that this sex difference is due to the inhibitory action of estrogens on the mycelium to yeast transformation necessary for infectivity. Only 3% of cases occur in children and 10% in adolescents.

32. What is the most common presenting complaint of paracoccidioidomycosis?

The lung is the primary site of infection. However, respiratory complaints are the least common presenting symptom. Painful mucosal ulcerations involving the mouth and nose are the most common findings. Patients may also have enlarged cervical lymph nodes and verrucous, crusted, edematous facial lesions. Hematogenous dissemination may also cause disease in the adrenals, spleen, liver, gastrointestinal tract and CNS.

33. Which organism is responsible for penicilliosis?

Penicilliosis is caused by the dimorphic fungus *Penicillium marneffei*. It is inhaled into the lungs and causes disease in both immunocompetent and immunocompromised patients, with a predilection to the latter.

34. Where is penicilliosis endemic?

Penicilliosis is endemic in southeast Asia, although there have been few case reports in other Asian countries. The increase in HIV-infected individuals in these areas has led to the emergence of this organism as a cause of infection.

35. How does penicilliosis present clinically?

Patients usually present with either localized pulmonary or disseminated disease. Most patients will have generalized lymphadenopathy, hepatosplenomegaly, fever, weight loss, and skin lesions that resemble molluscum contagiosum. These lesions are multiple, umbilicated papules located on the face and trunk and may ulcerate. Biopsy and culture are used for diagnosis and treatment is with itraconazole, or Amphotericin B in severe cases.

OPPORTUNISTIC FUNGAL INFECTIONS

36. Define opportunistic infection.

Opportunistic infections are caused by organisms that typically produce disease in a host with lowered resistance. Many opportunistic infections involve the skin. The three discussed in this chapter are cryptococcosis, aspergillosis, and mucormycosis.

37. Discuss the important epidemiologic factors of cryptococcosis.

Cryptococcosis is caused by *Cryptococcus neoformans*, a ubiquitous encapsulated yeast found in the soil, particularly soil contaminated with pigeon excreta. During the pre-AIDS era (prior to 1980), cryptococcal infections were rare and about 50% occurred in patients with lymphoreticular malignancies. Today cryptococcosis is the fourth leading cause of opportunistic infection and second leading cause of fungal infection in the AIDS population. It is the leading cause of fungal meningitis. The mortality rate of untreated disseminated cryptococcosis is 70–80%.

38. How is an infection with cryptococcosis acquired?

Infection occurs from inhalation of the organism leading to a primary lung infection. Immunocompetent patients generally present with a mild pulmonary infection. Disseminated disease via the hematogenous route occurs in 10–15% of immunosuppressed patients, with a predilection for the meninges. Other organs involved include the skin (10–20%), bone, prostate and kidney. There are a few rare reports of primary inoculation cutaneous disease, which manifests itself as a solitary papule/nodule. However, cutaneous disease is generally indicative of disseminated disease and a poor prognosis.

39. What are the cutaneous manifestations of disseminated cryptococcosis?

Cryptococcosis is a great simulator of a wide variety of cutaneous diseases. These include molluscum contagiosum–like lesions (Fig. 8), Kaposi sarcoma–like lesions, pyoderma gangrenosum–like lesions, herpetiform lesions, cellulitis, ulcers, subcutaneous nodules, and palpable purpura. Lesions are most commonly found on the head, neck and genitals, but can be found anywhere. Cutaneous lesions are found in 10–20% of HIV-infected patients.

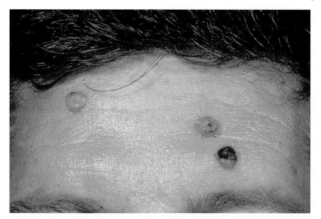

FIGURE 8. Disseminated cryptococcosis. Multiple papules and nodules that resemble molluscum contagiosum. (Courtesy of James E. Fitzpatrick, MD.)

40. What patient population is at increased risk of aspergillosis?

Neutropenia and corticosteroid therapy, especially when combined, are the two most important risk factors for aspergillosis. Solid organ transplant, bone marrow transplant recipients, and leukemic patients, in particular, are at high risk. Other at-risk patients include HIV-infected individuals, patients on broad-spectrum antibiotic use, and patients on immunosupression therapy.

41. How common are cutaneous lesions in aspergillosis?

Aspergillus species are ubiquitous saphrophytes in the air, soil, and decaying vegetation. It is primarily a respiratory pathogen, with the lungs and sinuses as the major sites of infection. Disseminated disease occurs in 30% of aspergillosis cases, and cutaneous lesions develop in less than 11%. There are several documented reports of primary invasive skin infections occurring in neutropenic patients associated with intravenous catheters and adhesive tape contaminated with spores (Fig. 9). Invasive disease is almost uniformly fatal.

42. Describe the cutaneous lesions in aspergillosis.

Patients may have single or multiple lesions that begin as a well circumscribed papule, which over several days enlarges into an ulcer with a necrotic base and surrounding erythematous halo. The organism has a propensity to invade blood vessels, causing thrombosis and infarction. The skin lesions can be very destructive and extend into cartilage, bone and fascial planes. Aspergillosis should be considered in the differential diagnosis of necrotizing lesions.

43. What opportunistic fungus is clinically and histologically similar to *Aspergillus*?

Patients with prolonged neutropenia, especially leukemia patients, are susceptible to infections with *Fusarium*. *Fusarium* is a filamentous mold found in soil and plants. Inhalation into the lungs is the primary route of infection, however, primary cutaneous infection from indwelling catheters may occur. The lung is the usual site of infection, however, 75% of patients have

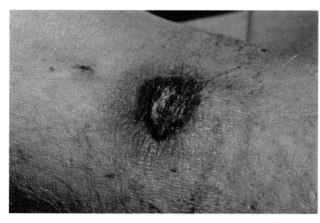

FIGURE 9. Aspergillosis cellulitis at the site of adhesive tape demonstrating erythematous plaques with pustules.

hematogenous spread with a predilection for the skin and sinuses. The cutaneous lesions caused by *Fusarium* are similar to aspergillosis. The typical presentation is a painful erythematous nodule with central ulceration and necrosis. Cellulitis and onychomycosis have also been reported. Histologically, the two are identical (septate hyphae with acute angle branching). The treatment of choice is amphotericin B and the prognosis is poor.

44. What are the most important predisposing factors for acquiring mucormycosis?

Mucormycosis is caused by rapidly growing molds from several genera, including *Mucor, Rhizopus, Absidia,* and *Rhizomucor*. These organisms are ubiquitous in decaying vegetation, fruit and bread. Approximately one third of patients have diabetes, and diabetics in ketoacidosis are at especially high risk. Other reported associations include malnutrition, uremia, neutropenia, corticosteroid therapy, burns, antibiotic therapy and HIV-infected individuals with a history of intravenous drug use. The neutrophil is the predominant component of host defense.

45. Discuss the clinical manifestations of rhinocerebral mucormycosis.

Rhinocerebral mucormycosis is the most common form of mucormycosis, although many other forms exist, including a cutaneous form. Most commonly the organism is deposited in the nasal turbinates or lung through inhalation. The majority of patients with rhinocerebral mucormycosis are diabetics (often in ketoacidosis) or have leukemia. Patients present with fever, headache, facial pain, orbital cellulitis and cranial nerve dysfunction. The patients may have loss of vision from retinal artery thrombosis. This form is often fatal. Treatment consists of rapid diagnosis with aggressive debridement and antifungal therapy.

46. Can mucormycosis be acquired from contaminated dressings?

Yes. Primary cutaneous mucormycosis can occur when the spores are directly inoculated into abraded skin. In the 1970s, there was a nationwide epidemic associated with contaminated elastic dressings. Patients presented with a cellulitis under the covered areas. Primary cutaneous mucormycosis has also been reported from gardening, arthropod bites, automobile accidents and burns.

47. What is the treatment of mucormycosis?

The treatment of mucormycosis includes rapid diagnosis in conjunction with correction of any underlying diseases, administration of amphotericin B, and aggressive surgical debridement of necrotic tissue in order to minimize mortality.

BIBLIOGRAPHY

1. Aristizabal BH: Morphological transition of *Paracoccidioides brasiliensis* conidia to yeast cells: In vivo inhibition in females. Infect Immunol 66:5587–5591, 1998.
2. Bethlem EP: Paracoccidioidomycosis. Curr Opin Pulmon Med 5:319–325, 1999.

3. Body BA: Cutaneous manifestations of systemic mycoses. Dermatol Clin 14:125–135, 1996.
4. Bradsher RW: Clinical features of blastomycosis. Semin Respir Infect 12:229–234, 1997.
5. Coccidioidomycosis—Arizona, 1990–1995. MMWR 45:1069–1073, 1996.
6. Conces DJ: Endemic fungal pneumonia in immunocompromised patients. J Thorac Imaging 14:1–8, 1999.
7. Cooper CR: Pathology of Penicillium marneffei: An emerging acquired immunodeficiency syndrome–related pathogen. Arch Pathol Lab Med 121:798–804, 1997.
8. Davies SF: Epidemiological and clinical features of pulmonary blastomycosis. Semin Respir Infect 12:206–218, 1997.
9. Davis JD: Recurrent mycetoma of the foot. J Foot Ankle Surg 38:55–60, 1999.
10. Durden FM: Cutaneous involvement with Cryptococcus neoformans in AIDS. J Am Acad Dermatol 30:844–848, 1994.
11. Fitzpatrick TB (ed): Dermatology in General Medicine, 5th ed. New York, McGraw-Hill, 1999.
12. Fothergill AW: Identification of dematiaceous fungi and their role in human disease. Clin Infect Dis 22(Suppl 2):S179–S184, 1996.
13. Galgiani JN: Coccidioidomycosis: A regional disease of national importance. Rethinking approaches for control. Ann Intern Med 130:293–300, 1999.
14. Gross ML: Deep fungal infections in the tropics. Dermatol Clin 12:695–700, 1994.
15. Kauffman CA: Sporotrichosis. Clin Infect Dis 29:231–236, 1999.
16. Lortholary O: Endemic mycoses: A treatment update. J Antimicrob Chemother 43:321–331, 1999.
17. Mandell GL: Principles and Practice of Infectious Disease. New York, Churchill Livingstone, 1995.
18. Mostafa WZ: Disseminated cryptococcosis with cutaneous lesions. J Dermatol 23:209–213, 1996.
19. Myskowski PL: Fungal disease in the immunocompromised host. Dermatol Clin 15:295–305, 1997.
20. Perfect JR: The new fungal opportunists are coming. Clin Infect Dis 22(Suppl):S112–S118, 1996.
21. Peterson KL: Rhinocerebral mucormycosis: Evolution of the disease and treatment options. Laryngoscope 107:855–862, 1997.
22. Sarosi GA: Concise review for primary care physicians: Therapy for fungal infections. Mayo Clin Proc 69:1111–1117, 1994.
23. Scully C: The deep mycoses in HIV infection. Oral Dis 3(Suppl 1):S200–S207, 1997.
24. Sirisanthana T: Epidemiology and management of penicilliosis in human immunodeficiency virus–infected patients. Int J Infect Dis 3:48–53, 1998.
25. Smego RA: Lymphocutaneous syndrome: A review of non-sporothrix causes. Medicine 78:38–63, 1999.

33. PARASITIC INFESTATIONS

Jeffrey J. Meffert, M.D., COL, MC, USAF

1. Where and how does one acquire cutaneous parasitic diseases?

Cutaneous parasitic infestations are a major source of morbidity, affecting millions worldwide. Tropical climates, crowding, poor nutrition, sanitation problems, and limited medical resources are all associated with increased variety and severity of parasitoses. Ecologically temperate climates and industrialized societies are also afflicted by significant parasitic infestations because of local vectors, distant vacations, and widespread travel to and from areas of endemic infection for business, political, humanitarian, or military purposes. Immunosuppression through drug or disease leads to cutaneous manifestations of parasitic diseases that often may be caused by remarkable organisms with exceptional severity.

2. What is "creeping eruption?"

Properly known as **cutaneous larva migrans** and popularly known as "sandworms," creeping eruption occurs when the larva of dog and cat hookworms (*Ancylostoma caninum* and *A. braziliense*) penetrate intact, exposed skin and begin migrating through the epidermis. The most common location for the eruption is the sole of the foot, although other sites such as the buttocks, backs, and thighs which may have rested on contaminated sand are susceptible. Lacking the enzymes necessary to penetrate and survive in the deeper dermis, the larvae wander a serpiginous route at a speed up to 3 cm/day. Clinically, the primary lesion is a pruritic, erythematous serpiginous burrow (Fig. 1). While the larvae usually die in 2–8 weeks, survival up to a year has been reported. Several cases of cutaneous larva migrans–related erythema multiforme have been reported.

A variety of other animal hookworm species may also cause creeping eruption. Human hookworms may briefly cause a similar eruption, but the better-adapted parasites soon find their way into the circulation.

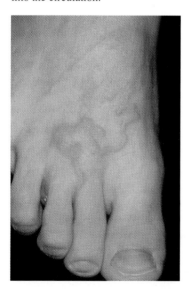

FIGURE 1. Creeping eruption. Cutaneous larva migrans due to canine hookworm.

3. How do you treat creeping eruption?

An older method was to freeze the leading point of the burrow. This sometimes produced significant tissue destruction and often missed the larva, which may be up to 2 cm ahead of the visible burrow. The treatment of choice is 10% topical thiabendazole suspension applied four times

236

a day for at least 2 days after the last sign of burrow activity. This regimen has a high cure rate and minimal toxicity. Rare cases may require oral thiabendazole. Oral ivermectine may have a role in the treatment of this disease.

4. What is different about larva currens?

Larva currens, or "racing larva," is caused by *Strongyloides stercoralis,* a nematode with a normal life cycle similar to the hookworm's (Fig. 2). *Strongyloides,* however, is unique in that it can complete its life cycle within the human host and bypass the obligate soil phase of the hookworms. Autoinfection may occur to a point of overwhelming infestation and host death, especially in immunocompromised victims.

The serpentine eruption of larva currens appears much the same as creeping eruption but is more likely to occur on the thighs, buttocks, or perineum due to larval penetration from the nearby colon. The eruption is more fleeting and lasts no more than a few days, during which the larva's migratory speed may be clocked at up to 10 cm/hour. A nonspecific rash or hives may also occur because of hypersensitivity to the parasite.

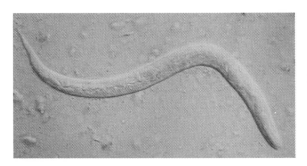

FIGURE 2. Larva currens (*Strongyloides stercoralis*).

5. Are there other nematode infestations that cause skin disease?

Enterobius vermicularis (pinworms) may cause a noisome perianal itch, but secondary complications including dermatitis, bacterial infections, and local abscesses can develop. Treatment is a single dose of mebendazole.

Trichinella spiralis, which is acquired by eating undercooked pork, may cause a diffuse rash, nailbed splinter hemorrhages, and a subtle but persistent periorbital edema.

6. How do filarial infections differ from other nematode infections?

All the filariae have an insect vector integral to their life cycle and live in pairs within their mammalian host. The microfilarial offspring of this couple are the primary source of morbidity. The most important filarial diseases are filariasis, loiasis, and onchocerciasis.

Parasitic Infestations of the Skin

PARASITIC INFESTATION	VECTOR OR MODE OF TRANSMISSION
Filariasis	Mosquito
Onchocerciasis	Black fly
Creeping eruption	Soil contact and larval penetration
African trypanosomiasis	Tsetse fly
American trypanosomiasis	Kissing bug
Leishmaniasis	Sand fly
Schistosomiasis	Water contact and cercarial penetration
Dracunculiasis, sparganosis	Ingestion of larva
Echinococcosis, cysticercosis	Ingestion of cysts
Amebiasis	Direct contact or ingestion of cysts
Loiasis	Horse and deer flies
Demodex	Person-to-person contact in childhood

7. Where is onchocerciasis most prevalent? How is it transmitted?

Onchocerciasis, a disease produced by the tissue nematode *Onchocerca volvulus,* affects millions of people in both Africa and Central and South America. The infective larval forms are transmitted to humans through the bite of the black fly (*Simulium*). The common term for onchocerciasis, **river blindness,** takes its name from its feared complication and the fast-flowing rivers where the parasite and vectors are found.

8. Does river blindness cause cutaneous manifestations?

As the larval forms of *Onchocerca* develop into adult worms at the site of the bite, they produce subcutaneous nodules called *onchocercomas,* where numerous microfilariae are produced. They migrate into the skin, inducing a secondary dermatitis, skin pigmentation changes, skin thickening, frank elephantiasis, and an often disabling itching. The microfilariae also may migrate into the tissue of the eye and produce blindness due to severe uveal and corneal inflammation.

9. What are some of the problems with onchocerciasis treatment?

Diethylcarbamazine is effective treatment for the microfilarial stage, but a hypersensitivity reaction to large numbers of dying parasites in the anterior chamber of the eye may cause irreversible blindness and, in some cases, death. A safer course, in otherwise asymptomatic victims, is periodic "nodulectomy," which removes the adult worms and significantly lowers the morbidity of onchocerciasis.

10. What is loiasis?

Loiasis, an infection endemic in the jungles of west and central Africa, is produced by the adult form of the tissue nematode, *Loa loa,* which is transmitted through the bite of various flies including deer flies (*Chrysops* species). Usually asymptomatic, this filarial disease may cause large areas of transient edema (**Calabar swelling**) as the worm migrates, and it may even migrate visibly across the conjunctiva. Subcutaneous nodules may also be seen in this disease, but the worm's unique migration habits lead to the common name "eyeworm."

11. What causes elephantiasis?

The term elephantiasis is applied to many dermatologic conditions that ultimately result in severe lymphatic obstruction and stasis. The affected limb may become massively enlarged, ini-

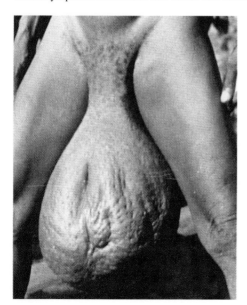

FIGURE 3. Marked scrotal enlargement in elephantiasis. (From Zaiman H, Jong EC: Parasitic diseases of the skin and soft tissue. In Stevens DL (ed): Atlas of Infectious Diseases, vol II. New York, Churchill Livingstone, 1995, ©Current Medicine, used with permission.)

tially with pitting edema but later with a woodlike induration. The skin becomes discolored, and patches of warty growths may eventually cover the entire affected area. Lymphangitis and mechanical obstruction from lymphatic filariasis is but one way of causing elephantiasis. Offending organisms include *Wuchereria bancrofti, Brugia malayi,* and *B. timori.* The *Brugia* species cause elephantiasis of the extremities most commonly, while *Wuchereria* is notorious for genital disease that may eventuate in massive scrotal enlargement (Fig. 3).

12. Can other filarial diseases affect the skin?

Dirofilaria tenuis, the raccoon heartworm, can cause subcutaneous nodules. *Dracunculus medinensis,* or guinea worm, wanders through the subcutaneous tissue as part of its life cycle and eventually settles down where it may cause nodules and ulceration. The native treatment is to snare the worm (up to 120 cm long in the female worm) through the skin and roll it up on a stick (the matchstick technique). Some medical historians believe that the caduceus, the symbol for a physician, has its origins from the ancient method of extracting the *Dracuncula* worm with a stick (Fig. 4).

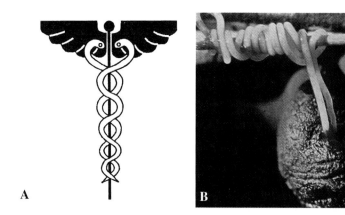

A   **B**

FIGURE 4. *A,* Caduceus. *B,* The classic matchstick recovery technique used in extracting the adult female worm. (From Zaiman H, Jong EC: Parasitic diseases of the skin and soft tissue. In Stevens DL (ed): Atlas of Infectious Diseases, vol II. New York, Churchill Livingstone, 1995. ©Current Medicine, used with permission.)

13. What is myiasis?

Myiasis is a disease in which various species of flies lay their eggs on or in human skin. When laid in an open wound such as a chronic leg or decubitus ulcer, the eggs hatch into larvae (maggots) that feed on damaged skin and complete their life cycle. This is called "wound myiasis" and causes mild to severe inflammation, depending upon the fly species and wound location.

14. What is a warble?

More properly called **furuncular myiasis** in humans, a warble occurs when fly eggs or larvae are introduced into intact skin. A large larva, more than 1 cm in length in some species, grows over time. Careful examination usually reveals a "snorkel" protruding through the skin of a boil that moves when the abscess is manipulated. Surgical extirpation is the treatment of choice, although other therapies including occlusion of the furuncle opening with petrolatum have been reported to be successful (Fig. 5A).

15. What is Congo floor maggot?

Unlike other forms of myiasis in which the larva feeds and pupates within the host tissue, the Congo floor maggot (*Auchmeromyia luteola*) lives in the soil or in the earthen floor of huts and crawls upon the host in the night for a blood meal. The larva, which may grow up to 18 mm long, requires 6–20 feedings before it pupates in the dirt. They carry no disease and may be avoided by sleeping on a raised bed.

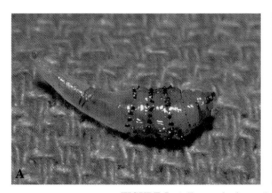
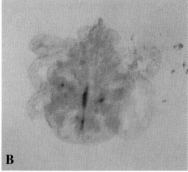

FIGURE 5. *A*, Furuncular larva. *B*, Trombiculid mite.

16. What is tungiasis?

The sand flea, *Tunga penetrans,* can burrow into the foot where the female lays eggs, causing painful abscesses. Treatment is best accomplished by killing the female with chloroform or surgical excision. While late lesions will spontaneously ulcerate, potential complications include secondary infection and tetanus.

17. What is the difference between a chigoe and a chigger?

Chigoe is another name for *Tunga penetrans*. The chigger is a trombiculid mite (Fig. 5B).

18. Do chiggers burrow into the skin to lay eggs like the sand flea?

They usually do not burrow beneath the skin but the larval forms attach via their mouth parts (adults do not bite) and feed on tissue juices and lymph. They may feed for a few days if not removed, although the intense itching usually starts within a few hours after attachment. In some parts of Asia, they are a vector of scrub typhus and may be discouraged from attachment by proper wear of clothing, permethrin repellents, and washing in hot soapy water.

19. What is leishmaniasis?

Leishmaniasis, also known as Baghdad boil, kala-azar, espundia, oriental sore, and a variety of other colorful terms, is caused by *Leishmania* species, a protozoan parasite with a multi-continental distribution. Biting sand flies (*Phlebotomus* species) spread the disease between humans and a large variety of wild and domestic animal reservoirs.

Several species and subspecies of *Leishmania* may produce infection, and the clinical manifestations and disease severity are generally species specific. Most forms cause nodules and chronic ulcerations of the skin that can spread lymphatically and lead to widespread cutaneous disease (Fig. 6).

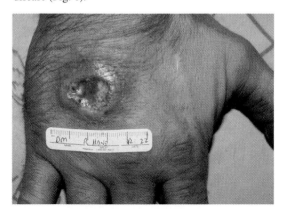

FIGURE 6. Cutaneous leishmaniasis.

20. Name the different types of leishmaniasis.

Leishmaniasis

SPECIES	DISEASE	DISTRIBUTION
L. donovani group	Visceral leishmaniasis, kala-azar	India, Asia, Middle East, Africa
L. tropica group	Old-world cutaneous leishmaniasis, oriental sore, newly discovered viscerotropic disease	India, Middle East
L. viannia group (*L. braziliensis* group)	New-world mucocutaneous leishmaniasis, espundia	Latin America
L. mexicana group	American cutaneous leishmaniasis	Mexico, Central America, Texas, South America

21. Can leishmaniasis be contracted in the United States?

While most cases of leishmaniasis seen in the United States are acquired elsewhere, a form of cutaneous disease caused by *L. mexicana* may be acquired in central Texas and has been nicknamed "Highway 90 disease" by those familiar with its distribution.

22. Do any other protozoan diseases affect the skin?

Entamoeba histolytica and several species of trypanosomes may also cause cutaneous disease.

23. How does cutaneous amebiasis, due to *Entamoeba histolytica*, present?

Usually the result of direct extension from hepatic or colorectal disease, cutaneous amebiasis presents with serpiginous, warty ulcers of the anogenital area called *amebomas*. These ulcers may produce extensive tissue loss and predispose to severe secondary bacterial infections. Less common presentations include infection by direct inoculation of the perineum in dysenteric infants wearing diapers and on the penis following anal intercourse with an infected person.

24. What are the skin findings in trypanosomiasis?

American trypanosomiasis, or Chagas' disease, is caused by the parasite *Trypanosoma cruzi,* which is introduced through the conjunctiva or skin following the bite of blood-sucking reduviid bugs (kissing bugs). This insect has the disgusting habit of defecating on the skin following its human blood meal, and the infected feces are inoculated into the conjunctiva or wound. A unilateral conjunctivitis and lid edema (**Romana's sign**) are usually the first clinical signs. Later, the patient may become systemically ill with various rashes and subcutaneous nodules, as well as cardiac and gastrointestinal lesions that may be fatal.

African trypanosomiasis, also called sleeping sickness, is due to *Trypanosoma gambiense* or *T. rhodesiense*. It may present with a trypanosomal chancre at the site of the bite, followed by nodules and a dermatitis. The cardiac and neurologic complications of both forms of trypanosomiasis are the most serious clinical concerns.

25. Describe the cutaneous manifestations of schistosomiasis as they relate to the parasite's life cycle.

Schistosomiasis is a trematode (fluke) infection produced by one of three species of the genus *Schistosoma*. Schistosomes have a complex life cycle that involves developing in freshwater snails (intermediate host) and the release of free-swimming cercariae that penetrate the human skin. Penetration produces a transient pruritus and burning followed by blisters, bruising, and crusted papules over the next few days. As the worm reaches maturity in the portal or caval venous system, the ova are released by the adult female and passed into the feces or urine. Some ova are deposited in the skin and may produce nodules, ulcers, and warty tumors. The anogenital region is most often involved through direct extension from the bladder or rectum, but spread through the bloodstream and lymphatics may produce lesions at other sites.

26. Are swimmer's itch and sea bather's eruption the same thing?

No. **Swimmer's itch,** also called clam digger's itch and bather's itch, is caused by the penetration of the skin by schistosome cercariae that normally infest birds. When first exposed, the

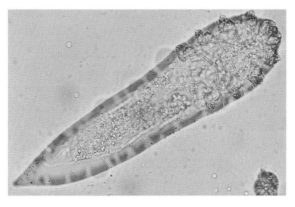

FIGURE 7. *Demodex folliculorum* (mineral oil preparation, original magnification 500X).

victim will have a prickly eruption within a few minutes of cercarial penetration that rapidly resolves. Repeated exposure, through an allergic response, leads to larger, longer lasting, and more pruritic papules that may cause pustules, blisters, and dermatitis. As with creeping eruption, the parasite cannot complete its life cycle since it cannot penetrate the epidermis.

Sea bather's eruption is caused by contact with larval forms of a marine jellyfish. In contrast to swimmer's itch, which presents with lesions in exposed areas, sea bather's eruption typically presents with pruritic macules and papules in areas covered by clothing. It is felt that the clothing holds the larvae close to the skin long enough to cause a small sting.

27. What is sparganosis?

Sparganosis is an infection produced by various species of the tapeworm *Spirometra,* which is seen most commonly in Asia and Southeast Asia. Sparganosis is typically acquired by drinking water containing infected copepods or the ingestion of inadequately cooked snake or frog meat. Clinically, it presents as pruritic or painful nodules that contain the encysted tapeworm. "Application sparganosis" occurs when an eye or ulcer is contaminated by a poultice made from these same animals and is characterized by similar nodules at the site of inoculation. Sparganosis is best treated by surgical removal of the tapeworm.

28. Can other tapeworms affect the skin?

Taenia solium (pork tapeworm) may produce **cysticercosis cutis,** which is acquired from the oral ingestion of eggs, usually due to poor sanitary habits. Clinically, it presents as painless subcutaneous nodules containing the larval stage of the tapeworm.

Echinococcus granulosus, a dog tapeworm, produces fluctuant, cystic tumors in the skin (**hydatid disease**) as well as generalized hives and itching. It is acquired from the ingestion of contaminated food or water.

29. What is *Demodex*?

These microscopic mites reside by the thousands in the hair follicles (*D. folliculorum*) and sebaceous glands (*D. brevis*) of adult humans. They resemble carrots with legs and live off sebum and squamous debris (Fig. 7).

30. Does *Demodex* cause skin disease?

The role of *Demodex* in facial eruptions, particularly rosacea, has been a topic of debate for decades. Many convincing reports describe a recalcitrant folliculitis, often seen in immunosuppressed patients, which responds to mite-killing topical therapy. The contribution of *Demodex* to garden-variety rosacea is less certain.

BIBLIOGRAPHY

1. Bonnar E, Eustace P, Powell FC: The *Demodex* mite population in rosacea. J Am Acad Dermatol 28:443–447, 1993.
2. Brown M, Hebert AA: Insect repellents: An overview. J Am Acad Dermatol 36:243–249, 1997.

3. Chaudry AZ, Longworth DL: Cutaneous manifestations of intestinal helminthic infections. Dermatol Clin 7:275–290, 1989.
4. Davies HD, Sakuls P, Keystone JS: Creeping eruption. Arch Dermatol 129:588–591, 1993.
5. Davis BR: Filariases. Dermatol Clin 7:313–321, 1989.
6. Elgart ML: Onchocerciasis and dracunculosis. Dermatol Clin 7:323–330, 1989.
7. Evans TG: Leishmaniasis. Infect Dis Clin North Am 7:527–546, 1993.
8. Freedberg IM, et al (eds): Fitzpatrick's Dermatology in General Medicine, 5th ed. New York, McGraw-Hill, 1999.
9. Furner BB: Cutaneous leishmaniasis in Texas: Report of a case and review of the literature. J Am Acad Dermatol 23:368–371, 1990.
10. Goddard J: Physicians' Guide to Arthropods of Medical Importance. Boca Raton, FL, CRC Press, 1996.
11. Kirchoff LV: Chagas disease. Infect Dis Clin North Am 7:487–502, 1993.
12. Kubba R: Leishmaniasis. Dermatol Clin 7:331–350, 1989.
13. Marsella R, Ruiz de Gopegui R: Leishmaniasis: A re-emerging zoonosis. Int J Dermatol 37:801–814, 1998.
14. Odom RB, James WD, Berger TG: Andrews' Diseases of the Skin. Philadelphia, W.B. Saunders, 2000.
15. Vaughan TK, English JC 3rd: Cutaneous larva migrans complicated by erythema multiforme. Cutis 62:33–35, 1998.
16. Vollmer RT: Demodex-associated folliculitis. Am J Dermatopathol 18:589–591, 1996.
17. Weber LA: Drug therapy of fungal and parasitic diseases. Dermatol Clin 7:387–396, 1989.

34. ARTHROPOD BITES AND STINGS

C. Paul Sayers, M.D.

1. What are arthropods?

Arthropods, the most successful group of all living animals, are invertebrates that arise from eggs and share three anatomic features:

1. Body segmentation (head, thorax, abdomen)
2. A hard outer exoskeleton
3. Paired, symmetrical, and jointed appendages (legs, antennae, mouthparts, sensory organs)

Insects and the arachnids are the most important members.

Classification of the Arthropods

Arachnids (spiders, ticks, mites, scorpions)
Insects (bees, lice, fleas, beetles, mosquitoes, butterflies, moths, etc.)
Millipedes
Centipedes
Crustaceans

2. Are most arthropods harmful to humans?

Despite our fear of insects and spiders, of the 1 million named species of arthropods, only 0.5% are injurious to man. Direct injury of the skin may occur from bites, stings, or contact. Tissue injury may result from allergic sensitization or reaction to venom. Arthropods are vectors of bacterial, viral, rickettsial, and protozoan diseases.

BITES AND STINGS

3. How do you diagnose a bite or sting reaction?

The annoyance of the mosquito or the immediate pain of a bee sting rarely poses a problem of recognition. Diagnostic problems arise when the arthropod is not seen or felt, but leaves a nonspecific rash, papules, pain, or swelling. Careful history, knowledge of local arthropod populations, and physical examination with a high index of suspicion are necessary. Investigation of the environment, including exposure to pets, pests such as rats and mice, and nesting birds and bats near or in the home or workplace, is occasionally necessary. Consultation with a veterinarian or entomologist may be beneficial in unusual cases.

4. Why are some bites and stings extremely painful or dangerous while others are simply itchy, red bumps?

The host reaction largely depends on whether the bite or sting is defensive, toxic, or for feeding. The highly visible, buzzing yellow bee or wasp stings primarily in defense of the hive. The venom is a mixture of polypeptides, enzymes, and low-molecular-weight vasoactive compounds such as histamine and serotonin that cause instant, severe pain for immediate negative feedback.

The bite of a spider, on the other hand, contains toxins and proteolytic, digestive enzymes that subjugate and then liquify the prey for food. Unfortunately, these venoms are often quite painful and destructive when injected into humans.

The bites of ectoparasites that require blood for nutrition or reproduction, such as mosquitoes, are almost always harmless and painless, unless allergic reaction takes place. These salivary products are often allergenic and cause itching and redness.

5. Do ectoparasites such as mosquitoes, ticks, fleas, and mites bite randomly?

No. Most arthropods are attracted to their hosts by a number of physical and chemical stimuli, such as warmth, moisture, carbon dioxide, and lipids on the skin. Thus, to arthropods, some human hosts are more attractive than others.

6. Why are bite reactions to ectoparasites different in different people?

Given the same environmental conditions, the severity of bug bite reactions depends on the immunologic status of the patient. In general, an immunologically sensitive, attractive patient with intense exposure will have widespread, symptomatic eruptions. However, a severely symptomatic eruption may result from only a few bites in a very sensitive person, while many bites may produce no symptoms at all in a person with an acquired immunologic tolerance.

7. List the five stages of immunologic reactivity to arthropod bites.

In clinical settings and experimental models, continuous exposure to biting arthropods will produce five stages of reactivity. Confusing clinical reactions may emerge because immunologic reaction may be nonreactive, severe, or even tolerant depending on the patient's immune status.

Stages of Reactions to Continuous Arthropod Biting

Stage 1	Bite is nonreactive in persons never exposed before.
Stage 2	Delayed red papule begins 24 hours after the bite and subsides within a week.
Stage 3	An immediate wheal after a bite, followed by the delayed papule 24 hours later.
Stage 4	Immediate wheal only, without the delayed papule, i.e., loss of delayed hypersensitivity.
Stage 5	Immunologic tolerance and no reaction after prolonged exposure.

8. How do you treat bee stings?

Most female bee stings cause transient swelling, redness, and pain at the site of the sting. The venom-containing stinger, if still present, should be removed by gently scraping the skin horizontally. Stinger removal with forceps compresses the venom gland, forcing more venom into the skin, and should be avoided. Rest, elevation, and ice to the area are helpful. Antihistamines may be used. Patients should be watched carefully for systemic signs of toxicity or allergic reactions.

9. What chemicals are in bee's venom?

Biochemical components of bee, ant, or wasp venoms fall into three main categories:

1. Small nonproteinaceous substances, such as serotonin, acetylcholine, and various catecholamines, induce redness, pruritus, pain, and vascular changes.

2. Small peptides account for immediate local swelling, pain, and tenderness, as well as for the hemolytic, neurotoxic, and lethal properties of venom.

3. Larger peptide molecules, which aid in spreading the venom and synergize the activity of other venom components, are strongly allergenic and account for the sensitization reactions.

10. What are the signs of serious systemic reactions to bee or wasp stings?

Profound, severe anaphylactic reaction may occur with nausea and vomiting, diarrhea, hypotension, shortness of breath, bronchospasm, generalized edema (especially around the mouth and throat), collapse, and even death.

11. How do you treat the anaphylactic syndrome from a bee sting?

If a reaction begins, treatment includes subcutaneous injection of epinephrine, 1:1000 in aqueous solution. In addition, intravenous diphenhydramine and cortisone as well as oxygen, fluids, vasopressors, and bronchodilators may be used as needed. Since most fatalities occur within the first hour, early intervention by the allergic patient with a self-administered epinephrine injection may prevent a reaction from developing. Emergency treatment kits may be prescribed and carried at all times (Ana-kit by Hollister-Stier or EpiPen/Epipen Jr.). Education in sting avoidance and evaluation for venom immune therapy should be considered.

12. When you are chased by bees, is it best to run or stand still to avoid being stung?

The best treatment for stings is prevention. Exposure to areas of wildflowers or clover fields should be avoided, especially if you are allergic. Brightly colored clothing, flowery designs, and the use of colognes, perfumes, and scented soaps should be minimized. When confronted by bees or wasps, avoid rapid movements and either stand still or withdraw very slowly to prevent agitation.

13. Do ants exhibit unique sting characteristics?

Different species of ants produce different sting reactions. The **harvester ant** leaves a small, yellow stinger in the wound. This sting is unusual in that the pain starts slowly and progressively gets worse over the next 6–24 hours. Piloerection and sweating also may occur around the sting site.

The bite of the imported **fire ant** can produce sterile pustules at the sting site. These stings are often grouped and cause severe pain of shorter duration than the honeybee sting. Unlike the venom from the other members of the order Hymenoptera, the fire ant venom consists of 0.1% protein, and the remainder is piperidine alkaloids and water. The alkaloids cause the pain and swelling. Treatment of ant stings is symptomatic.

14. What species of spiders are medically important?

The brown recluse and the female black widow are the most serious spiders in the United States. The hobo spider (*Tegenaria agrestis*) in the Pacific Northwest can produce necrotic arachnidism as well. Up to 60 other species may bite humans, causing a small amount of pain or even necrosis at the site, but these reactions are transient, self-limiting, and require little attention. Most species are too small and inject insignificant amounts of venom, or the biting mouthparts will not penetrate the human skin.

15. How do you diagnose and treat the black widow bite?

The female black widow produces a loose web, inhabits dark, quiet places, and bites when disturbed. The spider is 10–15 mm long and has a black globose abdomen, often with a red hourglass figure on the ventral surface. This spider is found in all 48 contiguous states.

The initial bite may sting slightly and then begins to burn. The skin changes may be minimal, but the systemic symptoms of pain and muscle cramping may become intense. Diaphoresis, dizziness, anxiety, salivation, and other neurotoxic symptoms may ensue.

Treatment should be prompt. Antisera is available and affords prompt relief, especially in the very young, old, or those with a history of heart disease or hypertension. Calcium gluconate, muscle relaxants, and pain medications also are used.

16. How do you diagnose and treat a brown recluse spider bite?

Unlike the black widow, the brown recluse produces a dermonecrotic toxin that can cause severe necrosis of the skin as well as a hemolytic toxin that causes severe, even life-threatening hemolysis.

The brown recluse is brown to yellow in color with a dark brown violin-like marking on the dorsum of the cephalothorax, hence the name fiddleback spider. This spider is reclusive, hiding in undisturbed places such as storage rooms, cracks and crevices, and under logs, stones, or furniture. The bite commonly occurs when a person is cleaning old storage areas or trying on clothes in storage. The initial bite may be painless but usually is sharp and stinging. Often, the spider is not seen or recovered. The initial stinging subsides in 6–8 hours and is replaced by a dull aching pain that gradually increases in intensity and is accompanied by itching. The bite then shows a central blue color (impending necrosis), a surrounding white area (vasospasm), and peripheral red halo (inflammation). Extension of this reaction demonstrates a gravitational spread to dependent areas. Over the next 2–4 days, the extent of the necrosis will be known. After 2–3 days, a rare but serious and life-threatening systemic reaction from venom may occur.

First aid measures are important and can be remembered by the mnemonic **RICE. R**est, **i**ce, **c**ompression, and **e**levation of the bite site tend to decrease the temperature and lower the enzymatic activity of the dermonecrotic toxin, a phospholipase. General wound care, tetanus toxicoid, antibiotics such as erythromycin or cephalexin, and observation for systemic problems may be necessary until the wound heals. Dapsone has been used to inhibit neutrophil function that amplifies the necrosis. The use of corticosteroioods and early excisional surgery for dermonecrosis is controversial. Systemic corticosteroids may be useful to modify the hemolysis of systemic loxoscelism.

INFESTATIONS

17. What is scabies?

Scabies is a contagious infestation caused by a mite that affects humans and other mammals, such as dogs, cats, horses, cows, pigs, and others. ***Sarcoptes scabiei*** var. ***hominis,*** the etiologic agent of human scabies, lives its entire life on the human host. The female mates, burrows into the upper epidermis, lays her eggs, and eventually dies after 1 month. The mite and its feces cause severe pruritus. Scabies infestations are typically transmitted from person to person by direct contact and, less commonly, by fomites.

18. How is scabies recognized clinically?

Scabies is characterized by the insidious onset of red, pruritic papulovesicular lesions that are associated with the mite. The itch is worse at night, and secondary cases involving other persons in the home are common. The rash consists of diagnostic linear burrows and pruritic papules located in the interdigital webs of the hands, the volar wrist, extensor elbows, axillary areas, central abdomen, genitalia, buttocks, and anterior thighs (Fig. 1A). Red nodules may also develop as well as large numbers of mite-free vesicles (Fig. 1B). The diagnosis is made by scraping the small (5-mm), linear, scaly burrows to reveal the female mite, her eggs, or fecal material under the microscope (Fig. 2).

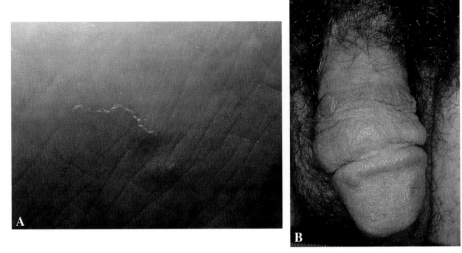

FIGURE 1. Scabies. *A*, Characteristic linear burrow. *B*, Nodular scabies most commonly presents in male genitalia as markedly pruritic papules. This lesion is almost diagnostic. (Courtesy of James E. Fitzpatrick, MD.)

19. Under what circumstances is the diagnosis of scabies obscured?

Atypical variants occur in the very young, the old, immunocompromised, partially treated, or excessively clean patient.

20. What is Norwegian scabies?

Crusted Norwegian scabies is a massive infestation with inordinate numbers of scabies mites due to inadequate host response. The large numbers of organisms cause a hyperplastic growth of the epithelium. Scratching is absent because itching is minimal. The condition is seen in debilitated patients, those with mental illness, sensory neuropathy, or paresis, and immunosuppressed patients (AIDS, post-transplantation, or topical/systemic corticosteroid therapy). Topical treatment with permethrin and keratolytics is difficult, so oral ivermectin (200 μg/kg) has been used with good success.

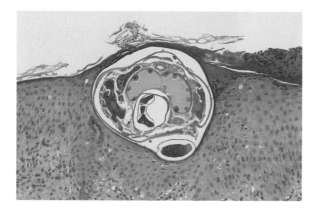

FIGURE 2. Biopsy of scabies demonstrating mite in burrow (Courtesy of James E. Fitzpatrick, MD.)

21. What agents are used to treat scabies?

Lindane 1% lotion—applied at night from the neck down; repeat in 4–5 days.

5% Permethrin cream—same as above.

5–10% Sulfur ointment—qd for 3 days (pregnant or lactating women and infants < 2 mo)

All close contacts should also be treated at the same time. Clothing and bed linens should be washed and dried.

22. Discuss the three varieties of lice that affect humans.

The **head louse** (*Pediculus humanus* var. *capitis*) is 2–4 mm long with three pairs of legs that are of equal length. The body is dorsoventrally flattened. The entire life cycle is spent in the scalp hair. Visible eggs or nits are deposited on the hair shaft, singly and close to the scalp. Pruritus of the scalp with secondary infection is common. Associated cervical and occipital lymphadenopathy is common. Head lice are more common in school-aged children, especially young females with longer hair.

The large **body louse** (*Pediculus humanus* var. *corporis*) resembles the head louse in configuration. It lives and reproduces in the lining of clothes and leaves the clothing for feeding only, being rarely found on the skin. The patient presents with pruritic papules and areas of hyperpigmentation. This problem occurs in a setting of poverty, overcrowding, and poor hygiene in individuals who rarely change or clean their clothes.

The **pubic louse** (*Phthirus pubis*), or crabs, is smaller, broad-shouldered, and has a narrow head. The miniature crab-like body is dorsoventrally flattened and has three pairs of legs. Eggs are found on the hair shaft. The pubic louse may also be found on short occipital scalp, body, eyebrow, eyelash, and axillary hair. One-third of sexually active patients with pediculosis pubis have other sexually transmitted diseases.

23. How should lice infestations be treated?

Head and pubic lice infestations are treated similarly. Standard treatment consists of lindane shampoo alone or regular shampoo followed by a 1% permethrin cream rinse. The rinse should be applied for 10 minutes after the area is dried. The treatment is repeated in 1 to 2 weeks if any viable nits are seen. If this should fail, a 5% permethrin cream (Elimite) could be used overnight with occlusion and repeated in 5 days. Finally, an oral dose of ivermectin 200μg/kg repeated in 10 days is highly effective. Removal of nits with a specially designed comb ensures that the infestation is cleared. All close contacts should also be treated.

Body lice are eliminated by thorough cleaning of the clothes. The patient needs symptomatic relief only and a fresh change of clothes.

24. How do you diagnose and treat a flea infestation?

The bites of the adult jumping flea are classically on the lower legs and ankles, particularly in females who wear no protective outer clothing (Fig. 3). The bite causes small, red, pruritic papules that may form vesicles or bullae.

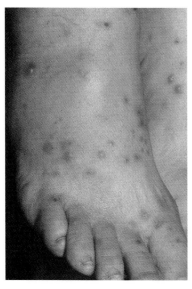

FIGURE 3. Flea bites. Papulovesicular lesions commonly found near the exposed ankles of women.

Treatment of the patient is symptomatic. The household pet and all animal contacts should be treated with insecticidal powders, shampoos, and dips. For each adult flea found on the animal, there are perhaps hundreds of adults, eggs, larvae, and pupae in the carpeting or bedding material of the host animal. Apply strict environmental controls: vacuum the pet's sleeping areas, wash or destroy the bedding, and apply an insecticide containing a residual pyrethroid and a growth regulator to the area.

25. What mite infestations of animals can affect humans?

Ornithonyssus sylviarum (northern fowl mite)	Chickens
Ornithonyssus bacoti (tropical rat mite)	Rats
Ornithonyssus bursa (tropical fowl mite)	Sparrows
Dermanyssus gallinae (poultry mite)	Chickens
Canine scabies	Dogs
Feline scabies	Cats
Cheyletiella	Dogs, cats, rabbits

26. How is *Cheyletiella* infestation recognized in humans? In animals?

Cheyletiella species are free-living, nonburrowing ectoparasitic mites of dogs, cats, and rabbits. The mite is about the same size as the scabies mite but can be easily differentiated by the presence of pincher-like palps tipped with strong claws used for grasping fur (Fig. 4). The eggs are attached to the hair shaft of the animal. The most common sources of the infestation are long-haired cats and new puppies. Animals are often asymptomatic, but a white dandruff-like scale on their backs and necks is seen on close examination.

Patients infested with the mite complain of a severe pruritic eruption, which is grouped or widespread, that involves the anterior arms and legs, chest, and abdomen, where the pet is held in close contact. The red papules may develop vesicles, pustules, and even necrosis. The severity and extent of the rash depend on the duration of contact with the pet. Diagnosis is made by examination of the pet and recovery of the organism by scraping. Treatment is directed toward the pet, pet contacts, and the environment. The patient requires symptomatic care only. *Cheyletiella* infestation often goes undiagnosed or unrecognized and is much more common than we think.

27. Where do bedbugs live? What do their bites look like?

The human bedbug, *Cimex lectularius,* is wingless, small, ovoid, dorsoventrally flattened, and reddish-brown in color (Fig. 5A). They feed rapidly and painlessly at night and live gregariously

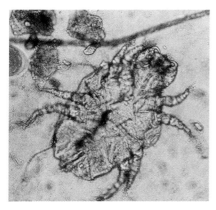

FIGURE 4. *Cheyletiella* mite resembles scabies in size but is identified by the hook-like palps anteriorly.

in dark closets, behind wall paper, or under furniture during the day and are not usually seen. Once thought to be associated only with unclean housing, bedbugs can be found even in pristine homes and may be passively brought in on luggage, clothing, or second-hand furniture.

The pruritic bites are grouped into a "breakfast, lunch, and dinner" pattern (Fig. 5B). They last for several days and then clear without treatment.

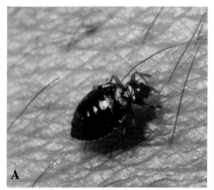
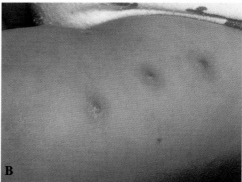

FIGURE 5. *A*, Human bedbug feeding on human skin. *B*, The bedbug bite typically occurs on the trunk and extremities in a generalized asymmetrical papular eruption that may be grouped into a "breakfast, lunch, and dinner" pattern.

28. Do species of bedbugs that parasitize other animals bite humans?

Yes. Close relatives of the human bedbug often inhabit the nests of birds or bats that are located in the attic or eaves of homes. They may bite humans, particularly if the natural host leaves the nest. In suspected arthropod bite reactions, a close search of the house for unwanted birds or bats should be made. Diagnosis is made by recovering and identifying the bug, followed by fumigating the house and cleaning out the nesting bird or bat if necessary.

INSECT VECTORS

29. What are assassin bugs? Why are they important?

Assassin bugs are true bugs that belong to the family Reduviidae. They are characterized by sucking mouthparts, generally in the form of a flexible beak. These bugs are primarily predators of other insects, but some are adapted to sucking blood from vertebrates, including humans.

In the United States, reduviid bugs such as the masked hunter, wheel bug, or black corsair produce a bite that is as painful as a hornet sting. The reactions usually persist for several hours, but occasional patients may get bullous reactions that last for days. The painful nocturnal bite is often confused with a spider bite.

The triatomids are a subfamily of the reduviids and are generally adapted to nocturnal, painless feedings on blood. They can live in the adobe dwellings in the U.S. Southwest. Initially, the bites form red, pruritic papules that last for weeks. Later, large patches of urticaria may develop as well as systemic anaphylactoid reactions.

In Central and South America, many triatomids, particularly the kissing bug, are infected with the etiologic agent of Chagas' disease (American trypanosomiasis), which is spread to humans from contamination of broken skin with the bug's feces.

30. How do tick bites affect humans?

Ticks are very familiar pests to those who frequent rural or wilderness areas. Ticks belong to the class Arachnida, along with spiders and scorpions, and are closely related to mites. All ticks are blood-sucking ectoparasites of mammals, birds, reptiles, and amphibians. Humans are an accidental host for ticks and react in various ways. The tick bite may cause a foreign-body reaction, allergic reaction to salivary proteins, reaction to a toxin (e.g., tick paralysis), or, more importantly, infectious disease carried by the tick (Fig. 6).

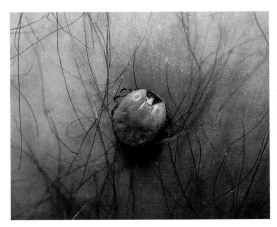

FIGURE 6. Attached feeding tick with an allergic host response manifesting as erythema and induration. (Courtesy of James E. Fitzpatrick, MD.)

31. What diseases are transmitted by ticks?

Tick-Borne Diseases of North America

Viruses	Colorado tick fever
	Tick-borne encephalitis
Rickettsia	Rocky Mountain spotted fever
	Ehrlichiosis
	Typhus
Bacteria	Lyme disease
	Relapsing fever
	Tularemia
Protozoa	Babesiosis

32. What is the most common vector-borne infectious disease in the U.S.?

Lyme disease. It is caused by *Borrelia burgdorferi*, a spirochete,and transmitted by the hard ticks, *Ixodes scapularis* (deer tick) and *I. pacificus* in the pacific states. Although Lyme disease occurs throughout the world, most cases occur in highly endemic areas in the northeast, midwest (Minnesota, Wisconsin), and pacific west. Most cases occur in late spring and early summer and present with fever and malaise associated with an annular erythema migrans around the site of a tick bite. Months later disseminated infections reveal cardiac, neurologic, and arthritic symptoms. Treatment consists of antibiotics such as amoxicillin or doxycycline.

33. If ticks may stay on a host for several days, why do they often go unnoticed?

The nymphal form of the tick is the most common type to bite humans and is roughly the size of the dot on the letter *i* on this page. In addition to the small size, the bite is painless due to the tick's salivary secretion of anesthetic, anticoagulant, and cement.

34. How are ticks removed once they attach to the skin?

Prompt removal of an attached tick may prevent transmission of disease. Suffocation techniques with petrolatum, heating with matches, or application of irritants should be avoided. Removal of the attached tick should be done by gentle, steady traction by forceps or glove-protected fingers that grip the tick near the head's attachment. Direct contact with the tick should be avoided to prevent contact with infectious organisms. The site and date of the tick removal should be recorded for future observations. The tick can be saved for identification and possible analysis for infectious disease.

35. How do you prevent tick bites?

1. Wear protective clothing, including long-sleeved shirts and pants tucked into the socks. The clothing should be white or light-colored to permit close and frequent inspection for ticks.

2. Permethrin-containing spray may be applied to the clothing, where it remains through several washings. This spray serves as a repellent as well as insecticide.

3. Apply repellent containing diethyltoluamide (deet) on exposed areas on hands and face. The concentration of deet in the newer preparations is in the 30–35% range to lessen concerns about systemic absorption and toxicity.

36. Name some important arthropod-borne diseases.

Selected Diseases Transmitted by Arthropods

DISEASE	VECTOR
Arboviruses (including yellow fever, dengue, encephalitis)	Mosquitoes, ticks
Babesiosis	Hard ticks
Boutonneuse fever (tick bite fever) (*Rickettsia conorii*)	Rabbit flea
Colorado tick fever	Hard ticks
Ehrlichiosis	Hard ticks
Endemic relapsing fever (*Borrellia duttoni*)	Soft ticks
Epidemic relapsing fever (*Borrellia recurrentis*)	Human body lice
Epidemic typhus (*R. prowazekii*)	Human body lice
Filiariasis (*Wuchereria bancrofti, Brugia malayi*)	Mosquitoes
Leishmaniasis (*Leishmania* spp.)	Phlebotomid flies
Loiasis (*Loa loa*)	Tabanid flies
Lyme disease (*Borrelia burgdorferi*)	Hard ticks
Malaria (*Plasmodium* spp.)	Mosquitoes
Murine typhus (*R. mooseri*)	Rat fleas, lice
Onchocerciasis (*Onchocerca volvulus*)	Black flies
Plague (*Yersinia pestis*)	Rat fleas
Q fever (*Coxiella burnetii*)	Hard ticks, fleas
Rickettsial pox (*R. akari*)	Mouse mites
Rocky Mountain spotted fever (*R. rickettsii*)	Hard ticks
Scrub typhus (*R. tsutsugamushi*)	Mites (chiggers)

From Braunstein WB: Ectoparasites. In Mandell GL, et al (eds): Principles and Practice of Infectious Diseases, 4th ed. New York, Churchill-Livingstone, 1995, p 2558; with permission.

37. What are the most effective insect repellents?

The most effective repellent for the prevention of bites from mosquitoes, chiggers, blackflies, midges, and fleas is deet. An 8–10% concentration is adequate for children and 20–50% for adults. A new preparation, Editar (an acronym for extended-duration topical arthropod repellent) provides a slow release and is marketed by 3M as Ultrathon and by Amway as Hour Guard. Permethrin aerosol (Permanone) applied to clothing is the best tick repellent.

BIBLIOGRAPHY

1. Alexander JOD: Arthropods and the Human Skin. Berlin, Springer-Verlag, 1984.
2. Brown M, Hebert AA: Insect repellents: An overview. J Am Acad Dermatol 36:243–249, 1997.
3. Burkhart CG, Burkhart CN, Burkhart KM: An assessment of topical and oral prescription and over-the-counter treatments for head lice. J Am Acad Dermatol 38:979–982, 1998.
4. Burns DA: The investigation and management of arthropod bite reactions acquired in the home. Clin Exp Dermatol 12:114–120, 1987.
5. Dahl MV: Cutaneous reactions to arthropod bites and stings. Clin Cases Dermatol 3:11–16, 1991.
6. Eads RB, Francy DB, Smith DB: The swallow bug, *O. vicarius* Horvath (Hemiptera:Cimicidae), a human household pest. Proc Entomtol Soc Wash 82:81, 1980.
7. Elston DM: Insect repellents: An overview. J Am Acad Dermatol 38:644–645, 1998.
8. Evans HE: The Pleasures of Entomology. Washington, D.C., Smithsonian Institution Press, 1985.
9. Feingold BD, Benjamini E: Allergy to flea bites: Clinical and experimental observation. Am Allergy 19:1275–1289, 1961.
10. Hewitt M, Walton GS, Waterhouse M: Pet animal infestations and human skin lesions. Br J Dermatol 85:215, 1971.
11. Jaramillo-Ayerbe F, Berrio-Munoz J: Ivermectin for crusted Norwegian scabies induced by use of topical steroids. Arch Dermatol 134:143–145, 1998.
12. Larrivee DH, Bengamini E, Feingold BF, et al: Histologic studies of guinea pig skin: Different stages of allergic reactivity and flea bites. Exp Parasitol 15:491, 1964.
13. Lee B: *Cheyletiella,* report of 14 cases. Cutis 47:11, 1992.
14. Muller GH, Kirk RW, Scott DW: Small Animal Dermatology, 4th ed. Philadelphia, W.B. Saunders, 1989.
15. Shapiro ED: Tick-borne diseases. Adv Pediatr Infect Dis 13:187-218, 1997.
16. Taplin D, Meinking TL, Porcelain SL, et al: Permethrin 5% cream: A new treatment for scabies. J Am Acad Dermatol 15:995–1001, 1986.
17. Wong RC, Hughes SE, Voorhees JJ: Spider bites. Arch Dermatol 123:98–104, 1987.

V. Cutaneous Manifestations of Internal Diseases

35. CUTANEOUS MANIFESTATIONS OF INTERNAL MALIGNANCY

John L. Aeling, M.D.

1. List the five criteria that establish an association between a skin disease and internal malignancy.

In the late 1950s, Helen Curth, while evaluating acanthosis nigricans, established five criteria necessary to make this association. These five criteria are called **Curth's postulates:**

1. Concurrent onset of the cutaneous disease and internal malignancy, or at the time of onset of the cutaneous disease, the internal malignancy is recognizable

2. Parallel course of the skin disease and internal malignancy

3. There is a specific type or site of malignancy associated with the skin disease

4. Sound statistical evidence that the malignancy is more frequent in patients with the skin disease than in age- and sex-matched controls

5. A genetic link between a syndrome with skin manifestations and an internal malignancy.

2. What is Sweet's syndrome?

Sweet's syndrome occurs mostly in women aged 30–60 and consists of characteristic skin lesions, fever, malaise, and leukocytosis. Less commonly, there is involvement of the joints, eyes, lungs, kidneys, and liver. Approximately 20% of cases have an association with a hematopoietic malignancy or, more rarely, a solid tumor.

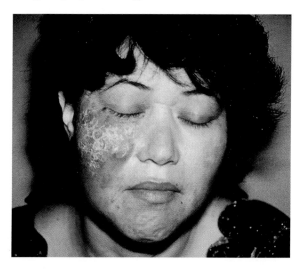

FIGURE 1. Sweet's syndrome in a woman with an inflammatory plaque and nodules on the face.

3. Describe the cutaneous lesions of Sweet's syndrome.

The clinical hallmark of Sweet's syndrome is the presence of sharply demarcated, painful plaques on the face, neck, upper trunk, and extremities (Fig. 1). The surface of the plaques have a mamillated (nipple-like) appearance and often show papulovesicles and pustules. Some lesions have a target-like appearance, and lesions on the lower extremities may resemble erythema nodosum. Oral mucous membrane and eye lesions can be seen. Skin lesions may develop at the site of minor skin trauma or needlesticks in a small subset of patients. This phenomenon is called **pathergy** and is also seen in pyoderma gangrenosum and Behçet's syndrome.

4. Are any laboratory abnormalities found in Sweet's syndrome?

Leukocytosis $> 10,000/mm^3$ is present in 60% of patients. Elevated sedimentation rates, increased numbers of segmented neutrophils, lymphopenia, anemia, and increased α_2-globulin and C-reactive protein levels can be seen. A handful of cases have been reported with anti-neutrophilic cytoplasmic antibodies.

5. What cancers are associated with Sweet's syndrome?

The most commonly associated malignancy is **myelogenous leukemia,** but lymphocytic leukemia, T- and B-cell lymphomas, polycythemia, and, rarely, solid tumors also have been reported. Male patients have had a greater frequency of associated malignancy. There are no clinical or histopathologic differences between patients with and without associated cancer. Patients with persistent laboratory abnormalities, especially anemia, thrombocytosis, and thrombocytopenia, require close observation and thorough diagnostic evaluation.

6. Describe the clinical appearance of acanthosis nigricans.

Acanthosis nigricans appears as a velvety, hyperpigmented, papillomatous, dirty-appearing skin. It is most frequently seen on the neck, axilla, groin, and dorsal hand surfaces. It is often associated with numerous skin tags and rarely affects mucosal surfaces (Fig. 2).

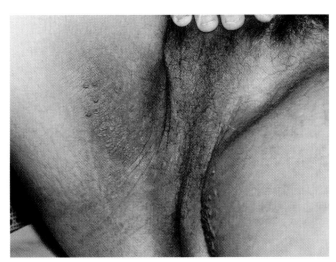

FIGURE 2. Acanthosis nigricans with hyperpigmented velvety skin lesions and small tags on the proximal thigh and groin.

7. What clinical disease states are associated with acanthosis nigricans?

Acanthosis nigricans is a common skin finding, reported in 7.1% of children aged 11–16, and is frequently associated with obesity. It is commonly found in association with diabetes and other endocrinopathies. Insulin resistance is a frequent underlying feature. Systemic corticosteroids, niacin, estrogen, pituitary extract, and testosterone have all been reported to induce acanthosis nigricans. At least 35 syndromes are reported to have acanthosis nigricans as an associated feature, and most of these have an underlying endocrinopathy.

Paraneoplastic acanthosis nigricans is rare and is most commonly associated with gastrointestinal cancer, especially gastric carcinoma. When associated with malignancy, it is usually abrupt in onset, severe, and may involve mucous membranes and palmar skin. When the cancer is in remission, paraneoplastic acanthosis nigricans will remit, and if the cancer recurs, it also returns.

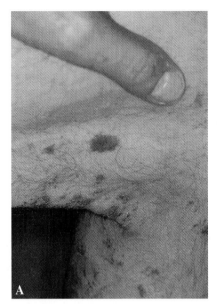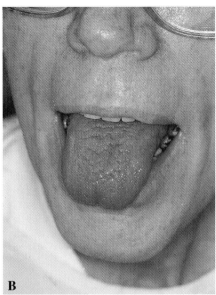

FIGURE 3. Glucagonoma syndrome. *A*, Erosive plaques on the leg. *B*, Atrophic glossitis.

8. What is necrolytic migratory erythema?

This characteristic skin eruption is associated with an alpha-cell tumor of the pancreas. It presents as erythema with superficial pustules and erosions, typically involving the face, intertriginous skin, and acral extremities (Fig. 3). Alopecia, weight loss, glossitis, stomatitis, nail dystrophy, anemia, and diabetes are frequent associations. The eruption tends to migrate and desquamate, and most patients have elevated glucagon serum levels (glucagonoma syndrome). Skin biopsy shows necrosis of the upper portion of the epidermis and is usually diagnostic. This unique skin disease is probably related to low serum amino acid levels.

9. What is hypertrichosis lanuginosa?

Hypertrichosis lanuginosa (malignant down) is an acquired excessive growth of lanugo hair. It usually begins on the face and ears and eventually can involve most hair-bearing skin. Glossitis is frequently an associated finding. If drug-related causes (such as minoxidil, diazoxide, and cyclosporine) can be excluded, there is a high association with internal malignancy. The most common associated cancers are lung, gastrointestinal, and carcinoid. This rare cutaneous finding has also been reported in patients with anorexia nervosa.

10. Where does Trousseau's sign typically present?

Trousseau's sign consists of recurrent and **migratory superficial thrombophlebitis,** affecting both large and small cutaneous veins, which is associated with an internal cancer. Crops of oval to linear, erythematous, tender skin lesions are seen most commonly on the **arms, legs, flanks, and abdomen.** Thrombosis of internal veins can also occur and lead to a variety of symptoms. Men are more commonly affected. The most common associated cancers are lung and pancreatic carcinoma.

Superficial migratory thrombophlebitis can also be seen in Behçet's syndrome and several coagulation factor deficiencies, including deficiencies of factor XII, antithrombin III, protein S and C, and plasminogen activating factor. Hypercoagulable states also occur in patients with anti-cardiolipin antibody syndrome, liver disease, nephritis, pregnancy, infection, and oral contraceptive use.

11. Describe the classical skin lesions of dermatomyositis.

The classic eruption of dermatomyositis is a reddish-purple erythema involving the face, typically the eyelids (**heliotrope sign**). The rash may be faint or quite inflamed and edematous (Fig. 4A).

In addition to the facial rash, lesions on the scalp, neck, upper trunk, and extensor extremities are common. As the lesions mature, scaling and atrophy may develop. The erythema on the hands occurs over the knuckles rather than over the phalanges, as is typical of lupus erythematosus. Cuticular telangiectasias can be seen in both lupus erythematosus and dermatomyositis. Frequently, flat-topped red-to-violaceous papules known as **Gottron's papules** develop over the knuckles of patients with dermatomyositis (Fig. 4B).

The skin lesions of dermatomyositis may precede clinical or laboratory evidence by weeks, months, or years. A few patients may never develop muscle dysfunction. The skin lesions are notoriously resistent to topical steroid therapy.

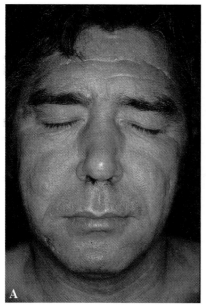

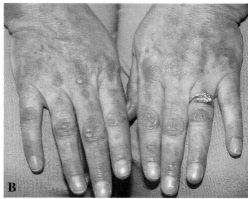

FIGURE 4. Dermatomyositis. *A*, Facial erythema and heliotrope sign. *B*, Classic hand lesions and Gottron's papules on the knuckles.

12. Is dermatomyositis associated with internal malignancy?

The true incidence of malignancy associated with dermatomyositis is difficult to define. In 153 patients with dermatomyositis, an associated malignancy was found in 8.5% of the total and 19.2% of the men. The cancer may occur before, during, or after the development of dermatomyositis. Most of the reported cases have been in patients > age 40, although cases in children have been reported.

The type of cancer reported to be associated with dermatomyositis parallels the incidence of cancer found in the general population. Thirty-seven percent of patients reported in the literature have had an associated malignancy; however, this figure has a significant selection bias. The association of malignancy with polymyositis is even less clear-cut. Patients newly diagnosed with dermatomyositis should not have extensive and expensive diagnostic work-ups for occult malignancy.

13. What are the three components of Sézary's syndrome?

As originally described, Sézary's syndrome represents a triad of findings: (1) cutaneous erythema; (2) lymphadenopathy; and (3) > 10–15% atypical mononuclear cells in peripheral blood.

This syndrome is a subset of cutaneous T-cell lymphoma (CTCL). Erythroderma can also be associated with drug reactions, psoriasis, and other cutaneous diseases. Patients with Sézary syndrome frequently have intolerable itching, often to the point that they are suicidal. Lymphadenopathy, nail dystrophy, and hair loss are common associated features. The diagnosis is established by a skin biopsy showing CTCL, the presence of at least 15% atypical mononuclear cells in peripheral blood, and the typical clinical picture. Approximately 10–15% of patients with erythroderma will have an associated lymphoma or, more rarely, leukemia.

14. What is paraneoplastic pemphigus?

Paraneoplastic pemphigus is a recently described blistering skin disease with a reported association with lymphoma, although a few cases are reported with solid tumors. The clinical picture may resemble pemphigus vulgaris, bullous pemphigoid, or erythema multiforme major (Stevens-Johnson syndrome). The disease responds poorly to immunosuppressive therapy and frequently is fatal.

15. Discuss the laboratory findings in patients with paraneoplastic pemphigus.

Skin and oral mucous membrane biopsy specimens reveal epidermal acantholysis, epidermal spongiosis, suprabasilar clefts, basal cell vacuolar changes, and dyskeratotic keratinocytes. Direct immunofluorescent examination reveals IgG and less commonly IgA with or without complement in the intracellular spaces and C3, IgG, or IgM at the basement membrane zone. Antibodies have been demonstrated against desmoplakins, proteins in keratinocyte attachment plaques (desmosomes), and against a 230 kd protein in the basement membrane (bullous pemphigoid antigen). Rat bladder is a useful substrate for indirect immunofluorescent examination and shows positive staining with serum from patients with paraneoplastic pemphigus but will be negative with serum from patients with classic pemphigus vulgaris.

16. What is the characteristic finding in erythema gyratum repens?

This rare skin eruption is characterized by a widespread, ever-changing pattern of skin lesions resembling **wood grain**. The erythematous circinate lesions may have a fine scale and move up to 1 cm a day. Almost all patients with this unique dermatoses have an associated malignancy. It was first reported in conjunction with breast cancer, which remains the most common association, but has also been reported with lung, bladder, cervical, and prostate cancers. The skin lesions clear within a few weeks after removal of the malignancy and usually recur if the cancer returns.

17. How do the lesions in Bazex syndrome (acrokeratosis paraneoplastica) progress?

This syndrome begins with acral violaceous erythema on the ears, nose, hands, and feet. Early lesions may show small vesicles. As the lesions progress, they become hyperkeratotic and psoriasiform, especially on the hands and feet. Paronychia and nail dystrophy are common. Later, the eruption may generalize, and lesions on the face may appear dermatitic or lupus-like. The syndrome is more common in men and is associated with squamous cell carcinoma of the upper aerodigestive tract.

There is another Bazex syndrome inherited as an autosomal dominant disease. This syndrome is characterized by acral follicular atrophoderma, early development of multiple facial basal cell carcinomas, and, in some patients, hypohidrosis.

18. Where does Paget's disease most commonly occur?

On the female breast, although cases have been reported in men. It begins as a small eczematous patch on the nipple that gradually spreads onto the areola and eventually to the skin of the breast. The borders of the lesion are sharply marginated, and the surface may be crusted, moist, erythematous, and/or scaly. Paget's disease of the breast invariably has an underlying ductal carcinoma, although often there is no breast mass and mammograms can be normal. Any chronic eczematous lesion on the nipple or areola that is unresponsive to topical therapy should have an excisional biopsy, which includes nipple ducts and underlying breast tissue. The associated ductal carcinoma may be small and focal and is easily missed by small punch or shave biopsy.

Extramammary Paget's disease occurs on the axilla, groin, or anogenital skin. The disease may present with solitary or multiple lesions. It is often associated with an underlying adnexal carcinoma, and about 20% of cases have carcinoma of the rectum or genitourinary tract.

19. Which disorder of protein metabolism is associated with skin lesions and malignancy?

Primary systemic amyloidosis. The cause of this disease is a plasma cell dyscrasia, even though bone marrow aspiration in some cases may be normal. The most common associated skin lesions are purpura or ecchymoses that are seen most frequently on thin skin areas, i.e., eyelids, neck, groin, axilla, umbilicus, or oral mucosa. The hemorrhagic lesions may occur on areas of clinically normal skin or in skin having waxy papules, plaques, nodules, or tumors. The intracutaneous bleeding is due to infiltration of blood vessel walls with amyloid protein. Other less common skin lesions include alopecia, nail dystrophies, scleroderma-like lesions, macroglossia, cutis verticis gyrata, bullous lesions, and dyspigmentation.

20. List the autosomal dominant diseases that have prominent skin findings and internal cancer.

Autosomal Dominant Diseases with Skin Findings and Malignancy

DISORDERS	SKIN FINDINGS	CANCER	ASSOCIATIONS
Cowden syndrome	Keratotic facial papules	Breast	Mucosal papules
	Acral keratosis	Thyroid	Fibrocystic disease of
	Soft tissue tumors		the breast
Torre's syndrome	Sebaceous tumors	Colon	Colon polyps
	Keratoacanthomas		
Gardner's syndrome	Epidermoid cysts	Colon	Colon polyps
			Osteomas
			Desmoids
			Abnormal dentition
Peutz-Jeghers syndrome	Pigmented macules on mucosa, face, acral extremities	Intestinal	Intestinal polyps
Multiple mucosal neuroma syndrome	Neuromas of lips, tongue, and oral mucosa	Thyroid	Pheochromocytoma Marfanoid habitus
Neurofibromatosis	Neurofibromas Café-au-lait macules	Neurofibrosarcoma (rare)	Lisch nodules Seizures Deafness

21. Describe the cutaneous features of Gardner's syndrome.

The cutaneous hallmark of the syndrome is epidermoid cysts, which often appear before puberty, frequently on the extremities. These cysts may be many or few. The syndrome is also characterized by osteomas (typically on facial bones), fibrous and desmoid tumors, abnormal dentition, lipomas, hypertrophy of retinal pigmented epithelium, and leiomyomas of the gastrointestinal tract. The syndrome is characterized by the early onset of colonic polyposis and has a very high incidence of colon cancer.

22. What are the clinical findings in Cowden syndrome (multiple hamartoma syndrome)?

This syndrome is characterized by a triad of findings: (1) small keratotic facial papules (Fig. 5A); (2) cobblestoning of the oral mucosa (Fig. 5B); and (3) acral keratotic skin lesions

These patients also have benign tumors of neural, fibrous, vascular, and epithelial origin. Multiple small tumors of facial hair follicles (trichilemmomas) are pathognomonic of this syndrome. Fibrocystic disease of the breast is common, and 30% of women will develop breast cancer. Many other associated cancers have been reported, with thyroid cancer being the second most common malignancy.

23. When do the characteristic skin lesions of Peutz-Jeghers syndrome appear?

Brown to blue-black macules (lentigines) are present at birth or early infancy on the lips, oral mucosa, nasal mucosa, palms, soles, dorsal hand surfaces, central face, and elbows. Polyps of the small intestine develop in 90% of patients; polyps may also occur in the stomach, colon, and rectum. There is an increased incidence of gastrointestinal malignancy, but it is not nearly as common as in patients with Gardner's syndrome. In one series, 16 fatal malignancies were seen in 72 cases, with an average age at death of 36 years. Intussusception occurs in about 50% of cases.

24. How does multiple mucosal neuroma syndrome typically present?

As the name implies, this syndrome is characterized by the development of multiple flesh-colored papules on the tongue, lips, and, occasionally, other mucosal surfaces early in life. These patients have a characteristic appearance with thick prominent lips and a marfanoid habitus. Ninety percent of these patients develop medullary thyroid carcinoma, and half will suffer from pheochromocytoma that is often multifocal and/or bilateral.

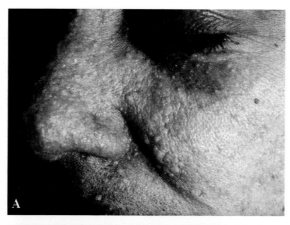

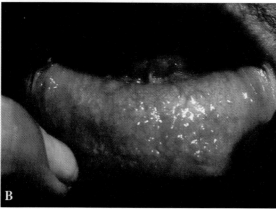

FIGURE 5. Cowden syndrome. *A,* Typical small keratotic papules on the face. *B,* Characteristic cobblestone papules on the mucosal surface of the lower lip.

25. What is Torre's syndrome (Muir-Torre's syndrome)?

This syndrome includes cutaneous sebaceous neoplasia and a high incidence of low-grade colon cancer. The sebaceous tumors include sebaceous adenomas, epitheliomas, and carcinomas. In addition, about one-third of patients develop keratoacanthomas. The sebaceous skin tumors may be few or many, but even one sebaceous adenoma should alert the clinician that the patient may have this syndrome.

26. Is the sign of Leser-Trélat (eruptive seborrheic keratoses) associated with internal malignancy?

This association remains controversial. Seborrheic keratoses are common in older patients and so is cancer. There have been many skin lesions and skin diseases reported to be associated with internal malignancy, but these are difficult to prove and probably represent spurious associations. Examples include dermatitis herpetiformis, bullous pemphigoid, pemphigus vulgaris (excluding paraneoplastic pemphigus), persistent erythemas (excluding erythema gyratum repens), cutaneous vasculitis, pruritus, scleroderma, and ichthyosis.

27. Is dry scaly skin associated with internal malignancy?

Yes. Acquired ichthyosis was first reported to be associated with Hodgkin's disease in the 1940s. In 32 patients with acquired ichthyosis Hodgkin's disease was reported in 80% of the cases and was the presenting symptom in a few patients. This association is also reported with T-cell lymphoma, leukemia, Kaposi's sarcoma, malignant histiocytosis, leiomyosarcoma, and multiple myeloma.

28. Which recessively inherited diseases have skin findings and associated internal malignancy?

Recessively Inherited Deseases with Skin Findings and Malignancy

DISORDER	INHERITANCE	CLINICAL FINDINGS	CANCER
Wiskott-Aldrich syndrome	X-linked recessive	Chronic dermatitis Thrombocytopenia Recurrent infections	Lymphoma, esp. non-Hodgkin's
Bloom's syndrome	Autosomal recessive	Photosensitivity Telangiectasia of sun-exposed skin Short stature Decreased serum Igs Recurrent infections Sister chromatid exchange	Lymphomas Leukemias
Ataxia-telangiectasia (Louis-Bar syndrome)	Autosomal recessive	Progressive cerebellar ataxia Telangiectasia Recurrent sinus and pulmonary infections Decreased/absent serum IgA	Lymphomas (increased cancer risk also seen in heterozygotes)
Dyskeratosis congenita	X-linked recessive (dominant also reported)	Skin atrophy and hyper-pigmentation Nail dystrophy Oral precancerous leukoker-atosis	Oral cancers Other malignancies

29. Can pyoderma gangrenosum be associated with internal malignancy?

Yes. Pyoderma gangrenosum (PG) is an ulcerative skin disease of unknown etiology. The lesions are painful, may rapidly enlarge, and are characterized by an erythematous or violaceous undermined border with a necrotic center (Fig. 6). The most common diseases associated with PG are inflammatory bowel disease, rheumatoid arthritis, and a small subset may have monoclonal IgA gammopathy. In a review of several studies PG was associated with internal malignancy in 7.2% of patients. Leukemia is the most frequently reported malignancy with myelocytic and myelomonocytic leukemia accounting for the majority of cases. Other reported hematologic cancers are multiple myeloma, polycythemia vera, and lymphoma. In two thirds of the cases associated with myelocytic leukemia the PG preceded or was concurrent with the diagnosis of the leukemia. There are rare sporadic reports of PG associated with solid tumors.

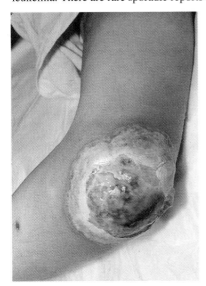

FIGURE 6. A young woman with acute-onset pyoderma gangrenosum.

30. Can you list any other skin diseases not discussed in this chapter that have been associated with internal malignancy?

The association of some skin diseases with internal malignancy remains controversial and may be related to selection bias or isolated case reports.

Several early reports associating **Bowen's disease** (carcinoma in situ of the skin) with internal malignancy stated an incidence of 15-30% of cases. Several more recent large, retrospective well documented studies found no association. **Porphyria cutanea tarda** (PCT) is a chronic blistering skin disease of sun-exposed skin with associated skin fragility, hypertrichosis, and late sclerodermoid skin changes. The disease is due to a defect in porphyrin metabolism and is often associated with chronic liver disease. There are reports of PCT associated with hepatomas, however most of these patients also have had cirrhosis of the liver and hepatomas are more common in patients with cirrhosis regardless of the etiology. **Erythromelalgia** is a rare skin disease characterized by erythematous, painful, burning of the feet, ankles, and lower extremities. The disease is aggravated by heat exposure and relieved by cooling. Many patients can find relief only by soaking their legs in ice water. The incidence of associated malignancy has been variably reported between 3 and 65% of cases. Some authors subdivide the disease into two subtypes: The idiopathic type which frequently begins in childhood and the secondary type associated with hematologic malignancies, usually polycythemia vera or essential thrombocythemia.

Generalized pruritus without skin lesions has been reported as a symptom of internal malignancy. Pruritus is reported as an initial symptom of Hodgkin's disease in 5-10% of patients and in 3% of those with non-Hodgkin's lymphoma. The relationship of this symptom to visceral solid cancers is far less clear. **Erythema annulare centrifugum** (EAC) is a chronic skin disease characterized by annular or polycyclic lesions that slowly enlarge or migrate. The disease is most commonly associated with infection or drugs and a large number of cases are idiopathic. Internal malignancy is reported in a minority of cases of EAC, usually as isolated case reports. Erythema gyratum repens, a characteristic skin disease previously discussed in this chapter, is highly specific for underlying cancer. **Vasculitis** is rarely associated with internal malignancy. In one large review of 200 patients with vasculitis and cancer 77.5% had a hematologic malignancy. There are small series and isolated case reports associating **bullous pemphigoid** with internal malignancy. However, a retrospective review of 73 patients with bullous pemphigoid compared to age- and sex-matched controls with psoriasis and contact dermatitis found no difference in the incidence of cancer. **Multicentric reticulohistiocytosis** is a rare disease characterized by multiple skin papules and nodules in patients with severe arthritis. Skin biopsy shows characteristic histology of a diffuse histiocytic cellular infiltrate with large multinucleate giant cells with ground glass cytoplasm. Associated malignancy was reported in 28% of the patients in 82 cases reported in the literature up to 1995. The disease preceded the development of cancer in 73% of the patients. This association is controversial, there was no consistent cancer reported, and there are no careful prospective studies.

BIBLIOGRAPHY

1. Anhalt GJ, Kim SC, Stanley JR, et al. Paraneoplastic pemphigus. N Engl J Med 323:1729–1735, 1990.
2. Botella-Estrada R, Sanmartin O, Oliver V, et al: Erythroderma: A clinicopathologic study of 56 cases. Arch Dermatol 130:1503–1507, 1994.
3. Callen JP: Skin signs of internal malignancy. Semin Dermatol 3:340–357, 1984.
4. Chuang TY, Reizner GT. Bowens disease and internal malignancy. A matched case control study. J Am Acad Dermatol 19:47–51, 1988.
5. Cohen PR, Kurzrock R: Cutaneous paraneoplastic syndromes. Clin Dermatol 3:1–187, 1993.
6. Cohen PR, Talpaz M, Kurzrock R. Malignancy-associated Sweet's syndrome: Review of the world literature. J Clin Oncol 6:1887–1897, 1988.
7. Giardiello FM, Welsh SB, Hamilton SR, et al: Increased risk of cancer in the Peutz-Jeghers syndrome. N Engl J Med 316:1511–1514, 1987.
8. Lober CW. Should the patient with generalized pruritus be evaluated for malignancy? J Am Acad Dermatol 19:350–352, 1988.
9. Schwartz RA: Acanthosis nigricans. J Am Acad Dermatol 31:1–19, 1994.
10. Von den Driesch P: Sweet's syndrome (acute febrile neutrophilic dermatosis). J Am Acad Dermatol 31:535–556, 1994.

36. CUTANEOUS MANIFESTATIONS OF ENDOCRINOLOGIC DISEASE

Carl Bigler, M.D.

1. How does endocrinologic disease cause skin disorders?

There are several mechanisms by which endocrinologic diseases produces cutaneous changes:

- Hormones interact with cell surface receptors to regulate cellular function. Many cell types in the skin have hormonal receptors. Deficient or excess hormone levels can alter skin metabolism. An example is the warm and moist skin associated with hyperthyroidism.
- Hormone deficiency or excess may affect the skin indirectly rather than through specific receptors. An example is the hyperglycemia of diabetes that results in increased cutaneous infections.

For some unusual skin disorders that are highly suggestive of endocrinologic disease, such as necrobiosis lipoidica diabeticorum and scleredema in diabetes mellitus and pretibial myxedema in hyperthyroidism, the pathogenesis is not understood.

2. What is necrobiosis lipoidica diabeticorum?

This disease most commonly occurs on the pretibial areas, although it may occur at other sites. Early lesions present as nondiagnostic erythematous papules and evolve into annular lesions that have a yellowish-brown color, dilated blood vessels, and central epidermal atrophy (Fig. 1). Developed pretibial lesions can be diagnosed by clinical appearance.

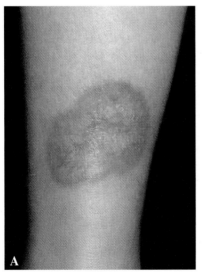 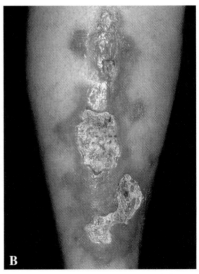

FIGURE 1. Necrobiosis lipoidica diabeticorum. *A,* Typical yellow-red plaque of a developed lesion. *B,* Late lesion, with central atrophy and extensive ulceration. (Courtesy of James E. Fitzpatrick, MD.)

3. Do all patients with necrobiosis lipoidica diabeticorum have diabetes?

No. In a study of 171 patients with necrobiosis lipoidica diabeticorum, about 60% had diabetes. Many other patients subsequently developed diabetes, had abnormal glucose tolerance tests, or a strong family history of diabetes. Only about 10% of patients were not in a high-risk group to develop diabetes. In a more recent study with 65 patients, 22% either had or developed diabetes. Patients with necrobiosis lipoidica diabeticorum should be screened for diabetes.

4. Is necrobiosis lipoidica diabeticorum common in patients with diabetes?

No. It occurs in 0.3% of patients with diabetes and may occur in both insulin-dependent and insulin-resistant diabetic patients.

5. What is scleredema?

Scleredema presents as a woody induration and thickening of skin involving the neck, back, and upper arms. Histopathologic examination reveals a thickened dermis with increased mucinous ground substance. Scleredema has been associated with preceding streptococcal infections, monoclonal gammopathy, and diabetes. In adults with scleredema (adultorum), insulin-resistant diabetes occurs with some frequency and is associated with a prolonged chronic course, in contrast to post-streptococcal scleredema which often resolves within 1–2 years.

6. Is insulin resistance associated with other skin findings?

Acanthosis nigricans. Insulin-like growth factors are produced by the liver in response to high levels of circulating insulin. These growth factors bind to epidermal growth factor receptors or other receptors and produce thickening of the epidermis and hyperkeratosis.

7. What does acanthosis nigricans look like?

Acanthosis nigricans presents as velvety, hyperpigmented plaques, most commonly in neck creases and axillae (Fig. 2). The patient may complain about "dirty skin" under the arms that is impossible to clean. The tops of knuckles may also demonstrate small papules.

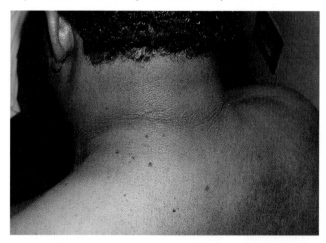

FIGURE 2. Velvety hyperpigmentation of the neck crease in a patient with classic acanthosis nigricans. (Courtesy of James E. Fitzpatrick, MD.)

8. Is diabetes the only condition associated with acanthosis nigricans?

No. There are many causes of insulin resistance and hyperinsulinemia. Endocrine diseases such as Cushing's syndrome with excess cortisol, acromegaly with excess growth hormone, or polycystic ovarian disease are also associated with acanthosis nigricans. Patients with familial obesity and acanthosis nigricans usually have associated hyperinsulinemia. Certain malignancies, most commonly gastrointestinal adenocarcinomas, may autonomously make insulin-like growth factors and thus produce acanthosis nigricans. Oral acanthosis nigricans suggests malignancy as the cause.

9. Describe the clinical manifestations of pretibial myxedema.

Pretibial myxedema is characterized by brawny, indurated plaques over the pretibial areas. These plaques may be skin-colored or have an unusual brownish-red color (Fig. 3). On biopsy, the skin is infiltrated by mucinous ground substance. Pretibial myxedema is specific for Graves' disease but occurs in only 3–5% of patients with the disease. Pretibial myxedema is often associated with Graves' ophthalmopathy that results in exophthalmos and acropachy (clubbed nails). Treatment of hyperthyroidism has no effect on pretibial myxedema.

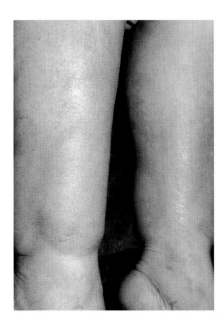

FIGURE 3. Large indurated skin-colored plaques of pretibial myxedema.

10. What bacterial infections are more common in diabetic patients?

Cutaneous bacterial infections are relatively more common and severe in patients with diabetes. Diabetic foot ulcers are a leading cause of morbidity and health care cost. Foot numbness from diabetic neuropathy prevents recognition of injury and hyperglycemia impairs white blood cell function, allowing bacterial infection. Staphylococcal folliculitis or skin abscesses are well described in diabetic patients and respond well to antibiotics and surgical drainage of abscesses. Diabetic patients may develop external necrotizing ear infections caused by *Pseudomonas aeruginosa.*

11. What are the most common fungal skin infections associated with diabetes?

Candidiasis, usually caused by *Candida albicans.* Mucocutaneous candidiasis is characterized by red plaques with adherent white exudate and satellite pustules. Candidal vulvovaginitis is extremely common. Perianal dermatitis in either men or women may be caused by *Candida.* Other mucocutaneous forms of candidiasis include thrush (infection of oral mucosa), perlèche (angular cheilitis), intertrigo (infection of skinfolds), erosio interdigitalis blastomycetica chronica (finger webspace infection), paronychia (infection of the soft tissue around the nailplate), and onychomycosis (infection of the nail). The mechanism appears to involve increased levels of glucose that serve as a substrate for *Candida* species to proliferate. Patients with recurrent cutaneous candidiasis of any form should be screened for diabetes.

12. Are there more dangerous fungal infections associated with diabetes?

Rarely, **mucormycosis** will complicate diabetic ketoacidosis. Mucormycosis is a severe and progressive infection of the soft tissues caused by saprophytic fungi such as *Mucor, Rhizopus,* and *Absidia* species. This infection is poorly responsive to systemic antifungals and is often fatal.

13. Why are diabetic patients in ketoacidosis especially prone to mucormycosis?

These fungi prefer an acid pH, grow rapidly in high glucose media, and are one of the few fungi that utilize ketones as a growth substrate. All these growth requirements are present in patients with diabetic ketoacidosis.

14. What other skin disorders are commonly encountered in diabetic patients?

Diabetic dermopathy (atrophic, scarred, hyperpigmented papules on the anterior leg), yellow skin and nails, skin tags, and diabetic thick skin occur commonly (> 30%). Bullous disease of diabetes (tense bullae of the lower extremities) and diabetic stiff hands are less common complications.

15. What are the skin manifestations of hypothyroidism?
Mild hypothyroidism: The skin is dry, scaly, cold, and pale. Dryness and scale may make the skin pruritic. The nails are brittle.
Severe and long-standing hypothyroidism: There may be yellow and diffusely thickened skin (Fig. 4), loss of the outer third of the eyebrows and enlarged and thickened lips and tongue.

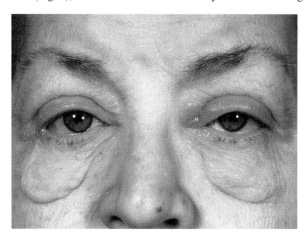

FIGURE 4. Patient with severe generalized myxedema demonstrating intensive periocular edema and very yellow skin. (Courtesy of James E. Fitzpatrick, MD.)

16. Why do hypothyroid patients have yellow skin?
The yellow skin is due to excess serum carotene that is deposited in the stratum corneum. Carotenemia results from impaired hepatic conversion of carotene to vitamin A in patients with hypothyroidism.

17. Why do hypothyroid patients have thickened skin?
There is increased dermal mucopolysaccharide or mucin within the skin (myxedema).

18. How does the myxedema of hypothyroidism differ from pretibial myxedema of Graves' disease?
Myxedema of hypothyroidism has smaller quantities of mucin with a generalized distribution over the entire surface area of skin. Pretibial myxedema often has dermal pools of mucin and is localized to the anterior legs.

19. Are the skin changes of hypothyroidism reversible with thyroid replacement?
Yes.

20. What are the skin manifestations of hyperthyroidism?
They are the opposite of hypothyroidism. Hyperthyroid skin is moist, warm, smooth, and erythematous. The skin may be pruritic. The nails may separate from the nailbed (onycholysis).

21. Which hormone gives the skin a darkened or tanned appearance?
Adrenocorticotropic hormone (ACTH) darkens the skin by stimulating melanocytes to produce melanin. In contrast to normal tanning, the darkening is often accentuated in palmar creases and mucous membranes. (A note of caution: dark skin creases and mucous membranes may be a normal variant in more darkly pigmented races.) The most common cause of elevated ACTH levels is Addison's disease, in which hypofunctioning adrenals and deficient serum cortisol remove the negative feedback inhibition of the pituitary gland that increases ACTH production.

22. What skin disease is associated with insulin-dependent diabetes, hypothyroidism, and Addison's disease?
Vitiligo. This is a trick question. Vitiligo is not caused by deficient hormones but is an autoimmune disease that results in the destruction of melanocytes and is associated with the

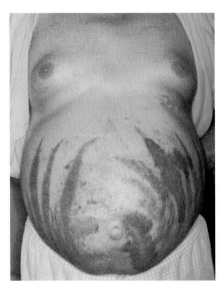

FIGURE 5. Cushing's syndrome (excess glucocorticoids), showing truncal obesity and abdominal striae. (Courtesy of James E. Fitzpatrick, MD.)

autoimmune endocrinopathies. Vitiligo presents clinically as white macules most commonly on the face and hands. Vitiligo is present in 4% of patients with insulin-dependent diabetes, 7% of patients with Graves' disease, and 15% of patients with Addison's disease. There is also a familial predisposition to this group of diseases.

23. What skin findings are associated with glucocorticoid excess or Cushing's disease?

The skin is generally thin and atrophic. Wound repair is inhibited, and striae develop in sites such as the abdomen, upper chest, and buttocks, where the skin is normally stretched. These striae are often large and purple in color, in contrast to idiopathic or pregnancy-induced striae (Fig. 5). The skin has a ruddy appearance, and telangiectasias may be prominent. The skin bruises and tears easily. These changes may also be seen in skin that has been treated with high-strength topical steroids for long periods of time. Broadened facial features (moon facies), increased subcutaneous fat on the upper back and neck (buffalo hump), and truncal obesity are also characteristic.

24. Are the skin changes caused by excess glucocorticoids reversible?

Partially. Striae and telangiectasias may fade but often do not disappear.

25. Which hormones have the greatest effect on sebaceous glands and hair?

The androgens. Androgens at the time of puberty induce sebaceous gland activity and the development of acne. Excess androgen in women may cause acne, hirsutism (increased facial hair), or alopecia (male- or female-pattern balding). Associated signs may include hyperpigmentation of genital and areolar skin and clitoromegaly. Possible causes of hirsutism and acne in women include adrenal and ovarian tumors, prolactin-producing pituitary tumors, polycystic ovarian disease, adrenal enzyme deficiencies, and familial acne and hirsutism that may be related to increased end-organ sensitivity to normal circulating levels of androgens. Most acne and hirsutism in women is benign and familial. Screening tests for tumors include serum prolactin, dehydroepiandrosterone sulfate (DHEAS) which is an androgen produced by the adrenal glands, and total testosterone.

26. Are there medications and nutritional supplements that may cause acne?

Yes. Supplements and medications that have androgen effects and can cause acne may not appear in the patient's list of medications. New-onset acne in a recreational weightlifter, either male or female, may result from the use of androgens. New-onset acne in a young woman may be the result of use of birth control. The progesterone-like hormone in many birth control pills and in all long-acting depository forms may have androgen effects. New-onset acne in a perimenopausal woman may result from small amounts of testosterone added to some estrogen supplements.

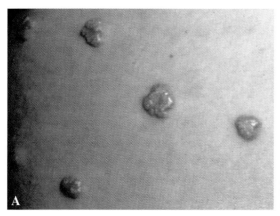
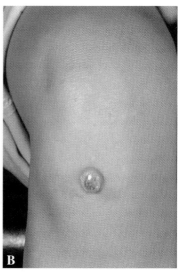
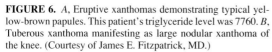

FIGURE 6. *A*, Eruptive xanthomas demonstrating typical yellow-brown papules. This patient's triglyceride level was 7760. *B*, Tuberous xanthoma manifesting as large nodular xanthoma of the knee. (Courtesy of James E. Fitzpatrick, MD.)

27. What are xanthelasma?

Xanthelasma are distinctive yellowish plaques on the eyelids and around the eyes. Histologically, these lesions appear similar to eruptive xanthomas. Unlike eruptive xanthomas, xanthelasma are not commonly associated with elevated triglycerides. Although people with xanthelasma may have normal total cholesterol and triglyceride levels, xanthelasma is a marker for tissue deposition of cholesterol that is important in the origin of coronary artery disease. More subtle lipid abnormalities, such as lower "good" HDL-C cholesterol, also can be found.

28 What are eruptive xanthomas?

Eruptive xanthomas are multiple, small, skin-colored to yellow-brown papules that occur in crops, most commonly on the buttocks, thighs, or elbows (Fig. 6A). On biopsy, there is accumulation of lipid within histiocytes and around blood vessels in the skin. These distinctive papules are a cutaneous sign of very high triglyceride levels. There is often associated lipemia retinalis on fundoscopic examination. These patients are at risk to develop pancreatitis that may be severe. Often eruptive xanthomas are precipitated by the new onset of diabetes.

29. How do eruptive xanthomas differ from tuberous xanthomas?

Tuberous xanthomas are larger and deeper than eruptive xanthomas and may be palpated as nodules similar to a large radish, small turnip, or other vegetable *tuber* or root within the deep dermis or subcutaneous fat (Fig. 6B). These xanthomas are the result of cholesterol accumulation within these tissues, in contrast to the smaller, papular, eruptive xanthomas which contain triglyceride. Tuberous xanthomas are a marker of high cholesterol levels, and these patients are at risk for coronary artery disease at a young age. Tendinous xanthomas (e.g., similar lesions attached to large tendons such as the Achilles tendon) may also be present.

30. What are the cutaneous features of acromegaly?

Acromegaly is the result of excess pituitary growth hormone. Bone thickening is prominent and results in coarse facies and enlarged hands. The skin changes are the result of the production of insulin-like growth factors and, thus, overlap with changes due to insulin resistance. The skin is hypertrophied and thickened, and acanthosis nigricans may be present. These changes may be accentuated on the scalp as whorled furrowing (cutis vertices gyrata).

31. How does panhypopituitarism affect the skin?

The skin in patients with panhypopituitarism appears pale, and there are fine wrinkles around the eyes and mouth. Body hair and genital hair are sparse. Sweat and sebum production are also diminished. The skin dryness and thickening are not as prominent as in primary hypothyroidism because there is some autonomous thyroid gland function in panhypopituitarism.

BIBLIOGRAPHY

1. Cruz PD Jr, Hud JA Jr: Excess insulin binding to insulin-like growth factor receptors: Proposed mechanism for acanthosis nigricans. J Invest Dermatol 98(6 suppl): 82S–85S, 1992.
2. Derksen J, Nagesser SK, Meinders AE, et al: Identification of virilizing adrenal tumors in hirsute women. N Engl J Med 331:968–973, 1994.
3. Diven DG, Gwinup G, Newton R: Skin signs of internal disease: The thyroid. Dermatol Clin 7:547–558, 1989.
4. Fatourechi V, Pajouhi M, Fransway AF: Dermopathy of Graves' disease (pretibial myxedema): Review of 150 cases. Medicine 73(1):1–7, 1994.
5. Feingold KR, Elias PM: Endocrine-skin interactions. J Am Acad Dermatol 17:921–940, 1987.
6. Huntley AC: Skin signs of internal disease: Cutaneous manifestations of diabetes mellitus. Dermatol Clin 7:531–546, 1989.
7. Lowitt MH, Dover JS: Necrobiosis lipoidica. J Am Acad Dermatol 25:735–748, 1991.
8. Matsuoka LY, Wortsman J, Goldman J: Acanthosis nigricans. Clin Dermatol 11:21–25, 1993.
9. Muller SA, Winkelmann RK: Necrobiosis lipoidica diabeticorum: A clinical and pathological investigation of 171 cases. Arch Dermatol 93:272–281, 1966.
10. O'Toole EA, Kennedy U, Nolan JJ, et al: Necrobiosis lipoidica: Only a minority of patients have diabetes mellitus. Br J Dermatol 140:283–286, 1999.
11. Parker F: Xanthomas and hyperlipidemia. J Am Acad Dermatol 13:1–30, 1985.
12. Perez MI, Kohn SR: Cutaneous manifestations of diabetes mellitus. J Am Acad Dermatol 30:519–531, 1994.
13. Plourde PV, Marks JG, Hammond JM: Acanthosis nigricans and insulin resistance. J Am Acad Dermatol 10:887–891, 1984.
14. Ramirez-Amador V, Esquivel-Pedraza L, Caballero-Mendoza E, et al: Oral manifestations as a hallmark of malignant acanthosis nigricans. J Oral Pathol Med 28:278–281, 1999.
15. Ribera M, Pinto X, Argimon JM, et al: Lipid metabolism and apolipoprotein E phenotypes in patients with xanthelasma. Am J Med 99:485–490, 1995.
16. Romano G, Moretti G, Di Benedetto A, et al: Skin lesions in diabetes mellitus: prevalence and clinical correlations. Diabetes Res Clin Pract 39:101–106, 1998.
17. Sperling LC, Heimer WL: Androgen biology as a basis for the diagnosis and treatment of androgenic disorders in women. J Am Acad Dermatol 28:669–683, 1993.

37. SKIN SIGNS OF GASTROINTESTINAL DISEASE

Paul M. Benson, M.D., COL, MC

1. What are some of the cardinal skin signs of disease of the digestive tract?

Jaundice, ascites, purpura, and spider angiomas are well-known cutaneous hallmarks of advanced cirrhosis of the liver. Other less-common clues include the freckling on the lips of patients with Peutz-Jeghers syndrome or the destructive lesions of pyoderma gangrenosum on the legs associated with inflammatory bowel disease. It is not surprising that many diseases of the skin also involve the oral and anal mucosa, because embryologically, the foregut (giving rise to the oral epithelium) and hindgut (developing into the anal mucosa) share a common ectodermal component in the first weeks of fetal development. As a consequence, the skin becomes a "mirror" of underlying pathology, both obvious and occult, in the GI system.

2. Why aren't all jaundiced patients yellow?

Jaundice (icterus) is the accumulation of bilirubin and various bile pigments in the skin and other organs. It may result from intrinsic disease of the liver, obstruction due to gallstones or tumors, or overproduction of bilirubin as with hemolysis. Bilirubin has a strong affinity for tissues rich in elastic tissue. It accumulates earliest in the sclera of the eye, the skin (especially the face), hard palate, and abdominal wall. Jaundice is best seen in bright daylight, and it is possible to overlook mild jaundice with indoor lighting. Clinically apparent jaundice is not noticeable until the serum bilirubin exceeds 2.5–3.0 mg/dl in the adult. Infants may have much higher levels of bilirubin in the serum (i.e., 6.0–8.0 mg/dl) before they become jaundiced.

3. What can jaundice tell me about the type of liver disease in a patient?

Jaundice comes in many "colors," some of which may be clinically useful. Bilirubin, of course, causes the **yellow** coloration in the skin. **Orange** shades come from xanthorubin (intrahepatic jaundice), and a **greenish** hue is due to biliverdin (obstructive jaundice). **Deep green** skin color is due to marked biliverdinemia and is characteristic of obstructive jaundice such as might be seen with pancreatic cancer. Patients with hepatobiliary disease, especially obstructive jaundice, often have severely itchy skin; constant scratching and rubbing result in hyperpigmentation secondary to increased melanin in the skin, and the combination of melanin and bile pigments imparts a **bronze** color to the skin. Bronze color is also seen in hemochromatosis.

4. What disorders are in the clinical differential of jaundice?

Do not forget exogenous plant pigments or other metabolic diseases when examining a patient who appears jaundiced. The differential diagnosis of jaundice includes carotenemia (excessive ingestion of carotenoids), lycopenemia (from tomato juice), and the sallow skin of myxedema.

5. What other clinical findings are suggestive of hepatic and biliary tract disease?

Common Skin Findings in Chronic Liver Disease

Jaundice	Purpura
Pigmentary changes	Loss of body hair
Spider angioma	Gynecomastia
Palmar erythema	Peripheral edema
Dilated abdominal wall veins	

Pruritus is common and may be severe. It is particularly intense in primary biliary cirrhosis, diseases caused by biliary tract obstruction, and cholestatic jaundice. Constant scratching may lead to excoriations, pigment disturbances, and thickening of the skin (lichenification).

Hepatobiliary diseases are associated with alterations of the vasculature, including spider angiomas, palmar erythema, and cutaneous varices. Spider angiomas (vascular spiders) are classically

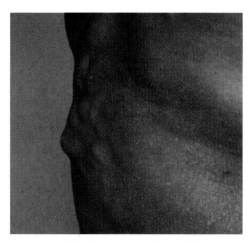

FIGURE 1. Profile view showing dilatation of the umbilical vein in the epigastrium. Enlarged abdominal wall veins reflect portal venous hypertension. The patient also had esophageal varices.

associated with chronic liver disease. However, these may be seen in other conditions including pregnancy and oral contraceptive use, and in normal persons, especially children. The vascular spider consists of a coiled central arteriole with smaller vessels radiating outward like the legs of a spider. In chronic liver disease, they are numerous and are found on the face, neck, upper chest, hands, and forearms. "Liver palms" refers to the mottled erythema and increased warmth of the palms, and sometimes the soles of the feet, in chronic liver disease. Palmar erythema also may be seen in pregnancy, lupus erythematosus, pulmonary disease, and hyperthyroidism.

Portal venous hypertension due to chronic liver disease leads to the development of collateral circulation. Esophageal varices are an example. In the skin, this is seen as dilatation of the veins of the abdominal wall (Fig. 1). "Caput medusae" (head of Medusa) refers to the dilated periumbilical veins and has been known for centuries as a marker of advanced liver disease.

In men with chronic liver disease, a "hyperestrogen state" leads to gynecomastia, testicular atrophy, loss of axillary, truncal and pubic hair, and a female pattern of pubic hair.

Purpura, ecchymoses, and gingival bleeding reflect impaired hepatic production of various clotting factors, especially the vitamin K-dependent factors. Peripheral edema and ascites indicate hypoalbuminemia (albumin is made in the liver) and/or portal venous hypertension.

6. Intestinal bleeding is an important clinical finding. What diseases associated with GI bleeding may also have clues in the skin?

Conditions Associated with GI Bleeding and Skin Lesions

Inflammatory conditions	Vascular malformations and tumors
Ulcerative colitis	Hereditary hemorrhagic telangiectasia (Osler-
Crohn's disease	Weber-Rendu)
Henoch-Schönlein purpura	Ehlers-Danlos syndrome
Polyarteritis nodosa	Blue rubber bleb nevus syndrome
Hereditary polyposis syndromes	Kaposi's sarcoma
Gardner's syndrome	Miscellaneous
Peutz-Jeghers syndrome	Pseudoxanthoma elasticum
Multiple hamartoma syndrome (Cowden's syndrome)	

7. What is pyoderma gangrenosum?

Pyoderma gangrenosum is a severe ulcerative condition most often affecting the lower legs (Fig. 2). It is one of the skin lesions associated with the abdominal pain and bleeding of inflammatory bowel disease. Pyoderma gangrenosum begins as a small tender pustule that breaks down to form an expanding ulcer with a violaceous undermined border. Lesions may develop at sites of minor trauma, a phenomenon known as **pathergy.** The ulcers of pyoderma gangrenosum may become quite large before healing with a thin, atrophic scar.

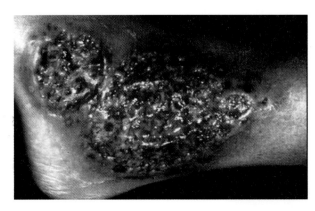

FIGURE 2. Pyoderma gangrenosum. Large necrotic undermined ulcer on the leg of a patient with active ulcerative colitis.

8. What causes pyoderma gangrenosum? Why is it important?

The exact cause of pyoderma gangrenosum is not known, but much else about the disease is well-established. Some feel it is a type of vasculitis in the skin. After the diagnosis of pyoderma gangrenosum is made, the next step should be to look for an underlying cause. Important conditions to search for include chronic infectious hepatitis, inflammatory bowel disease (ulcerative colitis, Crohn's disease), rheumatoid arthritis, lupus erythematosus, HIV infection, and leukemia.

About 5% of patients with ulcerative colitis have pyoderma gangrenosum, and the course of both illnesses may parallel each other. Patients may have pyoderma gangrenosum for several years before developing inflammatory bowel disease.

9. A patient with anemia and blood in the stools has red macules on the lips. What should I think of?

The most likely cause is **hereditary hemorrhagic telangiectasia** (HHT), also known as Osler-Weber-Rendu syndrome. This is an uncommon autosomal dominant condition. At puberty or later, affected individuals develop linear, punctate, and papular red lesions on the lips, face, mucous membranes, fingers, and toes. The entire GI tract may be affected with similar lesions. Bleeding may be minimal, causing a chronic iron-deficiency anemia, or massive, leading to acute severe blood loss. The mucous membranes, especially the nasal mucosa, are also involved. In children, an important early clue to the diagnosis is recurrent severe nosebleeds before the presence of other more typical findings. Patients continue to develop new lesions throughout life. Some individuals with HHT also have arteriovenous malformations of the lungs, liver (causing cirrhosis), CNS, and eye.

10. What is pseudoxanthoma elasticum (PXE)? How does this cause GI bleeding?

PXE is a group of closely related inherited disorders. The basic defect appears to be in the elastic tissue in various organs—the skin, blood vessels, eye, and heart. For unknown reasons, the elastic tissue swells, becomes fragmented and ultimately undergoes calcification. As a result, a major part of the structural framework in these tissues is weakened, leading to disastrous consequences.

Changes of PXE in the skin are of obvious importance and develop in adolescence or early adulthood. The skin lesions consist of yellowish pebbly plaques on the neck, axillae, antecubital fossae, abdomen, and thighs. It has a peculiar texture and color reminiscent of "plucked chicken skin."

Internally, the yellowish papules of PXE are seen in the mouth, esophagus, and stomach. Involvement of the elastic tissue of the gastric arteries may result in sudden, massive hemorrhage. Involvement of the eye, specifically Bruch's membrane, causes angioid streaks of the retina. Sudden hemorrhage with acute loss of vision may be a presenting sign. Involvement of large vessels results in claudication, hypertension, and angina at an early age.

11. Is there any clinical significance of pigmented macules on the lips?

A number of conditions have pigmented macules, or "freckling," of the lips. The most important one concerning the GI tract is Peutz-Jeghers syndrome. It is one of the "classic" polyposis syndromes with skin findings, intestinal polyps, and an increased risk of cancer. Peutz-Jeghers syndrome is inherited as an autosomal dominant disorder.

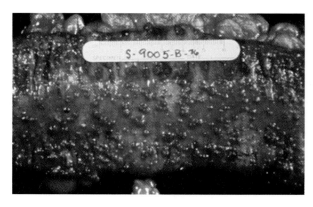

FIGURE 3. Segment of colon from a patient with Gardner's syndrome, demonstrating the immense numbers of premalignant polyps.

12. When do the pigmented macules of Peutz-Jeghers syndrome develop? How long do they last?

At birth or in infancy, small round to oval macules develop that vary from brown to blue-brown in color. They most often occur on the lips and buccal mucosa, but the nose, palms, soles, fingers, hard palate, and gingiva may also be affected. It is important to remember that the lip macules fade in adulthood, but those in the mouth persist. Be sure to examine the mouth! How many patients have you seen with freckles in the mouth?

13. What are the internal findings in Peutz-Jeghers syndrome (PJS)?

Aside from freckles in the mouth, individuals with PJS also have multiple polyps in the small intestine, most commonly the jejunum and ileum. When only a few polyps are present, there may be no symptoms. However, when present in large numbers, the polyps may bleed or cause intussusception or obstruction. The polyps are hamartomatous polyps, which means that they are composed of benign elements normally present in the gut. There is a 2% to 3% risk, however, of intestinal malignancy in patients with PJS. It is thought that lurking among the masses of benign polyps is the occasional adenomatous polyp that is a precursor lesion of intestinal cancer. In addition, it has been recently discovered that patients with this syndrome have a much greater risk of developing cancer of the ovary, breast, endometrium, and pancreas.

14. What is Gardner's syndrome?

Gardner's syndrome is another polyposis syndrome inherited in an autosomal dominant fashion. Patients with this syndrome have numerous epidermal inclusion cysts in the skin, various dental abnormalities including osteomas of the mandible, and innumerable premalignant adenomatous polyps throughout the colon (Fig. 3). The lifetime risk of colon cancer in untreated patients is 100%.

Features of Gardner's syndrome

Skin findings	Congenital retinal pigmentation
Epidermal cysts	Osteomas
Desmoid tumors	Dental abnormalities
Fibromas	Adenomatous colonic polyps (risk of cancer = 100%)

15. Describe some of the cutaneous signs of cancer in the gastrointestinal system.

The skin may be involved with GI tract malignancy in several ways.

1. The skin may be a site of metastasis from a primary GI tract cancer. This happens most frequently with adenocarcinoma of the colon (Fig. 4).

2. There is a large group of paraneoplastic dermatoses—i.e., a benign skin condition associated with an underlying malignancy. Examples include "malignant" acanthosis nigricans, superficial migratory thrombophlebitis, and glucagonoma syndrome. In a few instances, such as excess glucagon secretion in the glucagonoma syndrome, the link between the skin and gut is clear. In other cases (such as acanthosis nigricans), the skin condition may occur in many individuals without cancer, so a thorough evaluation of the patient is indicated.

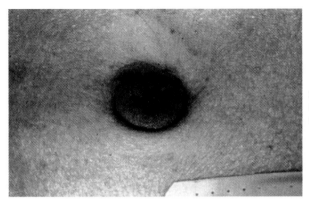

FIGURE 4. Sister Mary Joseph nodule. Metastatic lesion of colon cancer to the umbilicus.

16. What is "malignant" acanthosis nigricans?

There are many causes of acanthosis nigricans (AN), including endocrine disorders, obesity, medications, and underlying cancer. However, the sudden onset of widespread AN in an adult with weight loss should suggest an underlying malignancy (Fig. 5). Many cancers have been reported with "malignant" AN, but almost 60% of patients have adenocarcinoma of the stomach. In most of these cases, the tumor is present in an advanced stage at the time the AN develops. However, some patients have AN before or months after the discovery of the gastric malignancy. In some cases, successful resection of the adenocarcinoma leads to regression of the AN, suggesting the presence of an epidermal growth factor secreted by the tumor.

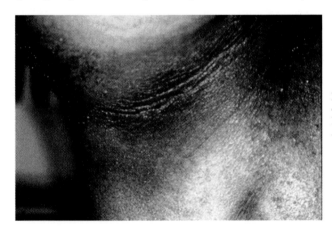

FIGURE 5. The axilla of an obese person showing velvety, hyperpigmented lesions of acanthosis nigricans.

17. What is superficial migratory thrombophlebitis?

Many conditions produce a state of increased blood coagulability, leading to venous thrombosis. One important GI-related cause is pancreatic cancer which may be asymptomatic at the time the thrombophlebitis develops. Trousseau described this sign of internal malignancy (Trousseau's sign). Ironically, he developed thrombophlebitis as a manifestation of his fatal gastric cancer.

Superficial migratory thrombophlebitis presents as tender erythematous linear cords along the course of superficial veins of the trunk and extremities. There may be multiple lesions that resolve, with new lesions developing elsewhere. The thrombophlebitis is remarkably resistant to anticoagulant therapy and the cause is unknown. It is essential that any patient presenting with superficial migratory thrombophlebitis undergo a thorough evaluation to rule out underlying malignancy.

18. What cancers are associated with superficial migratory thrombophlebitis?

Superficial migratory thrombophlebitis is not specific for gastrointestinal malignancies and has been associated with a variety of underlying disorders including other malignancies such as lung carcinoma, Hodgkin's disease, and multiple myeloma. Other nonmalignant associations include Behçet's disease and rickettsial infections.

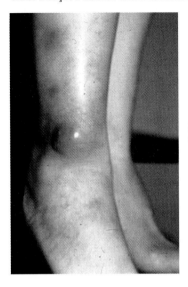

FIGURE 6. Pancreatic panniculitis. Tender erythematous fluctuant nodules on the lower legs of a patient with acute pancreatitis.

19. How is inflammation of the fat (panniculitis) associated with pancreatic disease?

The pancreas is both an exocrine (i.e., pancreatic digestive enzymes) and an endocrine (i.e., insulin, glucagon) organ. Almost 99% of the pancreas is dedicated to the production of pancreatic digestive enzymes. Acute pancreatitis caused by viral infection, drugs, alcohol, pancreatic cancer, or trauma leads to massive outpouring of these digestive enzymes.

Patients with pancreatitis are often extremely ill with fever, vomiting, and severe abdominal pain. They may develop tender red and fluctuant nodules on the lower legs (Fig. 6) associated with joint pain and swelling. They have elevated levels of lipase and amylase in the serum and elevated amylase in the urine. It is felt that these pancreatic enzymes cause autodigestion of the fat in the subcutaneous tissue and periarticular fat pads.

20. What metabolic liver disease causes blistering and scarring of the skin associated with photosensitivity?

Porphyria cutanea tarda (PCT) is a metabolic disease characterized by chronic blistering and scarring of the dorsal hands, forearms, ears, and face associated with photosensitivity to sunlight (Fig. 7). In addition to the blistering and scarring, skin findings include thickened coarse hairs (hypertrichosis) over the temples, forehead, and cheeks; occasional shiny, thickened scleroderma-like changes of the face, scalp, posterior neck, and torso; and hyperpigmentation or hypopigmentation.

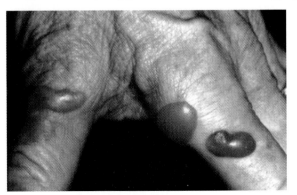

FIGURE 7. Vesicles and blisters, some hemorrhagic, on the digits of a patient with porphyria cutanea tarda.

PCT may be inherited in an autosomal dominant fashion or may be sporadic. There is a high incidence of liver disease in patients with PCT. Factors that may trigger attacks of PCT include alcohol abuse, hepatitis C infection, estrogens especially oral contraceptives, and HIV infection. The biochemical defect is a deficiency of the hepatic and red blood cells enzyme uroporphyrinogen decarboxylase. This is the fifth enzyme in the metabolic pathway of the synthesis of hemoglobin. An accumulation of porphyrin precursors that are photosensitizing compounds leads to the skin changes. A useful laboratory test that can be performed in the office is the demonstration of pink fluorescence of the patient's urine when exposed to ultraviolet light. A Wood's light emitting ultraviolet A (UVA) can be used for this test. Patients also have increased total body iron stores reflected in increased serum iron and ferritin levels. Quantitative measurement of urine porphyrins in a 24-hour urine specimen will confirm the diagnosis.

Treatment of PCT includes elimination of alcohol and other incriminating medications, photoprotection, phlebotomy, and low-dose antimalarial therapy.

21. What chronic skin disease is associated with a gluten-sensitive enteropathy?

Dermatitis herpetiformis (DH) is considered one of the autoimmune blistering skin diseases. Patients develop intensely itchy papules, papulovesicles and occasionally tense blisters in a symmetric distribution over the scalp and posterior neckline, shoulders and back, elbows, knees, and the lumbosacral area (Fig. 8). Lesions on the palms may be seen but the mucous membranes are only rarely involved. A high percentage (up to 70%) of patients will have histologic evidence of a gluten-sensitive enteropathy manifested as villous atrophy of the jejunum associated with a chronic lymphocytic inflammation.

The disease in the skin and the intestinal tract (small intestine) appears to be triggered by dietary gluten found in many grains but not in rice, corn, and oats. There are usually no abdominal symptoms but an occasional patient may complain of bloating, cramping and diarrhea. A diet completely free of gluten will slowly clear the skin and intestinal tract lesions. However, this diet is difficult for many patients to adhere to. The disease is characterized by the accumulation of polymorphonuclear neutrophils (PMNs) and granular deposits of IgA in the tips of the dermal

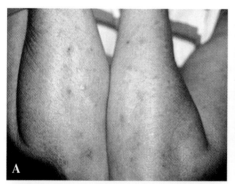
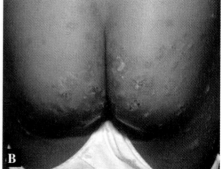
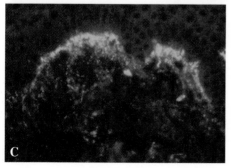

FIGURE 8. Dermatitis herpetiformis. *A*, Papules and vesicles with excoriations in a symmetric distribution on the elbows and knees are typical of dermatitis herpetiformis. *B*, Excoriations and secondary infection due to intense itching and scratching are common. Lesions may be confused with scabies and folliculitis. *C*, Direct immunofluorescence of lesional skin in dermatitis herpetiformis showing granular deposits of IgA in the tips of dermal papillae.

papillae of the skin. These two findings are considered diagnostic of DH. In addition, most patients express HLA-B8 and have an increased frequency of HLA-DR3 and HLA-DQw2.

Treatment includes strict adherence to a gluten-free diet and the use of either dapsone (diaminodiphenylsulfone) or sulfapyridine. Dapsone is the more effective of the two listed drugs. The condition is lifelong with only rare periods of brief remission.

BIBLIOGRAPHY

1. Callen JP, Jorizzo JL, Greer KE, et al (eds): Dermatologic Signs of Internal Disease, 2nd ed. Philadelphia, W.B. Saunders, 1994, pp 219–244.
2. Graham-Brown RAC, Rathbone B, Marks J: The skin and disorders of the alimentary tract. In Freedberg IM, Eisen AZ, Wolff K, et al (eds): Fitzpatrick's Dermatology in General Medicine, 5th ed. New York, McGraw-Hill, 1999, pp 1909–1918.
3. Graham-Brown RAC, Sarkany I: The hepatobiliary system and the skin. In Freedberg IM, Eisen AZ, Wolff K, et al (eds): Fitzpatrick's Dermatology in General Medicine, 5th ed. New York, McGraw-Hill, 1999, pp 1918–1929.
4. Gregory B, Ho VC: Cutaneous manifestations of gastrointestinal disorders: Parts I and II. J Am Acad Dermatol 26:153–166, 371–383, 1992.
5. Odom RB, James WD, Berger TG (eds): Andrew's Diseases of the Skin, 9th ed. Philadelphia, W.B. Saunders, 2000, pp 599–601, 653–655.
6. Poole S, Fenske NA: Cutaneous markers of internal malignancy: I. Malignant involvement of the skin and the genodermatoses. J Am Acad Dermatol 28:1–13, 1993.
7. Poole S, Fenske NA: Cutaneous markers of internal malignancy. II. Paraneoplastic dermatoses and environmental carcinogens. J Am Acad Dermatol 28:147–163, 1993.
8. Ward SK, Roenigk HH, Gordon KB: Dermatologic manifestations of gastrointestinal disorders. Gastroenterol Clin North Am 27:615–636, 1998.

38. CUTANEOUS MANIFESTATIONS OF RENAL DISEASE

Kathleen M. David-Bajar, M.D., COL, MC

1. What types of skin changes are associated with renal disease?

There are three main categories of skin disease associated with renal diseases:

1. Cutaneous manifestations of renal failure—skin changes are found in nearly all patients
2. Systemic diseases with prominent renal and cutaneous manifestations (e.g., Henoch-Schönlein purpura)
3. Diseases affecting the kidney in which skin biopsy may be helpful in making the diagnosis, even when cutaneous findings are not prominent (e.g., primary systemic amyloidosis)

2. What cutaneous findings occur in renal failure?

Cutaneous Findings in Chronic Renal Failure

FINDING	% AFFECTED	FINDING	% AFFECTED
Changes in cutaneous pigmentation	70%	Nail changes	66%
Yellowish tinge	40%	Half-and-half nails	39%
Hyperpigmentation of palms, soles	30%	Pale nails	23%
Hyperpigmentation, diffuse or photodistributed	22%	Splinter hemorrhages	11%
		Xerosis (dry skin)	Most
Pallor	8%	Pruritus	63%
Cutaneous infections	70%	Keratotic pits of palms, soles	14%
Onychomycosis	52%	Perforating disorder	4%
Tinea pedis	25%	Finger pebbles	86%
		Calcinosis cutis	1%

3. What cutaneous findings are present in patients being treated with dialysis?

Many of the skin changes described in patients with chronic renal failure are also found in patients with renal failure undergoing treatment with either peritoneal dialysis or hemodialysis. A high percentage of patients receiving dialysis complain of pruritus that may be severe. In some instances, the pruritus worsens with dialysis. Patients on renal dialysis may develop a bullous eruption similar to porphyria cutanea tarda (Fig. 1A). Acne has been described in association with dialysis and therapy with testosterone.

Several perforating diseases are associated with chronic renal failure, with or without renal dialysis, including Kyrle's disease, reactive perforating collagenosis, and perforating folliculitis. Some authors group all of the perforating diseases seen in these patients under one term–**acquired perforating dermatosis of chronic renal failure.** The pathogenesis of these conditions is not understood. Dialysis patients may also develop cutaneous complications from this treatment, such as infections or contact dermatitis in the area of the peritoneal cannula or arteriovenous fistula.

4. Describe the nail changes in chronic renal failure.

Both half-and-half nails and Muehrcke's nails are associated with chronic renal failure. In **half-and-half nails,** the proximal half of the nail is white, and the distal portion retains the normal pink color (Fig. 1B). This is believed to be due to edema of the nail bed.

Muehrcke nails are associated with hypoalbuminemia and have two transverse parallel white bands, separated from each other and from the lunula by areas of normal pink nail.

5. What is uremic frost?

Although a rare finding today, this discoloration of the face was originally described as a classic manifestation of chronic renal failure. Whitish deposits were noted about the face and neck, believed to be due to deposition of crystallized urea from sweat.

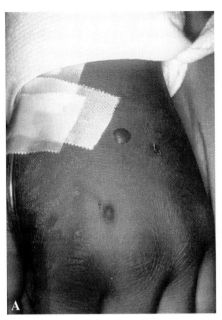 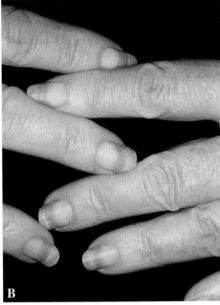

FIGURE 1. Cutaneous findings. *A,* Tense vesicle on the dorsal hand of a patient undergoing renal dialysis. *B,* Half-and-half nails in a patient with chronic renal failure.

Abnormalities of Skin Color Associated with Renal Failure

SKIN FINDING	COLOR	DISTRIBUTION	ETIOLOGY
Uremic frost	White	Face, nostrils, neck	Deposition of crystallized urea from sweat
Pallor	Yellowish	Generalized	Anemia, urochrome deposition
Hyperpigmentation	Brown	Photodistributed or generalized	Increased β-melanocyte stimulating hormone
Bruising	Red-purple-green-yellow-brown	Sites of trauma	Hemostatic abnormalities

6. What causes the pallor of chronic renal failure?

This pallor is due mainly to the anemia that invariably accompanies chronic renal failure. In addition, a yellowish cast may be noted and is believed to be due to urochrome deposition in the skin.

7. What causes the pigmentary changes of the skin seen in chronic renal failure?

It is the result of increased amounts of melanin present in the basal layer of the epidermis and superficial dermis. It has been proposed that such patients have decreased metabolism of β-melanocyte-stimulating hormone (β-MSH) by diseased kidneys, leading to elevated plasma levels of β-MSH, a hormone that stimulates melanocytes to produce more melanin.

8. Is pruritus a common finding in all renal failure?

No. Patients with acute renal failure do not develop pruritus. However, it is common in patients with chronic renal failure. Also, some patients with chronic renal failure treated with dialysis have exacerbation of their pruritus. The precise cause of uremic pruritus is unknown. One study suggests that uremic patients have a histamine-releasing factor in their sera that is depleted or diminished by ultraviolet B light. Another study found a reduction in the total number of skin nerve terminals in uremic patients and proposed that skin innervation is altered in chronic renal failure patients, possibly as a consequence of neuropathy. Secondary hyperparathyroidism, which sometimes develops in chronic renal failure, may also induce pruritus.

9. How is the pruritus of renal failure treated?

First of all, a specific diagnosis should be sought. Patients with renal failure may develop other skin conditions associated with pruritus, such as scabies or allergic contact dermatitis. Also, reactions to medications may be associated with pruritus. Xerosis is often present and can be treated with avoidance of irritants, use of mild or no soap for cleansing the skin, and the frequent use of emollients. When pruritus is believed to be due to secondary hyperparathyroidism, surgical therapy may be indicated. When no specific cause for pruritus is found, treatment with ultraviolet B (UVB) light may be beneficial.

10. Discuss the perforating disorders of the skin.

These are a group of diseases in which altered components of skin are eliminated via the epidermis, a process termed **transepidermal elimination.** Several different perforating diseases have been associated with chronic renal failure, including Kyrle's disease, reactive perforating collagenosis, and perforating folliculitis.

Because features of more than one type of perforating disorder have been noted in skin biopsies from patients with chronic renal failure, it has been suggested that this condition be referred to as the **acquired perforating dermatosis of chronic renal failure.** This eruption occurs in up to 10% of patients on dialysis but has also developed in patients with renal failure even without dialysis treatment. The lesions consist of keratotic papules and nodules on the trunk and extremities (Fig. 2). They occur more commonly in black patients. Skin biopsy confirms the diagnosis. This eruption may resolve spontaneously over a period of months.

Kyrle's disease is a controversial entity, with some authorities doubting its existence. As originally defined by Kyrle, it is a disease in which an abnormal clone of keratinocytes perforates through the epidermis into the dermis.

Reactive perforating collagenosis is a disease in which presumably abnormal collagen is being extruded from the dermis through the epidermis. **Perforating folliculitis** is a disease characterized by follicular plugs and curled-up hairs that perforate through the follicle into the dermis.

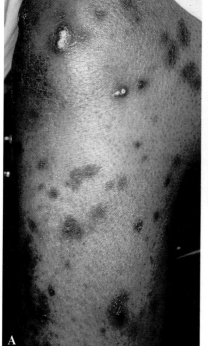

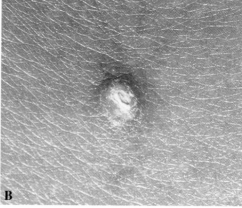

FIGURE 2. Perforating disease of chronic renal failure. *A,* Small erythematous papules with central crusts or scale are seen on the lower leg. Central umbilication of the papules can be seen, the area of "perforation." The hyperpigmented macules are areas of prior involvement. *B,* Close-up of hyperatotic papule demonstrating cell area of "perforation." (Courtesy of James E. Fitzpatrick, MD.)

11. Describe the porphyria-like eruption of dialysis.

Patients with chronic renal failure on dialysis sometimes develop skin fragility, blisters, hyperpigmentation, and hypertrichosis that is indistinguishable from the cutaneous lesions seen in porphyria cutanea tarda. Although most of these patients do not have elevated levels of porphyrins, some do. When these patients are anuric, plasma and fecal specimens are submitted for porphyrin studies.

12. What is Fabry's disease?

Fabry's disease (angiokeratoma corporis diffusum universale) is the result of defective activity of a lysosomal enzyme, α-galactosidase A, which leads to deposition of neutral glycosphingolipids, particularly trihexosyl ceramide, in many cells and tissues of the body. It is inherited in an X-linked recessive pattern, with nearly all patients being male. Heterozygous females are generally asymptomatic, although they often have characteristic corneal opacities.

13. Describe the skin lesions in Fabry's disease.

Angiokeratomas are the skin lesions seen in Fabry's disease. They begin as pinpoint erythematous to purplish macules or flat papules with slight scaling and often start in early childhood with progressive increase in size and number. They are typically distributed in the "bathing suit area"—the area between the waist and the knees. These lesions may be quite subtle. A skin biopsy may aid in establishing the diagnosis since special stains such as Sudan black B, scarlet red, or periodic acid–Schiff may demonstrate glycolipid deposition in the skin. Electron microscopy is frequently used to help establish the diagnosis because it demonstrates characteristic cytoplasmic glycolipid deposits (typically within endothelial cells).

Other findings in patients with Fabry's disease include acute attacks of severe pain, particularly in the palms and soles, often beginning in childhood. In adult life, cardiac ischemia and infarcts, transient ischemic attacks, stroke, and progressive kidney failure may develop.

14. What vasculitic diseases frequently involve both the kidneys and skin?

Leukocytoclastic vasculitis	Polyarteritis nodosa	Wegener's granulomatosis
Henoch-Schönlein purpura	Microscopic polyarteritis	

When skin lesions suggestive of vasculitis occur, a skin biopsy should be done to confirm the diagnosis and determine the type of vessel and inflammation involved (see also Chapter 15). Vessel involvement may vary from small postcapillary venules (leukocytoclastic vasculitis) to medium-sized arteries (polyarteritis nodosa). If vasculitis is confirmed, testing should be done to determine if the kidneys are also involved.

15. How should skin biopsy be used for the diagnosis of systemic amyloidosis?

In primary systemic amyloidosis, immunoglobulin light chain proteins are deposited in skin, tongue, heart, spleen, joints, peripheral nerves, and carpal ligaments. Cutaneous changes may be present, including purpura of the upper trunk, face, and neck and eyelid purpura, which is very characteristic of primary systemic amyloidosis. Waxy papules, particularly on the palms and fingertips, have also been reported.

Even when there are no cutaneous changes present, skin biopsy may help make a diagnosis of primary systemic amyloidosis. Clinically normal skin, abdominal fat, tongue, and rectal biopsies have been used to confirm the diagnosis, thus avoiding the need for more invasive biopsies of internal organs.

BIBLIOGRAPHY

1. Clayton BD, Jorizzo JL, Sherertz E: Cutaneous changes in renal disorders. In Freedberg IM, et al (eds): Fitzpatrick's Dermatology in General Medicine. New York, McGraw-Hill, 1999.
2. Desnick RJ, Eng CM: Fabry disease: A galactosidase A deficiency. In Freedberg IM, et al (eds): Fitzpatrick's Dermatology in General Medicine. New York, McGraw-Hill, 1999.
3. Fabrizio F, Baraldi A, Sevignani C, et al: Cutaneous innervation in chronic renal failure patients: An immunohistochemical study. Acta Derm Venereol (Stockh) 72:102–105, 1992.
4. Fuchs E, Lynfield Y: Dialysis acne. J Am Acad Dermatol 23:125, 1990.

5. Goicoechea M, de Sequera P, Ochando A, et al: Uremic pruritus: An unresolved problem in hemodialysis patients. Nephron 82:73–74, 1999.
6. Muehrcke RC: The finger-nails in chronic hypoalbuminaemia: A new physical sign. BMJ 1327–1328, 1956.
7. Myrick SR, Radomski JS, Cohn HE: Surgical treatment of secondary hyperparathyroidism in patients with chronic renal failure by sub-total parathyroidectomy. Am Surg 60:638–640, 1994.
8. Patterson JW: The perforating disorders. J Am Acad Dermatol 10:561–581, 1984.
9. Pico MR, Lugo-Somolinos A, Sanchez JL, Burgos-Calderon R: Cutaneous alterations in patients with chronic renal failure. Int J Dermatol 31:860–863, 1992.
10. Poh-Fitzpatrick MB, Masullo AS, Grossman ME: Porphyria cutanea tarda associated with chronic renal disease and hemodialysis. Arch Dermatol 116:191–195, 1980.
11. Smith AG, Schuster S, Thody AJ, et al: Role of the kidney in regulating plasma immunoreactive beta-melanocyte stimulating hormone. BMJ 1:874–876, 1976.
12. Szepietowski JC, Schwartz RA: Uremic pruritus. Int J Dermatol 37:247–253, 1998.
13. Wong CK, Wang WJ: Systemic amyloidosis. A report of 19 cases. Dermatology 189:47–51, 1994.

39. CUTANEOUS MANIFESTATIONS OF AIDS

George W. Turiansky, M.D., LTC, MC, and
William D. James, M.D.

1. How significant is the occurrence of skin disease in the setting of HIV infection?

Dermatologic diseases are frequently encountered in HIV-infected patients. In one study of 100 serial outpatients, a 92% prevalence of skin disease was noted. Skin disease may also be the first manifestation of HIV disease and may suggest HIV infection because of increased severity of presentation, atypical clinical appearance, or increased resistance to treatment. In addition, mucocutaneous disease may be the initial sign of a systemic process, such as an infection or neoplasm, in an HIV-infected patient. Highly active antiretroviral therapy (HAART) was introduced in 1997and has significantly decreased the occurrence and severity of many skin conditions associated with HIV infection.

2. Outline the clinical spectrum of cutaneous disease associated with HIV infection.

Mucoutaneous Diseases Seen in HIV Infection

Neoplastic diseases	Infectious diseases
Kaposi's sarcoma	Bacterial
Lymphoma	*Staphylococcus aureus* infections
Squamous cell carcinoma	Syphilis
Basal cell carcinoma	Bacillary angiomatosis
Papulosquamous diseases	Fungal
Seborrheic dermatitis	*Candida, Penicillium marneffei*
Xerosis/acquired ichthyosis	Dermatophytosis
Psoriasis vulgaris	Cryptococcosis
Reiter's syndrome	Histoplasmosis
Miscellaneous diseases	Viral
Eosinophilic folliculitis	Human papillomavirus (HPV)
Drug eruptions	Molluscum contagiosum
Hyperpigmentation	Herpes simplex virus (HSV)
Photoeruptions	Varicella-zoster virus (VZV)
Pruritus	Cytomegalovirus (CMV)
Lipodystrophy	Epstein-Barr virus
Granuloma annulare	Arthropods
Aphthosis	Scabies

3. What are the most common dermatoses associated with HIV infection?

Papulosquamous dermatoses are among the most commonly seen cutaneous manifestations of HIV infection, and these include seborrheic dermatitis (Fig. 1) and xerosis. Other common dermatologic conditions include **bacterial infections,** such as *Staphylococcus aureus* skin infections. **Fungal infections,** such as mucocutaneous candidiasis (oropharyngeal and vulvovaginal) and dermatophytosis (tinea pedis, tinea cruris, tinea manuum, and onychomycosis), are also commonly encountered. Frequently seen **viral infections** include human papilloma virus infections (condyloma acuminata, common and plantar warts) as well as infections with herpes simplex virus, varicella-zoster virus, molluscum contagiosum, and Epstein-Barr virus (oral hairy leukoplakia).

4. Can mucocutaneous changes occur as a result of primary HIV infection?

Yes. The earliest cutaneous sign of HIV infection is an exanthem consisting of discrete, erythematous macules and papules that usually measure 10 mm or less. They are located primarily over the trunk but also are seen on the palms and soles. These lesions may become hemorrhagic. The exanthem of acute HIV infection is not clinically or histologically specific. Mucosal changes described include oral, genital, and anal ulcers. These changes are associated with an acute febrile illness.

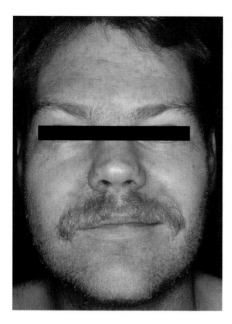

FIGURE 1. Seborrheic dermatitis: Erythematous patches with yellow scale are present on the forehead, nose, and paranasal areas of an HIV-positive patient. (Courtesy of James E. Fitzpatrick, MD.)

5. What is the most common bacterial pathogen in HIV disease? How does it manifest itself?

Staphylococcus aureus is the most common cutaneous bacterial pathogen in HIV disease. Cutaneous infections due to *S. aureus* most commonly present as a **superficial folliculitis.** Less common manifestations include impetigo, ecthyma, furunculosis, cellulitis, abscesses, and botryomycosis. In addition, *S. aureus* can secondarily infect underlying primary dermatoses such as eczema, scabies, herpetic ulcers, and Kaposi's sarcoma or colonize intravenous catheter sites. Staphylococcal colonization (carriage) of the nose and flexures (perineal, toe webspaces) is known to be increased in HIV disease and may account for the increased incidence of cutaneous infections.

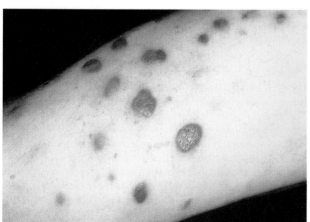

FIGURE 2. Kaposi's sarcoma. Multiple violaceous papules and plaques. (Courtesy of James E. Fitzpatrick, MD.)

6. What is the most common cutaneous malignancy in HIV disease?

Kaposi's sarcoma, or more specifically epidemic Kaposi's sarcoma. The incidence has decreased from >40% in males with AIDS in 1981 to <20% in 1989. Most cases occur in homosexual or bisexual men with HIV disease. However, Kaposi's sarcoma has been reported in HIV-negative homosexual males. Human herpesvirus 8 is associated with epidemic as well as other types of Kaposi's sarcoma.

7. What are the cutaneous clinical features of epidemic Kaposi's sarcoma?

Epidemic Kaposi's sarcoma has a widespread, symmetrical distribution of rapidly progressive macules, patches, nodules, plaques, and tumors. Common areas of involvement include the trunk, extremities, face, and oral cavity. Early lesions consist of erythematous macules, patches, or papules that may have a bruise-like halo. Lesions enlarge at different rates and tend to be oval or elongated in shape, following the lines of skin cleavage. Lesions can vary in color from pink to red, purple, or brown and can easily mimic purpura, hemangiomas, nevi, sarcoidosis, pityriasis rosea, secondary syphilis, lichen planus, basal cell carcinoma, and melanoma. Lesions can become hyperkeratotic, ulcerated, or hemorrhagic.

Disfigurement and pain secondary to edema can occur, especially on the face, genitals, and lower extremities. Koebnerization, or formation of new lesions at sites of trauma, can be seen. Secondary bacterial infection can also occur. Lesions can be arranged in several known patterns, such as a follicular (clustered) pattern (Fig. 2), pityriasis rosea-like pattern, or dermatomal pattern.

8. How is Kaposi's sarcoma is treated?

Treatment of localized disease includes intralesional vinblastine, radiotherapy, liquid nitrogen cryotherapy, surgical excision, and topical alitretinoin. Treatment of more extensive disease includes α-interferon as well as single- or multiple-agent chemotherapy with vinblastine, vincristine, bleomycin, or liposomal doxorubicin.

9. Is the course of syphilis altered in HIV-infected individuals?

Although the course of syphilis in most HIV-infected patients is not different from that in a normal host, it may differ in several ways.

- Altered clinical manifestations of syphilis, including the usual painless chancre becoming painful secondary to bacterial infection. Lues maligna, a rare manifestation of secondary syphilis, can occur and consists of pleomorphic skin lesions with pustules, nodules, and ulcers with necrotizing vasculitis.
- Altered serologic tests for syphilis, with limited or absent antibody tests for syphilis including repeatedly negative reagin and treponemal antibody tests. Seronegative secondary syphilis as well as exaggerated antibody responses have been reported. Loss of treponemal antibody positivity has also been noted.
- Concurrent coinfection with another sexually transmitted disease.
- Decreased latency period with accelerated development of tertiary syphilis within months to years.
- Lack of response to antibiotic therapy with relapses.

10. How does syphilis increase the risk for HIV infection?

The syphilitic chancre can itself serve as a source of HIV transmission in the HIV-infected person. An HIV-negative patient with a genital ulcer, such as in primary syphilis, can be at increased risk for acquiring HIV if exposed to an HIV-positive sexual partner.

11. What is oral hairy leukoplakia?

Oral hairy leukoplakia, which is predictive for development of AIDS, is primarily seen in HIV-infected patients but also has been described rarely in HIV-negative immunosuppressed organ transplant recipients. It is due to Epstein-Barr virus replication within clinical lesions. Oral hairy leukoplakia occurs primarily on the lateral edges of the tongue as parallel, vertically oriented, white plaques, producing a corrugated appearance (Fig. 3A). It can infrequently also involve the dorsal and ventral aspects of the tongue, the buccal or labial mucosa, and soft palate. The plaque in this condition does not rub off with scraping (unlike candidal thrush) and is usually asymptomatic. Histologically, parakeratosis, acanthosis, and ballooning cells (koilocytes) are seen. *In situ* Epstein-Barr virus DNA hybridization of lesional scrapings or tissue sections show positive nuclear staining within epithelial cells. Lesions may respond to acyclovir, zidovudine, podophyllin, tretinoin, or excision but do not respond to anticandidal treatment.

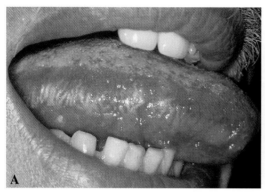

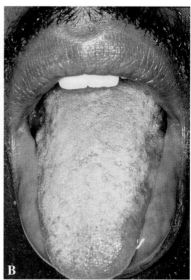

FIGURE 3. Oral changes. *A*, Oral hairy leukoplakia: Vertically oriented white plaques with a corrugated appearance are seen on the lateral edge of the tongue. *B*, Hyperplastic candidiasis: A white coating that does not scrape off is present on the dorsal surface of the tongue in this HIV-positive patient.

12. Name the four types of oropharyngeal candidiasis that can be seen in HIV disease.

Pseudomembranous candidiasis appears as whitish, cottage-cheese-like or creamy plaques at any site in the oropharynx. These are removable when scraped and may leave a reddish surface. **Erythematous candidiasis** appears as well-demarcated patches of erythema on the palate or dorsal tongue. Lesions of erythematous candidiasis on the tongue can look smooth and depapillated. **Hyperplastic candidiasis** appears as a white coating on the dorsum of the tongue that persists with scraping (Fig. 3B). **Angular cheilitis** consists of erythema, cracking, and fissuring of the mouth corners. More than one type of oropharyngeal candidiasis can coexist.

13. What is HIV-associated eosinophilic folliculitis?

HIV-associated eosinophilic folliculitis is a chronic, pruritic dermatosis of unknown etiology characterized by discrete, erythematous, follicular, urticarial papules on the head and neck, trunk, and proximal extremities (Fig. 4). Most cases occur in males, but the disease has been reported in females. Bacterial cultures are negative, and the eruption does not resolve with antistaphylococcal treatment. It is associated with peripheral eosinophilia, an elevated serum IgE level, and advanced HIV infection (CD4 counts < 250 cells/mm³). Eosinophilic folliculitis is not specific for HIV infection, as it has rarely been described in association with hematologic malignancies.

Transverse histologic sections are superior to vertical sections in the diagnosis of this disease. Histopathologic findings include a perivascular and perifollicular mixed infiltrate with variable numbers of eosinophils and spongiosis of the follicular infundibulum or sebaceous gland with a mixed infiltrate. Treatment options include potent topical corticosteroids, antihistamines, ultraviolet B phototherapy, itraconazole, oral metronidazole, permethrin cream, and isotretinoin.

14. Is the incidence of drug eruptions increased in HIV disease?

Definitely, and especially with sulfonamides and amoxicillin clavulanate. About half of HIV-infected patients with *Pneumocystis carinii* pneumonia treated with intravenous trimethoprim-sulfamethoxazole develop a widespread macular or papular erythematous eruption within weeks of initiating treatment. In HIV disease, sulfonamides are commonly used in the prophylaxis and treatment of *P. carinii* pneumonia and CNS toxoplasmosis. More severe drug reactions, such as Stevens-Johnson syndrome and toxic epidermal necrolysis, have also been reported in HIV patients.

15. Describe clinical features of molluscum contagiosum infection in the HIV-infected host.

Molluscum contagiosum, a poxvirus infection, is seen in approximately 8–18% of patients with symptomatic HIV disease and AIDS. Although molluscum lesions often appear as dome-

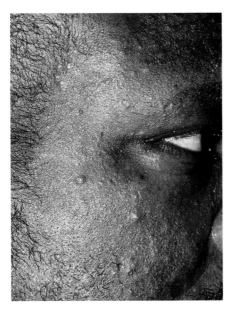

FIGURE 4 Eosinophilic folliculitis: Multiple, pruritic, firm, urticaria-like pink papules are present on the face of this HIV-positive patient.

shaped, flesh-colored umbilicated papules, they can have an unusual appearance, involve atypical sites, and be widespread.

In HIV disease, molluscum lesions tend to occur on the face, trunk, intertriginous areas, and buttocks as well as in the genital area. Beard area lesions are commonly seen, and these are probably spread by shaving. Lesions can be large (> 1 cm, giant molluscum) or hyperkeratotic, can simulate skin cancers, common and genital warts, and keratoacanthomas, and can become confluent. Lesions can also involve the follicular epithelium with sparing of the interfollicular epithelium. Molluscum lesions can be associated with a localized chronic dermatitis surrounding a centrally located lesion (molluscum dermatitis). With progressive immune dysfunction, lesions increase in number and become diffuse. Disseminated cryptococcosis, histoplasmosis, and *Penicillium marneffei* infection can mimic facial molluscum contagiosum.

16. How is molluscum contagiosum treated?

Treatment options include liquid nitrogen cryotherapy, curettage, electrodessication, trichloroacetic acid, topical wart preparations, laser ablation, tretinoin, topical fluorouracil and imiquimod, and topical or intravenous cidofovir. However, treatment of widespread lesions in advanced HIV disease is problematic, as lesions are numerous and tend to recur.

17. Is the prevalence of common and genital warts increased in HIV infection?

The prevalence of human papillomavirus (HPV) infections is increased in HIV disease, including verruca vulgaris (common warts) and condyloma acuminata (genital warts). Lesions can be numerous, large, confluent, and resistant to standard treatment with increasing immunodeficiency. Condyloma acuminata occur in the genital and perianal areas, where it is associated with receptive anal intercourse. In HIV disease, the incidence of HPV-associated intraepithelial neoplasia of the cervix and of the anus in homosexual men is increased. Resolution of recalcitrant hand warts temporally related to protease inhibitor–containing antiretroviral therapy has been reported.

18. What causes bacillary angiomatosis?

Bacillary angiomatosis is a gram-negative rickettsial-like bacillary disease caused by the *Bartonella* species *B. henselae* and *B. quintana*. The disease can involve the skin as well as the liver, spleen, lymph nodes, and bone. Cutaneous lesions consist of solitary or multiple red-to-violaceous, vascular-appearing papules and nodules that can simulate hemangiomas, pyogenic granulomas, and Kaposi's sarcoma. Organisms can be demonstrated in lesional biopsies by Warthin-Starry stain. An association between bacillary angiomatosis in humans and traumatic exposure to cats having *B. henselae* blood infection has been shown. Treatment is with erythromycin or doxycycline.

19. How does varicella-zoster virus infection present in the HIV-positive patient?

Primary infection with the varicella-zoster virus (VZV, chickenpox) in HIV disease may be associated with complications such as pneumonia, encephalitis, hepatitis, profuse eruption, and even death. **Reactivation** of latent VZV infection is increased in HIV disease. Reactivation usually manifests itself as a typical unidermatomal eruption, but with advanced immunodeficiency, multidermatomal and disseminated eruptions can occur. These eruptions may be vesiculobullous, hemorrhagic, necrotic, or poxlike and may be very painful. Chronic, painful verrucous and ecthymatous (pox-like) lesions can occur and appear as hyperkeratotic warty nodules and necrotic ulcerations, respectively.

20. Do any photosensitive dermatoses occur in HIV disease?

Various photosensitive dermatoses have been described in HIV disease, and these include porphyria cutanea tarda, lichenoid photoeruptions, and chronic actinic dermatitis. Photosensitivity may, in fact, be the presenting sign of HIV infection.

Most cases of **porphyria cutanea tarda** (PCT) in HIV infection are acquired and many are associated with historical or serologic evidence of hepatitis B or C infection as well as with elevated transaminase levels and history of alcohol abuse. Patients present with blisters, erosions, crusting, scarring, and increased skin fragility on the face and dorsal hands. In one study, urinary and stool porphyrin excretion patterns classic for PCT occurred in hepatitis C–positive AIDS patients without any clinical evidence of porphyria.

Lichenoid photoeruptions in HIV infection occur most often in black individuals with advanced HIV disease and may be associated with photosensitizing drug use. Patients present with pruritic, violaceous plaques that begin on the face, neck, dorsal hands, and arms that may hyperpigment and may extend to non-sun-exposed sites. Histopathologic features are primarily those of lichenoid drug eruption or hypertrophic lichen planus, but some patients have findings of lichen nitidus. Patients may improve or clear with discontinuation of a photosensitizing drug, sun avoidance, and sunscreen use.

Chronic actinic dermatitis has been described in markedly immunosuppressed patients and presents as a chronic pruritic and idiopathic eczematous dermatitis in a photodistribution. Phototesting shows increased sensitivity to ultraviolet B. Histologic findings demonstrate eczematous, lymphoma-like, and psoriasiform changes.

21. What is known about granuloma annulare in the setting of HIV infection?

A recent study of 34 consecutive HIV-positive patients with a clinical and histologic diagnosis of granuloma annulare revealed that the generalized form of granuloma annulare was a more common clinical pattern than the localized form of granuloma annulare. In this study, two patients with localized granuloma annulare had perforating lesions both clinically and histologically. Although granuloma annulare can occur in all stages of HIV infection, it is slightly more common in patients with AIDS. Generalized granuloma annulare lesions appear as multiple, discrete, skin-colored dermal papules distributed on the trunk and extremities. Localized granuloma annulare lesions present as solitary or few discrete papules or annular plaques on one area of the body. The histologic findings of HIV-associated granuloma annulare are similar to those of non–HIV-infected persons. There are no known cases of diabetes mellitus reported in association with HIV and granuloma annulare.

22. Describe some of the potential cutaneous side effects of antiretroviral therapy.

A syndrome of lipodystrophic changes is temporally associated with use of protease inhibitors and includes benign symmetric lipomatosis, enlargement of the dorsocervical fat pad ("buffalo hump"), breast hypertrophy, visceral abdominal fat accumulation ("crix belly," "protease paunch") (Fig. 5), peripheral fat wasting with prominence of the superficial veins, and loss of the buccal fat pad. Lipodystrophic changes have been associated with hypertriglyceridemia, hypercholesterolemia, hyperglycemia, insulin resistance, and hyperinsulinemia. Evidence of

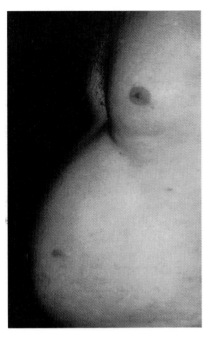

FIGURE 5. Lipodystrophy: Visceral abdominal fat accumulation is seen in this HIV-positive patient who was taking indinavir for 3 years.

associated Cushing's syndrome or disease is lacking. Lipodystrophic changes have occasionally been reported in patients not taking protease inhibitors. Histologic findings include atrophy of the subcutaneous fat, fat lobules with variably sized and often large adipocytes, prominent capillary vascular proliferation, and focal lymphocytic infiltrate and lipogranuloma formation. The exact mechanism involved in these changes is not clear to date. In addition, antiretroviral therapy has recently been temporally associated with symptomatic angiolipomatosis. Also, painful periungual inflammation (paronychia) of the fingernails and toenails has been reported with use of indinavir and lamuvidine.

DISCLAIMER

Opinions and assertions contained herein are the private views of the authors and are not to be considered as official or as reflecting the views of the U.S. Army, the Department of Defense, or the U.S. Government.

BIBLIOGRAPHY

1. Alam M, Scher RK: Indinavir-related recurrent paronychia and ingrown toenails. Cutis 64:277–278, 1999.
2. Basarab T, Jones RR: HIV-associated eosinophilic folliculitis: Case report and review of the literature. Br J Dermatol 134:499–503, 1996.
3. Berger TG: Lichenoid photoeruption in immunodeficiency virus infection. Arch Dermatol 130:609–613, 1994.
4. Berger TG, Heon V, King C, et al: Itraconazole therapy for human immunodeficiency virus–associated eosinophilic folliculitis. Arch Dermatol 131:358–360, 1995.
5. Blauvelt A, Harris HR, Hogan DJ, et al: Porphyria cutanea tarda and human immunodeficiency virus infection. Int J Dermatol 31:474–479, 1992.
6. Blauvelt A, Plott RT, Spooner K, et al: Eosinophilic folliculitis associated with the acquired immunodeficiency syndrome responds well to permethrin. Arch Dermatol 131:360–361, 1995.
7. Buckley R, Smith K: Topical imiquimod therapy for chronic giant molluscum contagiosum in a patient with advanced human immunodeficiency virus I disease. Arch Dermatol 135:1167–1169, 1999.
8. Carr A, Samaras K, Thorisdottir A, et al: Diagnosis, prediction, and natural course of HIV I protease inhibitor–associated lipodystrophy, hyperlipidaemia, and diabetes mellitus: A cohort study. Lancet 353:2093–2099, 1999.

9. Chang Y, Cesarman E, Pessin MS, et al: Identification of herpesvirus-like DNA sequences in AIDS-associated Kaposi's sarcoma. Science 266:1865–1869, 1994.

10. Cockerell CJ: Cutaneous manifestations of HIV infection other than Kaposi's sarcoma: Clinical and histologic aspects. J Am Acad Dermatol 22:1260–1269, 1990.

11. Conant M, The International and North American Panretin Gel KS Study Groups: Topical alitretinoin gel as treatment for cutaneous lesions of AIDS-related Kaposi's sarcoma: Results of multicenter, double-blind, vehicle-controlled trials. Presented at the 6th Conference on Retroviruses and Opportunistic Infections, Chicago, 1999.

12. Costner M, Cockerell CJ: The changing spectrum of the cutaneous manifestations of HIV disease. Arch Dermatol 134:1290–1292, 1998.

13. Dank JP, Colven R: Protease inhibitor–associated angiolipomatosis. J Am Acad Dermatol 42:129–131, 2000.

14. Dover JS, Johnson RA: Cutaneous manifestations of human immunodeficiency virus infection: Parts 1 and 2. Arch Dermatol 127:1383–1391, 1549–1558, 1991.

15. Friedman-Kien AE, Saltzman BR: Clinical manifestations of classical, endemic African, and epidemic AIDS-associated Kaposi's sarcoma. J Am Acad Dermatol 22:1237–1250, 1990.

16. Gregory N: Clinical manifestations of photosensitivity in patients with human immunodeficiency virus infection. Arch Dermatol 130:630–633, 1994.

17. Gregory N, Sanchez M, Buchness MR: The spectrum of syphilis in patients with human immunodeficiency virus infection. J Am Acad Dermatol 22:1061–1067, 1990.

18. James W (ed): AIDS: A ten-year perspective. Dermatol Clin 9:391–615, 1991.

19. Lo JC, Mulligan K, Tai VW, et al: "Buffalo hump" in men with HIV I infection. Lancet 351:867–870, 1998.

20. Lobo DV, Chu P, Grekin RC, et al: Nonmelanoma skin cancers and infection with the human immunodeficiency virus. Arch Dermatol 128:623–627, 1992.

21. Mastrolorenzo A, Urbano FG, Salimbeni L, et al: Atypical molluscum contagiosum infection in an HIV-infected patient. Int J Dermatol 37:378–380, 1998.

22. Meadow KP, Tyring SK, Pavia AT, et al: Resolution of recalcitrant molluscum contagiosum virus lesions in HIV-infected patients treated with cidofovir. Arch Dermatol 133: 987–990, 1997.

23. Myskowski PL: Molluscum contagiosum: New insights, new directions. Arch Dermatol 133:1039–1041, 1997.

24. O'Connor WJ, Murphy GM, Darby C, et al: Porphyrin abnormalities in acquired immunodeficiency syndrome. Arch Dermatol 132:1443–1447, 1996.

25. Otley CC, Avram MR, Johnson RA: Isotretinoin treatment of human immunodeficiency virus–associated eosinophilic folliculitis. Arch Dermatol 131:1047–1050, 1995.

26. Pappert A, Grossman M, DeLeo V: Photosensitivity as the presenting illness in four patients with human immunodeficiency viral infection. Arch Dermatol 130:618–623, 1994.

27. Penneys NS: Skin Manifestations of AIDS, 2nd ed. St. Louis, Mosby, 1995.

28. Piantanida EW, Turiansky GW, Kenner JR, et al: HIV-associated eosinophilic folliculitis: Diagnosis by transverse histologic sections. J Am Acad Dermatol 38:124–126, 1998.

29. Pujol RM, Domingo P, Xavier-Matias-Guiu, et al: HIV-I protease inhibitor–associated partial lipodystrophy: Clinicopathologic review of 14 cases. J Am Acad Dermatol 42:193–198, 2000.

30. Resnick L, Herbst JS, Raab-Traub N: Oral hairy leukoplakia. J Am Acad Dermatol 22:1278–1282, 1990.

31. Rosenthal D, LeBoit PE, Klumpp L, et al: Human immunodeficiency virus-associated eosinophilic folliculitis: A unique dermatosis associated with advanced human immunodeficiency virus infection. Arch Dermatol 127:206–209, 1991.

32. Simpson-Dent SL, Fearfield LA, Staughton RCD: HIV associated eosinophilic folliculitis: Differential diagnosis and management. Sex Transm Infect 75:291–293, 1999.

33. Smith KJ, Skelton HG, Yeager J, et al: Cutaneous findings in HIV-1-positive patients: A 42-month prospective study. J Am Acad Dermatol 31:746–754, 1994.

34. Smith KJ, Skelton HG, Yeager J, et al: Metronidazole for eosinophilic pustular folliculitis in human immunodeficiency virus type I–positive patients. Arch Dermatol 131:1089–1091, 1995.

35. Spach DH, Colven R: Resolution of recalcitrant hand warts in an HIV-infected patient treated with potent antiretroviral therapy. J Am Acad Dermatol 40:818–821, 1999.

36. Toro JR, Chu P, Yen T-S B, et al: Granuloma annulare and human immunodeficiency virus infection. Arch Dermatol 135:1341–1346, 1999.

37. Tosti A, Piraccini BM, D'Antuono A, et al: Paronychia associated with antiretroviral therapy. Br J Dermatol 140:1165–1168, 1999.

38. Walmsley S, Northfelt DW, Melosky B, et al: Treatment of AIDS-related cutaneous Kaposi's sarcoma with topical alitretinoin (9-cis-retinoic acid) gel. Panretin Gel North American Study Group. J Acquir Immune Defic Syndr 22:235–246, 1999.

39. Weinburg JM, Mysliwiec A, Turiansky GW, et al: Viral folliculitis: Atypical presentations of herpes simplex, herpes zoster, and molluscum contagiosum. Arch Dermatol 133:983–986, 1997.

40. CUTANEOUS SIGNS OF NUTRITIONAL DISTURBANCES

Carl W. Demidovich, M.D.

1. When do skin abnormalities occur in association with nutritional disturbances?

Skin manifestations occur when structural or enzymatic processes are affected by a deficiency or excess of a particular nutrient. This can be seen with dietary insufficiency or excess, malabsorption, drug interference, catabolic states, and metabolic, renal, hepatic, and inherited disorders. Nutrients include protein, carbohydrate, fat, vitamins, minerals, and trace elements.

2. Do nutritional disturbances involve the skin exclusively?

Absolutely not. Nutritional disorders are generalized conditions that cause multisystem disorders. Inadequate diet usually causes multiple nutrient deficiencies, with the resulting clinical picture a combination of these deficiencies. Clinical history, review of systems, and physical examination are of utmost importance when attempting to determine the underlying etiology of skin findings suggestive of a nutritional disorder.

3. Which skin changes are seen with protein and calorie deprivation in adults?

In clinical observations and prospective experiments, adults with starvation demonstrate rough, inelastic, pallid, gray skin with pigmentary changes in the malar and periorificial areas. Hair is thinned and growth of nails is slow. Nails may also demonstrate fissuring. There is decreased subcutaneous fat and, with time, muscle wasting.

4. What is marasmus?

Marasmus (from the Greek meaning *wasting*), or **childhood caloric malnutrition,** is a combined or proportional energy and protein deficiency with resultant catabolism and utilization of muscle and fat. There are no specific or significant skin findings. Infants often demonstrate a "monkey facies" due to loss of buccal fat that normally gives the face a rounded appearance.

5. What is kwashiorkor?

Kwashiorkor (Ga language of Ghana meaning "sickness of the weanling"), or **childhood protein malnutrition,** is a result of protein deficiency with concurrent normal to excessive carbohydrate intake. It is a common affliction worldwide, and is seen in developed countries in association with poverty, neurologic disease, and malabsorption. There is muscle wasting with preservation of normal fat stores. The low ratio of protein to energy is felt to disrupt the body's usual hypometabolic response to caloric deficiency and is biochemically manifest as markedly increased lipis peroxidation. Clinically, edema, hypoalbuminemia, growth retardation, fatty liver, psychomotor changes, and prominent skin findings are seen.

6. Describe the skin findings in kwashiorkor.

In black children, initial circumoral pallor progresses to diffuse depigmentation. In white children, there is diffuse blanching erythema that rapidly progresses to dusky nonblanching purple macules and papules. Classic findings include **mosaic skin** (dry, fine areas of desquamation with cracking along skin lines) and **enamel paint dermatosis** (Fig. 1), which evolves into large areas of erosion and desquamation. Hair in affected patients is sparse, thin, fragile, and depigmented. This hair depigmentation may produce the **flag sign,** which is alternating pigmented and depigmented bands seen along the hair shafts corresponding to periods of normal and inadequate nutrition.

7. How can I remember the differences in skin findings associated with kwashiorkor and marasmus?

Kwashiorkor, or **P**rotein malnutrition may be memorized by thinking of "**KP,**" the military term for kitchen patrol. **K**washiorkor is associated with peeling skin, as are hands of dish**wash**ers.

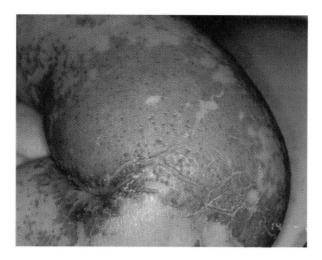

FIGURE 1. Enamel paint dermatosis in a child with kwashiorkor. (Courtesy of William Weston, MD.)

8. Do skin abnormalities occur with fat deficiency?

Essential fatty acid deficiency occurs with deficiency of linoleic acid, a precursor of arachidonic acid. It is seen primarily with malabsorption syndromes and with prolonged total parenteral nutrition. Skin findings consist of a periorificial or generalized dermatitis caused by increased transepidermal water loss due to loss of the barrier function of the skin. Periorificial dermatitis cannot be clinically differentiated from lesions seen in acrodermatitis enteropathica (see question 17). Dietary or intravenous linoleic acid supplementation is curative, although adults often respond to only topical application.

9. Are any skin findings associated with fat excess?

Yes. Obesity researchers have documented an increased incidence of plantar hyperkeratosis (thickened soles), acanthosis nigricans, striae, and skin tags in patients overweight by more than 100%. Excess fat deposition predisposes to **intertrigo,** a dermatitis occurring between skinfolds, sometimes associated with secondary bacterial or candidal infection.

10. Which water-soluble vitamin abnormalities have skin findings?

Nearly all of the water-soluble vitamins demonstrate skin findings in deficiency states. There is considerable overlap in the skin findings, especially among the B-complex deficiencies, which is expected since they all function as coenzymes or cofactors in redox, carboxylation, or transamination reactions. Common clinical findings in riboflavin (B_2), pyridoxine (B_6), cobalamin (B_{12}), and biotin deficiencies include angular cheilitis, periorificial dermatitis, and glossitis.

11. Name the four "D's" of pellagra.

Diarrhea   Dermatitis   Dementia   Death

Pellagra (Italian, *pelle-* skin and *agra-* sharp burning or rough) is a deficiency of niacin that manifests clinically in classic form as the "four D's." Great variability is seen in the extent and type of gastrointestinal, neurologic, and skin manifestations. Niacin is available in animal products, enriched wheat flour, and is synthesized from tryptophan. Pellagra is most commonly seen in alcoholics and in patients on isoniazid therapy, which interferes with tryptophan metabolism.

12. Describe the dermatitis in pellagra.

The dermatitis is characteristically but not invariably photodistributed. Acutely, it is erythematous and may be associated with either pruritus or burning. Within 2–3 weeks, it becomes dry, scaly, and thickened. **Casal's necklace** is a term used to describe sharply demarcated dermatitic lesions that develop around the neck and clinically resemble a necklace (Fig. 2). Dermatitic lesions also occur in the perineal and genital areas, over bony prominences, and on the face. The skin abnormalities in pellagra respond rapidly to niacin supplementation and heal in a centrifugal fashion.

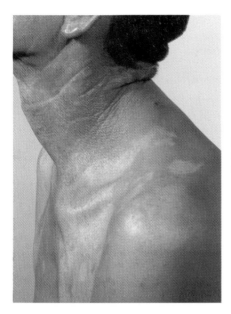

FIGURE 2. Pellagra, showing the typical photodistributed dermatitis on the neck and chest known as Casal's necklace. (Courtesy of Richard Gentry, MD.)

13. Does scurvy still exist?

Yes, but it is rare. Vitamin C present in fresh fruit and vegetables is a necessary cofactor in collagen synthesis. Deficiency states initially demonstrate enlargement and keratosis of hair follicles with development of corkscrew hairs. Within weeks, there is a proliferation of blood vessels around hair follicles and in the interdental papillae of gingiva with hemorrhage (Fig. 3). Impaired collagen synthesis results in poor wound healing. Recent reports also describe clinical findings of purpura mimicking vasculitis and extensive ecchymoses on the lower extremities.

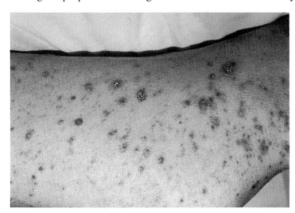

FIGURE 3. Scurvy. Characteristic perifollicular hemorrhage and follicular hyperkeratosis.

14. Do deficiencies of the fat-soluble vitamins occur?

Yes, but less commonly because these vitamins have significant storage depots. Vitamin K deficiency is seen with malabsorption syndromes and in the newborn period prior to bacterial colonization of the intestine. Clinical lesions range from petechiae to massive hemorrhages. Vitamin D and E deficiencies are not associated with skin findings.

15. What abnormalities occur with vitamin A deficiency?

This disorder primarily involves the skin and eyes. **Phrynoderma,** the name applied to the cutaneous eruption of vitamin A deficiency, is a keratotic follicular eruption that initially appears on the proximal extremities. It eventually extends to the trunk, back, abdomen, buttocks, and neck. Facial lesions may resemble large comedones of acne. Eye symptoms include **nyctalopia** (delayed dark adaptation, the earliest finding), **night blindness,** and **xerophthalmia.** Objective findings are **Bitot's spots,** which are areas of shed corneal epithelium, and in severe disease, **keratomalacia.** Vitamin A deficiency is most commonly caused by malabsorption disorders.

16. Is vitamin A excess toxic?

Yes. Hypervitaminosis A may develop either acutely or chronically. Acute toxicity is rare but is most commonly due to vitamin A overdose. It has also been documented in Arctic explorers consuming polar bear livers, which are rich in vitamin A. Clinically, it presents as large areas of desquamation associated with headache and vomiting. Chronic toxicity is more common and displays features associated with side effects of retinoid therapy—alopecia, exfoliation, and skin dryness. Pseudotumor cerebri with papilledema may occur early before any other signs. All symptoms and signs resolve in days to weeks following cessation of supplementation.

17. What is acrodermatitis enteropathica?

Acrodermatitis enteropathica is a rare autosomal recessive disorder of intestinal zinc absorption. Zinc is normally incorporated into multiple types of enzymes present in all body tissues but is concentrated five- to sixfold in the epidermis. Deficiency of this trace element results in dramatic findings. The classic triad consists of **acral dermatitis, alopecia,** and **diarrhea.** Growth failure, anemia, impaired wound healing, and mental and emotional disturbances are also seen. The periorificial and acral dermatitis (Fig. 4) was considered to be pathognomonic in the past, but more recent reports have described similar cutaneous eruptions in essential fatty acid deficiency, biotin deficiency, and infants treated for organic acidurias. Acrodermatitis enteropathica develops in days to weeks after birth in bottle-fed infants and shortly after weaning in breastfed infants. Uncommonly, signs and symptoms are first noted at puberty.

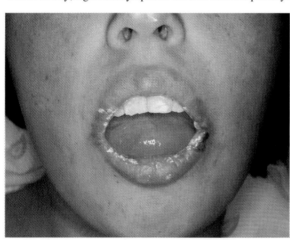

FIGURE 4. Periorificial dermatitis in a patient with acrodermatitis enteropathics. (Courtesy of James E. Fitzpatrick, MD).

18. How is acrodermatitis enteropathica diagnosed and treated?

Diagnosis is made by demonstrating low plasma or serum zinc levels. Hair zinc levels reflect only long-term status and may not reflect early deficiency. Oral or intravenous zinc supplementation promotes rapid improvement, with reversal of most clinical manifestations in hours to days. Untreated infants develop failure to thrive, with progressive deterioration and death.

19. Can zinc deficiency be acquired?

Yes, in association with diabetes mellitus, collagen vascular disease, pregnancy, Crohn's disease, nephrotic syndrome, dialysis, renal tubular disease, burns, antimetabolite drugs, alcoholism, malabsorption syndromes, and HIV infection. Clinical findings are similar to those of the inherited form of acrodermatitis enteropathica.

20. What is carotenoderma?

Carotenoderma is a yellow or orange skin discoloration most prominent on the palms, soles, and central face. It is more common in children and is associated with ingestion of carotene found in carrots, oranges, squash, spinach, yellow corn, butter, eggs, pumpkin, yellow turnips, sweet potatoes, and dried seaweeds. It is clinically apparent when serum carotene levels are three to four times normal. The discoloration spares the sclera and mucosal surfaces, which can be used to differentiate this benign condition from jaundice (Fig. 5). Elimination of the offending food results in normalization of skin color in 2–6 weeks. Carotenemia also occurs in diabetes mellitus and hypothyroidism due to impaired hepatic conversion of carotene to vitamin A. It has been reported in anorexia nervosa with undetermined etiology.

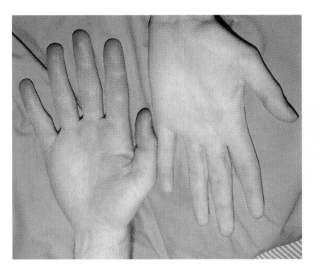

FIGURE 5. Characteristic yellow discoloration of skin in a patient with carotenoderma contrasted with normal skin color. This patient was eating up to one bunch of carrots per day. (Courtesy of James E. Fitzpatrick, MD).

21. Has supplementation with micronutrients or homeopathic remedies been associated with any cutaneous disorders?

Yes. Ginkgo, reported to increase mentation, memory, and energy levels, has been documented to increase bleeding time and has been associated with intraoperative bleeding and postoperative hematoma and ecchymosis. Certain Chinese herbal supplements and proprietary medicines have been reported to contain inorganic arsenic. This has caused chronic arsenicism, clinically manifest as Bowen's disease (squamous cell carcinoma in situ) and arsenical keratoses on the palms and soles.

BIBLIOGRAPHY

1. Barthelemy H, Chouvet B, Cambazard F: Skin and mucosal manifestations in vitamin deficiency. J Am Acad Dermatol 15:1263–1274, 1986.
2. Bleasel NR, Stapleton KM, Lee MS, Sullivan J: Vitamin A deficiency phrynoderma due to malabsorption and inadequate diet. J Am Acad Dermatol 41:322–324, 1999.
3. Danbolt N, Closs K: Acrodermatitis enteropathica. Acta Derm Venereol (Stockh) 23:127–169, 1942.
4. De Raeve L, De Meirleir L, Ramet J, et al: Acrodermatitis enteropathica-like cutaneous lesions in organic aciduria. J Pediatr 124:416–420, 1994.
5. Eastlack JP, Grande KK, Levy ML, Nigro JF: Dermatosis in a child with kwashiorkor secondary to food aversion. Pediatr Dermatol 16:95–102, 1999.
6. Garcia-Hidalgo L, Orozco-Topete R, Gonzalez-Barranco J, et al: Dermatoses in 156 obese adults. Obes Res 7:299–302, 1999.
7. Ghorbani AJ, Eichler C: Scurvy. J Am Acad Dermatol 30:881–883, 1994.
8. Gonzalez-Gay MA, Garcia-Porrua C, Lueiro M, et al: Scurvy can mimick cutaneous vasculitis: Three case reports. Rev Rhum Engl Ed 66:360–361, 1999.

9. Hendricks WM: Pellagra and pellagralike dermatoses: Etiology, differential, diagnosis, dermatopathology and treatment. Semin Dermatol 10:282–292, 1991.
10. Horrobin DF: Essential fatty acids in clinical dermatology. J Am Acad Dermatol 20:1045–1053, 1989.
11. Keys A: The Biology of Human Starvation. Minneapolis, University of Minnesota Press, 1950.
12. Lenhartz H, Ndasi R, Anninos A, et al: The clinical manifestation of the kwashiorkor syndrome is related to increased lipid peroxidation. J Pediatr 132:879–881, 1998.
13. McLaren DS: Skin in protein energy malnutrition. Arch Dermatol 123:1674–1676, 1987.
14. Miller SJ: Nutritional deficiency and the skin. J Am Acad Dermatol 21:1–30, 1989.
15. Myung SJ, Yang SK, Jung HY, et al: Zinc deficiency manifested by dermatitis and visual dysfunction in a patient with Crohn's disease. J Gastroenterol 33:876–879, 1998.
16. Nakjang Y, Yuttanavivat T: Phrynoderma: A review of 105 cases. J Dermatol 15:531–534, 1988.
17. Nishimura Y, Ishii N, Sugita Y, Nakajima H: A case of carotenodermia caused by a diet of the dried seaweed called Nori. J Dermatol 25:685–687, 1998.
18. Prendiville JS, Manfredi LN: Skin signs of nutritional disorders. Semin Dermatol 11:88–97, 1992.
19. Rossouw JE: Kwashiorkor in North America. Am J Clin Nutr 49:588–592, 1989.
20. Sasaki G, Satoh T, Yokozeki H, et al: Confluent ecchymoses on the lower extremities of a malnourished patient. J Dermatol 26:399–401, 1999.

VI. *Benign Tumors of the Skin*

41. BENIGN MELANOCYTIC TUMORS

Patrick Walsh, M.D.

1. What is a mole?

A small burrowing mammal of the family Talpidae. It is also a term commonly used to describe a melanocytic nevus.

2. What is a nevus?

Derived from the Latin term meaning spot or blemish, *nevus* was originally used to describe a congenital lesion or birthmark (mother's mark). In modern usage, the term describes a cutaneous hamartoma, or benign proliferation of cells. However, when the term is used without a descriptive adjective, it is usually referring to a melanocytic nevus. Other examples of nevi include the epidermal nevus and nevus sebaceus.

3. Are there different types of melanocytic nevi?

Yes. Melanocytic nevi can be classified according to their histology (junctional, compound, or intradermal location of the nevus cells) or appearance (e.g., halo nevi or blue nevi). In addition, there are congenital melanocytic nevi and acquired nevi.

4. Explain the natural developmental history of melanocytic nevi.

Melanocytes arise from the neural crest in embryonic life and migrate to their final location in the skin, eye, and brain during fetal life. The melanocytes that migrate to the skin take up residence on the epidermal side of the dermal/epidermal junction. Melanocytic nevus cells are derived from these skin melanocytes but differ from normal epidermal melanocytes in a number of ways. They are no longer dendritic, they do not distribute melanin to surrounding keratinocytes, and they are less metabolically active.

Melanocytic nevi begin as a proliferation of nevus cells along the dermal/epidermal junction (forming a junctional nevus, Fig. 1A). With continued proliferation of nevus cells, they extend from the dermal/epidermal junction into the dermis (forming a compound nevus). The junctional component of the melanocytic nevus may resolve, leaving only an intradermal component (intradermal nevus, Fig. 1B). New melanocytic nevi may form naturally, possibly due to ultraviolet light exposure, from the ages of 6 months to 40 years and later. They may also resolve spontaneously. However, the appearance or disappearance of any melanocytic lesion should be brought to the attention of a physician.

5. What is a halo nevus?

Halo nevus, also known as Sutton's nevus or leukoderma acquisitum centrifugum, is a melanocytic nevus with a surrounding area of depigmentation (Fig. 1C). Halo nevi can be solitary or multiple, most commonly occur before age 20 years, and can be associated with vitiligo. The pathogenesis is poorly understood, but the depigmentation has been shown to involve the immunologically mediated destruction of nevus cells and nearby melanocytes. The halo nevus may represent the early stages of regression and involution of a melanocytic nevus. It may also represent an immunologic reaction against cells that have undergone malignant transformation.

Although most pigmented lesions with halos are benign, malignant melanoma can rarely be seen with an associated halo. If a pigmented lesion has an irregular border or halo or shows other atypical features, it should be biopsied.

6. What is a congenital nevus?

A melanocytic nevus that is present at birth. For the purpose of management, any melanocytic nevus that arises during the first year of life is considered "congenital." Congenital melanocytic nevi (CMN) are usually characterized as small, large, or giant. Small CMN are usually defined as <1.5 cm in diameter, large CMN as >1.5 cm but <20 cm in diameter, and giant CMN as >20 cm in diameter. Another scheme for classifying small, large, and giant CMN considers the ease of surgical removal and repair of the resulting surgical defect. Still another classification scheme describes giant CMN as being as large as two of the patient's palms for lesions on the trunk and extremities or one palm for lesions on the face or neck (Fig. 1D).

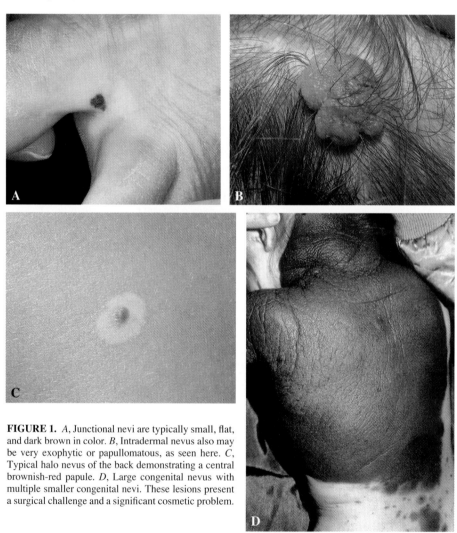

FIGURE 1. *A,* Junctional nevi are typically small, flat, and dark brown in color. *B,* Intradermal nevus also may be very exophytic or papullomatous, as seen here. *C,* Typical halo nevus of the back demonstrating a central brownish-red papule. *D,* Large congenital nevus with multiple smaller congenital nevi. These lesions present a surgical challenge and a significant cosmetic problem.

Although there is little agreement about the risk of developing melanoma within a CMN, some general guidelines can be stated. The risk appears to relate to the size of the CMN. A small CMN does not appear to have a significantly greater risk for melanoma than a noncongenital melanocytic nevus. There is about a 4–6% chance of developing melanoma in a giant CMN.

7. What is a blue nevus?

It is a melanocytic nevus characterized by the deep dermal accumulation of melanin-producing, melanocytic, and often dendritic nevus cells. The deep dermal location of the pigment-producing cells, and therefore the pigment, causes the lesion to have its blue, black, or gray appearance (the Tyndall effect). The three commonly identified varieties of blue nevi are the common blue nevus, cellular blue nevus, and combined blue nevus–melanocytic nevus.

8. Can blue nevi become malignant?

Yes. Malignant blue nevi can develop de novo, in existing cellular blue nevi, or in a nevus of Ota. Most commonly, the lesion presents as an expanding dermal nodule that may ulcerate. As with other forms of cutaneous melanoma, metastases may develop. However, malignant blue nevi are rare, and often there is controversy regarding their histopathologic diagnosis.

9. What is a combined melanocytic nevus?

A combined melanocytic nevus is a blue nevus with an overlying melanocytic nevus. The blue nevus may be a common or cellular blue nevus. The overlying melanocytic nevus can be junctional, compound, or intradermal.

10. In which age group does a Spitz nevus typically develop?

A Spitz nevus is a melanocytic nevus that most commonly occurs in **children,** but it may occur at any age. Histologically, it is composed of nevus cells that are pleomorphic and cytologically atypical; these cells typically demonstrate a spindle or epithelioid appearance. The lesion has been called benign juvenile melanoma, reflecting the fact that some of these lesions have histologic characteristics similar to melanoma. The lesion usually presents as a small, pink nodule on the face or lower extremities.

11. How does a nevus of Ota differ from a nevus of Ito?

The **nevus of Ota** (also called nevus fuscoceruleus ophthalmomaxillaris) is characterized clinically as a blue to gray hyperpigmentation of the skin, mucosa, and conjunctiva in the distribution of the trigeminal nerve. Histologically, it is composed of heavily melanized dendritic dermal melanocytes in the upper dermis. The **nevus of Ito** is similar in histology to the nevus of Ota but is distributed along the neck and shoulder.

12. Where do Becker's nevi occur?

A Becker's nevus is characterized by an area of hyperpigmentation and often hypertrichosis, most commonly on the upper back, shoulder, or chest of males (Fig. 2). The lesions usually become noticeable at puberty. Histologically, there is an increased number of melanocytes, dermal melanophages, terminal hairs, and hyperpigmentation of the epidermal basal layer. Some lesions can also show increased smooth muscle and have been called smooth muscle hamartomas.

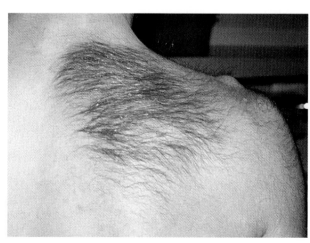

FIGURE 2. A Becker's nevus on the upper back of a young man. This lesion has no potential for malignant degeneration.

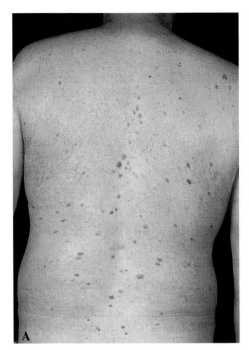

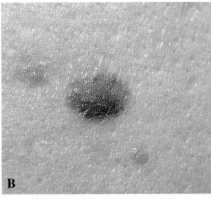

FIGURE 3. Atypical nevi. *A*, Patient with familial atypical melanocytic nevus syndrome demonstrating numerous atypical nevi. *B*, An atypical nevus demonstrating marked variegation in color and loss of normal symmetry.

13. What is a dysplastic melanocytic nevus?

Dysplastic nevus is a term that is generally discouraged for lack of a precise definition. However, it has been commonly used to describe an atypical-appearing melanocytic nevus believed to have increased potential for malignant transformation. Since this lesion was first described, the dysplastic nevus has been the subject of controversy. Argument has centered around the criteria for its histopathologic diagnosis, the incidence of melanoma developing in the lesion, and the histopathologic association of melanoma arising in a dysplastic nevus. The quoted incidence of this association is reported as low as 1% and as high as 40%.

Even the terminology used for this lesion is the subject of controversy. *Dysplastic nevus* was first coined by Green et al. in 1980. Three years earlier, Clark and Elder described families with an increased incidence of melanoma and multiple atypical melanocytic nevi, which they called the *familial atypical mole-melanoma syndrome*. Other names for this have come and gone—the B-K mole, precancerous melanosis, atypical melanocytic hyperplasia, Clark's nevus, active junctional nevus, and melanocytic nevus with architectural disorder and cytologic atypia. A recent NIH consensus conference has recommended discontinuing use of the term dysplastic nevus and replacing it with **atypical nevus.** The conference also recommended replacing dysplastic nevus syndrome with **familial atypical melanocytic nevus syndrome.**

14. How common are atypical melanocytic nevi?

The exact incidence is unknown, but it is estimated that 2–8% of the population have one or more atypical nevus.

15. Is there a difference between an atypical nevus and melanoma in situ?

Yes. The difference is determined by the histopathology. An atypical nevus has atypical melanocytic nevus cells at the dermal-epidermal interface, whereas melanoma in situ has atypical melanocytes both singly and in small nests scattered through all levels of the epidermis (pagetoid pattern). Recommended treatment for melanoma in situ is complete full-thickness excision with a minimum of a 0.5-cm margin of normal skin. Treatment for an atypical nevus is complete full-thickness excision with a minimum 0.2-cm margin of normal skin. Melanoma in situ has a greater tendency to develop a vertical growth phase and become invasive malignant melanoma.

16. Describe the clinical appearance of atypical nevi.

Atypical nevi are usually larger than ordinary nevi (>6 mm) and have slightly irregular borders that fade into the surrounding normal skin (Fig. 3). Variation of color within lesions is common, with varying shades of brown, tan, and light red. The lesions typically are located on the upper trunk and proximal extremities and often have a "fried-egg" appearance, with a dark center surrounded by pigment which has poor margination.

17. Is there a difference between a liver spot and a freckle?

Yes. Liver spot is the term commonly used to refer to a **solar** or **senile lentigo**. A lentigo is a hyperpigmented (usually brown or black) macule that is characterized histopathologically by increased numbers of melanocytes at the dermal-epidermal junction and increased amounts of melanin in both the melanocytes and basal keratinocytes. These lesions commonly arise on the dorsal aspects of the hands and face. Although solar lentigines are induced by ultraviolet radiation, they do not increase in pigmentation with exposure to the sun. **Freckles** (ephelides) are hyperpigmented macules limited to sun-exposed skin. Microscopically, they show increased amounts of melanin in basal keratinocytes, but not increased numbers of melanocytes. Freckles characteristically darken with sun exposure and lighten when the affected areas are protected from ultraviolet radiation.

18. What is a mongolian spot?

A mongolian spot is a congenital hyperpigmented spot found in the sacrococcygeal region. Most frequently found in black or Asian infants, it also occurs in infants of other races. The pigmentation often disappears spontaneously in the first 3–5 years of life but may persist into adulthood. These lesions are believed to represent the delayed disappearance of dermal melanocytes. The deep blue pigmentation is another example of the Tyndall effect.

19. What is a café au lait macule?

Café au lait macules (CALMs) are uniformly light-brown (the color of coffee with cream) macules that vary in size from 2 to >20 cm and often have irregular borders. They are characterized by increased melanin in both melanocytes and keratinocytes and by giant melanosomes. They may be a marker of multisystem disease, most importantly neurofibromatosis.

20. What is a nevus spilus?

A nevus spilus is an irregularly shaped, light-brown macule with darkly pigmented macules or papules scattered randomly within the macule (Fig. 4). The light areas demonstrate the microscopic

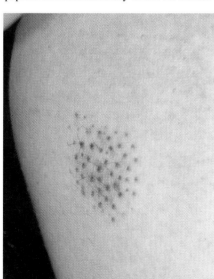

FIGURE 4. Nevus spilus showing a large café-au-lait macule with multiple small pigmented lesions.

changes of a café au lait macule, and areas of increased melanin with darker pigmentation show the histology of lentigos or junctional nevi. It is unclear if there is an association between these lesions and neurofibromatosis.

21. Can melanocytic nevi arise in locations other than the skin?

Yes. Melanocytic nevi can occur on the retina, conjunctiva, and oral (and other) mucosal surfaces.

22. What is a labial lentigo?

Labial lentigo is a hyperpigmented macule that develops on the lip. Seen most commonly in young women, there is thickening of the epidermis and increased melanin in the basal keratinocytes.

BIBLIOGRAPHY

1. Hashimoto K, Mehregan A: Tumours of the Epidermis. Boston, Butterworths, 1990.
2. Rhodes AR: Benign neoplasias and hyperplasias of melanocytes. In Freedberg IM, Eisen AZ, Wolff K, et al (eds): Dermatology in General Medicine, 5th ed. New York, McGraw-Hill, 1999.
3. Rhodes AR: Dysplastic melanocytic nevi. In Freedberg IM, Eisen AZ, Wolff K, et al (eds): Dermatology in General Medicine, 5th ed. New York, McGraw-Hill, 1999.

42. VASCULAR NEOPLASMS

Joseph G. Morelli, M.D.

1. Which is the most common benign vascular neoplasm of childhood?

Hemangioma, which is a benign tumor of vascular endothelium. This tumor typically presents at ages 2–8 weeks and then goes through a rapid growth phase during the first year of life. It then begins to regress, with complete regression in 50% of patients by age 5. Regression does not necessarily imply return of the skin to normal.

2. What are the clinical subtypes of hemangioma?

(1) Superficial—bright red papules; (2) deep—soft blue nodule (Fig. 1); and (3) mixed—combination of the above.

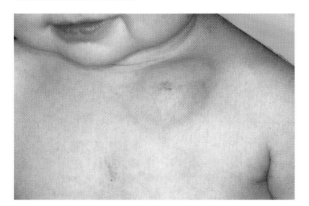

FIGURE 1. Deep hemangioma.

3. Name the complications of hemangiomas.

Obstruction of a vital function (such as vision, breathing, eating, defecation, or urination), ulceration followed by bleeding and infection, and high-output cardiac failure.

4. What is the most common complication of hemangiomas?

Ulceration is the most frequent complication and occurs predominantly in hemangiomas found in the diaper area (Fig. 2).

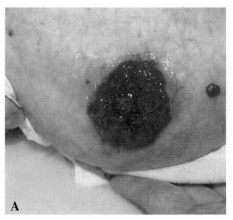
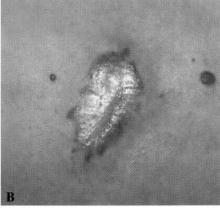

FIGURE 2. *A,* Ulcerated hemangioma. *B,* Same hemangioma 3 months following one pulsed dye laser treatment.

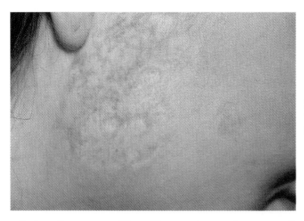

FIGURE 3. Scarring, hypopigmentation, and telangiectasia following regression of a hemangioma.

5. Are there any residua of hemangiomas after regression?

Hypopigmentation, telangiectasia, excess skin, fibrofatty deposits, and if ulceration occurred, scarring (Fig. 3).

6. Port wine stains and lymphangiomas are not neoplasms, but what are they?

They are vascular malformations.

7. What are blue-black hyperkeratotic vascular papules?

Angiokeratomas. There are five types of angiokeratomas:

1. Localized angiokeratomas—usually solitary and found on an extremity
2. Angiokeratoma circumscriptum—presents at birth as unilateral plaques on an extremity (Fig. 4)
3. Angiokeratoma of Mibelli—develops in childhood or adolescence over the dorsal surface of the hands or feet
4. Angiokeratoma of Fordyce—most commonly seen on the scrotum
5. Angiokeratoma corporis diffusum (Fabry's disease)—an X-linked recessively inherited disease in which ceramide trihexoside accumulates in vascular endothelium. Multiple skin lesions are found between the umbilicus and knees. Patients frequently develop hypohidrosis, paresthesias, cardiac and renal disease.

8. Where and in whom are cherry angiomas most commonly seen?

Cherry angiomas are extremely common, acquired, 1–5-mm, red to purple papules primarily located on the trunk and upper extremities (Fig. 5). They are most commonly seen in the middle-aged and elderly. In one study, 75% of the patients over age 64 had cherry angiomas.

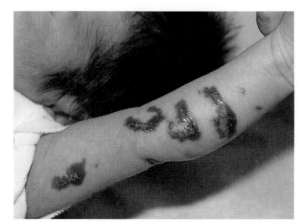

FIGURE 4. Angiokeratoma circumscriptum.

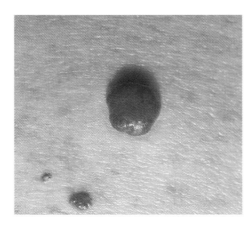

FIGURE 5. Multiple cherry angiomas. (Courtesy of James E. Fitzpatrick, MD.)

9. Where do you find venous lakes?

These are dark blue, slightly raised papules occuring on sun-exposed skin surfaces of elderly patients, most commonly located on the ears, lips, and face. They may be mistaken for melanoma. Twelve percent of patients over age 64 have one or more venous lakes.

10. What is the most common presenting feature of a pyogenic granuloma?

Pyogenic granulomas are 5–10-mm soft red papules that **bleed easily with minor trauma** (Fig. 6). They are most common on the skin but may also occur on mucosal surfaces or, rarely, within blood vessels. Granuloma gravidarum is a variant that occurs on the gingiva during pregnancy. The pathogenesis is unknown, but approximately one-third will occur after local trauma.

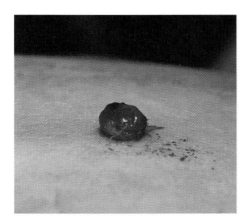

FIGURE 6. Pyogenic granuloma.

11. Where are you likely to find a lesion of angiolymphoid hyperplasia?

These lesions usually are found on the head and neck. They appear clinically as red-brown papules. Histologically, they demonstrate clusters of vessels with prominent endothelial cells, often accompanied by a nodular lymphocytic infiltrate that may appear as lymphoid follicles. The lesions are at times associated with a peripheral eosinophilia. The etiology is unknown.

12. What vascular tumor is associated with the Sucquet-Hoyer canal?

The Sucquet-Hoyer canal is the arterial segment of the glomus body and may give rise to **glomus tumors.** A solitary glomus tumor is a painful, purple nodule measuring a few millimeters in diameter. Multiple glomus tumors are inherited in an autosomal dominant fashion, may be much larger than the solitary form, and have been confused with the blue-rubber bleb nevus syndrome.

13. Mat-like telangiectasias on the face, lips, tongue, ears, hands, and feet associated with internal bleeding is known as what syndrome?

Osler-Weber-Rendu syndrome, or hereditary hemorrhagic telangiectasia. Most patients present with epistaxis. Gastrointestinal telangiectasias are common, and genitourinary, pulmonary, CNS, and hepatic lesions may also occur. It is inherited as an autosomal dominant disease.

14. What is the most common cause of acquired facial telangiectasia?

Chronic ultraviolet light exposure is the leading cause of acquired facial telangiectasia. Other common causes include rosacea, connective tissue disease, and abuse of potent topical steroids.

15. Which benign acquired vascular disease is often initially confused with Kaposi's sarcoma?

Acroangiodermatitis—an eruption of purple macules, papules, and plaques usually associated with chronic venous insufficiency. Similar skin lesions can be found overlying arteriovenous malformations.

BIBLIOGRAPHY

1. Alcalay J, Sandbank M: The ultrastructure of cutaneous venous lakes. Int J Dermatol 26:645–646, 1987.
2. Cox NH, Paterson WD: Angioma serpiginosum: A simulator of purpura. Postgrad Med J 67:1065–1066, 1991.
3. Fetsch JF, Weiss SW: Observation concerning the pathogenesis of epithelioid hemangioma (angiolymphoid hyperplasia). Mod Pathol 4:449–455, 1991.
4. Heys SD, Brittenden J, Atkinson P, Eremin O: Glomus tumour: An analysis of 43 patients and review of the literature. Br J Surg 79:345–346, 1992.
5. Imperial R, Helwig EB: Angiokeratoma: A clinicopathological study. Arch Dermatol 95:166–175, 1967.
6. Morelli JG, Tan OT, Yohn JJ, Weston WL: Management of ulcerated hemangiomas in infancy. Arch Pediatr Adol Med 148:1104–1108, 1994.
7. Peery WH: Clinical spectrum of hereditary hemorrhagic telangiectasias (Osler-Weber-Rendu disease). Am J Med 82:989–997, 1987.
8. Yi JU, Lee CW. Acroangiodermatitis: A clinical variant of stasis dermatitis. Int J Dermatol 29:515–516, 1990.

43. FIBROUS TUMORS OF THE SKIN

Martin B. Giandoni, M.D., and James E. Fitzpatrick, M.D.

1. What are tumors of fibrous tissue?

Tumors of fibrous tissue are mesenchymal tumors composed of fibroblasts or their variants. Fibroblasts produce normal structural components of the dermis, including collagen, elastin, and ground substance (dermal mucin). Most tumors of fibroblast origin produce collagen, but they also may produce dermal mucin or elastin as the primary product. Some tumors are composed primarily of myofibroblasts, specialized fibroblasts that demonstrate contractile properties because of cytoplasmic actin filaments. Other specialized fibroblasts may demonstrate phagocytosis, and tumors demonstrating this characteristic are referred to as fibrohistiocytic tumors. Tumors of fibrous tissue are conventionally divided into those that are fibrous and those that are fibrohistiocytic.

Fibrous Tumors of the Skin

Benign fibrous tumors	Malignant fibrous tumors
Acquired digital fibrokeratoma	Fibrosarcoma
Acrochordons	Benign fibrohistiocytic tumors
Connective tissue nevus (collagenoma, elastoma)	Fibrous papule
Dermatomyofibroma	Dermatofibroma
Desmoids (extra-abdominal and abdominal	Reticulohistiocytoma (solitary and multiple)
fibromatosis)	Xanthogranuloma (including juvenile xan-
Fibrous hamartoma of infancy	thogranuloma)
Infantile digital fibromatosis	Malignant fibrohistiocytic tumors
Knuckle pads	Atypical fibroxanthoma*
Nodular fasciitis	Dermatofibrosarcoma protuberans
Keloid	Malignant fibrous histiocytoma

*Some dermatologists consider atypical fibroxanthoma to be a benign fibrohistiocytic tumor, but this is controversial.

2. What is an acrochordon?

An acrochordon (skin tag, fibroma durum) is a soft, flesh-colored to dark brown, often pedunculated, cutaneous papule usually located on the neck, axilla, or groin. It is probably the most common mesenchymal neoplasm. Acrochordons are often multiple, usually 1–4 mm in size, but occasionally 3 cm or larger in diameter. The larger baglike lesions are called soft fibromas or fibroepithelial polyps (Fig. 1).

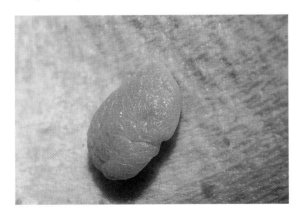

FIGURE 1. Typical acrochordon demonstrating skin-colored soft pedunculated papule. Exophytic seborrheic keratoses and nevi may resemble acrochordons.

3. Is there a known cause for acrochordons?

An exact cause is not known. The frequent association of acrochordons with diabetes mellitus, obesity, pregnancy, menopause, acanthosis nigricans, and certain endocrinopathies suggests

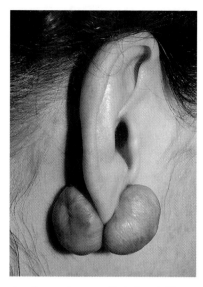

FIGURE 2. "Dumbbell" keloids of the earlobe following ear piercing.

that they are hormonally induced. However, the ubiquitous nature of these lesions in healthy older adults has been interpreted by some authorities as simply a manifestation of skin aging.

4. Are any complications associated with acrochordons?

Yes. The most common complications are recurrent **trauma** to individual lesions (e.g., laceration with a shaving razor) or spontaneous **torsion** and **infarction** of a pedunculated lesion. When a pedunculated lesion twists on its stalk, the blood supply is compromised and tissue ischemia occurs. Usually, sudden pain, swelling, necrosis, and even secondary infection result. Often, this sequence of events results in disappearance of the lesion.

5. Are acrochordons associated with intestinal polyposis?

Several widely reported studies asserted a statistically significant association between the presence of acrochordons and colonic polyps. However, other investigators, using methodology that better accounted for the fact that 60–70% of the elderly have acrochordons, demonstrated no statistical association. Most dermatologists believe that acrochordons are not a marker for colonic polyps but are simply more common in the elderly population that is predisposed to colonic polyposis.

6. How can acrochordons be treated?

The simplest way to treat acrochordons is scissors-snip excision (usually without anesthesia). Smaller lesions can be rapidly treated by electrodesiccation or even cryotherapy (beware of postinflammatory dyspigmentation with cryotherapy). Larger lesions (> 2 cm) can be shaved off after local anesthesia or excised.

7. What is a hypertrophic scar?

A hypertrophic scar represents excessive collagen deposition at a site of wound healing. Typically, the scars are initially red, raised, firm, and often pruritic. With time, they flatten and become white. Hypertrophic scars do not extend beyond the limits of the original trauma. Scars, including hypertrophic scars, are not usually considered to be neoplasms since they are reactive and eventually regress with time.

8. What is a keloid?

A keloid also represents excessive collagen deposition at a site of wound healing. Clinically, a keloid can be indistinguishable from a hypertrophic scar, though the excess collagen deposition of a keloid is usually more exaggerated. Microscopically, developed keloids can be differentiated from hypertrophic scars by the presence of large eosinophilic collagen fibers and more abundant mucin. Also, unlike hypertrophic scars, keloids rarely undergo involution, and they frequently proliferate well beyond the bounds of the original trauma. Some keloids, particularly on the sternum or upper back, even seem to develop without preceding trauma.

9. List the clinical features useful in distinguishing hypertrophic scars from keloids.

In early lesions it may be impossible to make this distinction, but in developed lesions the following features are useful:

Clinical Features that Distinguish Hypertrophic Scars from Keloids

HYPERTROPHIC SCAR	KELOID
Any age group, especially children	Adolescents and young adults
All racial and ethnic groups	Blacks and Asians > Caucasians
No familial tendency	Familial tendency
Limited to sites of trauma	Sites of trauma or spontaneous
Onset within 2 months	Onset within 1 year
Any anatomic site	High-risk anatomic site
Dome-shaped lesions	Dome-shaped, exophytic, or crab-like extensions
Confined to site of trauma	Extends into normal skin
Improved by corrective surgery	Often worsened by surgery
Spontaneous regression	No spontaneous regression

10. Do any factors predispose to hypertrophic scars and keloids?

Many factors can predispose individuals to develop hypertrophic scars and keloids.

1. Certain drugs (e.g., isotretinoin) predispose to hypertrophic scarring, and most dermatologic surgeons defer any elective surgery for at least 1 year following discontinuation of isotretinoin.

2. The type of injury and degree of tissue injury also play a role. Thermal burns with their associated severe tissue damage commonly produce hypertrophic scars or keloids.

3. Regional variations exist. Skin that is continuously under tension or tightly stretched over bony protuberances and other anatomic peculiarities predispose to the development of hypertrophic scarring and keloids.

4. Dark-skinned races are more prone to both hypertrophic scarring and keloid formation. Blacks are 2–19 times and Asians 3–5 times more likely than Caucasians to develop keloids.

5. Certain genodermatoses such as Ehlers-Danlos syndrome, Rubinstein-Taybi syndrome, osteogenesis imperfecta, and progeria have all been reported to have increased risk for the development of keloids.

11. List the anatomic regions of the body that are most at risk to develop keloids.

Presternal area, upper back, upper arms, especially over deltoids, beard area, especially over mandibular angle, and earlobes (Fig. 2).

12. Are there effective treatments for hypertrophic scars and keloids?

Various traditional and novel modalities for therapy exist. In general, **hypertrophic scars** respond well to less-aggressive therapy, such as potent topical steroids, intralesional steroids, chronic pressure dressings, and even chronic occlusive dressings with medical Silastic gel sheeting. Some cases may require surgical revision or dermabrasion.

Keloids demand more aggressive therapy with long-term precautions to prevent recurrence. Surgical excision, corticosteroid injection, and cryotherapy alone can be used but are often not effective. Radiation has been employed with good results but should be used with caution and only by an experienced physician. Laser excision has theoretical advantages, but long-term studies have not demonstrated an advantage over conventional surgery. Combination approaches appear to work best. Cryosurgery followed by corticosteroid injection is effective in some patients. Surgical excision with subsequent steroid injection is probably the most effective approach. One regimen calls for steroid injection to the surgical site 1–4 weeks postoperatively and then monthly for 6 months.

13. What is an acquired digital fibrokeratoma?

These solitary, firm, hyperkeratotic papules most commonly occur around interphalangeal joints but may occur on any site of the hands or feet. They are typically pedunculated and often

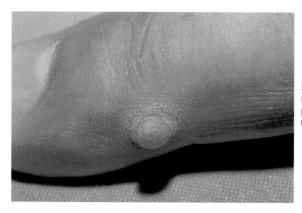

FIGURE 3. Typical acquired digital fibrokeratoma demonstrating an exophytic firm papule with a hyperkeratotic collarette.

demonstrate a collarette of hyperkeratosis at the base (Fig. 3). Often, they are mistaken clinically for warts or supernumerary digits. Histologically, they demonstrate overlying hyperkeratosis and thickened collagen bundles.

14. Has a cause been identified for acquired digital fibrokeratoma?

Some authorities believe that these lesions arise as a reaction to recurring **trauma.** Often, a history of an activity with recurring trauma to the affected area (e.g., guiding a knitting needle) can be elicited; however, many patients do not recall trauma to the site.

15. How can an acquired digital fibrokeratoma be treated?

Saucerization with secondary healing and simple excision are both effective. Hard cryotherapy is sometimes effective but may require multiple treatments.

16. What is nodular fasciitis?

Nodular fasciitis (pseudocarcinomatous nodular fasciitis) is a rare, benign, fibroblastic tumor that many consider to be a pseudoneoplastic or reactive growth. It may occur at any age but most commonly presents in young adults as a solitary, rapidly growing, subcutaneous nodule on the extremities. The nodule may be painful, is typically 1–3 cm in size, and may adhere to the underlying fascia. Simple excision is curative, but untreated lesions have been documented to regress spontaneously. The importance of this lesion is that, histologically, it may be confused with malignant fibrous neoplasms, because the fibroblasts are large and pleomorphic and mitotic figures are relatively common.

17. What is a connective tissue nevus?

Connective tissue nevus is a term used for cutaneous hamartomas composed primarily of collagen (collagenomas), elastin (elastomas), or a combination of these two. While these are produced by fibroblasts, connective tissue nevi are typically no more cellular than normal dermis. Clinically, they present as one or more dermal papules or plaques. Connective tissue nevi composed primarily of collagen are skin-colored, while those composed primarily of elastin may be skin-colored or yellowish.

18. Why are connective tissue nevi important?

Connective tissue nevi usually do not produce problems, although large lesions may be distressing to the patient for cosmetic reasons. Other patients may become concerned because numerous collagenomas (**eruptive collagenomas**) develop over a short period of time (Fig. 4). However, some of these nevi serve as cutaneous markers for other systemic syndromes. Collagenomas called **shagreen patches** are frequently seen in patients with tuberous sclerosis. Multiple connective tissue nevi called **dermatofibrosis lenticularis disseminata** are composed primarily of elastic fibers and are the cutaneous marker for Buschke-Ollendorff syndrome. Buschke-Ollendorff syndrome is an autosomal dominant disorder that presents with osteopoikilosis of the bones and connective tissue nevi.

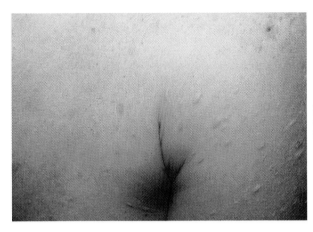

FIGURE 4. Multiple small skin-colored papules in a patient with eruptive collagenomas.

19. What is infantile digital fibromatosis?

Infantile digital fibromatosis is a rare tumor composed of myofibroblasts that develops in infancy and early childhood on the fingers and toes. The primary lesion is a skin-colored or red tumor usually located on the lateral or dorsal surface of the digit. Histologically, they consist of myofibroblasts with characteristic eosinophilic cytoplasmic inclusions composed of actin filaments.

20. Describe the natural history of infantile digital fibromatosis.

The tumors of infantile digital fibromatosis may grow up to 2 cm but will eventually regress over a period of years. Occasionally, large lesions may produce functional impairment or joint deformities. The recurrence rate is very high, with up to two-thirds of all cases recurring following surgical removal. The importance of this tumor is that physicians not familiar with the natural history of this tumor may become overly aggressive and amputate a digit.

21. What is a dermatofibroma?

A dermatofibroma, or fibrous histiocytoma, is the most common fibrohistiocytic tumor of the skin. Usually, these are small, firm, flat, or exophytic papules on the lower extremities of adults. Though most commonly 2–4 mm in diameter, they can occasionally grow to 2–3 cm. They may be skin-colored but more commonly demonstrate tan or brown hyperpigmentation and hypertrophy of overlying epidermis. Nondermatologists frequently mistake them for nevi. Other common locations include the sides of the trunk and upper arms.

Microscopically, most dermatofibromas are composed primarily of fibroblasts that produce abundant collagen. Within some but not all dermatofibromas, there are often cellular areas composed of cells with round nuclei that phagocytize lipid or hemosiderin. Multinucleated giant cells may also be present. Dermatofibromas that phagocytize abundant hemosiderin are sometimes referred to as hemosiderotic dermatofibromas or sclerosing hemangiomas.

Dermatofibromas characteristically demonstrate a positive "dimple" sign, which is a dimpling of the skin produced when lateral pressure is applied to the dermatofibroma between the thumb and forefinger. This is also called the Fitzpatrick sign, in honor of Dr. Thomas Fitzpatrick (Fig. 5).

22. Do dermatofibromas transform into skin cancer?

Dermatofibromas are considered to be benign fibrohistiocytic tumors that do not demonstrate a malignant potential. Though dermatofibromas share clinical and some general histologic similarities with a malignant neoplasm called dermatofibrosarcoma protuberans, histochemical markers show the two are distinct. Although the dermatofibroma itself does not progress into malignancy, the overlying epidermis demonstrates a slight risk to develop into basal cell carcinoma.

23. What is the best way to treat a dermatofibroma?

In general, it is best to avoid treating a dermatofibroma. When a lesion is distressing in appearance, painful, or frequently traumatized, simple excision may be indicated. Several authors

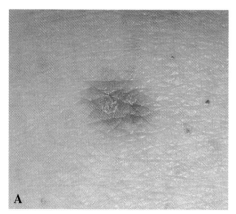
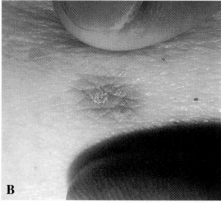

FIGURE 5. *A*, Characteristic light brown dermatofibroma that is not sharply demarcated. *B*, "Dimple" or Fitzpatrick sign demonstrating tendency of dermatofibromas to dimple when compressed laterally.

have reported successful treatment with cryotherapy. The anticipated benefit of treatment should be weighed against the predictable cosmetic outcome of the therapeutic modality.

24. Are multiple dermatofibromas associated with any internal diseases?

Multiple dermatofibromas have been associated with systemic lupus erythematosus and, less commonly, myasthenia gravis. Both of these associations are rare, and patients presenting with isolated dermatofibromas should not be routinely evaluated for these conditions.

25. What is a "fibrous papule of the nose"?

A fibrous papule of the nose is a relatively common, small (usually 2–3 mm), dome-shaped, asymptomatic papule usually located on the lower portion of the nose. The color is variable and may be skin-colored, white, or red. Less commonly, it may occur on other parts of the face. Microscopically, fibrous papules are composed of fibroblasts that may be fusiform, stellate, or multinucleated, and are associated with abundant thick collagen bundles that are oriented around hair follicles or dilated blood vessels. Their greatest significance lies in their clinical similarity to an early basal cell carcinoma. Fibrous papules of the nose are histologically identical to the angiofibromas found in patients with tuberous sclerosis, and most authorities regard fibrous papules to be a solitary form of angiofibroma.

26. How is a fibrous papule of the nose best treated?

Superficial shave excision, cryotherapy, or simple excision are effective modalities.

BIBLIOGRAPHY

1. Bernstein KE, Lattes R: Nodular (pseudosarcomatous) fasciitis, a nonrecurrent lesion: Clinicopathologic study of 134 cases. Cancer 49:1668–1678, 1982.
2. Fitzpatrick TB, Gilchrist BA: Dimple sign to differentiate between benign and malignant neoplasms. N Engl J Med 296:1518, 1977.
3. Kawaguchi M, Mitsuhashi Y, Hozumi Y, Kondo S: A case of infantile digital fibromatosis with spontaneous regression. J Dermatol 25:523–526, 1998.
4. Kobus RJ, Lubbers LM, Coleman CR: Connective tissue nevus and osteopoikilosis in the hand: The Buschke-Ollendorff syndrome. J Hand Surg 14A:535–538, 1989.
5. Lin RY, Landman L, Krey PR, et al: Multiple dermatofibromas and systemic lupus erythematosus. Cutis 37:45–49, 1986.
6. Niessen FB, Spauwen PH, Schalkwijk J, Kon M: On the nature of hypertrophic scars and keloids: A review. Plast Reconstr Surg 104:1435–1458, 1999.
7. Phillips JC, Knautz MA, Sangueza OP, Davis LS: Familial cutaneous collagenoma. J Am Acad Dermatol 40:255–257, 1999.
8. Vinson RP, Angeloni VL: Acquired digital fibrokeratoma. Am Fam Physician 52:1365–1367, 1995.

VII. Malignant Tumors of the Skin

44. COMMON CUTANEOUS MALIGNANCIES

Milton J. Schleve, M.D.

1. How are skin cancers classified?

Primary cutaneous cancers are classified on the basis of their cell of origin within the skin. Skin cancers are most commonly derived from keratinocytes (e.g., squamous cell carcinoma) or melanocytes (e.g., malignant melanoma), which are normal components of the epidermis. Less commonly, they arise from other cells within the epidermis, dermis, or subcutis.

Classification of Cutaneous Malignancies

	CELL OF ORIGIN
Premalignancies (in situ)	
Actinic keratosis	Keratinocyte
Bowen's disease (squamous cell carcinoma)	Keratinocyte
Malignant melanoma	Melanocyte
Lentigo maligna (Hutchinson's freckle)	Melanocyte
Common cutaneous malignancies	
Basal cell carcinoma	Debatable—follicular keratinocyte, basal keratinocyte, primary germ cell
Squamous cell carcinoma	Keratinocyte
Keratoacanthoma	Follicular keratinocyte
Melanomas	
Malignant melanoma	Melanocyte
Lentigo maligna melanoma	Melanocyte
Uncommon cutaneous malignancies	
Sweat gland carcinoma (numerous variants)	Apocrine or eccrine sweat gland/duct
Follicular carcinomas (several variants)	Follicular epithelial cells
Extramammary Paget's disease	Unknown—apocrine
Trabecular cell carcinoma (Merkel cell tumor)	Fibroblast or dermal dendrocyte
Atypical fibroxanthoma	Fibroblast
Dermatofibrosarcoma protuberans	Fibroblast
Fibrosarcoma	Fibroblast
Angiosarcoma	Endothelial cell
Kaposi's sarcoma	Endothelial cell
Hemangiopericytoma	Pericyte
Malignant peripheral nerve sheath tumors	Schwann cells
Liposarcoma	Lipocyte

2. What are the most common nonmelanoma skin cancers (NMSC)?

Basal cell carcinoma and squamous cell carcinoma. In the United States, about 1 million cases of NMSC occur yearly, which makes these the most common of all "cancers." Keratoacanthomas are also listed as NMSC, but this classification is debatable and some authorities consider them to be benign epithelial neoplasia. Common nonmelanoma skin premalignancies include actinic keratosis, actinic cheilitis, and Bowen's disease.

3. What is the most important cause of NMSC?

The overwhelming majority of precancerous and cancerous skin lesions are caused by **sun exposure.** Several observations and epidemiologic studies support the role of ultraviolet light in the production of skin cancers:

1. Most NMSC develop on skin chronically exposed to the sun, with 85% or more occurring on the head and neck.

2. The incidence of NMSC is lower in more polar latitudes (e.g., Minneapolis) than equatorial latitudes (e.g., Hawaii).

3. Studies have demonstrated that Japanese emigrants to Hawaii have a higher incidence of NMSC than Japanese who have grown up in Japan, which has a higher polar latitude.

4. Epidemiologic studies clearly demonstrate that NMSC are more common in individuals with lighter skin than individuals with darker skin.

5. NMSC can be induced on animal models by solar irradiation and prevented by the use of sunscreens.

4. Are there any other causes of NMSC?

Arsenic ingestion
Chronic ulcers and scars (e.g., burn wounds)
Environmental pollutants
Genetic factors (e.g., xeroderma pigmentosum)
Local prolonged heat exposure

Topical exposure to tars and oils
Viral infection (e.g., some strains of
human papillomavirus)
Radiation treatment (e.g., acne treatment)

5. How are are NMSC diagnosed?

A cutaneous malignancy should always be considered in any patient who reports a new cutaneous lesion, particularly in sun-exposed skin. NMSC are usually, but not always, clinically distinct, although there is considerable overlap in appearance within NMSC. Ultimately, the diagnosis is established by shave, punch, incisional, or excisional biopsy, with the choice of biopsy technique depending on the size and location of the suspected malignancy.

6. What are basal cell carcinomas?

Basal cell carcinomas (BCC, epitheliomas) are the most common cutaneous malignancy and outnumber squamous cell carcinomas by a 4:1 ratio. They are low-grade malignancies of the skin and are microscopically composed of basaloid cells with characteristic peripheral palisading of the nuclei. These basaloid tumor islands usually demonstrate connections to the overlying epidermis or follicular epithelium. BCCs are locally invasive tumors that rarely metastasize.

The origin of these common tumors is controversial. The most accepted theories are that they originate from either undifferentiated cells in the basal cell layer or from follicular epithelium. Recent immunohistochemical studies have suggested that most BCCs demonstrate at least some degree of follicular differentiation.

7. Describe the clinical and histologic appearance of basal cell carcinomas.

BCCs may have more than one clinical or histologic appearance. The most common presentation are as **nodular** BCCs, which are typically slow-growing lesions with a smooth or pebbly surface. They characteristically appear translucent or pearly and often demonstrate dilated vessels (Fig. 1A). They can gradually break down, bleed, and form ulcers (**nodulo-ulcerative** BCC, Fig. 1B). **Superficial spreading** BCC are thin lesions that demonstrate a horizontal growth pattern. They present as erythematous, minimally indurated, slow-growing plaques with variable scale that are most commonly located on the trunk (Fig. 1C). They can be confused with tinea corporis, nummular dermatitis, or other NMSC such as Bowen's disease.

Morpheaform (also desmoplastic or sclerosing) BCC are a type of infiltrative lesion that may resemble scars or even normal skin. Microscopically, they are composed of narrow cords and strands of basaloid cells that infiltrate between the collagen bundles. This variant can easily be missed, even by experienced dermatologists. Their true extent is often much greater than the appearance suggests.

Basal cell carcinomas can also be completely or focally pigmented and mistaken for malignant melanoma. A rare variant of BCC looks like a large skin tag or fibroma. This variant is usually found on the trunk of older men and is called a **Pinkus tumor** or fibroepithelioma of Pinkus.

8. What do typical squamous cell carcinomas look like clinically?

Squamous cell carcinomas (SCC) may resemble basal cell carcinomas, actinic keratoses, or warts, but often the initial appearance is as an ill-defined, red lesion with a rough surface (Fig. 2A). SCC are more likely to demonstrate overlying scale than BCC. At times, the scale may

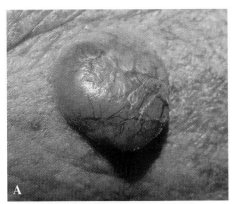

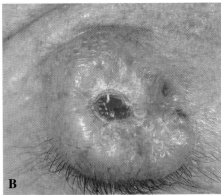

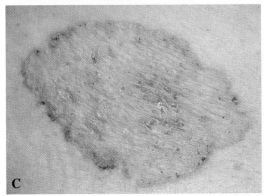

FIGURE 1. Variants of basal cell carcinoma (BCC). *A*, Nodular BCC demonstrating characteristic dilated blood vessels. *B*, Nodulo-ulcerative BCC above the eyebrow, demonstrating pearly appearance and central ulceration. (*A–B* courtesy of James E. Fitzpatrick, MD). *C*, Large superficial spreading BCC demonstrating multiple small papules with focal scale and crust.

project above the skin surface, producing a cutaneous horn. Larger lesions may break down and ulcerate. **Verrucous** carcinomas are a variant of SCC that look like warts and are often misdiagnosed (Fig. 2B). Like warts, they often occur on hands and feet but can also appear on the anogenital epithelium and oral mucosa.

SCC are more aggressive than BCC and more likely to metastasize. SCC arising from actinic keratoses are estimated to metastasize in 0.5% of cases, while those arising from the lower lip metastasize in 16% of cases. Tumors arising in burn scars, draining sinuses, and modified epithelium (e.g., glans penis, vulva) and in immunocompromised patients are also more likely to metastasize.

9. What are keratoacanthomas?

Keratoacanthomas are relatively common epidermal tumors that almost invariably appear on sun-exposed skin. There is controversy as to whether this lesion should be considered as benign or malignant. Microscopically, the tumor is composed of well-differentiated but cytologically atypical keratinocytes that are difficult for pathologists to separate from squamous cell carcinoma. The mitotic rate may be very high. Clinically, however, keratoacanthomas usually behave in a benign fashion and spontaneously regress over a period of weeks or months if left untreated. Clouding the issue is the fact that approximately 10% of lesions that clinically resemble keratoacanthomas develop into invasive SCC. It is not clear whether these are SCC from their inception, keratoacanthomas that have developed into SCC, or more aggressive keratoacanthomas. The site of origin of keratoacanthomas is uncertain, but experimental and epidemiologic studies implicate follicular epithelium.

10. How do keratoacanthomas present clinically?

Keratoacanthomas are usually easy to recognize. They appear suddenly, typically on sun-exposed skin, as skin-colored domes that develop a central keratin-filled plug (Fig. 3). They grow at a faster rate than squamous cell carcinomas and usually reach a size of 1–2 cm before regressing. Rarely, they may attain a size of 5 cm or more (giant keratoacanthomas).

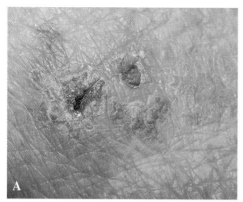

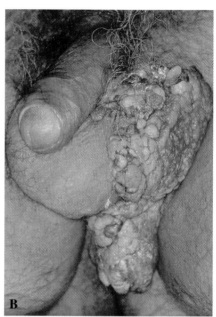

FIGURE 2. Variants of squamous cell carcinoma (SCC). *A,* Early SCC arising in an actinic keratosis. *B,* Large verrucous carcinoma of the genitalia. Verrucous carcinomas often reach large sizes before diagnosis since they are often treated as warts.

11. What is an actinic keratosis?

Actinic keratoses (solar keratoses) are sun-induced precancerous lesions of the skin. They are very common in elderly patients with light skin color and significant sun exposure. Microscopically, actinic keratoses are characterized by a proliferation of cytologically atypical keratinocytes that bud off of or replace the bottom of the epidermis. The atypical cells do not involve the full thickness of the epidermis. A definitive prospective study has never been done, but epidemiologic and retrospective studies suggest that 2–5% of actinic keratoses progress into squamous cell carcinomas if left untreated.

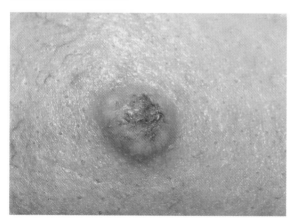

FIGURE 3. Keratoacanthoma demonstrating a crateriform nodule with a central keratin plug. (Courtesy of James E. Fitzpatrick, MD.)

12. What do actinic keratoses look like?

Actinic keratoses initially appear as tiny, palpable bumps on normal sun-exposed skin that gradually enlarge and become red and scaly (Fig. 4). The overlying scale may be extensive to the point that markedly exophytic cutaneous horns are produced. Less common variants include atrophic and pigmented actinic keratoses. **Actinic cheilitis** is a term used for actinic keratoses that present on the sun-exposed vermilion lip. Many patients who complain of chronic dry lower lips actually have extensive actinic cheilitis.

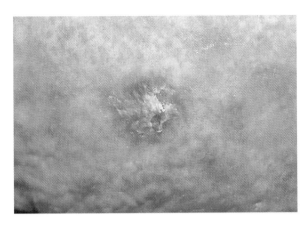

FIGURE 4. Typical actinic keratosis demonstrating scaly papule on an erythematous base.

13. What is Bowen's disease?

Bowen's disease is a form of squamous cell carcinoma in situ that may appear on any skin surface, including non-sun-exposed skin (Fig. 5A). Microscopically, it demonstrates full-thickness cytologic atypia of the keratinocytes. Actinic keratoses that progress into full-thickness atypia are often referred to as **bowenoid actinic keratoses**. SCC in situ occurring on the male genitalia has also been described under the name **erythroplasia of Queyrat**. Clinically, Bowen's disease presents as persistent, erythematous, slightly indurated plaques with variable scale (Fig. 5B). It may resemble mammary Paget's disease, extramammary Paget's disease, and superficial spreading basal cell carcinoma. Pigmented Bowen's disease is an uncommon variant that may resemble malignant melanoma.

14. How should premalignant lesions, such as actinic keratoses and actinic cheilitis, be treated?

We should probably first ask, "Why should premalignant lesions be treated?" While a small percentage of actinic keratoses disappear spontaneously, 2–5% develop into squamous cell carcinoma. Clinically, small SCC are difficult to separate from actinic keratoses. The smallest SCCs are picked up when a suspected actinic lesion does not respond to treatment or a lesion appears in a treated area.

Since actinic lesions can vary from tiny, barely palpable lesions to an entire lip or scalp, treatment modalities depend on the size and location of lesions. Small, individual papules can be treated by cryosurgery or by curettage (usually after local anesthesia). Larger areas can be treated by cryosurgery, curettage, dermabrasion, chemical peels, and topical 5-FU. Laser ablation (CO_2 laser) and excision with mucosal advancement are reserved for extensive involvement of the lip.

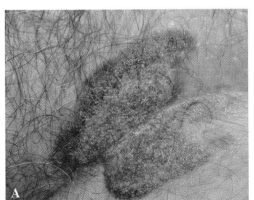
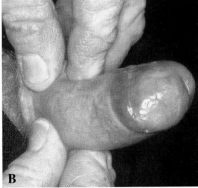

FIGURE 5. *A,* Pigmented Bowen's disease presenting as an eroded plaque of the groin. *B,* Bowen's disease of the penis (erythroplasia of Queyrat) presenting as an erythematous, minimally indurated plaque.

15. What factors should you consider in treating NMSC?

The method of destruction depends upon the degree of invasion, location, health of the patient, potential for recurrence or metastasis, and availability of various methods.

Management of Cutaneous Premalignancies and Malignancies

LESION	TREATMENT
Actinic keratosis	Cryosurgery
	Curettage ± electrosurgery
	Fluorouracil, topical
	Chemical peel
	Dermabrasion
Actinic cheilitis	Cryosurgery
	Electrosurgery
	Chemical peel
	Laser ablation
	Lip shave and advancement
Basal cell carcinoma (BCC)	
Superficial spreading	Cryosurgery
	Curettage ± electrosurgery
	Laser ablation
	Imiquimod
Nodular	Cryosurgery
	Curettage ± electrosurgery
	Excision
	Radiation therapy
	Mohs surgery
Morpheaform, aggressive BCC, or recurrent BCC	Excision with margin control
	Mohs surgery
Nonresectable lesions	Cryosurgery
	Radiation therapy
	Chemotherapy
Keratoacanthoma	Deep shave plus curettage
	Curettage plus desiccation
	Intralesional 5-Fluorouracil
	Cryosurgery
	Excision
Bowen's disease (SCC in situ)	Curettage ± electrosurgery
	Fluorouracil, topical
	Imiquimod
	Curettage plus fluorouracil
	Cryosurgery
	Laser
	Excision
Squamous cell carcinoma (SCC)	
Small, nonaggressive	Curettage ± electrosurgery
	Cryosurgery
	Excision
Large or aggressive	Excision with margin control
	Mohs surgery
	Radiation therapy
	Lymph node dissection

16. How frequently do NMSC occur?

The exact incidence of NMSC is unknown because they are not routinely entered into tumor registries. It is estimated that 1 million new cases of NMSC occur each year in the United States, making them by far the most common cancers in the United States. In 1990, skin cancer accounted for >2.7 million outpatient visits, which represented 0.4% of all outpatient visits in the United

States. The lifetime risk of developing NMSC is 1 in 5. Statistically, if a patient develops one NMSC, the risk of another new lesion in 5 years is 30–50%.

17. How can NMSC be prevented?

The easy answer is to avoid sun exposure, particularly during childhood. It has been estimated that 75–80% of the total lifetime dose of solar radiation is received before the age of 20. If children and adolescents received adequate sun protection, the incidence of NMSC would drastically decrease. Sun protection techniques for children and adults alike include avoidance of the midday sun, liberal use of sunscreens, and wearing of protective clothing. Tans, whether received from natural sunlight or tanning booths, represent damaged skin that is more likely to develop NMSC. It is important for health care providers to nurture the idea that pale skin is more attractive than tanned skin. In the future we will be able to identify people with deficiencies in UV-induced DNA repair mechanisms and eventually be able to correct the deformity.

BIBLIOGRAPHY

1. Dodson JM, DeSpain JE, Clark P: Malignant potential of actinic keratoses and the controversy over treatment. Arch Dermatol 127:1029–1030, 1991.
2. Dufresne RG Jr, Curlin MU: Actinic cheilitis: A treatment review. Dermatol Surg 23:15–21, 1997.
3. Fleming ID, Amonette R, Fleming MD: Principles of management of basal and squamous cell carcinoma of the skin. Cancer 75:699–704, 1995.
4. Gloster HM Jr, Brodland DG: The epidemiology of skin cancer. Dermatol Surg 22:217–226, 1996.
5. Grossman D, Leffell DJ: The molecular basis of nonmelanoma skin cancer: new understanding. Arch Dermatol 133:1263–1270, 1997.
6. Guercio-Hauer C, Macfarlane DF, Deleo VA: Photodamage, photoaging, and photo protection of the skin. Am Fam Physician 50:327–332, 334, 1994.
7. Marks R, Rennie G, Selwood T: The relationship of basal cell carcinomas and squamous cell carcinomas to solar keratoses. Arch Dermatol 124:1039–1042, 1988.
8. Olbricht SM: Treatment of malignant cutaneous tumors. Clin Plast Surg 20:167–180, 1993.
9. Rose LC: Recognizing neoplastic skin lesions: A photo guide. Am Fam Physician 58:873–884, 887–888, 1998.
10. Schwartz RA: Keratoacanthoma. J Am Acad Dermatol 30:1–19, 1994.
11. Schwartz RA: The actinic keratosis. A perspective and update. Dermatol Surg 23:1009–1019, 1997.
12. Shriner DL, McCoy DK, Goldberg DJ, Wagner RF Jr: Mohs micrographic surgery. J Am Acad Dermatol 39:79–97, 1998.
13. Skidmore RA Jr, Flowers FP: Nonmelanoma skin cancer. Med Clin North Am 82:1309–1323, 1998.
14. Taylor CR, Sober AJ: Sun exposure and skin disease. Annu Rev Med 47:181-91, 1996.
15. Voss N, Kim-Sing C: Radiotherapy in the treatment of dermatologic malignancies. Dermatol Clin 16:313–320, 1998.

45. MALIGNANT MELANOMA

Patrick Walsh, M.D., and Stephen J. Hoffman, M.D., Ph.D.

1. What is melanoma?

Melanoma is a malignancy of melanocytes and nevus cells. In terms of incidence, melanoma is the most rapidly increasing form of cancer in the United States. It is now the most common cancer in young women aged 25–29 years. The estimated chance of developing melanoma is expected to increase from approximately 1 in 100 for individuals born in 1990 to 1 in 75 for individuals born in the year 2000. Cutaneous melanoma is differentiated from ocular melanoma, a malignancy of ocular pigment cells.

2. What causes melanoma?

Although all of the causes of melanoma are not known with certainty, epidemiologic studies suggest that brief, intense exposure to **ultraviolet A** (long-wave UV radiation) contributes to the development of melanoma. Other potential causes include mutations in, or loss of, tumor suppressor genes.

3. List the high-risk groups for developing melanoma.

1. Individuals with fair complexions (i.e., those with skin types I and II, who burn easily and never tan) and who are in sunlight for short, intense periods of time have a higher incidence of melanoma.

2. Individuals with numerous atypical-appearing melanocytic nevi or large congenital melanocytic nevi are also at increased risk.

3. Persons who have had melanoma previously or have had an immediate family member diagnosed with melanoma have an increased risk.

4. Describe the clinical appearance of melanoma.

Cutaneous melanoma can have a number of different appearances. Malignant melanomas often begin in preexisting melanocytic nevi.The exact percentage of malignant melanomas arising in preexisting nevi versus arising de novo is controversial. When this happens, the nevus usually demonstrates a change in appearance, such as an increase in size or change in shape, or it may bleed easily when traumatized. Classically, early melanoma lesions are characterized by containing different colors, such as different hues of brown, black, red, and blue. Melanoma may also appear as a brown or black discoloration of the nail or as a skin ulcer that does not heal.

5. What are the ABCDs of melanoma?

The development of a new or changing pigmented lesion is the classic initial presentation of melanoma. A lesion that demonstrates a noticeable increase in size over a period of weeks to months or development of pigment irregularity (black, hues of brown, red, blue, or white) should be evaluated by a physician and biopsied. The **ABCDs** of melanoma are a helpful guideline for determining which moles could be suspicious for melanoma:

A—Asymmetry. Any mole that appears unusual or shows asymmetry in shape should be evaluated.

B—Border and bleeding. The border of any melanocytic nevus should be relatively smooth, with a clear demarcation between the nevus and surrounding normal skin. Nevi that develop irregular or ill-defined borders should be evaluated. **B** is also for bleeding, and any mole that bleeds needs careful evaluation.

C—Color. Most moles have a homogeneous tan or brown color. Moles that develop pigment variegation within an otherwise homogeneous background should be evaluated.

D—Diameter. Most melanomas are >6 mm in diameter, but an otherwise suspicious lesion that is small might also be malignant.

The most important consideration in evaluating any melanocytic nevus is whether the nevus has changed in terms of the ABCDs over a relatively short time (weeks to months). Furthermore, the ABCDs are meant strictly as guidelines and cannot take the place of a thorough evaluation.

6. Where on the body does melanoma most commonly arise?

Melanoma can arise on any part of the body. Primary tumors are most common on the trunk in men and on the lower extremity in women.

7. Are there different types of melanoma?

There are several different types of melanoma and each may appear somewhat differently.

Superficial spreading malignant melanoma (SSMM) is the most common form of melanoma in whites. It is a slowly enlarging brown (usually) or black spot that may have both a macular and papular component. The lesion may show color variegation and irregular borders (Fig. 1A).

Nodular melanoma is a pigmented (usually brown or black) papule that slowly enlarges and frequently ulcerates. Nodular melanomas may ulcerate, presenting as a nonhealing skin ulcer (Fig. 1B).

Acral lentiginous melanoma is the most common form of melanoma in blacks, Asians, and Hispanics (Fig. 2). It usually appears as brown or black macules arising on the glaborous (non-hair-bearing) skin of an extremity (palms, soles, or nailbeds).

Lentigo maligna melanoma usually presents as an irregularly shaped, flat, pigmented lesion on actinically damaged skin. It is seen most frequently on the face or other sun-exposed sites. More advanced lesions can develop papules or nodules, indicating the lesion has developed a vertical or downward growth component.

Amelanotic melanoma is usually considered a non-pigment-producing variant of nodular melanoma. Amelanotic melanoma can be confused with other benign skin lesions, such as pyogenic granuloma.

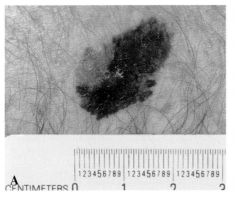 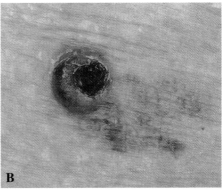

FIGURE 1. Superficial spreading malignant melanoma. *A*, This lesion shows asymmetry, notched borders, and shades of light brown, dark brown, and tan. *B*, Superficial spreading malignant melanoma that has developed a nodular melanoma. (Courtesy of James E. Fitzpatrick, MD.)

8. What are Clark's levels?

A system used to describe the depth of invasion of a melanoma that was originally described by Dr. Wallace H. Clark, Jr. The system provides a helpful means to determine the probability of developing progressive disease. Primary tumors are classified according to the degree of invasion into the various anatomic levels of the skin. This classification scheme has been shown to correlate well with 5-year survival rates.

> Level I—tumor cells in epidermis only (melanoma in situ)
> Level II—tumor cells extend from epidermis into (but do not fill) papillary dermis
> Level III—tumor cells extend from epidermis into and fill papillary dermis
> Level IV—tumor cells extend into reticular dermis
> Level V—tumor cells extend through the dermis into underlying subcutaneous fat

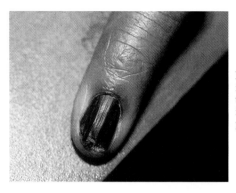

FIGURE 2. Acral lentiginous malignant melanoma in situ arising in the nail bed of a black woman. Note the presence of pigment in the periungual tissue (positive Hutchinson's sign). (Courtesy of James E. Fitzpatrick, MD.)

9. How do Clark's levels correlate with prognosis?

The survival for patients with melanoma relates to the thickness of the primary tumor. Melanoma in situ, or Clark's level I melanoma, is nearly 100% cured with adequate excision. Patients with tumors extending to Clark's level II have a survival of >95% at 5 years, and those with tumors extending to Clarks's level III have a >90% survival rate. Thicker lesions have a greater tendency to recur and metastasize. Patients with Clark's level IV melanoma have approximately a 75% 5-year survival rate, while those with Clark's level V have a <50% 5-year survival.

Correlation of Primary Tumor Thickness and Survival Rates for Cutaneous Melanoma

CLARK'S LEVEL		BRESLOW'S DEPTH			
LEVEL	5-YEAR SURVIVAL RATE	DEPTH (MM)	5-YEAR SURVIVAL RATE	DEPTH (MM)	5-YEAR SURVIVAL RATE
II	99%	<0.85	99%	<0.75	95–99%
III	95%	0.86–1.69	94%	0.76–1.49	90–95%
IV	75%	1.70–3.64	78%	1.50–4.00	60–75%
V	39%	>3.64	42%	>4.00	<50%

10. What is Breslow's depth?

A more precise assessment of the level of invasion of the primary malignant melanoma. An ocular micrometer is used to directly measure the distance that tumor cells have invaded. The distance of invasion is measured from the granular layer of the epidermis to the point of deepest invasion by the tumor cells. This measurement appears to be more easily reproducible among institutions and more objective than Clark's levels.

11. How do Clark's levels and Breslow's depth correlate?

In terms of prognostic value in helping to predict 5-year survival rates, the two measurement schemes correlate well (see table above).

12. How is melanoma treated?

The standard of care for treating melanoma is to:
1) Establish a histologic diagnosis of the suspect lesion,
2) Completely excise the tumor with adequate margins,
3) Assess for the presence of detectable metastastic disease, and
4) Conduct follow-up evaluations for the rest of the patient's life.

To establish a **histologic** diagnosis, the suspect lesion should be completely excised to the depth of the subcuticular fat. If this is not possible due to anatomic location or size of the lesion, an incisional biopsy or punch biopsy to the depth of the subcuticular fat should be performed on the thickest or most atypical portion of the lesion.

Once a diagnosis of melanoma is established, wide local **excision** of the primary tumor to the muscle fascia is recommended. Baseline evaluations then should be performed to determine if any detectable second primary tumor, local extension of the first primary, or possible **metastatic** disease is present. These evaluations include a complete physical examination, including complete skin evaluation and lymph node exam, baseline laboratory tests that may include a complete blood count and liver function tests, and a chest x-ray. Any abnormality detected with these exams is more fully investigated with the proper diagnostic procedure (e.g., a fine-needle aspirate to assess an enlarged lymph node or CT of the abdomen for abnormal liver chemistry).

13. How wide should surgical margins be?

There is ongoing controversy regarding the width of normal-appearing skin that should be excised. At one time, 5.0-cm margins were recommended. A National Institutes of Health Consensus Conference on Melanoma has recommended surgical margins based on the depth of invasion of the primary tumor. Malignant melanoma in situ should be excised with a 0.5-cm border of normal skin. Lesions that have a Breslow's depth of <1.0 mm should have wide local re-excision with 1.0-cm margins. Lesions that are 1–2 mm thick should be excised with 1–2-cm margins (2 cm if primary closure can be achieved or no significant difference exists in reconstruction between a 1- and 2-cm margin of excision). Lesions that are intermediate, 2–4 mm thick, are excised with 2-cm margins. Lesions >4.0 mm thick should be excised with 3.0-cm margins. These recommendations are meant only as general guidelines, and individual patient considerations must be taken into account.

14. Does a biopsy of melanoma increase the risk of spreading tumor cells or causing metastases?

Two independently conducted studies of this question have concluded that incisional biopsies of melanoma do not cause the tumor to spread locally or metastasize.

15. Which tests or examinations are conducted during the routine follow-up of patients who have had melanoma?

During the follow-up evaluations, patients should receive a physical exam directed toward the detection of a local recurrence of the primary, the development of metastatic disease in the surrounding skin or the draining lymphatic system, or development of a second primary melanoma. As in the initial staging evaluation, any abnormality detected by physical exam, review of systems, or laboratory tests is more fully investigated. If no abnormalities are detected by routine physical exam and review of systems, repeat laboratory tests and chest x-ray are usually obtained every year.

16. How is melanoma staged for systemic disease?

The literature can be confusing because there are two staging systems for widespread disease. The old but still quoted method is:

Stage I—resected primary tumor, no metastases
Stage II—regional cutaneous or lymph node metastases
Stage III—visceral metastases

The current and preferred staging system for melanoma is that of the American Joint Commission on Cancer (AJCC) from 1992. It is based on the TNM (tumor, lymph node, metastasis) system, which allows the assessment of patients based on the thickness of the primary tumor and whether lymph node or other metastases are present.

Staging and Survival Rates for Cutaneous Melanoma

STAGE	DEPTH (MM)	TUMOR	NODE	METASTASIS	5-YEAR SURVIVAL
Ia	<0.75	T1	N0	M0	
Ib	0.76–1.50	T2	N0	M0	95%
IIa	1.51–3.00	T3	N0	M0	
IIb	>3.00	T4	N0	M0	78%
III	—	Any T	In-transit	M0	
			N1	M0	52%
IV	—	Any T	Any N	M1	18%

17. Describe the recommended follow-up for a patient with melanoma.

Routine follow-up evaluations vary depending on the depth of the primary tumor. It is important to stress that unlike many malignancies, melanoma has a tendency to recur many years after the primary tumor is removed. Therefore, patients at high risk for recurrence need to be followed very closely for long periods of time.

Recommended Follow-Up Schedules for Patients with Early-Stage Melanoma

STAGE	FOLLOW-UP	DURATION	THEREAFTER
Ia	Every 6–12 mos	2 yrs	Variable
Ib	Every 6–12 mos	5 yrs	Variable
II	Every 3–6 mos	2–3 yrs	Every 6–12 mos for life

18. What is elective lymph node dissection (ELND)? When is it indicated?

ELND is the dissection of the draining lymph node basin in patients with deep primary melanomas who are felt to be at high risk for development of metastasis to the lymph nodes. Since melanoma is known to spread by both the lymphatic and hematogenous routes, surgical excision of all involved nodes in patients who present or relapse with stage III disease involving regional nodes has been the standard of treatment. However, the overall 5-year survival rate for surgery alone in large series is 36% and varies from 17% to 51% depending on the number of nodes involved. These results led to the concept that elective lymph node dissection may benefit patients with deep primary melanomas at high risk for microscopic lymph node involvement. The rationale was that for some patients early removal of this microscopic disease would prevent this being a source for more distant metastases and result in improved survival. However, several large randomized trials have failed to support this concept, and most large melanoma centers do not routinely perform elective lymph node dissections.

19. What is sentinel lymph node biopsy? When is it indicated?

In 1990 Morton introduced intraoperative lymphatic mapping and selective lymph node (SNL) dissection or sentinel lymph node biopsy as an alternative to elective lymph node dissection for melanoma patients. He showed that the histology of the SLN reflects the histology of the entire lymph node basin, because when it is negative the other lymph nodes within that basin are almost always also negative. The initial data from large series show substantial differences in the survival curves of patients depending on their SLN status and in multivariate analysis the status of the sentinel node has been confirmed as the most important prognostic factor for patients with primary melanoma.

Intraoperative lymphatic mapping and sentinel node biopsies are now being performed in clinical practice in several centers in the U.S. and abroad. However, it is still considered an experimental procedure and several points need to be emphasized. First, SLN biopsies require close collaboration between the nuclear radiologist, surgeon, and pathologist. Patient selection is also paramount. This procedure cannot be carried out accurately if a wide excision has been performed; therefore, patients considered candidates should be referred for this procedure prior to the wide excision, which can be carried out simultaneously with the SLN biopsy. At the University of Colorado, SLN biopsies are performed on all primary melanomas that measure >1 mm or Clark's levels IV and V.

20. What is linear melanonychia?

A linear pigmented streak of the nail (Fig. 3). Among the many potential causes, subungual melanoma is the most serious. A biopsy of the nail matrix is required if melanonychia develops rapidly, if it involves only a single digit, or if other causes of the abnormal pigmentation cannot be determined. This is a more common presentation of melanoma in blacks than in whites.

Note that longitudinal pigmented nail bands are commonly seen in darkly pigmented patients but are less common in light-skinned patients. If a pigmented nail band involves only one nail, occurs in a middle-aged or elderly white patient, shows progressive widening or darkening, or has extension of pigment onto the surrounding nailfold, a biopsy is indicated to rule out melanoma.

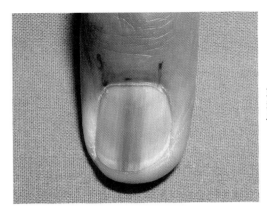

FIGURE 3. Linear melanonychia demonstrating linear brown streak of pigment. (Courtesy of James E. Fitzpatrick, MD.)

21. What is Hutchinson's sign?

The development of pigmentation at the base of linear melanonychia involving the proximal nailfold and periungual skin (Fig. 3). This sign is felt to be a very specific indication that the linear melanonychia is due to melanoma.

22. What is Hutchinson's freckle?

Lentigo maligna, the precursor lesion of lentigo maligna melanoma. The lesion appears as a relatively large (>1.0 cm), irregularly shaped, hyperpigmented macule that arises on sun-damaged skin (Fig. 4).

23. Are there any new ways to assess prognosis in patients with melanoma?

Some recently reported experimental tests may prove helpful in the early detection of metastatic disease. One such test is a **reverse transcriptase polymerase chain reaction** test used to detect circulating melanoma cells in the peripheral blood. Two groups have found that this test correlates positively with stage of disease and may be helpful in identifying patients who will eventually develop metastasis. Another test being developed is a **positron emission tomography**

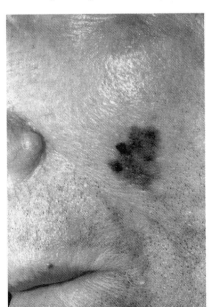

FIGURE 4. Lentigo maligna. These lesions remain superficial at the dermal-epidermal interface, often for many years, before they develop a vertical growth phase and become lentigo maligna melanoma. They are most commonly seen in elderly patients on sun-exposed skin.

using a glucose analog coupled to a positron emitter. This test also is capable of identifying clinically undetectable lymph node and visceral metastases. Both of these tests may allow earlier detection and thereby more successful treatment of metastatic disease.

24. What forms of chemotherapy are used in the treatment of metastatic melanoma?

There are currently no curative forms of therapy for patients with metastatic disease, and response rates with standard forms of chemotherapy average only about 20%. **Dacarbazine** has shown some efficacy as single-agent therapy. Response rates average around 20%, with durations averaging <6 months and a complete response rate of about 5%. **Cisplatin** has been shown to be somewhat effective as single-agent therapy, but it has significant toxicities. Other studies have shown that the **nitrosoureas** (carmustine, lomustine, and semustine) have an overall response rate ranging from 13–18%. Similarly, tubular **toxins** such as vinblastine, vincristine, and taxol have led to response rates of between 12–15%.

25. How effective is immunotherapy in malignant melanoma?

Monoclonal antibody therapy has been investigated using a variety of monoclonal antibodies linked with ricin-A toxin. As with most therapies in malignant melanoma, occasional dramatic responses have been seen and recorded in patients, but the overall efficacy is quite limited and responses have been noted in only 10–12% of treated patients (unpublished data).

The use of **biologic response modifiers,** such as interferon (IFN) and other cytokines, has had modest success. The use of IFN-alfa as a single-agent treatment has yielded response rates of 15–20% and complete response rates in up to 5% of patients. Rosenberg et al. have reported that the systemic administration of interleukin-2 (IL-2), with or without concomitant administration of tumor-infiltrating lymphocytes, has had limited success. Combining chemotherapy with biologic response modifiers may prove to be a more efficacious systemic therapy, and clinical trials are currently underway.

Combination therapy with the chemotherapeutic drugs dacarbazine and cisplatin, along with immunotherapeutic agents such as IFN-alfa and IL-2, has yielded significantly higher response rates, variously reported in the 40–50% range. Most of these cases, however, were limited to metastases involving soft tissues, including lymph nodes and subcutaneous tissue or the lung. Very few responses have been recorded in patients with liver or other visceral metastases. Furthermore, there has been little prolongation of survival with the use of combination therapy.

26. Does gene therapy offer any better results?

Several different strategies are being explored that are generically termed "gene therapy." One strategy involves the genetic modification of tumor-infiltrating lymphocytes to make them more effective at killing tumor cells. Another strategy involves the genetic modification of the tumor cells so that they produce immunostimulatory cytokines, which attract and stimulate cells involved in the immune response. Yet another approach involves the in situ genetic modification of tumor nodules so that they produce non-self HLA antigens; the immune system recognizes and rejects these modified tumor nodules in a manner similar to that in which transplanted organs are rejected. All three approaches have generated promising results in laboratory and/or clinical trials, but all are still in the early investigational phases.

27. How about local perfusion?

The treatment of localized cutaneous and lymphatic metastases by isolated hyperthermic limb perfusion using a combination of chemotherapeutic and immunotherapeutic agents has generated renewed interest following a successful European trial. In this treatment, the circulation of the affected limb is isolated, the blood slowly heated, and then it is returned to the limb along with high doses of melphalan with or without tumor necrosis factor or gamma-interferon. Because the circulation of the limb is isolated from the remaining systemic circulation, much higher doses of the therapeutic agents can be administered than what could be tolerated systemically.

BIBLIOGRAPHY

1. American Joint Committee on Cancer: AJCC Manual for Staging of Cancer, 4th ed. Philadelphia, J.B. Lippincott, 1992.
2. Balch CM, Cascinelli N, Sim FH, et al: Elective lymph node dissection: Results of a prospective randomized surgical trial. In Balch CM, Houghton AN, Sober AJ, Soong S-J (eds): Cutaneous melanoma, 3rd ed. St. Louis, MO, Quality Medical Publishing, 1998.
3. Barnhill RL, Mihm MC Jr, Fitzpatrick TB, Sober AJ: Neoplasms: Malignant melanoma. In Fitzpatrick TB, Eisen AZ, Wolff K, et al (eds): Dermatology in General Medicine, 4th ed. New York, McGraw-Hill, 1995.
4. Buzaid AC, Ross MI, Soong S-J: Predictive factors that influence melanoma outcomes: Classification and staging. In Balch CM, Houghton AN, Sober AJ, Soong S-J (eds): Cutaneous melanoma, 3rd ed. St. Louis, MO, Quality Medical Publishing, 1998.
5. Clark WH Jr: A classificiation of malignant melanoma in man correlated with histogenesis and biologic behavior. In Montagna W (ed): Advances in Biology of the Skin, vol VIII: The Pigmentary System. New York, Pergamon, 1967.
6. Johnson TM, Smith JW II, Nelson BR, Dhang A: Current therapy for cutaneous melanoma. J Am Acad Dermatol 32:689–707, 1995.
7. Lederman JS, Sober AJ: Does biopsy type influence survival in clinical Stage I cutaneous melanoma? J Am Acad Dermatol 86:983–987, 1985.
8. Reintgen DS, et al: Lymphatic mapping and sentinel lymphadenectomy. In Balch CM, Houghton AN, Sober AJ, Soong S-J (eds): Cutaneous melanoma, 3rd ed. St. Louis, MO, Quality Medical Publishing, 1998.

46. LEUKEMIC AND LYMPHOMATOUS INFILTRATES OF THE SKIN

John L. Aeling, M.D.

1. Define lymphoma.

A lymphoma is a malignancy of the immune system that is characterized by an abnormal proliferation of lymphocytes and related cell types. Most lymphomas begin in lymph nodes and are divided into Hodgkin's and non-Hodgkin's lymphomas. The non-Hodgkin's lymphomas are further subdivided into T-cell and B-cell subtypes.

MYCOSIS FUNGOIDES

2. Is there a lymphoma that begins in the skin?

Yes. Mycosis fungoides begins in the skin and often remains localized there for many years. Rarely, other T- and B-cell lymphomas also can present with skin lesions.

3. What type of lymphoma is mycosis fungoides?

Mycosis fungoides is a low grade T-cell lymphoma. Histologically, it has a polymorphous cellular infiltrate with polymorphonuclear leukocytes, eosinophils, lymphocytes, and atypical mononuclear cells. The atypical mononuclear cells are moderately large and have a folded (cerebriform) nucleus. These cells are typically seen within the epidermis either singly or in small clusters (Pautrier's microabscesses). The mycosis cells are primarily CD4-positive, helper T cells.

4. How common is mycosis fungoides?

It accounts for 2–3% of all lymphomas.

5. How does mycosis fungoides begin?

Typically, mycosis fungoides begins with persistent scaly patches (Fig. 1A) that respond poorly to topical therapy with emollients and topical steroids. In the early stages, skin biopsy is frequently not diagnostic. The average time from onset of skin lesions to diagnosis is 7 years. In this early phase of the disease, a diagnosis of parapsoriasis en plaque is often made. In time the patches thicken and become plaques. Eventually, skin tumors develop (Fig. 1, B–C) and the lymph nodes can become involved. Visceral disease is a late occurrence in this low-grade lymphoma. Median survival for persons with patch- and plaque-stage disease is 12 years; for tumor stage disease, it is 5 years; and for nodal or visceral disease, it is 3 years.

6. What is parapsoriasis?

The skin diseases included under this diagnosis are poorly understood and encompass a morass of confusing terms. The "splitters" have described over a dozen varieties of parapsoriasis, while the "lumpers" limit this designation to only a few types. This discussion supports the "lumpers" viewpoint.

Small-plaque parapsoriasis is characterized by chronic, well-marginated, mildly scaly, slightly erythematous, and round to oval skin lesions measuring <4–5 cm in diameter. The long axes of the lesions are arranged in a parallel configuration, and the lesions occur on the trunk and proximal extremities in a pityriasis rosea-like pattern. The lesions have been likened to fingerprints and reported under the descriptive term of **digitate dermatoses**. This form of parapsoriasis does not progress to lymphoma.

Large-plaque parapsoriasis presents as palm-sized or larger lesions located most frequently on the thighs, buttocks, hips, lower abdomen, and shoulder girdle areas (Fig. 2). The lesions may be pink, red-brown, or salmon-colored. They often have fine scale and show epidermal atrophy with cigarette-paper wrinkling. Some patients may have lesions with a netlike or reticular pattern

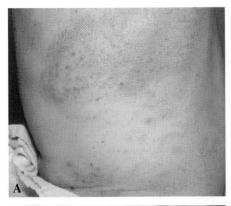

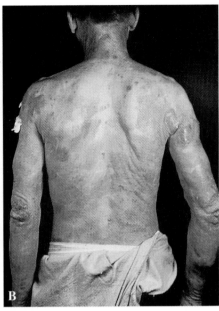

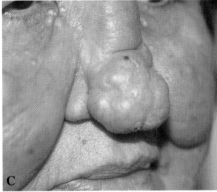

FIGURE 1. Mycosis fubgoides. *A*, A 12-year-old boy with extensive patch-stage mycosis fungoides. *B*, A patient with extensive patch, plaque, and tumor stage mycosis fungoides. *C*, Tumor-stage mycosis fungoides. This patient had skin lesions for 18 years before tumors developed and a diagnosis was made.

with telangiectasia and fine scale. This clinical type of lesion is referred to as **retiform parapsoriasis** or **poikiloderma atrophicans vasculare.** Fifteen to 20% of patients with large-plaque parapsoriasis eventually develop mycosis fungoides.

7. What type of skin lesions are seen in patients with mycosis fungoides?

Although the classic skin lesions are scaly patches, plaques, and tumors, a wide variety of skin lesions have been reported, such as follicular papules and pustules with or without alopecia (alopecia mucinosa). Bullous, erythrodermic, hypopigmented, vasculitic, and hyperkeratotic lesions also have been described.

A rare variant of mycosis fungoides is granulomatous slack skin disease (Fig. 3). This disorder is characterized by the slow development of lax erythematous skin which eventually develops large pendulous folds of redundant integument. Histologic examination shows a dense atypical granulomatous infiltrate with destruction and phagocytosis of elastic tissue.

8. What is the TNM classification of mycosis fungoides (T=skin lesions, N=lymph node involvement, and M=visceral disease)?

IA	Skin patches or plaques with < 10% skin surface involvement
IB	Skin patches or plaques with > 10% skin surface involvement
IIA	Skin patches or plaques with palpable lymph nodes
IIB	Skin tumors with or without palpable lymph nodes
III	Generalized erythroderma with or without palpable lymph nodes
IVA	Skin disease with histopathologic lymph node disease
IVB	Visceral disease with or without lymph node involvement

9. List the treatments for mycosis fungoides.

There are many treatments for mycosis fungoides. Although permanent cures are unusual, complete remissions are common, especially in early-stage disease:

Topical corticosteroids	Extracorporeal photophoresis
Psoralen photochemotherapy (PUVA)	Electron-beam therapy (total body and spot radiation)
Topical nitrogen mustard (HN$_2$)	Oral retinoids
Topical nitrosourea (carmustine, BCNU)	Interferons
Phototherapy with ultraviolet B	Single and multidrug chemotherapy

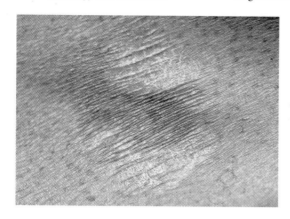

FIGURE 2. Large-plaque parapsoriasis. The lesion was unresponsive to topical treatment.

10. Describe topical nitrogen mustard (HN$_2$) therapy.

This treatment is one of the most common for mycosis fungoides in the United States, and it has been used extensively in this disease since the early 1960s. It is easy to learn, can be applied by the patient at home, and has few side effects. The treatment consists of the topical application of 10 mg of nitrogen mustard in 60 ml of water every day to the entire skin surface except the eyelids and genitalia. Complete response rates for stage I disease are over 50%. The treatment is well tolerated with few side effects and no severe systemic side effects. Over 50% of patients will develop allergic contact dermatitis to the topical medication, and there is a long-term risk for basal and squamous cell carcinoma. Some physcians prefer to use the medication in an ointment base.

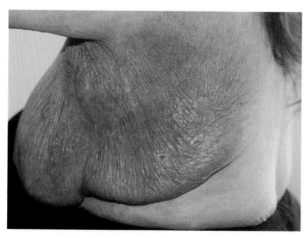

FIGURE 3. A young woman with granulomatous slack skin, a rare variant of mycosis fungoides.

11. If a patient develops allergic contact dermatitis to topical nitrogen mustard, does the treatment have to be permanently discontinued?

No. The medication should be temporarily discontinued, and the dermatitis treated with either topical or systemic steroids. When the dermatitis has cleared, the patient can then be restarted on dilute HN$_2$. Usually, the patient will tolerate 10 mg of HN$_2$ in 1 gallon of water. The concentration of the HN$_2$ can be slowly increased over several months without a flare of the dermatitis. A rare patient may develop immediate contact urticaria to topical HN$_2$, requiring discontinuation of treatment.

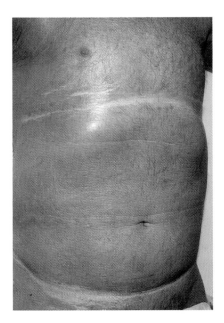

FIGURE 4. A patient with Sézary syndrome.

12. What is extracorporeal photophoresis?

After an oral dose of 8-methoxypsoralen, leukophoresis is performed and the patient's leukocytes are exposed to extracorporeal phototherapy with ultraviolet A. Treatments are given on two consecutive days at monthly intervals. The response rate is about 65% in uncontrolled studies. The treatment is expensive, requires the availability of specialized equipment, and is administered on an outpatient basis in a hospital setting. It is the only FDA-approved treatment for mycosis fungoides.

13. Is photochemotherapy an effective treatment of mycosis fungoides?

Yes. The response rates to psoralen plus ultraviolet A (PUVA) are at least equal to those with topical nitrogen mustard. A recent study from Sweden, where PUVA is the treatment of choice, showed a 50% decrease in mortality from mycosis fungoides after the introduction of PUVA. This retrospective study looked at a 30-year period, comparing pre-1979 to post-1979 death rates.

14. Is chemotherapy an effective treatment of mycosis fungoides?

Yes. Both partial and complete remissions can be achieved with both single-drug and multidrug chemotherapy protocols. However, the remissions are short-lived, and no one drug or combination of drugs appears to be superior. In a large blinded study, 103 patients randomized to 3000 cGy of electron-beam therapy followed by chemotherapy with cyclophosphamide, daunorubicin, etoposide, and vincristine were compared to a group of patients treated with topical HN_2 progressing to PUVA if necessary. After a median follow-up of 75 months, there was no difference in response rates or survival in the two groups.

15. Are interferons effective in treating mycosis fungoides?

Yes. Of the interferon group of drugs, recombinant interferon-alfa has been the most promising. Both complete remissions and partial remissions have been reported. Low-dose treatment protocols are as effective as high-dose and have fewer side effects. The recommended dose is 3 million units, given subcutaneously, three times weekly.

16. Describe the three subtypes of mycosis fungoides.

Sézary syndrome (Fig. 4) presents with the classic triad of erythroderma, lymphadenopathy, and atypical circulating mononuclear cells (Sézary cells). These cells are moderately large mononuclear cells with hyperconvoluted nuclei. These cells resemble activated T cells, and when >15% of circulating lymphocytes are atypical, it is considered significant, with 10–15% being considered borderline. However, the finding of circulating Sézary cells must be evaluated in context with the clinical picture and skin biopsy. Severe pruritus, ectropion, nail dystrophy, peripheral edema, alopecia, and keratoderma of the palms and soles are common associated features. The disease tends to wax and wane and generally progresses faster and is more resistant to treatment than typical mycosis fungoides.

Pagetoid reticulosis (Woringer-Kolopp disease) is characterized by a single or grouped hyperkeratotic skin lesion(s). Skin biopsy shows striking epidermotropism, with numerous atypical mononuclear cells, both singly and in clusters, scattered through all levels of the epidermis. The disease tends to be slowly progressive and responds well to local radiation.

The **tumor d'emblee** form was initially thought to be a type of mycosis fungoides that began with skin tumors without the usual progression through a patch-and-plaque stage. Recent reports suggest that some of these cases are B-cell primary cutaneous lymphomas and some represent Ki-1-positive primary cutaneous T-cell lymphomas.

OTHER LYMPHOMAS AND LEUKEMIAS

17. Outline the Ann Arbor clinical staging system for Hodgkin's disease.
Stage I—Single lymph node or extralymphatic site
Stage II—Two or more lymph node regions on the same side of the diaphragm or nodal involvement with a contiguous extralymphatic site
Stage III—Nodal involvement on both sides of the diaphragm, with or without a contiguous extralymphatic site
Stage IV—Multiple extralymphatic tissue sites, with or without nodal involvement.

18. What is a Reed-Sternberg cell?
It is a large cell with two mirror-image nuclei with large distinct nucleoli, often with surrounding halos (owl's eye cells). It is considered to be the malignant cell of Hodgkin's disease, and its presence confirms the histologic diagnosis. The origin of the cell is debated, with marker studies having shown both T- and B-cell immunoenzymatic staining.

19. What are the histologic classes of Hodgkin's disease?
Nodular sclerosis is the most common type, accounting for 35% of all patients with Hodgkin's disease. It is more common in women and has a relatively good prognosis. It is characterized by a particular type of Reed-Sternberg cell, called the **lacunar cell,** which is a large cell with a hyperlobulated nucleus and multiple nucleoli surrounded by a clear space (lacunae).

Mixed cellularity represents a histologic type that is intermediate between lymphocyte-predominance and lymphocyte-depletion types. It is the second most common type. Reed-Sternberg cells are prominent.

Lymphocyte-predominance type has a diffuse or slightly nodular histologic pattern (popcorn pattern). Reed-Sternberg cells are rare. It is the most common pattern found in young men, and the prognosis is excellent.

Lymphocyte-depletion pattern is characterized by a paucity of lymphocytes and numerous Reed-Sternberg cells or their variants. There is a diffuse fibrotic and a reticular variant of the lymphocyte-depleted subtype. This type tends to occur in older patients, with disseminate involvement and a poor prognosis.

20. Does Hodgkin's disease occur in the skin?
Yes, but very rarely. One series of 1800 cases reported a 0.5% incidence of specific skin lesions in patients with Hodgkin's disease. Many of the early reports of Hodgkin's disease presenting with skin lesions with no nodal involvement probably represent Ki-1-positive, T-cell lymphomas. Nonspecific skin lesions are common and include pruritus, pigmentation, prurigo, ichthyosis, alopecia, and herpes zoster.

21. How are cells immunophenotyped? What does the CD nomenclature mean?
CD stands for cluster designation and is a nomenclature for identification of specific cell sur-

face antigens defined by monoclonal antibodies. The procedure can be applied to both formalin-fixed and frozen tissue. It is very helpful in identifying subpopulations of T- and B-cell lymphocytes.

Cells Marked by CD Antigens

CD2	50% of natural killer (NK) cells (E rosette receptor)
CD3	T-cell receptor for antigen recognition
CD4	Helper T cells
CD5	Mature thymocytes, some B-cell subsets
CD7	T cells, NK cells
CD8	Suppressor T cells, NK cells
CD10	Pre-B cells, lymphoblastic leukemia cells
CD14	Monocytes
CD15	Reed-Sternberg cells, myeloid cells
CD19	Pan-B cells
CD20	Pan-B cells, dendritic cells
CD21	Receptor for complement 2 and Epstein-Barr virus
CD23	Activated B cells, monocytes, eosinophils, and platelets
CD25	Activated T and B cells, monocytes (interleukin-2 receptor)
CD30	Ki-1-related cells (antibody is BER-H2)
CD34	Lymphoid and myeloid precursor cells
CD43	T cells, myeloid cells
CD45	Leukocytes
CD45R	T cells, myeloid cells
CD74	HLA-invariant chain
CD75	Follicular center cells

22. What is lymphomatoid papulosis?

This chronic recurrent skin eruption is characterized by papules and/or nodules that frequently crust or ulcerate and self-heal, often with atrophic scars (Fig. 5). There are two histopathologic types. Type A has large Reed-Sternberg–like cells which are often CD30 (Ki-1)-positive. Type B has moderately large atypical cells with cerebriform nuclei similar to the cell type found in mycosis fungoides. These cells are usually CD30-negative. About 15–20% of patients with lymphomatoid papulosis will develop a lymphoma.

23. Are CD30-positive cells specific for lymphomatoid papulosis?

No. The monoclonal antibody CD30 (Ki-1) was first described in 1982 with positive staining of Reed-Sternberg cells of Hodgkin's disease. Positive staining was also found in the paracortical cells of reactive lymph nodes. Ki-1 positivity can be seen in primary T-cell lymphomas,

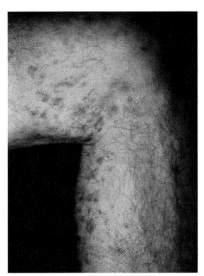

FIGURE 5. Lymphomatoid papulosis. The lesions occur in crops and self-heal.

large-cell anaplastic lymphomas, regressing atypical histiocytosis, and occasionally pityriasis lichenoides et varioliformis acuta (Mucha-Habermann disease). Ki-1-positive primary cutaneous lymphomas have a better prognosis than Ki-1-negative primary cutaneous lymphomas.

24. What is HTLV-1 virus? What is its significance?

HTLV-1 is a type C retrovirus associated with T-cell lymphoma and leukemia. It was initially isolated from a patient diagnosed with mycosis fungoides. The virus is endemic in Japan, the Caribbean, and northeastern South America, and a few cases have been reported in the United States. It can be transmitted by blood transfusions, intravenous drug abuse, breast feeding, and, less commonly, sexual contact. A small subset of patients who are HTLV-1-antibody-positive (<5%) will develop lymphoma or lymphocytic leukemia. The disease is characterized by immunosuppression, lymphadenopathy, cutaneous lesions, hypercalcemia, and a rapid downhill course.

25. Can multiple myeloma present with skin lesions only?

Yes. However, it is extremely rare for myeloma to begin with only skin lesions. Extraosseous lesions in association with osseous myeloma are common, and the skin is one of the extraosseous sites. There are many skin diseases associated with monoclonal gammopathy, including pyoderma gangrenosum, scleromyxedema, scleredema adultorum, leukocytoclastic vasculitis, collagen-vascular disease, xanthomas, Waldenström's macroglobulinemia, subcorneal pustular dermatosis, pustular psoriasis, and even urticaria. The diagnosis of multiple myeloma is confirmed when there are lytic bone lesions, anemia, hypercalcemia, M-protein > 3.5 gm/dl, urine protein > 500 mg/24 hrs, and bone marrow plasma cells exceeding 10%.

26. What is pseudolymphoma of the skin?

This term represents several clinical entities that probably have multiple etiologies. Included are lymphocytoma, Spiegler-Fendt sarcoid, lymphadenosis benigna cutis, and Jessner's benign lymphocytic infiltrate. In most cases, the etiology is unknown, although chronic arthropod bite reactions are an etiologic stimulus in some cases. The lesions present as indolent single or grouped, red or purple nodules or plaques on the head, neck, and upper trunk, and other anatomic sites can be involved. The infiltrate may show either B- or T-cell predominance. Some cases can be difficult to differentiate from lymphoma, and the patient must be followed before a definite diagnosis can be made.

27. What is actinic reticuloid?

This condition was first described in 1969. The patients are typically middle-aged or elderly men who have severe photosensitivity. The sun-exposed skin is markedly thickened, pruritic, and erythematous. Skin biopsy shows a dense, atypical, superficial and deep lymphocytic dermal infiltrate, often strikingly similar to the histopathologic changes found in mycosis fungoides. Some patients have been reported to develop T-cell lymphoma. The disease is chronic and difficult to treat. Some patients require continuous treatment with systemic steroids and/or azathioprine. These patients can react to low doses of ultraviolet A or B and even visible light.

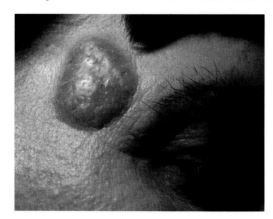

FIGURE 6. A patient with purely cutaneous B-cell lymphoma presenting with a single purple nodule on the temple.

28. Can B-cell lymphomas present with skin lesions?

Yes. Most benign and malignant cutaneous lymphocytic infiltrates are predominantly T cell in origin. Cutaneous involvement occurs in <5% of patients with B-cell nodal lymphoma. The lesions present as solitary or multiple, red to violaceous nodules or plaques (Fig. 6). Ulcerative lesions are uncommon and usually a late occurrence. Rarely, B-cell lymphomas can present with skin lesions only, and in these, the prognosis is better than with B-cell nodal lymphoma with secondary skin lesions. The treatment of choice is local radiation therapy.

29. What is the most common type of leukemia in adults?

Chronic lymphocytic leukemia. It is the most common cause of specific leukemic skin lesions, which are usually multiple and may present with papules, nodules, plaques, erythema, and, rarely, bullae (Fig. 7A). This neoplastic proliferation of lymphocytes is usually B cell in origin.

30. Can leukemia present with specific skin lesions?

Yes. Although uncommon, skin infiltration with neoplastic leukemia cells can be a presenting finding and precede the leukemic phase of the disease by several months. This is most common with the granulocytic leukemias. Often, this phenomenon is preceded by a myelodysplastic syndrome. The skin lesions may present as red or purple papules, nodules, or plaques.

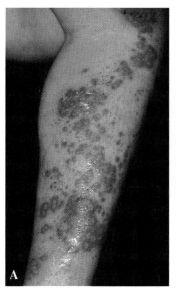
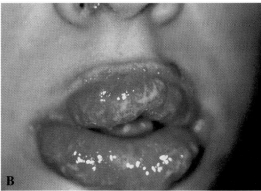

FIGURE 7. Cutaneous manifestations of leukemia. *A*, A patient with lymphocytic leukemia and multiple nodules on the lower extremity. *B*, A young child with myelomonocytic leukemia and severe gingivostomatitis.

31. What are some nonspecific skin lesions seen in patients with leukemia?

Nonspecific skin lesions are quite common in patients with all types of leukemia and preleukemia. The most common skin findings are petechiae, purpura, pruritus, papular eruptions, vasculitis, urticaria, herpes zoster, and erythroderma. Approximately 5–10% of patients with pyoderma gangrenosum have or will develop leukemia, usually of the myelocytic type. Gingival hyperplasia is a common association with acute myelomonocytic leukemia (Fig. 7B).

32. Are there any new treatments for cutaneous T-cell lymphoma?

Yes. Denileukin diftitox (Ontak, DAB/389) is interleukin-2 conjugated with a 389-amino acid portion of diphtheria toxin. The drug is given intravenously only to patients whose malignant cells express CD25, the IL-2 receptor. The drug can be associated with significant toxicity, including capillary leak syndrome, acute hypersensitivity-type reactions, hypoalbuminemia, and hypotension. It should be reserved for patients with advanced disease. Partial responses are reported in 30% and complete responses in 10% of patients.

Bexarotene (Targretin) is a synthetic retinoid that selectively activates retinoid X receptors. The drug is given orally at a recommended dose of 300 mg/m^2. Like other retinoid drugs, Targretin is teratogenic and should not be given to pregnant women. In a study of 58 patients with patch and plaque stage disease, side effects included hyperlipidemia in 78%, elevated liver enzymes in 10%, neutropenia in 38%, central hypothyroidism in 64% (41% of patients required thyroid replacement), and headache in 25% of patients. Partial response rate (50% improvement) was 67% and complete response occurred in 7% of patients. The drug is also available in a topical form (Targretin gel) and FDA-approved for treatment of Kaposi's sarcoma.

BIBLIOGRAPHY

1. Aractingi S, Bachmeyer C, Miclea J, et al: Unusual specific cutaneous lesions in myelodysplastic syndromes. J Am Acad Dermatol 33:187–191, 1995.
2. Duvic M, Martin AG, Kim Y, et al: Oral Targretin (bexarotene) capsules are safe and effective in refractory or persistent early-stage cutaneous T-cell lymphoma: Results of the phase 2-3 clinical trial. Presented at the American Society of Hematology Annual Meeting, New Orleans, 1999.
3. Epstein E, Levin D, Croft J, et al: Mycosis fungoides: Survival, prognostic features, response to therapy, and autopsy findings. Medicine 51:61–72, 1972.
4. Hoppe R, Wood G, Able E: Mycosis fungoides and the Sézary syndrome: Pathology, staging, and treatment. Curr Probl Cancer 14:295–371, 1990.
5. Kaye F, Bunn P, Steinberg S, et al: A randomized trial comparing combination electron-beam radiation and chemotherapy with topical therapy in the initial treatment of mycosis fungoides. N Engl J Med 321:1784–1790, 1989.
6. Kim YH, Bishop K, Varghese A, et al: Prognostic factors in erythrodermic mycosis fungoides and the Sézary syndrome. Arch Dermatol 131:1003–1008, 1995.
7. Lamberg SI: Clinical staging for cutaneous T-cell lymphoma. Ann Intern Med 100:187–192, 1984.
8. Rijlaarsdam JU, Scheffer E, Meijer CJLM, et al: Cutaneous pseudo-T-cell lymphomas: A clinicopathologic study of 20 patients. Cancer 69:717–724, 1992.
9. Santucci M, Pimpinelli N, Arganini L: Primary cutaneous B-cell lymphoma: A unique type of low-grade lymphoma. Cancer 67:2311–2326, 1991.
10. Swanbeck G, Roupe G, Sandstrom MH: Indications of a considerable decrease in the death rate in mycosis fungoides by PUVA treatment. Acta Derm Venereol (Stockh) 74:465–466, 1994.
11. Vonderheid E, Tan E, Kantor A, et al: Long-term efficacy, curative potential, and carcinogenicity of topical mechlorethamine chemotherapy in cutaneous T-cell lymphoma. J Am Acad Dermatol 20:416–428, 1989.
12. Wang HH, Myers T, Lach LJ, Hsieh CC, Kadin ME: Increased risk of lymphoid and nonlymphoid malignancies in patients with lymphomatoid papulosis. Cancer 86:1240–1245, 1999.
13. Willemze R: New concepts in the classification of cutaneous lymphomas. Arch Dermatol 131:1077–1080, 1995.

47. RARE MALIGNANT TUMORS OF THE SKIN

J. Ramsey Mellette, M.D., and John G. LeVasseur, M.D., MAJ, MC, USAF

EPITHELIOID SARCOMA

1. What is an epithelioid sarcoma?

It is the most common soft tissue sarcoma of the hand. The histogenesis of epithelioid sarcoma has not been established. It is important clinically because it can be mistaken for a benign inflammatory process (granulomatous or infectious). The origin of this malignancy is controversial but the clinical presentation, microscopic appearance, and tumor markers suggest it may be a variant of synovial sarcoma.

2. Why is it called "epithelioid" sarcoma?

Epithelioid describes the large plump epithelium-like cells that are characteristically seen histologically. These epithelioid or fusiform cells are arranged in nodules or palisade with necrosis in the center of the tumor nodule.

3. How does epithelioid sarcoma present?

This malignant tumor typically occurs on the distal extremity of young adults. It presents as a firm slow-growing intradermal or subcutaneous nodule or multinodular mass on the volar surface of the fingers, palms, forearms, or feet. It may ulcerate and the male-to-female ratio is approximately 2:1. They tend to be painless.

4. How are epithelioid sarcomas treated?

Early radical local excisional surgery is required, but a local recurrence rate of about 77% is encountered. Multiple recurrences are common because the tumor spreads insidiously along tendons, fascial planes, nerves, or blood vessels.

5. Can epithelioid sarcoma metastasize?

Yes. The recurrent spreading tumor can develop nodules and plaques along the forearm. Forty-five percent of patients develop metastases, mostly to the lymph nodes and lungs.

ANGIOSARCOMA

6. What is angiosarcoma?

Angiosarcoma of the skin is a highly malignant tumor of vascular endothelial cells.

7. Is there more than one type of angiosarcoma?

Yes. The three types are:
- Angiosarcoma of the face and scalp in the elderly
- Angiosarcoma associated with chronic lymphedema; it most commonly occurs in the upper extremity following radical mastectomy (Stewart-Treves syndrome)
- Post-irradiation angiosarcoma

8. How does angiosarcoma of the scalp and face in the elderly present?

Erythematous or hemorrhagic bruise-like macules and plaques develop in the scalp or less commonly on the face (Fig. 1). There is often extensive infiltration and the extent of the tumor is often underestimated clinically.

9. What is the clinical course and prognosis for angiosarcoma?

In the largest reported series of 72 patients, only 12% survived for 5 years. Metastases to the cervical nodes and hematogenous metastases to the lungs, liver, and spleen occur. The prognosis is best for lesions < 5 cm in diameter that are excised early.

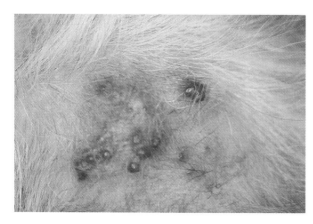

FIGURE 1. Angiosarcoma of the scalp in the elderly.

10. Is there an effective treatment for angiosarcoma?

Early diagnosis and complete surgical excision offer the best chance of survival. However, because the lesions tend to be multicentric, extensive, and rapidly growing over the face and scalp, surgical excision is rarely successful.

11. What is the clinical presentation of angiosarcoma arising in chronic lymphedema?

In the setting of an edematous upper extremity (Stewart-Treves syndrome), angiosarcoma occurs only rarely. It presents as cutaneous and subcutaneous nodules. The tumor develops a mean of 10 years following mastectomy and lymphadenectomy but ranges from 1 to 30 years. It is less commonly associated with filarial, congenital, traumatic, or idiopathic lymphedema.

12. What is the clinical course and prognosis?

The tumors increase in number and size rapidly and they often ulcerate. Radical surgery is required and metastases occur early, especially to the lungs, pleura, and chest wall. Death usually occurs within 1–2 years after the onset of the tumor.

MERKEL CELL CARCINOMA

13. What is Merkel cell carcinoma (MCC)?

Merkel cell carcinoma (MCC) is an aggressive malignant neoplasm first described by Toker in 1972. The Merkel cell is located in or near the basal cell layer of the epidermis (mostly in the digits) and is thought to function as a receptor of mechanical stimuli. It has not been proven that the cell of origin is the Merkel cell. Some authorities prefer the term neuroendocrine carcinoma or small cell carcinoma of the skin because of its microscopic appearance.

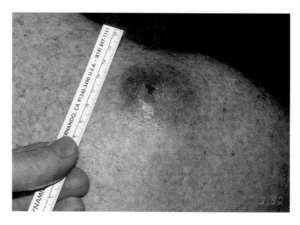

FIGURE 2. Merkel cell carcinoma presenting on the trunk.

14. Describe the clinical presentation of MCC.

Over 50% of patients present with a solitary erythematous nodule approximately 0.5–5.0 cm in diameter on the head, face, and neck. Other areas may be involved, including the extremities and trunk (Fig. 2). The tumor tends to grow rapidly and it is often indistinguishable from other skin cancers. Most cases are in whites, but tumors have been documented in blacks and Polynesians.

15. Is there a predilection for MCC?

Yes. MCC is predominantly a tumor of the elderly, occurring in patients 65 years and older, but the age range is 7–97 years.

16. Can any other tumors be microscopically confused with MCC?

Yes. MCC is composed of undifferentiated basaloid small cells that may be confused with metastatic oat-cell carcinoma of the lung, malignant lymphoma, sweat gland carcinoma, metastatic carcinoid tumors, and Ewing's sarcoma. Electron microscopy may be helpful since it demonstrates dense core neurosecretory granules.

17. What special stains are available to diagnose MCC?

MCC often has a characteristic paranuclear "dot" that stains with cytokeratin. MCC also stains positively for epithelial membrane antigen and synaptophysin, neuron-specific enolase, and chromogranin A.

18. How do you treat MCC?

Wide local excision with surgical margins up to 3.0 cm has been recommended. Other considerations at the time of surgery include assessment of regional lymph nodes (lymph node dissection) and irradiation. Local recurrences occur in 40% of patients.

19. Does MCC metastasize?

Yes. Up to 75% of patients develop regional lymph node metastases at some time during the course of their disease. Distant metastases occur to the lungs and other sites in 30–40%.

20. What is the overall prognosis?

Reported overall 5-year survival rates range from 30–64%. All patients need close follow-up after excision.

MICROCYSTIC ADNEXAL CARCINOMA

21. What are the clinical features of microcystic adnexal carcinoma?

Described in 1982, microcystic adnexal carcinoma (MAC) is a slow-growing tumor that histologically shows evidence of both follicular and sweat duct differentiation. The most common presentation is a slow-growing plaque or nodule on the upper lip. However, other sites, especially on

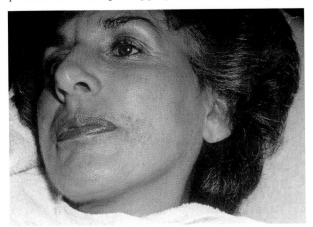

FIGURE 3. Middle-aged women with a typical microcystic adnexal carcinoma.

the face, have been reported (Fig. 3). The tumor is typically firm and ill-defined. Histologically it may be confused with morpheaform basal cell carcinoma, desmoplastic trichoepithelioma, or syringoma.

22. How is MAC treated?

Surgical excision by the Mohs technique is the treatment of choice for MAC. Frequent recurrences are seen without the type of microscopic control offered by the Mohs technique, primarily because of perineural invasion.

23. What is the prognosis?

Excellent with adequate excision. Metastases have not been reported.

DERMATOFIBROSARCOMA PROTUBERANS

24. What is dermatofibrosarcoma protuberans?

Dermatofibrosarcoma protuberans (DFSP) is a firm locally aggressive multinodular tumor that exhibits massive proliferation of spindle cells in the dermis and subcutaneous fat. These cells form intersecting bundles with a characteristic storiform (cartwheel) arrangement on the microscopic exam. The cell of origin is controversial. A rare pigmented variant of DFSP is called Bednar tumor.

25. Is a special stain available to identify DFSP?

Yes. DFSP stains positively for the human hematopoietic progenitor cell antigen CD-34, which helps to differentiate it from other fibrous tumors.

26. Describe the clinical features of DFSP.

DFSP presents as a slow-growing, elevated, and indurated plaque that is flesh-colored to red-brown or bluish color. The plaque may give rise to one or more nodules (Fig. 4). It may occasionally present as an atrophic lesion and be mistaken for a scar. It most commonly occurs on the trunk and extremities on young to middle-aged adults, but it may be seen on the head and neck.

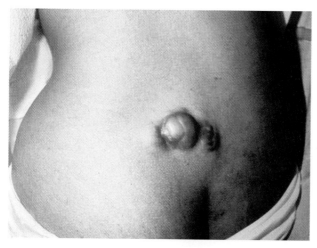

FIGURE 4. Multinodular dermatofibrosarcoma protuberans in a young woman.

27. Do DFSPs have a tendency to recur?

Yes. Local recurrence occurs following incomplete removal. Metastases occur in recurrent lesions but are rare.

28. How is DFSP treated?

Adequate local excision is the treatment of choice. Because of the high incidence of local recurrence, Mohs surgery is recommended by many dermatologic surgeons with cure rates > 95%.

ATYPICAL FIBROXANTHOMA

29. What is an atypical fibroxanthoma?

Atypical fibroxanthoma (AFX) is a superficial dermal tumor that microscopically shows large bizarre nuclei. AFX is thought to be a superficial form of malignant fibrous histiocytoma with a benign biologic behavior.

30. What is the clinical course?

Like most soft tissue tumors the clinical features are not unique and the diagnosis is made histologically following biopsy. It most commonly presents as a solitary nodule in sun-damaged skin of the head and neck or dorsum of the hands of the elderly (Fig. 5).

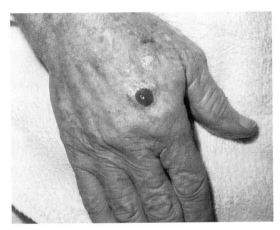

FIGURE 5. Atypical fibroxanthoma arising on a sun damaged hand.

31. What is the treatment and the prognosis?

Complete surgical excision is usually curative. Mohs micrographic surgery has been used to successfully treat these lesions.

MALIGNANT FIBROUS HISTIOCYTOMA

32. What is a malignant fibrous histiocytoma?

Malignant fibrous histiocytoma (MFH) is a tumor arising in the deep soft tissue. It is the most common soft tissue tumor in adults.

33. Do they arise in the skin?

Yes, about 10% arise in the superficial subcutis. Several histologic subtypes are recognized. The tumor primarily arises from the deep fascia or skeletal muscles on the extremities or from the retroperitoneum.

34. What is the prognosis and treatment?

Small superficial tumors have a much better prognosis than the deep ones. Ten percent of the superficial tumors above the fascia metastasize. Adequate surgical excision is necessary.

EXTRAMAMMARY PAGET'S DISEASE

35. What are the clinical features of extramammary Paget's disease?

Extramammary Paget's disease is an epidermal malignancy arising most commonly in the anogenital region as erythematous patches or plaques (Fig. 6). It may be confused with dermatitis. It occurs in older adults.

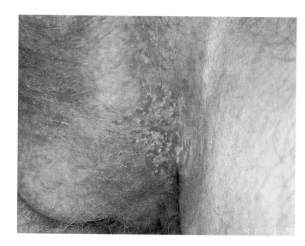

FIGURE 6. Typical extramammary Paget's disease arising in the groin.

36. Is it associated with underlying malignancies?

Yes, but in the minority of patients. An evaluation for underlying gastrointestinal and genitourinary adenocarcinoma is necessary.

37. How is it treated?

Surgical excision with careful margin control. Mohs micrographic surgery can be useful but the tumor can be multifocal and local recurrences occur.

SEBACEOUS CARCINOMA

38. Where do sebaceous carcinomas occur?

Sebaceous carcinomas occur in both ocular and extraocular sites. Ocular tumors are most common and they often arise from the meibomian glands of the eyelid.

39. How do they present?

Ocular tumors present as firm nodules more commonly in the upper eyelid than the lower eyelid (Fig. 7). It may be mistaken for a chalazion, therefore persistent or unusual lesions should be biopsied. Extraocular tumors occur only rarely and have been found on the head and neck of the elderly. Sebaceous carcinoma is more common in Asians.

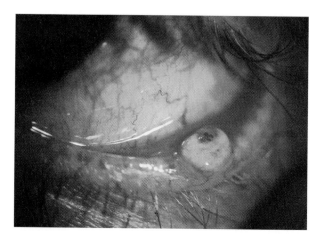

FIGURE 7. Sebaceous gland carcinoma on the lower eyelid.

40. What is the treatment and prognosis?

Treatment is complete surgical excision. Up to one third of patients with ocular tumors develop metastases to cervical lymph nodes. Muir-Torre syndrome should be considered.

LEIOMYOSARCOMA

41. What is leiomyosarcoma?

It is a malignant tumor primarily involving smooth muscle. Dermal tumors occur in erector pill muscles, dartos muscle (scrotum), and in vascular smooth muscle.

42. Describe dermal leiomyosarcoma.

The clinical appearance is not characteristic. The tumor is solitary, ranging from 0.5 cm to > 3.0 cm and is often found on the extremities.

43. What histologic stains help identify leiomyosarcoma?

Stains that highlight smooth muscle, such as Masson, trichrome, and muscle-specific actin and desmin stains.

44. What is the treatment and prognosis?

Early detection and adequate surgical excision is necessary. Dermal tumors only rarely metastasize, whereas subcutaneous tumors metastasize in about one third of patients.

BIBLIOGRAPHY

1. Arndt KA, et al (eds): Cutaneous Medicine and Surgery. Philadelphia, W.B. Saunders, 1996.
2. Barnhill RL: Textbook of Dermatopathology. New York, McGraw-Hill, 1998.
3. Cook TF, Fosko SW: Unusual cutaneous malignancies. Semin Cutan Med Surgery 17:114–132, 1998.
4. Enzinger FM, Weiss SW: Soft Tissue Tumors, St. Louis, Mosby, 1995.
5. Farmer EF, Hood AF: Pathology of the Skin. New York, McGraw-Hill, 2000.
6. Stadler FJ, Scott GA, Brown MD: Malignant fibrous tumors. Semin Cutan Med Surg 17:141–152, 1998.
7. Weedon D: Skin Pathology. San Francisco, Churchill-Livingstone, 1997.

48. METASTATIC TUMORS

Martin B. Giandoni, M.D., and James E. Fitzpatrick, M.D.

1. How often do internal malignancies metastasize to the skin?

Cutaneous metastases of internal malignancies are relatively uncommon. An autopsy study done on 7500 patients with internal malignancies demonstrated cutaneous metastases in 9% of patients. Most cases occur late in the course of the disease, but cutaneous metastasis may also be the initial presentation of an internal malignancy.

2. By what three mechanisms do internal malignancies metastasize to the skin?

They extend by local infiltration, lymphatic spread, or hematogenous spread. Breast carcinoma and oral cancer are the most likely to demonstrate direct extension into the skin. It is assumed that the fundamental mechanisms are similar to those of metastasis to parenchymal organs, but this has not been investigated.

3. What are the most common cancers that metastasize to the skin in women?

Different gender and age groups are affected by somewhat different metastatic malignancies. In a large study done at the Armed Forces Institute of Pathology in the early 1970s, the most common etiologies of cutaneous metastases in women were:

Breast carcinoma	69%	Ovary	4%
Colon	9%	Lung	4%
Malignant melanoma	5%		

Because of the rapid increase in the incidence of lung carcinoma and malignant melanoma in women, it is likely that metastatic disease from these two malignancies is now more common than reported in this study.

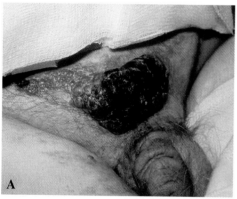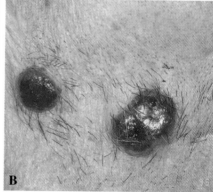

FIGURE 1. *A,* Large metastatic nodule of prostate carcinoma. The lower abdomen and pubic area are common sites for metastases of genitourinary cancers. *B,* Lung carcinoma metastatic to the chest wall, which is the most common site (courtesy of Paul Thompson, MD).

4. What are the most common cancers that metastasize to the skin in men?

In the same study, the five most common causes of skin metastases in men were:

Lung	24%	Oral squamous cell carcinoma	12%
Colon	19%	Kidney	6%
Malignant melanoma	13%		

In a more recent study malignant melanoma was the most common cause of cutaneous metastases, accounting for 32% of all cases.

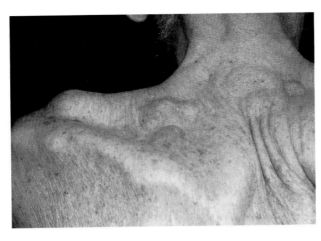

FIGURE 2. Metastatic adeno-carcinoma of the gastrointestinal tract presenting as skin-colored dermal and subcutaneous nodules.

5. Do metastases to the skin typically occur in random patterns?

No. Different tumors demonstrate characteristic patterns of metastases. As a rule, cutaneous metastases usually appear in skin that is near the primary tumor (Fig. 1). Most regional metastases are probably through the lymphatic system, while distant metastases are more likely to occur via the hematogenous route.

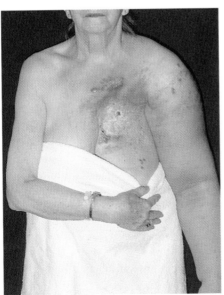

FIGURE 3. Inflammatory breast carcinoma presenting as an erythematous plaque on the anterior chest wall and red dermal papules on the shoulder.

Characteristic Sites of Cutaneous Metastases

PRIMARY TUMOR	SITE OF METASTASES
Oral squamous cell carcinoma	Head and neck
Thyroid carcinoma	Neck
Lung	Chest wall
Breast	Anterior chest wall
Renal cell carcinoma	Head
Gastrointestinal carcinoma	Abdomen
Genitourinary carcinoma	Lower abdomen

6. Describe the most common presentations of malignancies metastatic to the skin.

Cutaneous metastases most commonly present as a cutaneous nodule or group of nodules that may be movable or fixed to underlying structures. Less commonly, they may present as indurated plaques. They may be skin-colored (Fig. 2), violaceous, erythematous, or, rarely, pigmented (malignant melanoma). The overlying epidermis is usually intact, but large metastatic lesions may be eroded or ulcerated. Clinically, they may mimic primary cutaneous lesions, including epidermoid cysts, lipomas, primary cutaneous malignancies, neurofibromas, scars, pyogenic granulomas, cellulitis, and even dermatitis. Metastatic breast carcinoma may uncommonly present with distinct patterns, including carcinoma erysipelatoides (inflammatory carcinoma, Fig. 3), carcinoma telangiectaticum (a variant of inflammatory carcinoma), and carcinoma en cuirasse (a sclerodermoid pattern).

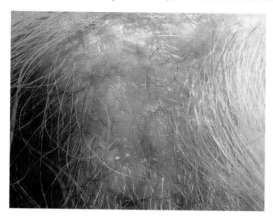

FIGURE 4. Alopecia neoplastica secondary to metastatic breast carcinoma. On palpation, the lesion was firm and indurated.

7. What is alopecia neoplastica?

The scalp appears to be a unique site for cutaneous metastasis, and often cutaneous metastases to the scalp are a presenting sign for internal malignancy. One characteristic clinical presentation is that of an isolated, indurated plaque in the scalp with associated alopecia (Fig. 4). Biopsy of this site will demonstrate cutaneous metastasis of a visceral malignancy and loss of hair follicles. The most common tumors to metastasize to the scalp are those of the breast, lung, and kidney.

8. What is a Sister Mary Joseph's nodule?

It is a nodular umbilical metastatic tumor (Fig. 5). This sign is named in recognition of Sister Mary Joseph, who was the superintendent of St. Mary's Hospital in Rochester, Minnesota, and served as the first surgical assistant to Dr. W.J. Mayo. She is credited with recognizing that patients with this finding had a poor prognosis.

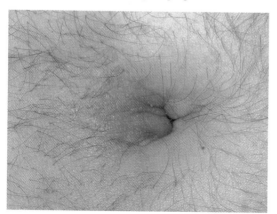

FIGURE 5. Sister Mary Joseph's nodule of the umbilicus. The primary malignancy was never detected.

9. Which tumors usually present as a Sister Mary Joseph's nodule?

The four most common tumors to present with this sign are stomach (20%), large bowel (14%), ovary (14%), and pancreatic tumors (11%). In about one-fifth of patients, the primary site cannot be determined.

10. How do you diagnose a cutaneous metastasis?

The diagnosis is best established by doing an excisional, incisional, or punch biopsy and submitting the specimen in formalin for routine processing. In addition to H&E stains, the pathologist can perform special histochemical stains (e.g., mucicarmine for mucin, Fontana-Masson for melanin) or immunoperoxidase studies (e.g., prostate-specific antigen for prostate cancer and calcitonin for medullary thyroid carcinoma). Problematic cases may require submission of part of the tumor for electron microscopy or frozen for immunoperoxidase studies that cannot be done on formalin-fixed tissue. Less commonly, the tumor specimen is obtained by a fine-needle aspiration.

11. What is the prognosis of a patient with a cutaneous metastasis?

Cutaneous metastasis is usually a poor prognostic sign and often reflects preexisting widespread internal metastasis. In one study, the average life expectancy after development of skin metastases was only 3 months. The prognosis is ultimately dependent on the primary tumor, and some patients do survive for years.

BIBLIOGRAPHY

1. Brownstein MH, Helwig EB: Spread of tumors to the skin. Arch Dermatol 107:80–86, 1973.
2. Lookingbill DP, Spangler N, Helm KF: Cutaneous metastases in patients with metastatic carcinoma: A retrospective study of 4020 patients. J Am Acad Dermatol 29:228–236, 1993.
3. Pitman KT, Johnson JT: Skin metastases from head and neck squamous cell carcinoma: Incidence and impact. Head Neck 21:560–565, 1999.
4. Powell FC, Cooper AJ, Massa MC, et al: Sister Mary Joseph's nodule: A clinical and histologic study. J Am Acad Dermatol 10: 610–615, 1984.
5. Reingold IM: Cutaneous metastases from internal carcinoma. Cancer 19:162–168, 1966.
6. Spencer PS, Helm TN: Skin metastases in cancer patients. Cutis 39:119–121, 1987.

49. SUNSCREENS AND PREVENTION OF SKIN CANCER

Joseph Yohn, M.D.

1. Describe the adverse effects of excess sun exposure.

Adverse effects of sun exposure can be both acute and chronic.

Acute effects	Sunburn
	Transient immune suppression
	Drug-induced phototoxic reactions
	Exacerbation of an underlying photosensitivity disorder (such as lupus erythematosus)
Chronic effects	Skin wrinkles
	Abnormal pigmentation
	Precancers (actinic keratoses)
	Impaired immune survelliance of pre-skin cancer and skin cancer
	Cataracts
	Basal cell carcinoma
	Squamous cell carcinoma
	Melanoma (see also Chapters 45 and 46).

2. Are there any health benefits of solar radiation exposure?

Health benefits of solar radiation are few. Skin exposure to ultraviolet B is necessary for the conversion of 7-dehydrocholesterol into previtamin D_3 that then isomerizes to vitamin D_3. Periodic exposure to the visible spectrum of solar radiation is believed to enhance psychological well-being. Lastly, the ultraviolet spectrum of solar radiation is used for the treatment of skin disorders such as psoriasis, eczema, and cutaneous T-cell lymphoma.

3. What are the spectra of ultraviolet (UV) radiation and their effects on human skin?

Sunlight is broken down into bands of light according to its physical characteristics and biologic effects.

- **UVC:** 100–290 nm wavelength. High-energy radiation that damages cells through direct DNA damage and through the generation of free radical species. Fortunately, UVC radiation is filtered by atmospheric ozone and does not reach the earth's surface.
- **UVB:** 290–320 nm. Mid-range radiation that is not completely filtered by atmospheric ozone, called the "burning" rays because it causes sunburn. UVB injures skin cells primarily through formation of DNA thymine dimers and DNA 6–4 photoproducts that, if not repaired properly, cause gene mutations and lead to altered cell function and carcinogenesis.
- **UVA:** 320–400 nm. Long-wave radiation that is the lowest energy spectrum of ultraviolet. UVA is not filtered by atmospheric ozone, and a 150-fold greater amount of UVA strikes the surface of the earth compared to UVB. UVA damages skin cells predominantly through the formation of free radicals. UVB penetrates to the basal layer of the epidermis, whereas UVA penetrates to the middermis. Skin wrinkling following chronic sun exposure is due to UVA injury of dermal fibroblasts resulting in altered collagen and elastin synthesis.

Combined, UVB and UVA are carcinogenic, and thus it is imperative to warn patients about the damaging effects of ultraviolet radiation and how to properly protect against its adverse effects.

4. List some of the important facts about skin cancer.

1. The sun causes at least 90% of all skin cancers.
2. One in six Americans will develop skin cancer during his or her lifetime.
3. In the United States, over 760,000 new cases of skin cancer are diagnosed annually, afflicting more people than any other cancer.
4. This year, >33,000 Americans will develop malignant melanoma and >6,000 will die.
5. Approximately 30% of melanomas occur in individuals <45 years of age.
6. Melanoma is the most common cancer in women aged 25–29 and the second most common (after breast cancer) for women aged 30–34.
7. The incidence of melanoma is increasing at a rate faster than that of any other cancer, having nearly doubled in the last decade.
8. Most people receive 50–80% of their cumulative lifetime sun exposure before age 18.

5. How does skin type affect the risk for skin cancer?

Anyone can get skin cancer, although some people are at greater risk than others. The skin phototype (SPT) system was developed to identify people who are prone to develop skin cancer. The SPT system is a six-point scale based on a person's skin color and ability to tan. Individuals who fall into SPT groups I and II are at highest risk for the development of skin cancer. These two groups of people are especially prone to develop basal cell and squamous cell carcinoma and are at high risk for developing melanoma. Skin types III and IV are less prone for developing basal cell and squamous cell carcinoma but are still at risk for developing melanoma. Basal cell carcinoma, squamous cell carcinoma, and melanoma are rare in skin types V and VI. If patients in groups V and VI develop melanoma, it usually occurs on the palms and soles (acrolentiginous melanoma) or on mucosal surfaces, such as in the mouth or on the genitalia.

Human Skin Phototypes

SKIN PHOTOTYPE*	UNEXPOSED SKIN COLOR	SUN RESPONSE HISTORY
I	White	Always burns, never tans
II	White	Always burns, tans minimally
III	White	Burns minimally, tans gradually and uniformly
IV	Light brown	Burns minimally, always tans well
V	Brown	Rarely burns, tans darkly
VI	Dark brown	Never burns, tans darkly

*Based on the first 30–60 minutes of sun exposure of untanned skin after the winter season.

6. What are the other risk factors for skin cancer?

The number of blistering sunburns and the total amount of sun exposure in a lifetime. **Sunburns** are directly related to melanoma risk. One study reported a 2.5–6.3-fold increased melanoma risk for a person with a history of three or more blistering sunburns. For this reason, indoor workers such as health care professionals and office workers who experience intense, intermittent sun exposure are more prone to developing melanoma.

Lifetime cumulative sun exposure directly correlates with basal cell and squamous cell carcinoma risk. Individuals who are exposed to the sun on a daily basis, such as farmers, fishermen, and construction workers, are at high risk for developing nonmelanoma skin cancer.

7. Do hereditary factors affect skin cancer risk?

Skin cancer appears to have a hereditary component. The prototype syndrome of genetically determined increased skin cancer risk is **xeroderma pigmentosum** (XP). XP patients suffer from an autosomal recessive defect in DNA repair that results in sun sensitivity and early onset of basal cell carcinoma, squamous cell carcinoma, and melanoma. While much of the molecular genetics of XP is understood, further study is necessary to better understand the genetics of other types of skin cancer-prone families. However, a useful recommendation is to have all first-degree relatives (parents, siblings, and children) of a skin cancer patient examined for skin cancer and taught sun-protection measures.

8. Are age or sex factors important in skin cancer risk?

Yes. Basal cell and squamous cell carcinoma incidences peak in the seventh decade of life. Melanoma incidence peaks around age 50.

Overall, men develop more skin cancer than women, but in the third and fourth decade of life, almost as many women develop skin cancer as men. Melanoma occurs most frequently on the chest, shoulders, and back in men, whereas in women, it develops more often on the legs. For both sexes, basal cell and squamous cell carcinoma develop most often on sun-exposed areas, including the head, neck, shoulders, arms, and hands. One caveat: patients should have a total skin exam because skin cancer of all types can occur on infrequently sun-exposed or non-sun-exposed areas.

9. What should physicians teach patients about skin cancer prevention?

Basically, two things: sun protection and the self-skin exam.

10. What warning signs of possible skin cancer should be looked for in the self-skin exam?

The self-skin exam is an important part of skin cancer prevention for two reasons: studies have shown that abnormal skin lesions are frequently discovered first by the patient, and skin cancer, when treated early, is curable.

Patients should be encouraged to examine their entire skin surface on a monthly basis, remembering to include the scalp and normally non-sun-exposed sites, including the buttocks, genitalia, and feet. Warning signs of a possible skin cancer include:

An open sore that does not heal in 3 weeks

A spot or sore that persistently itches, burns, stings, crusts, scabs, or bleeds

Any mole or brown spot that changes in size, thickness, or texture or develops an irregular border

A skin lesion that increases in size and appears pearly, translucent, tan, brown, black, or multicolored

11. List the 13 basic facts regarding sun protection.

All patients should know several basic facts about sun protection:

1. Sun damage is cumulative. Each dose of ultraviolet radiation (UVR), large and small, adds up, leading to skin wrinkling, dyspigmentation, and skin cancer.

2. There is no such thing as a "healthy tan." Skin tanning is a response to skin injury by UVR.

3. Avoid sun exposure between the hours of 10 am to 2 pm (11 am to 3 pm daylight savings time), when UVB is most intense. Plan outdoor activities for the early morning or late afternoon.

4. Protect the skin with clothing first, and apply sunscreen to any remaining unprotected skin.

5. Beware of high-altitude sun exposure. There is less atmosphere to absorb UVR, and therefore the risk of sunburn is greater.

6. UVR is stronger near the equator, where the sun's rays strike the earth most directly.

7. Use protective clothing and apply sunscreens even on overcast days. Although UVR is less intense on overcast days, it is still present and adds to cumulative skin damage.

8. UVR is reflected off of sand, concrete, and snow and adds to the total UVR exposure. Because UVR is reflected and scattered, sitting in the shade is not protective and sunburn can occur.

9. Do not use tanning beds. Although tanning beds emit primarily UVA, overexposure can cause sunburn, and their use enhances skin aging and the risk for skin cancer.

10. People at high risk for skin cancer (persons with skin types I and II, outdoor workers, and persons with a history of skin cancer or a photosensitivity disorder) should apply sunscreens daily.

11. Some medications (sulfonamides, tetracyclines, and birth control pills as well as over-the-counter products) and cosmetic ingredients (lime oil) can be photosensitizing.

12. Keep infants and children out of the sun. Begin using sunscreens on children after they learn to walk, and then allow sun exposure with moderation.

13. Teach children sun protection early.

12. What type of clothing is considered sun-protective?

Optimal sun protection includes wearing a hat, sunglasses, a long-sleeved shirt, and long pants. Be sure to choose the correct type of clothing for sun protection. Weave and construction of the fabric is more important than the fiber. Choose tightly woven materials for greater protection from UVR.

13. What are sunscreens?
In the broadest terms, sunscreens are agents that block ultraviolet radiation absorption by the skin. Sunscreens can be in the form of clothing, hats, sunglasses, or chemical or physical agents, including lotions, creams, pastes, and gels.

14. Compare the advantages and disadvantages of the physical and chemical sunscreens.
Physical sunscreens are agents that scatter and reflect UVR, while chemical sunscreens absorb UVR through a photochemical reaction. Physical sunscreens include zinc oxide and titanium dioxide and have advantages over chemical sunscreens. Physical sunscreens are inert, they do not break down over time, and they do not cause contact dermatitis or photodermatitis. They block both UVB and UVA. However, physical sunscreens have one drawback: they leave a slight makeup base appearance to the skin that some people find unappealing.

Titanium Dioxide-Containing Sunscreens (Physical Sunscreens)

PRODUCT	SPF	MANUFACTURER
Advanced Suncare Sunblock	15	Estee Lauder
Banana Boat Chemical-Free Sunblock	15, 25	Sun Pharmaceuticals
Basic Block Non-Chemical Sunscreen	21	Elizabeth Arden
Let The Sun Shine	21	Origins (Estee Lauder)
NatureBlock	15	Chanel
Outdoor Protection	15	Prescriptives
Spa for the Face Sunscreen	15	Elizabeth Arden
Special Defense Sunblock	25	Clinique
Sun Care	15	Shisheido
Sundown Sport	15	Johnson and Johnson

Although chemical sunscreens do carry a risk for contact dermatitis and photodermatitis, the risk is quite low (0.1%–2.0%). Another disadvantage of chemical sunscreens is that they degrade with sun exposure, requiring reapplication every 2 hours. However, for many people, the advantages of chemical sunscreens outweigh the disadvantages. Chemical sunscreens are available in a plethora of formulations, such as cream, lotion, and gels. There are formulations for use on the face, lips, and small children. Today, there are chemical sunscreen formulations that block both UVB and UVA, and these formulations should be recommended to patients.

Chemical Sunscreens That Block UVB and UVA

PRODUCT NAME	SPF	MANUFACTURER
Ban de Soleil Waterproof Sunblock Lotion	30	Proctor and Gamble
Clinique Sunblock	25	Clinique
Dura Screen	15	Reed and Carnick
Hawaiian Tropic Sunblocks	15, 30	Tanning Research
Photoplex	15	Herbert Laboratories
Pre Sun Moisturizing Sunscreen	25	Bristol Myers
Pre Sun Sensitive Skin Sunscreen	29	Bristol Myers
Shade UVA/UVB Sunblock Lotion	30	Schering-Plough
Shade UVA/UVB Sunblock Oil-Free Gel	25	Schering-Plough
Solbar	15, 30	Person and Covey
Sun Essentials Sunblock	15	Mary Kay
Sundown Sunblock Lotion	15, 30	Johnson and Johnson
Sunseekers Ultra Sunblock Lotion	15, 30	Avon

Sunscreens for Children

PRODUCT NAME	SPF	MANUFACTURER
Baby Sunblock	15, 25	Chesebrough Ponds
Bain de Soleil All Day for Kids	30	Proctor and Gamble
Banana Boat Baby Kote	30	Sun Pharmaceutical
Bull Frog	18	Chatten
Estee Lauder Baby Block	25	Estee Lauder
Hawaiian Tropic Baby	15	Tanning Research
Johnson's Baby Sunblock Lotion	15, 30	Johnson and Johnson
Pre Sun for Kids	29	Bristol Myers
Sun Seekers Children's Sunblock	15	Avon
Water Babies Sunblock Lotion	15, 30	Schering-Plough

15. What chemicals are used in chemical sunscreens?

	CONCENTRATION USED (%)
2-Ethylhexyl 2-cyano-3,3-diphenylacrylate	7–10
2-Ethylhexyl salicylate	3–5
2-Ethylhexylmethoxycinnamate	2–7.5
2-Phenylbenzimidazole-5-sulfonic acid	1–4
Cinoxate	1–3
Diethanolamine-*para*-methoxycinnamate	8–10
Digalloyl trioleate	2–5
Dioxybenzone	3
Glycerol *para*-Aminobenzoic acid	2–3
Homosalate	4–15
Menthyl anthranilate	3.5–5
Oxybenzone	2–6
Padimate O	1–4–5
para-Aminobenzoic acid (PABA)	5–15
Red petrolatum	80–100
Sulisobenzone	5–10
Triethanolamine salicylate	5–12

16. What factors should be considered in selecting a sunscreen?

1. The sunscreen should block both UVB and UVA and have a sun protection factor (SPF) rating of 15 or greater.

2. Avoid sunscreens that contain fragrance, as this can be a source of contact dermatitis or photodermatitis. *Para*-Aminobenzoic acid (PABA) also can cause contact dermatitis; many sunscreen products are now PABA-free.

3. Although some sunscreens claim to be waterproof and rub-proof or offer "all-day protection," these sunscreens should be reapplied after sweating or swimming.

17. How is an SPF determined?

Sunscreen SPF is defined as the ratio of the minimal dose of sunlight to cause redness of sunscreen-protected skin divided by the minimal dose of sunlight to cause redness of unprotected skin. An SPF of 15 effectively reduces UV skin absorption by 94%.

18. How much sunscreen should be applied? How often should it be reapplied?

Warn your patients that most people apply too little sunscreen. To cover the face, arms, legs, and upper torso of an average-sized adult requires 1 oz of sunscreen, which is generally a handful. A smaller person or child needs proportionally less. Sunscreen should be applied evenly and rubbed into all exposed skin. It should be applied 30–60 minutes before sun exposure and, under normal conditions, reapplied every 2 hours. Sunscreen should be reapplied more often if swimming, sweating, or rubbing has removed some of the product. Warn patients that reapplication does not double the SPF and to not rely on redness as a signal to reapply sunscreen. Skin damage occurs before sunburn appears.

19. Can sunscreens be safely used in children?

Yes. Most major cosmetic and pharmaceutical companies make sunscreen products for children. All recommendations for sunscreen use in adults should be followed for children. However, sunscreens should not be used in children <9 months of age. Any child who has not yet learned to walk should be protected with long sleeves, long pants, and a hat and should be kept away from direct sunlight.

20. Why are sunglasses included in sun-protection recommendations?

Sunglasses protect the eyelids, sclera, cornea, and lens from UVR injury. Intense, acute UVR eye injury results in sunburn of the eyelids, sclera, and cornea, whereas chronic sun exposure causes cataracts and skin cancer of the periorbital skin. Patients should be instructed to buy sunglasses that absorb UVB and UVA. Also, a large frame area better protects the skin around the eyes.

21. Are tanning pills safe to use?

No. Canthaxanthin, the active ingredient in most tanning pills, is not approved by the U.S. Food and Drug Administration. Side effects include nausea, diarrhea, pruritus, skin eruptions, night blindness, and drug-induced hepatitis. There has been one reported death due to aplastic anemia in a woman who took tanning pills.

22. What about "tan-in-a-bottle" lotions?

Self-tanning lotions are skin dyes and are safe to use. However, skin-coloring agents do not protect the skin from UVR injury. Therefore, sun-protection measures must be followed by people using self-tanning products.

23. If UVB is required for vitamin D metabolism, how will I maintain normal vitamin D levels with restricted sun exposure? How much sun exposure is necessary?

A daily short UVB exposure (10 minutes) of a small area of skin (face, hands and arms) will supply ample vitamin D for the body's needs. In the United States, proper vitamin D levels also can easily be maintained by eating a healthy diet. Many foods, such as milk and bread, are fortified with vitamin D, and most multivitamins contain vitamin D.

24. What is proper sunburn treatment?

- Take aspirin as soon as sunburn is detected to help reduce inflammation and control pain. Tylenol helps control pain but is not as effective as aspirin in reducing inflammation.
- Cool, wet compresses or tub soaks for 20 minutes four or five times daily will help with pain control.
- Do not use butter or heavy ointments, as they can cause skin irritation, and do not use benzocaine sprays, as they can cause contact dermatitis.
- Increased fluid loss can occur through sunburned skin. Therefore, fluid replenishment with an isotonic sport drink is recommended.
- Sun exposure should be avoided until the skin completely heals in 1–2 weeks. Sun-damaged skin is more susceptible to subsequent burns.

BIBLIOGRAPHY

1. Adam JE: Sun-protective clothing. J Cutan Med Surg 3:1–4, 1998.
2. Crane LA, Schneider LS, Yohn JJ, et al: "Block the sun, not the fun": Evaluation of a skin cancer prevention program for child care centers. Am J Prev Med 17:31–37, 1999.
3. Cummings SR, Tripp MK, Herrmann NB: Approaches to the prevention and control of skin cancer. Cancer Metastasis Rev 16:309–327, 1997.

4. Gasparro FP, Mitchnick M, Nash JF: A review of sunscreen safety and efficacy. Photochem Photobiol 68:243–256, 1998.
5. Gies PH, Roy CR, Toomey S, McLenman A: Protection against solar ultraviolet radiation. Mutat Res 422:15–22, 1998.
6. Gilchrest BA, Eller MS, Geller AC, Yaar M: The pathogenesis of melanoma induced by ultraviolet radiation. N Engl J Med 340:1341–1348, 1999.
7. Lim HW, Cooper K: The health impact of solar radiation and prevention strategies. J Am Acad Dermatol 41:81–99, 1999.
8. Naylor MF, Farmer KC: The case for sunscreens: A review of their use in preventing actinic damage and neoplasia. Arch Dermatol 133:1146–1154, 1997.
9. Schauder S, Ippen H: Contact and photocontact sensitivity to sunscreens: Review of a 15-year experience and of the literature. Contact Dermatitis 37:221–232, 1997.
10. Shea CR, Prieto VG: Recent developments in the pathology of melanocytic neoplasia. Dermatol Clin 17:615–630, 1999.
11. Sunscreen Drug Products for Over-the-Counter Human Use: Final Monograph. Food and Drug Administration, Final rule. Federal Registry 64(98):27666-93, 1999.
12. Ullrich SE, Kim TH, Anamthaswamy HN, Kripke ML: Sunscreen effects on UV-induced immune suppression. J Invest Dermatol 4:65–69, 1999.
13. Weinstock MA: Do sunscreens increase or decrease melanoma risk: An epidemiologic evaluation. Invest Dermatol 4:97–100, 1999.

50. TOPICAL CORTICOSTEROIDS

John L. Aeling, M.D.

1. When were corticosteroids discovered? When were they first used therapeutically?

1935 — Discovery of compound E (cortisone)

1948 — First reported use of cortisone and ACTH in the treatment of rheumatoid arthritis

1951 — First report of cortisone and ACTH used in the treatment of inflammatory dermatoses

1952 — First report of using compound F (hydrocortisone) topically

Since the mid-1950s, there have been numerous modifications of the corticosteroid molecule, with halogenation, esterification, hydroxylation, modification of side chains, and improvements in delivery systems that have dramatically increased the anti-inflammatory activity of this topical therapy. As the potency of the molecule has increased, so have the side effects.

2. Describe the basic steroid nucleus.

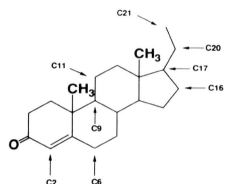

FIGURE 1. The basic steroid nucleus.

3. How is the potency of topical steroid medications determined?

The **vasoconstrictor assay** is the standard for determining the anti-inflammatory properties of topical steroid medications. The test medications are applied in serial dilutions to the forearms of volunteers for a standard length of time. Although the assay measures only one biologic function of the molecule, the amount of vasoconstriction correlates with the clinical effectiveness. The vagaries of the test can be minimized by using standardized lighting, trained observers, and large numbers of test subjects. Well-controlled clinical trials comparing topical steroid medications in different skin diseases is a better measure of efficacy, although these studies are time-consuming and expensive.

4. How many topical steroid medications are available in the United States?

The 1995 *PDR* lists 87 products available for topical use.

5. With so many products available, how do you decide which product to prescribe for your patient?

A multitude of decisions must be made each time a topical steroid is prescribed. Considerations include the disease being treated, anatomic site, patient age, vehicle, cost, amount, frequency of application, side effects, number of refills, and the specific medication.

When prescribing super-, high-, and mid-potency topical steroids, add directions to the prescription that the medication should *not* be used on the face, axilla, or groin unless otherwise recommended. It is common for patients to pass their medication to other family members or friends or save it for use on another skin problem in the future.

6. Why is the vehicle important when recommending a topical corticosteroid?

The choice of vehicle is of utmost importance when choosing a topical steroid. A steroid molecule in an ointment base will result in the most potent preparation, followed by emollients, gels, creams, lotions, solutions, and sprays. This difference in potency relates to several factors, including occlusion, bioavailability, lipid solubility, and the partition coefficient of each product.

The dilution or addition of ingredients to a proprietary product should be discouraged. This practice can affect the stability and/or bioavailability of a product. There have been reports that some generic medications have less bioavailability than their corresponding brandname products due to differences in formulations.

7. Are certain vehicles preferred for particular types or sites of lesions?

Ointments work best on chronic thickened skin lesions and should be avoided when the dermatosis is acute, vesicular, and weeping. Solutions, lotions, gels, or sprays are recommended for dermatoses in hairy areas. Creams or lotions are best for intertriginous locations. Gels and sprays can be used to treat inflammatory lesions on mucosal surfaces.

8. How are topical corticosteroids classified as to potency?

Many authors in the United States classify topical corticosteroids into seven categories of potency: 1) super potency, 2) high potency, 3) high mid-potency, 4) mid-potency, 5) low mid-potency, 6) mildly potent, and 7) low potency. The author prefers to rank them into four classes of potency.

Topical Steroid Potency*

Group I: Super potent (anti-inflammatory activity >1500)
    Clobetasol diproprionate 0.05% (Temovate)
    Betamethasone diproprionate 0.25% (Diprolene)
    Halbetasol proprionate 0.05% (Ultravate)
    Diflorasone diacetate 0.05% (Psorcon)
Group II: High potency (anti-inflammatory activity=100–500)
    Fluocinonide 0.05% (Lidex)
    Halcinonide 0.05% (Halog)
    Amcinonide 0.05% (Cyclocort)
    Desoximetasone 0.25% (Topicort)
Group III: Mid-potency (anti-inflammatory activity=10–100)
    Fluocinolone acetonide 0.01–0.2% (Synalar, Synemol, Fluonid)
    Hydrocortisone valerate 0.2% (Westcort)
    Hydrocortisone butyrate 0.1% (Locoid)
    Triamcinolone acetonide 0.01–0.5% (Kenalog, Aristocort)
    Betamethasone valerate 0.1% (Valisone)
    Clocortolone pivalate 0.1% (Cloderm)
    Flurandrenolide 0.05% (Cordran)
    Betamethasone benzoate 0.028% (Benisone, Uticort)
    Mometasone furoate 0.1% (Elocon)
    Diflorasone diacetate 0.05% (Florone, Maxiflor)
    Fluticasone proprionate 0.005% (Cutivate)
    Betamethasone diproprionate 0.005% (Maxivate)
Group IV: Low potency (anti-inflammatory activity=1–10)
    Hydrocortisone acetate 0.25–2.5% (1% is OTC; >1% is prescription)
    Desonide 0.05% (DesOwen, Tridesilon)
    Aclometasone 0.05% (Aclovate)
    Prednisolone 0.5% (Meti-Derm)
    Dexamethasone 0.1% (Decadron)
    Methylprednisolone 1% (Medrol)

---

*The individual steroid molecules can be moved up or down in the potency ranking by changing the base of the topical formulation.

9. How do topical steroids inhibit cutaneous inflammation?

The anti-inflammatory effects of topical steroids are many and complex. One of the most important actions is indirect. The steroid molecule binds to specific cytoplasmic steroid receptors and is transported to the cell nucleus, where it interacts with high-affinity binding sites on nuclear

DNA. Steroid-induced proteins, called **lipocortins,** are then synthesized by the target cells. There is good evidence that these proteins inhibit phospholipase A_2, an enzyme necessary for arachidonic acid formation. This inhibition results in the decreased formation of several potent inflammatory mediators, including protaglandins, leukotrienes, and platelet-activating factor. These proteins have also been shown to decrease vascular permeability.

The steroid molecule can bind to cell membranes, altering their function. This may be the method by which steroids cause abnormal cell adherence, reduced cell phagocytosis, and inhibited lysosomal enzyme release. Another immediate effect of topical steroids is to produce vasoconstriction, thus decreasing tissue edema, erythema, and heat. Topical steroids also produce profound effects on inflammatory cells. Polymorphonuclear leukocytes show decreased migration, phagocytosis, adherence, and numbers at sites of inflammation. Monocytes, lymphocytes, and Langerhans cells also show decreased function and numbers at sites of inflammation.

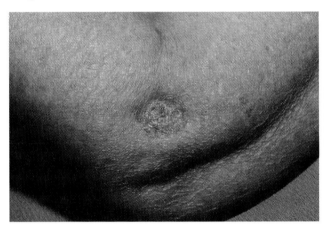

FIGURE 2. Cutaneous atrophy and slight hypopigmentation from intralesional steroids. (Courtesy of James E. Fitzpatrick, MD.)

10. What are the effects of topical steroids on the epidermis?

Thinning of the epidermis can occur within 7 days of use of superpotent topical steroids. After 3 weeks of potent topical steroid use, all layers of the epidermis are reduced in thickness by about one-half. The thinning of the epidermis, particularly the stratum corneum, impairs the barrier function of the epidermis, thus increasing transepidermal water loss and skin irritancy.

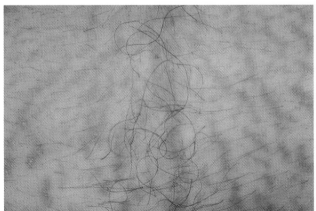

FIGURE 3. Striae associated with mid-potency topical steroid use.

11. What are the effects of topical steroids on the dermis?

Within 1–3 weeks of using superpotent topical steroids, the dermal volume is measurably reduced. This is due to decreased fibroblast production of dermal ground substance, primarily hyaluronic acid, and decreased dermal water content. After many weeks of topical steroid use, abnormal synthesis of collagen and elastin results in dermal atrophy (Fig. 2), skin fragility, striae (Fig. 3), telangiectasias, poor vascular support with skin purpura, and decreased wound healing.

12. How expensive are topical steroids?

Sales of topical steroids in the United States generate over $500 million per year. In 1994, the average retail cost for brandname topical steroids prescribed in large tubes (45–60 gm) was:

      Superpotent 86–98¢ per gm   Mid-potency 40–45¢ per gm
      High potency 65–70¢ per gm   Low potency 41–51¢ per gm

The price is even higher when smaller units are prescribed. A patient with atopic dermatitis with 50% skin involvement who is prescribed a mid-potency topical steroid to be applied twice daily for 1 month will spend $400–500.

13. Are there systemic side effects of topical steroid therapy?

With the introduction of more potent topical steroids, systemic side effects have become a very real concern. The superpotent topical steroids are over a thousand times more potent than hydrocortisone. Infants and children are more at risk for systemic side effects because they have greater surface-to-body ratio than adults and they may not be able to metabolize the steroid molecule efficiently.

Systemic side effects include suppression of the hypothalamic-pituitary-adrenal (HPA) axis, Cushing's syndrome, growth retardation, failure to thrive, cataracts, and glaucoma. Adults can show HPA axis suppression within 3–4 days of using as little as 7.5 gm of superpotent topical steroid daily. However, it is rare to see clinical Cushing's syndrome in an adult patient. Superpotent topical steroids are not recommended for children under age 12.

14. What are the local cutaneous side effects of topical steroids?

Local cutaneous side effects are the most common problem associated with topical steroids. Atrophy of the epidermis and dermis can occur quickly with potent topical steroids, especially when applied to thin-skinned or intertriginous areas, and lead to skin fragility, striae, telangiectasias, purpura, and increased skin irritability. One of the most frequent side effects is the production or aggravation of acne and acneiform skin lesions. Perioral dermatitis is frequently associated with the inappropriate use of topical steroids (Fig. 4). It occurs most commonly in adult women and is characterized by inflammatory follicular papules and pustules with a background of erythema and scaling. Most of the patients are fair-skinned Caucasians. Lesions are present on the chin, perioral, and perinasal skin, and less commonly on the eyelids. Most patients respond well to discontinuation of the topical steroid and oral antibiotics of the tetracycline class for 4–6 weeks. Some patients flare when the steroid is discontinued and some have recurrences.

Local Cutaneous Side Effects of Topical Steroids

Epidermal atrophy	Hirsutism
Steroid addiction syndrome	Perioral dermatitis
Dermal atrophy	Acne vulgaris
Striae	Acne rosacea
Purpura	Exacerbation of skin infections
Telangiectasia	Exacerbation of psoriasis
Hypopigmentation	Delayed wound healing

15. Are there really topical steroid addicts?

The topical steroid addiction syndrome is a frustrating side effect that occurs most commonly on the face or anogenital skin when high- or mid-potency topical steroids are used for several weeks, but on occasion, it can also occur with low-potency topicals. The typical patient complains of burning and stinging of involved skin with very few objective findings. Initially, the patient is treated for a mild dermatitis and responds well. However, when the topical steroid is discontinued, the symptoms quickly return and are more profound. Thus, the patient is reluctant to discontinue the steroid use despite the perpetuation of the syndrome.

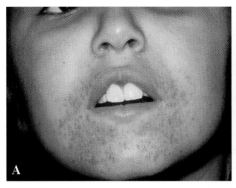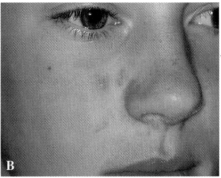

FIGURE 4. Perioral dermatitis (steroid rosacea). *A,* A prepubertal child with typical perioral dermatitis. *B,* A prepubertal child with perioral dermatitis and steroid vasoconstriction related to a mid-potency topical steroid. (Courtesy of William L. Weston, MD.)

This syndrome is due to thinning of the stratum corneum and epidermis, making the patient sensitive to irritants. Topical moisturizers, soaps, sunscreens, and makeup are poorly tolerated. The treatment is to discontinue all topical steroid medications and treat the patient with bland emollients, such as petrolatum. The patient should be warned that the symptoms will flare with the discontinuation of the steroid medication and may take weeks or even months to completely clear.

16. List some common mistakes that are made when prescribing a topical steroid.

Just as there are many decisions to be made when prescribing a topical, there are many opportunities for mistakes:

1. Prescribing too much or too little medication
2. Incorrect diagnoses
3. The condition being treated is not steroid-responsive
4. Using the medication for too long or too short a period of time
5. Recommending a product that is either too potent or too weak
6. Failure to recognize topical steroid side effects
7. Recommending the wrong vehicle
8. Use of air-tight occlusion

17. What skin diseases are not topical steroid-responsive?

Topical steroids are expensive, may have side effects, and may aggravate some skin conditions. Some skin diseases which do not respond to topical steroids or may be worsened by their use:

Acne and acneiform skin diseases	Large-vessel vasculitis
Skin infections (fungal, viral, and bacterial)	Panniculitis
Dry skin and ichthyosis	Deep granulomatous skin diseases
Pityriasis rosea	Parapsoriasis
Erythema multiforme	Pityriasis rubra pilaris
Urticaria	

18. What is tinea incognito?

The symptoms produced by tinea infections are due to the body's immune response to the offending fungal organism. Topical steroids decrease the inflammatory response to the offending organism. They initially help the symptoms associated with dermatophyte infections, but in decreasing the body's defense mechanisms, they allow the organism to proliferate. They also alter the typical clinical picture, thus delaying the correct diagnoses. Potent topical steroids have no place in the treatment of superficial fungal infections.

19. Can topical steroid medications cause contact dermatitis?

Yes. Contact dermatitis can be either irritant or allergic. **Irritant reactions** are frequent and most commonly are due to the propylene glycol content of the topical preparation. The patient complains of immediate burning or stinging after application. Irritant reactions are more common with cream bases than with ointments.

True **allergic contact dermatitis** is less frequent but more problematic. It can be due to the vehicle, preservative, fragrance, or the steroid molecule itself, and there is often cross-reactivity between steroid molecules. Allergic contact dermatitis should be suspected when a patient who has a steroid-responsive skin problem does not respond or has worsened with appropriate topical steroid therapy. Patch testing can help sort out this problem. Contact allergies are most common with hydrocortisone, budesonide, and tixocortol and are least common with betamethasone, clobetasol, mometasone, and triamcinolone.

20. Mrs. Jones brings her 9-month-old infant with moderate atopic dermatitis to your office. What topical steroid do you prescribe?

A low-potency ointment. Once-daily application on areas of active inflammation after bathing is often sufficient, and the product should not be used more than twice daily. Skin lubrication is a very important part of the treatment, and a lubricating ointment should be applied to the entire skin surface after every bath to prevent rapid evaporation and transepidermal water loss. Only low-potency steroids should be used in children under age 1.

21. A 40-year-old woman presents with a 5-year history of chronic dermatitis on her palms. What topical steroid do you prescribe?

Superpotent topical steroid. There is a big difference in absorption of topical medications based on regional skin differences. (A relative comparison of absorption differences reveals significant anatomic differences: forearm=1, back=1.7, sole=0.14, palm=0.83, scalp=3.5, cheek=13, eyelid and scrotum=42.) The medication should be used twice daily for 2 weeks with a 1-week rest period. This cycle can be repeated two or three times, and then the patient should be downgraded to a high- or mid-potency topical. Proper lubrication and hand protection from irritants is also an important part of the therapy. If the patient requires prolonged treatment with high or superpotent topical steroids, then alternate therapies such as topical tar or phototherapy should be considered.

22. A 35-year-old woman with moderate psoriasis presents with scalp, facial, and body plaque lesions. What topical steroid do you prescribe?

Often, it is necessary to prescribe more than one topical steroid for a patient. A high-potency topical steroid lotion or solution would be recommended for the scalp, a low-potency cream for the face, and a high- or superpotent ointment for the trunk and extremities. Once- or twice-daily application is recommended after a tub bath or shower and shampoo. When the psoriasis improves, the steroid can be downgraded to a lower potency product or fewer applications. Resistance to treatment (tachyphylaxis) is a common problem when treating psoriasis. Topical steroid holidays or alternate treatments, such as anthralin, tar, vitamin D analog (Dovonex), or phototherapy, should be considered for difficult chronic cases.

23. Mrs. Smith brings her 6-month-old infant with a 2-week history of diaper dermatitis to your office. What topical steroid do you prescribe? Would you recommend any other topical therapy?

For the diaper area, use only a low-potency topical steroid applied three times daily for no more than 7–10 days. The diaper area has air-tight occlusion, and any mid- or high-potency topical steroid can cause skin atrophy, striae, ulceration, aggravation of secondary bacterial infections, suppression of the HPA axis, and **granuloma gluteale** (a condition characterized by persistent reddish-purple nodules and plaques in the diaper area). Although the exact etiology of granuloma gluteale is debated, most agree that the inappropriate use of topical steroids and secondary candidiasis play important roles. Any diaper dermatitis that has persisted >3 days should be treated for secondary candidial infection.

24. How much topical steroid should you prescribe?

Topical medications are frequently under- or over-prescribed. One rule of thumb is that 1 gm of medication will treat four adult palm sizes. One palm size represents slightly less than 1% of adult skin surface area. It takes 30–45 gm of medication to treat the entire skin surface area (twice-daily [BID] application for 2 weeks = 840–1260 gm); 1 gm will treat the hands, scalp, face, and groin (BID application for 2 weeks = 60 gm); 3 gm will treat the arm or half the trunk (BID application for 2 weeks = 80 gm); and 4 gm will treat one leg (BID application for 2 weeks = 120 gm).

25. Your patient needs instruction on how much topical medication to apply. How can you instruct this patient?

There are numerous studies showing great variability and compliance problems when patients are treated with topical medications. Often, the patient is given a prescription or a few office samples and told, "We'll see you in 2 weeks."

It is very helpful for the physician or nurse to actually demonstrate on the patient how much medication to apply and the proper way to apply it. An excellent guideline for using topical medications is the **fingertip** unit. This is the amount of medication expressed from a tube with a 5-mm opening that extends from the tip of the index finger to the first joint on the palmar aspect of the finger. One fingertip unit equals 0.5 gm of medication and will treat two palm sizes in the average adult.

The Fingertip Unit*

Groin or hand	1 FTU	0.5 gm
Face or foot	2 FTU	1.0 gm
One arm	3 FTU	1.5 gm
One leg	6 FTU	3.0 gm
Trunk, front and back	14 FTU	7.0 gm

*One fingertip unit (FTU) will cover two palm sizes.

26. Is perioral dermatitis common in prepubertal children?

Yes. A retrospective review done at the University of Colorado over an 8-year period (1991–1998) evaluated 106 children (46 boys and 60 girls) under age 13 with perioral dermatitis, 29 of whom were under age 3. The mean age of onset was 7.04 years. A family history of rosacea was found in 20% of cases. Many authors use the term steroid rosacea when the eruption is triggered or aggravated by topical steroids. After abruptly stopping topical steroids and instituting oral erythromycin, 86% cleared within 4 weeks and 100% cleared by 8 weeks. Surprisingly, 54% of patients developed lesions while using the lowest-potency preparations, including 1% hydrocortisone. This finding contradicts the strategy that recommends tapering the patient off topical steroid medications. Only 3% of patients were using a superpotent product. Perinasal lesions were seen in 95%, perioral in 99%, and lower eyelids were involved in 44% of patients.

BIBLIOGRAPHY

1. Bode HH: Dwarfism following long-term topical steroid therapy. JAMA 244:364–370, 1980.
2. Cornell RC, Stoughton RB: Correlation of the vasoconstrictor assay and clinical activity. Arch Dermatol 121:63–67, 1985.
3. Finlay AY, Averill RW: The rule of hand: 4 hand areas = 2 FTU = 1 gm. Arch Dermatol 128:1129, 1992.
4. Hepburn D, Aeling JL, Weston WL: A reappraisal of topical steroid potency. Pediatr Dermatol 13:239–245, 1996.
5. Kligman AM: Topical steroid addicts. JAMA 235:1550, 1976.
6. Lepoittevin JP, Drieghe J, Dooms-Goossens A: Studies in patients with corticosteroid contact allergy. Arch Dermatol 131:31–37, 1995.
7. Olsen EA, Cornell RC: Topical clobetasol-17-proprionate: A review of its clinical efficacy and safety. J Am Acad Dermatol 15:246–255, 1986.
8. Stoughton RB: Are generic formulations equivalent to trade name topical glucocorticoids? Arch Dermatol 123:1312–1314, 1987.
9. Thompson EB: The structure of the human glucocorticoid receptor and its gene. J Steroid Biochem 27:911–919, 1977.
10. Weston WL, Fennessey PV, Morelli J, et al: Comparison of hypothalamus-pituitary-adrenal axis suppression from superpotent topical steroids by standard endocrine function testing and gas chromatography mass spectrometry. J Invest Dermatol 90:532–535, 1988.
11. Weston WL, Morelli JG: Steroid rosacea in prepubertal children. Arch Pediatr Adolesc Med 154:62–64, 2000.
12. Yohn JJ, Weston WL: Topical glucocorticosteroids. Curr Probl Dermatol 2:31–63, 1990.

51. CRYOSURGERY

Milton J. Schleve, M.D.

1. What is cryosurgery?

It's probably easiest to think of cryosurgery as controlled frostbite. A light touch of frostbite may produce a little pain, the skin gets red and swells, and fine desquamation develops within several days. With a deeper freeze, blisters are produced. Prolonged exposure to freezing conditions may result in the loss of fingers and toes. With cryosurgery, specific areas are necrosed and also the degree of necrosis is controlled.

2. Who uses cryosurgery?

A variety of physicians. It has applications in neurosurgery, oncology, gynecology, urology, and ophthalmology.

3. How does cryosurgery cause injury?

Freezing causes intracellular and extracellular ice crystals to form and the vascular stasis causes tissue anoxia and necrosis. The most efficient technique employs a rapid freeze and slow thawing. Multiple shorter freezes produce more damage than a longer freeze.

4. Which agents are used for cryosurgery?

Most cryosurgeons use liquid nitrogen. It is readily available, inexpensive, easy to store, and easy to use, and it works quickly. Less commonly used cryogens are Freon 12, Freon 22, solid CO_2, liquid N_2O (nitrous oxide), and liquid helium.

Because a colder cryogen causes deeper destruction, the Freons, solid CO_2, and nitrous oxide are used only for topical anesthesia and superficial destruction. Liquid nitrogen is the only agent that is reliable for deeper destruction.

Cryogens used in Cryosurgery

CRYOGEN	BOILING POINT (°C)
Liquid nitrogen	−195.8
Nitrous oxide, liquid	−89.5
Carbon dioxide, solid	−78.5
Chlorodifluoromethane (Freon 22)	−40.8
Dichlorofluoromethane (Freon 12)	−27.8
Dichlorotrifluoroethane (Freon 114)	3.8

5. Do you need a lot of expensive equipment to use cryosurgery?

No. Compared to other surgical techniques, the amount of equipment needed is modest. First, you need a reservoir for the liquid nitrogen. This is normally a 20–30-liter thermos (Dewar flask). From here, the liquid nitrogen (LN_2) is transferred to smaller containers.

For basic cryosurgery, you might only use various-sized cotton swabs to apply the LN_2. Most dermatologists use small, hand-held thermoses that spray the LN_2 directly on the skin. There are also various probes, neoprene cones, and thermocouple-pyrometer systems to treat malignant lesions.

6. What can you treat with cryosurgery?

Both benign and malignant lesions can be treated by cryosurgery. The most common lesions are warts, actinic keratoses, seborrheic keratoses, and molluscum contagiosum. Cryosurgery can be used for skin resurfacing.

Benign Lesions Treatable by Cryosurgery

Acne	Lentigo simplex
Actinic cheilitis	Molluscum contagiosum
Actinic keratosis	Myxoid cyst
Angioma	Pyogenic granuloma
Chondrodermatitis nodularis helicis	Sebaceous hyperplasia
Dermatofibroma	Seborrheic keratosis
Genital warts	Warts
Hypertrophic scar	Keloid

Malignant Lesions Requiring Monitoring During Cryosurgery

Basal cell carcinoma	Keratoacanthoma
Bowen's disease	Lentigo maligna
Kaposi's sarcoma	Metastatic skin lesions (palliative)
Squamous cell carcinoma	

7. How is cryosurgery accomplished?

There are several ways to apply cryogens. Various sizes of **swabs** can be dipped in LN_2 and touched to the lesion to freeze it. With a larger swab, there is more cryogen and the effects are faster and deeper. Swabs are not used to treat malignancies. It is best to use a separate swab and cup of cryogen for each patient to avoid cross-contamination.

The **spray** technique uses modified thermoses that allow the LN_2 to spray out of a nozzle. The degree of freezing is changed by the nozzle size, the pressure in the thermos, the distance to the lesion, and, of course, the length of freeze. This apparatus can be used for several hours, and contamination is not an issue. It also can treat very large lesions. A modification of this technique is to use neoprene cones to confine the LN_2, causing a more concentrated freeze.

Some cryosurgeons use **probes** for freezing. A probe is a metal object that is cooled by the cryogen and applied to the lesion. The probe is usually the size of the lesion, but it can be applied multiple times for larger lesions. A probe can vary from a diameter of a few millimeters to a hollow brass door knob. The disadvantages are that it is slower than the spray technique, a variety of sizes and shapes of probes are needed, and contamination can occur.

8. How are benign skin lesions treated?

The basic concept of all cryosurgery is that the amount of freezing beyond the lesion (lateral spread of freeze) is equal to the depth of freeze. Freezing 1–2 mm beyond the lesion will give a wound 1–2 mm deep, which is adequate for most benign lesions. Warts can be deeper, so either a deeper freeze or multiple smaller freezes can be used. Thick seborrheic keratoses can be frozen lightly and quickly curetted. For benign lesions, you do not want to cause a scar, so it is always better to undertreat until you are experienced.

9. How do you treat malignant lesions?

In treating cancers, we need to be very sure we treat them adequately. Most importantly, you should be able to clinically identify the margins of the lesion. Second, you must know the histology of the cancer to be sure cryosurgery is appropriate. Third, you must have equipment that ensures you reach a temperature of -50 to $-60°C$ beyond the peripheral extent and depth of the cancer. Many cryosurgeons use a second treatment to ensure tumor killing. Some cryosurgeons curette or shave tumors first to delineate and debulk the lesion.

The treatment of cutaneous cancers by cryosurgery is not accepted by all dermatologists. In general, surgically oriented dermatologists feel that the demonstration of negative surgical margins is preferrable to cryosurgery for significant cancers. Cryosurgeons argue that the cure rates achieved by cryosurgery are comparable to those of other surgical modalities, especially when margins of the tumor can be identified.

10. What are the cure rates of cryosurgery for malignant lesions?

Experienced cryosurgeons who treat many skin cancers report cure rates of 95–98% for primary basal cell carcinomas. These rates are comparable to those in surgery and radiation therapy. The cure rates using cryosurgery, radiation therapy, or excisional surgery for aggressive or recurrent skin cancers are significantly worse. In these cases, Mohs micrographic surgery is often recommended.

11. Are there contraindications to cryosurgery?

People with cold-related conditions, such as cryoglobulinemia, cryofibrinogenemia, cold urticaria, and Raynaud's disease, should not be treated with cryosurgery. Patients with heavily pigmented skin should be treated with caution since they are more likely to heal with hyperpigmented or hypopigmented scars.

12. For which patients is cryosurgery better than other methods?

Cryosurgery can be used for patients with bleeding disorders and in elderly patients in nursing homes. It avoids cross-contamination in patients with warts, hepatitis, and HIV.

13. What are the complications of cryosurgery?

After using cryosurgery, the wound is allowed to heal by itself (second intention). A normal cryosurgery wound can blister, ooze, form an eschar, and take 1–6 weeks to heal. Complications are uncommon and include infection, hypertrophic scars, nerve damage, and unacceptable scars.

BIBLIOGRAPHY

1. Dufresne RG Jr, Curlin MU: Actinic cheilitis: A treatment review. Dermatol Surg 23:15–21, 1997.
2. Fewkes JL, Cheney ML, Pollack SV: Cryosurgery. In Illustrated Atlas of Cutaneous Surgery. New York, Gower Medical Publishing, 1992.
3. Gage AA: History of cryosurgery. Semin Surg Oncol 14:99–109, 1998.
4. Gage AA, Baust J: Mechanisms of tissue injury in cryosurgery. Cryobiology 37:171–186, 1998.
5. Goncalves JC: Fractional cryosurgery: A new technique for basal cell carcinoma of the eyelids and periorbital area. Dermatol Surg 23:475–481, 1997.
6. Graham GF: Cryosurgery. Clin Plastic Surg 20:131–147, 1993.
7. Graham GF: Cryosurgery for benign, premalignant, and malignant lesions. In Wheeland RG (ed): Cutaneous Surgery. Philadelphia, W.B. Saunders, 1994.
8. Hocutt JE Jr: Skin cryosurgery for the family physician. Am Fam Physician 48(3): 445–452, 455–456, 1993.
9. Jester DM: Office procedures: Cryotherapy of dermal abnormalities. Prim Care 24:269–280, 1997.
10. Kuflik EG: Cryosurgery for cutaneous malignancy: An update. Dermatol Surg 23:1081–1087, 1997.
11. Kuflik EG, Gage AA: Cryosurgical Treatment for Skin Cancer. New York, Igaku-Shoin, 1990.
12. Sinclair RD, Dawber RP: Cryosurgery of malignant and premalignant diseases of the skin: A simple approach. Australas J Dermatol 36:133–142, 1995.
13. Torre D, Lubritz RR, Kuflik EG: Practical Cutaneous Cryosurgery. Norwalk, CT, Appleton & Lange, 1988.
14. Young R, Sinclair R: Practical cryosurgery. Aust Fam Physician 26:1045–1047, 1997.

52. MOHS SURGERY

J. Ramsey Mellette, M.D., and John G. LeVasseur, M.D., MAJ, MC, USAF

1. What is Mohs surgery?

In 1936 Dr. Frederic Mohs of the University of Wisconsin developed a precise method to remove cancers that became known as Mohs "chemosurgery." His technique provided controlled, serial, microscopic examination of tissue that had been chemically fixed applying zinc chloride paste directly to the tumor. The excised tissue was systematically mapped and examined by means of frozen sections. These steps were repeated in the areas demonstrated to be cancerous until a complete tumor-free plane was reached. The goals of Mohs surgery are to completely remove the tumor and maximize tissue conservation.

2. Is Mohs surgery still performed with the zinc chloride chemical paste?

Rarely! The technique has evolved to use fresh tissue methods. Frozen sections of fresh tissue effectively eliminate the need for zinc chloride paste.

3. When is Mohs surgery indicated?

Mohs micrographic surgery is now recognized as the more precise method of removing skin cancer. It is especially effective in treating **basal cell and squamous cell carcinomas of the face** and other cosmetically sensitive areas, because it can eliminate the cancer while sparing surrounding normal skin. It is also ideal for the removal of **recurrent skin cancers.** In these tumors, cancer cells persist in areas of scar tissue, and the clinical margins of the recurrent tumor are often indistinct. With the Mohs technique, all tumor nests can be identified and removed with a high degree of accuracy. Cure rates are 99% for primary basal cell cancers and 95% for recurrent tumors.

Other considerations in choosing Mohs surgery include:

1. Basal cell carcinomas with aggressive or elusive histopathologic features, such as morpheaform or sclerotic (desmoplastic), micronodular, multicentric, and infiltrating. These subtypes often extend beyond visualized margins.

2. Excessively large or deeply invasive cancers.

3. Primary basal cell or squamous cell carcinomas with poorly defined borders and in locations known to have high recurrence rates (nasolabial fold, nasal ala, medial canthus, pinna, and postauricular sulcus).

4. Any basal cell or squamous cell carcinoma within an orifice, such as nostrils or ear canals.

5. Any location where maximum preservation of normal tissue is paramount (e.g., nasal tip, nasal ala, lips, eyelids, ears, genitalia, fingers).

6. Tumors with positive margins after standard excision.

7. Tumors arising in immunosuppressed patients.

8. Less common contiguous tumors such as dermatofibrosarcoma protuberans and microcystic adnexal carcinoma.

4. Is Mohs surgery appropriate for all basal and squamous cell carcinomas?

Basal and squamous cell carcinomas are epidemic in the United States, with recent estimates of over 1 million cases per year. Standard treatments, including excisional surgery, electrodessication and curettage, cryosurgery, and radiation therapy, have cure rates in selected series near 90%. Mohs surgery may be time-consuming and more expensive because it requires special training and expertise. The procedure usually should be limited to indications outlined in question 3.

5. How is Mohs micrographic surgery performed today?

The first step is debulking of the cancer with curette or scalpel. A saucer-shaped piece of tissue is then excised from the cancerous area by beveling the surgical blade at about a 45° angle. This is in contrast to traditional surgical techniques in which the incision is made perpendicular

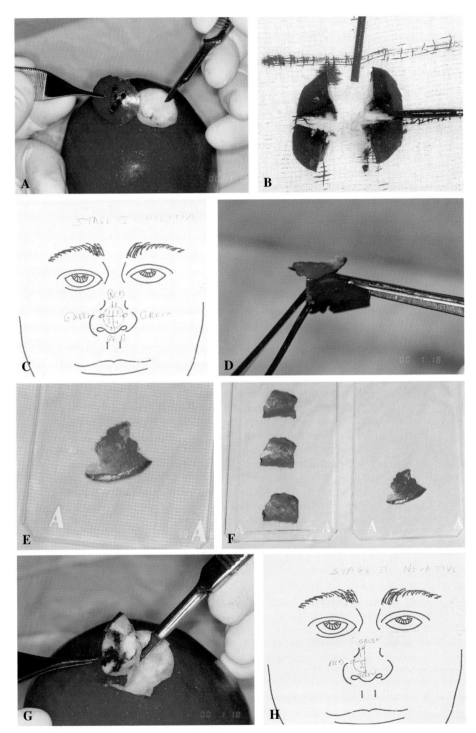

FIGURE 1. Apple model with tumor. *A*, Cancerous tissue is excised with blade beveled. *B*, Tissue is sectioned and color-coded. *C*, Anatomic map is labeled. *D–F*, Horizontal frozen sections are obtained to allow examination of the entire excision margin. *G–H*, Residual tumor is excised until the margins are clear.

to the skin. The specimen is then cut into pieces as if a pie. These slices are color-coded and placed in a petri dish. Using an anatomic cartoon representation of the site, a map is drawn to precisely label the area from which the tumor is taken. The tissue is then submitted to the Mohs histotechnician, who prepares frozen tissue sections under the supervision of the Mohs surgeon. These sections are obtained by cutting the undersurface in a horizontal plane so that the depth and most peripheral skin edge will be available for microscopic examination. Theoretically, 100% of the margin is examined, in contrast to routine histologic processes. If tumor is identified, the map is used as a guide to obtain additional tissue layers until a tumor-free plane is reached. Various steps of the procedure are illustrated in Figure 1 using an apple model.

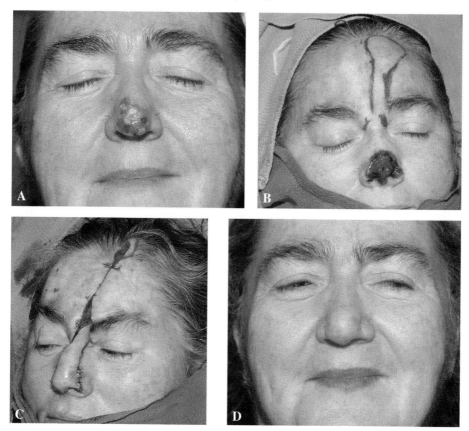

FIGURE 2. *A,* Preoperative basal cell carcinoma of the nasal tip. *B,* Defect of the nose following Mohs micrographic surgery. Paramedian forehead flap designed. Note preservation of cartilaginous skeleton. *C,* Paramedian forehead flap attached to reconstruct the nose. Forehead defect is closed. Pedicle is divided at 2 weeks. *D,* Long-term result.

6. Where is Mohs micrographic surgery performed?

It is usually performed in an **outpatient facility** under local anesthesia. Surgery begins early in the morning and is finished the same day unless the tumor is unusually extensive. In extreme cases with deeply invasive tumors, the Mohs surgeon may choose to have at least some of the Mohs procedure performed in an operating room under general anesthesia.

7. Is Mohs micrographic surgery time-consuming?

It often is. Because the Mohs technique is usually applied to problematic tumors, several stages may be required. Each step from the layer-by-layer removal to the laboratory preparation and examination under the microscope is delicate and requires precision.

8. Is the patient required to stay in the surgery suite between stages of Mohs surgery?

No. The wound is covered with a temporary dressing and the patient is placed in a comfortable waiting room area. The average waiting time between stages is approximately 1 hour, so patients are instructed to bring reading material, knitting, or other hobbies to help pass the time.

9. How extensive are scars after Mohs surgery?

The precision of Mohs surgery allows for maximum preservation of tissue, often resulting in smaller defects requiring less complex reconstruction (Fig. 2). Also, Mohs surgeons, especially those who have served fellowships, are well-trained and experienced in aesthetic reconstruction.

10. Who performs Mohs surgery?

The American College of Mohs Micrographic Surgery and Cutaneous Oncology currently recognizes about 50 training centers in the United States where qualified applicants receive comprehensive training in Mohs micrographic surgery. The period of training is 1–2 years, during which time the dermatologist acquires extensive experience with all aspects of the technique. Once training is completed, the physician becomes eligible for membership in the College.

Many dermatologists know the basic techniques and employ them in their practices. However, when patients require more extensive surgery, they usually are referred to a member of the College.

BIBLIOGRAPHY

1. Gross KG, Steinman HK, Rapini RP: Mohs Surgery Fundamentals and Techniques. St. Louis, Mosby, 1999.
2. Mikhail GR: Mohs Micrographic Surgery. Philadelphia, W.B. Saunders, 1991.
3. Shriner DL, McCoy DK, Goldberg DJ, Wagner RF Jr: Mohs micrographic surgery. J Am Acad Dermatol 39:79–97, 1998.

53. LASERS IN DERMATOLOGY

Stephen W. Eubanks, M.D.

1. What does the term *laser* stand for?

LASER is an acronym for **L**ight **A**mplification by **S**timulated **E**mission of **R**adiation.

2. What does "stimulated emission of radiation" mean?

In order to understand laser physics, one must first look at some basics of quantum mechanics. All atoms have electrons circling the nucleus in well-defined orbits. The electrons are usually stable in these orbits and seldom move between levels. The exceptions are the outermost electrons, which may move between the orbits by adding or subtracting distinct amounts of energy. This energy is usually in the form of a photon of light.

Stimulated absorption occurs when a single photon of light enters an atom and energizes a single electron to move into a higher orbit. The new electron is somewhat unstable at this new energy level and has a tendency to fall back to its resting state. **Spontaneous emission** occurs when that excited electron spontaneously falls back to the resting orbit, releasing a photon of light from the atom. The energy of this photon is equal to the energy difference between the two electron orbits.

While these two concepts appear to be simple, the concept basic to laser light may not be as straightforward. **Stimulated emission** takes place in the unnatural state of **population inversion.** This is a population where more atoms have excited electrons than have resting electrons. The difficulty of designing a laser system is to establish a medium in which many electrons are excited but still possess overall stability. Stimulated emission involves a photon of light entering an atom with an excited electron, and this electron actually falls to a lower orbit and two identical photons leave the system. These two photons are then able to enter two other atoms with excited electrons, allowing for rapid multiplication of photons in a process similar to a chain reaction. All of the generated photons are identical. This process accounts for the **S**timulated **E**mission of **R**adiation used in the acronym LASER.

3. How is the light amplified in the laser system?

The laser system uses an **optical resonator** to amplify and orient the light. This is a cylindrical chamber filled with the laser medium, with mirrors on each end and an absorptive lining. The photons of light are reflected between the mirrors, and the lining will absorb any light that is not perfectly parallel. These parallel photons continue to enter additional atoms, producing more photons by stimulated emission. By this process the laser **L**ight is **A**mplified. One end of the optical resonator has a mechanism to release the light periodically from the chamber.

4. What types of medium are used in laser systems?

The ability of an atom to be used in a laser system is a complicated function of quantum mechanics and the physical characteristics of the lattice in which it is constructed. The basic component of any medium is to be able to support a population inversion so that there may be stimulated emission.

Solids	**Ruby crystal:** composed of aluminum oxide [Al_3O_2] with scattered atoms of chromium [Cr] replacing some aluminum atoms in the crystal lattice
	Nd:YAG: (neodymium:yttrium-aluminum-garnet) with scattered atoms of neodymium replacing some yttrium atoms in the crystal lattice
	Er:YAG: (erbium:yttrium-aluminum-garnet) with scattered atoms of erbium replacing some yttrium atoms in the crystal lattice
Gases	Carbon dioxide (CO_2)
	Argon (Ar)
	Copper (Cu) vapor
Dyes	Fluorescent liquid dye (often rhodamine)
Other	Electrical diodes

5. What are the special features of laser light?

Laser light is unique because of three inherent features:

1. **Coherence.** There are two types of coherence, spatial and temporal. Spatial coherence is the property that represents a uniform wave front—i.e., the peaks and valleys of the waves are aligned as the light exits the laser, which allows the light to be in phase and focused to very small areas.

2. **Monochromaticity** (temporal coherence). This means all light waves have the same wavelength. Some lasers produce more than one wavelength of light, but these are predictable and the laser still produces only those specific wavelengths of light expected by the laser medium used.

3. **Collimation.** This means that all of the light exiting the laser is parallel and will not diffuse over distances.

6. Why is it helpful that laser light is monochromatic?

Many lasers target specific chromophores, which are biological structures with a specific absorption spectrum. This may be a relatively large structure such as a blood vessel, the hemoglobin within the red blood cell, or a specific subcellular organelle such as a melanosome. The **absorption spectrum** is the amount of light absorbed at various wavelengths. The idea is to match a peak absorption wavelength with the wavelength of the laser.

A good example is the laser targeting of hemoglobin, the primary absorptive entity within the blood found in target vessels of telangiectasias or port-wine stains. Oxyhemoglobin has large absorptive peaks at 488 and 517 nm, and there are small absorptive peaks at 550 nm and 585 nm. Logic would suggest targeting at lower wavelengths of 488 or 517 nm, but there is heavy absorption by melanin at these wavelengths. Therefore, a smaller but less "competitive" absorptive wavelength of 585 is more effective in treating blood and vascular lesions.

7. What is selective photothermolysis?

This incorporates the specific absorption chromophore of the target tissue and the duration of the laser pulse. The theory of selective photothermolysis assumes the laser light will pass through tissue until it targets the specific chromophore with an absorption spectrum corresponding to the wavelength of the laser. The target then absorbs the light, generating the heat in the target tissue.

The determination of the necessary amount of time the laser should operate to destroy the target but not the surrounding tissue involves the concept of **thermal relaxation**. Thermal relaxation is the amount of time necessary for 50% of the peak heat to diffuse out of the target. Each microscopic chromophore and each vessel have a specific thermal relaxation time. It is important for a laser to not exceed the thermal relaxation time or the heat will diffuse out into surrounding tissue, causing damage and possibly scarring.

8. What is the wave mode of a laser?

Lasers are either pulsed or continuous wave. **Pulsed light** is generated in a set of surges separated by some distinct amount of time. This time varies from 1 nsec to 300 μsec. Other laser light is generated **continuously,** and the laser mechanics must chop the light into smaller segments. As a rule, the continuous wave lasers have more of a potential to nonselectively heat the target and may cause scarring and damage to surrounding tissue.

9. What is Q-switching?

Q-switching is a way of obtaining short, powerful pulses of laser radiation. The Q refers to the **quality factor** of the optical resonator. A high-Q cavity in the optical resonator is one with a low energy loss, whereas a cavity with a high loss has a low Q. Q-switching refers to the abrupt change in the cavity loss.

To envision what this may do in a laser system, think of pumping energy into a laser medium where the loss is high. Laser action is precluded even when there is high-energy input to the system because the energy is "lost." If the loss is suddenly decreased in the face of the high-energy input there is a rapid growth of laser intensity within the cavity. A short, intense pulse is generated. This pulse could be as short as 10^{-7}–10^{-8} seconds. It is far quicker to change the "loss" of the system than to change the energy input. There are a variety of methods to Q-switching using mirrors, electro-optical switches, or absorbing devices.

10. How are the types of dermatologic lasers classified?

Dividing the lasers by their function is the most effective method of separating the lasers in a useful, fairly easy to remember format.

Lasers to resurface the skin	Carbon dioxide laser
	Erbium:YAG laser
Lasers to remove vascular lesions	Argon laser
	Krypton laser
	Flashlamp-pulsed dye laser
	Nd:YAG laser
	KTP laser
Lasers to remove pigmented lesions	Flashlamp-pulsed dye pigment lesion laser
	Green light copper vapor laser
	Green krypton laser
	Frequency-doubled Q-switched Nd:YAG laser
Lasers to remove hair	Nd:YAG laser
	Long-pulse Ruby laser
	Long-pulse alexandrite laser
Lasers to remove tattoos	Q-switched ruby laser
	Q-switched alexandrite laser
	Q-switched Nd:YAG laser

RESURFACING LASERS

11. Discuss the basic features and operation of the carbon dioxide laser.

The CO_2 laser has often been thought of as the dermatologist's laser due to low cost, office-based location, and wide variety of dermatologic uses. The CO_2 laser emits radiation at 10,600 nm, in the far-infrared region. All water in tissue absorbs this wavelength of light, and this absorption is not dependent on selective absorption by any biologic tissue. As the water absorbs energy, the temperature rapidly rises, vaporizing the tissue. The amount of tissue damage is related to the energy setting and the amount of time the laser impacts on the target.

The standard delivery system for the CO_2 laser is an articulated arm, which comprises a series of rigid tubes with mirrored joints capable of rotating in all directions. The light CO_2 laser is invisible and therefore must use a helium-neon laser as an aiming beam. The CO_2 laser operates in a range between 1–30 W of power. The mechanical pulses are set between 0.01–0.1 seconds, but the laser may also operate in a continuous wave mode. CO_2 lasers are usually used in either a focused or defocused mode, the former for high intensity use such as cutting and the latter for low-power destructive uses.

The new super-pulser and ultra-pulsed CO_2 lasers have powers up to 60 Watts and pulse duration in the range of 250 μsec and 1 msec.

Carbon Dioxide Laser

10,600 nm (far-infrared spectrum)	Surgical cutting
Energy absorbed by water	Low cost
General tissue vaporization	

12. What are some uses for the standard carbon dioxide laser?

Warts, xanthelasma, digital mucous cysts, leukoplakia, other premalignant lesions of lips, and surgical cutting. In the **defocused mode**, a variety of benign lesions of the skin may be removed. Treatment of warts has been the hallmark of CO_2 laser therapy. Large plantar and periungual warts are effectively treated, but the overall cure rate with CO_2 laser is not better than with more standard aggressive approaches. The main advantage of CO_2 laser treatment in these larger warts is the ability to decrease the bleeding during the laser excision and a slight decrease in scarring.

CO_2 laser in a **high-power focused mode** is very effective at surgical cutting, especially in patients on anticoagulants or those with other bleeding disorders.

13. How is CO_2 laser used for resurfacing?

The ultra-pulsed CO_2 laser effectively removes the top layers of the epidermis and causes collagen contraction in the superficial dermis. This combination of effects allows for the treatment of moderate facial wrinkles and sun damage. This treatment is often performed with the patient under conscious sedation. A variety of dressings have been proposed for the postoperative care, but hydrogel dressings such as Vigilon and SecondSkin are very effective. It may take up to 2 weeks before the surface has resurfaced with new, smoother skin.

14. Are there side effects of CO_2 laser resurfacing?

The initial risks are those of infection. Both bacteria and herpes simplex are potential risks that must be treated both pre- and postoperatively in all patients. Scarring is a risk if too much energy is used. Late-onset hypopigmentation is a fairly common and very serious risk with CO_2 laser. Postoperative erythema is common but usually resolves with time.

15. Are there hazards with the CO_2 laser?

The main precaution with the CO_2 laser is smoke evacuation. During the procedure, the laser generates a large amount of smoke that may harbor viral particles. A recent study has demonstrated an apparent increased incidence of nasopharyngeal warts in CO_2 laser surgeons, who probably acquire infection by inhalation of the laser plume. Other studies have suggested the presence of live viral particles or genetic material of both hepatitis viruses and HIV. Adequate vacuum devices and surgical masks are a must for use with this laser. The CO_2 laser will also burn any cloth or paper that it contacts; therefore, appropriate fire precautions must be observed. Clear plastic or glass eyewear is adequate to protect the eyes from this wavelength of laser light.

16. Discuss the basic features and operation of the erbium:YAG laser.

The erbium:YAG laser has some of the atoms of yttrium replaced with erbium atoms. This laser output is at 2490 nm. This wavelength is absorbed by water ten times better than the 10,600 nm light of CO_2 lasers. This more efficient effect leads to little collateral damage surrounding collagen and more efficient actual ablation of tissue. The clinical result is less effect on wrinkles but a smoother, faster-healing resurfacing procedure. By itself, erbium:YAG laser has been used to treat mild facial sun damage, some sun damage on necks and hands, and acne scarring. The latter uses the ability of the laser to plane down the edges of acne scars.

17. What are the risks of erbium:YAG laser resurfacing?

There is still a risk of bacterial or herpes simplex infection. The risks of scarring and hypopigmentation are reduced with this laser.

18. How are the resurfacing lasers now used in clinical practice?

Most practitioners now use a combination of the CO_2 and the erbium:YAG laser to perform a resurfacing procedure. The first passes over the face are made with the CO_2 laser for most of the epidermal removal and some of the collagen contraction. The erbium:YAG laser is then used to smooth out the surface. The healing is faster and it appears that side effects are lessened.

VASCULAR LESION LASERS

19. Which lasers are used to treat vascular lesions?

Vascular Lesion Lasers

LASER TYPE	WAVELENGTH	USE
Argon	488 nm, 514 nm	Telangiectasias, venous lesions, thick port-wine stains
Krypton, yellow	568 nm	Telangiectasias, thick port-wine stains
Copper vapor, yellow	578 nm	Telangiectasias, thick port-wine stains
Argon-pumped tunable dye	585–690 nm	Telangiectasias, thick port-wine stains
Flashlamp pulsed dye	585 nm	Telangiectasias, thin port-wine stains, especially in children, leg veins
Long-pulsed Nd:YAG	1064 nm	Leg veins
Long-pulsed KTP	532 nm	Facial telangiectasias, leg veins

20. What is the major disadvantage of the argon laser?

The argon laser was one of the first lasers to attempt to match a particular wavelength to a target tissue. The argon laser emits six wavelengths of light, but >80% is within the bands of 488 nm (blue) and 514.5 nm (green). These wavelengths correspond to a large absorption peak of oxyhemoglobin, but melanin also absorbs heavily in this range. In clinical applications, the melanin in the epidermis often heats up and causes epidermal damage while the dermal vascular target is being treated. Using the power necessary to destroy the deeper target may lead to scarring of the surface levels. This has dramatically curtailed the usefulness of the argon laser, and the newer, more selective lasers have replaced it.

Argon Laser

488 nm (blue) and 514.5 nm (green)
Continuous mode
Absorbed by oxyhemoglobin and melanin
Used to treat venous lesions and some thick port-wine stains
Mostly replaced by newer lasers
Moderate cost

21. Are there any advantages to using the argon laser?

At one time, the lower cost of the argon laser was attractive, but the newer pulsed dye lasers are making this less of an issue. Argon lasers are useful for vascular lesions with larger diameter vessels, such as venous lakes of the lips, and hypertrophied vascular nodules found in mature port-wine stains.

22. Discuss the krypton lasers.

Krypton Laser

520-nm (green) and 568-nm (yellow) wavelengths
Continuous-mode, thermal laser
Operates similar to photothermolysis
Green for epidermal pigmentation, yellow for thick vascular lesions
Problem with heat production
Low cost

The biggest problem with the krypton laser is scatter and heating of the surface. Cooling of the skin prior to and during the procedure is recommended. Because of the wavelength and the continuous-wave nature of this laser, it is more effective on larger-diameter vessels, such as those found in adult port-wine stains. In most cases this laser has been replaced by either pulsed dye or KTP lasers.

23. Describe the copper vapor laser.

Copper vapor lasers are continuous-wave thermal lasers that use electrical energy to heat metallic copper in a neon gas to the point that the metal vaporizes. The copper generates dual wavelengths of 511 nm (green light) and 578 nm (yellow light). A simple filter is switched to emit one or the other wavelength of light. The green light is used to treat pigmented lesions, and the yellow light to treat vascular lesions. The lasers have a high output with a very short pulse duration in the range of 20–30 nsec. In order to achieve the necessary energy levels to damage the target vessels, the laser is gated mechanically into "larger" pulses between 10 msec and 1 sec. The copper vapor laser has a small spot size of 0.7 mm that increases the treatment time unless used with a scanner, which is a computerized delivery device allowing the laser to automatically scan over and treat a large area more quickly and accurately than manual applications.

Copper Vapor Laser

511-nm (green) and 578-nm (yellow) wavelengths
Continuous-mode, thermal laser
Operates similar to photothermolysis
Green light good for epidermal pigmentation
Yellow light good for moderately thin port-wine stains
Good facial telangiectasias
Moderately expensive

24. How is the copper vapor laser used to treat vascular lesions?

Although the copper vapor laser is a continuous-wave thermal laser, it still operates on the same concept of selective photothermolysis. The 578-nm light is absorbed selectively by the oxyhemoglobin within small vessels. Even though the physics are different when contrasted to the pulsed dye laser, this laser compares well in effectiveness.

The major advantages of the copper vapor lasers are the lack of post-treatment purpura and larger diameter, deeper vessels that may be treated. Since the copper vapor laser has an effective pulse duration of 10 msec and 1 sec, there is usually more surrounding tissue damage than with the shorter-duration pulsed dye lasers, leading to some scarring and post-inflammatory hyperpigmentation. In most cases this laser has been replaced by either pulsed dye or KTP lasers.

25. What are the main features of the argon-pumped tunable dye laser?

Argon-Pumped Tunable Dye Laser

577 nm or 585 nm (yellow light)
Continuous mode, thermal laser
Treatment of port-wine stains
Small spot size is a problem
Moderate cost

26. What are pulsed dye lasers?

The various lasers that are "pulsed" use a variety of techniques to generate the laser light. The most common pulsed dye laser uses a **flashlamp** to energize the laser. The dye is a fluorescent dye, often rhodamine, as the active medium. This will generate a wavelength of 200–700 nm. The vascular lesion pulsed dye lasers use either 577 or 585 nm as the preferred wavelength, corresponding to a small peak in the oxyhemoglobin absorption spectrum in an area that does not have much competition from melanin. Newer pulsed dye lasers offer wavelengths that range from 585 to 600 nm. The flashlamp generates pulses with a duration of 300–500 μsec in older lasers and up to 40 msec in newer lasers.

Pulsed Dye Vascular Lesion Laser

585, 590, 595, 600 nm light
Flashlamp-excited fluorescent dye
Pulsed mode
Selective photothermolysis
High cost

27. What conditions has the flashlamp pulsed dye vascular lesion laser been useful in treating?

The pulsed dye lasers may be the most effective lasers in treating the thin, lightly colored **port-wine stains,** especially those in children. These lesions have been treated without scarring in children as young as 1 month of age. Increasing the wavelength to 595 nm allows for the treatment of many port-wine stains that were resistant to treatment with the shorter wavelengths. Pulsed dye laser treatment is effective for facial telangiectasias, cherry angiomas, childhood hemangiomas, poikiloderma of Civatte (a mottled vascular condition on the necks of adults), warts, scars, and possibly stretch marks. Leg veins under 1 mm in diameter are also effectively treated with pulsed dye lasers using 595–600 nm light and pulse duration of up to 20 msec.

Uses of Pulsed Dye Lasers

CONDITION	WAVELENGTH
Childhood port-wine stains	595 nm
Childhood proliferative angiomas	595 nm (every 2 weeks)
Facial telangiectasias, poikiloderma of Civatte	585 nm
Cherry angiomas	595 nm
Warts	585 nm (high energy)
Scars	595 nm
Stretch marks	585 nm (low energy)
Leg veins	595–600 nm

28. What are the disadvantages of the pulsed dye laser?

The pulsed dye lasers are not very useful in treating thicker vascular lesions, because the short pulse duration is not usually sufficient to damage the target vessels without increasing the power to a level that could lead to generalized damage and scarring. These lasers are not effective in treating venous lesions. There is significant post-treatment purpura that takes 7–10 days to resolve. This purpura results from the explosive optico-acoustic pulse generated by the pulsed dye lasers. This is a cosmetic problem that limits the use of the laser in some patients. As with all of the lasers mentioned, pulsed dye lasers are expensive to purchase, operate, and maintain.

29. How is the long-pulsed Nd:YAG laser used to treat leg veins?

The long-pulsed Nd:YAG lasers have a 1064-nm wavelength with pulse duration of up to 16 msec. The fluences are also very high, at ranges over 100 J/cm^2. The theory is to pulse the larger, deeper veins with multiple pulses separated by 20–30-msec delays. This apparently has the ability to damage larger vessels (up to 3 mm) without causing significant epidermal damage. A recent preliminary study showed moderate improvement with the only reported side effect being hypopigmentation lasting 3 months in 28% of the treated patients.

30. What is the KTP laser and how is it used to treat vascular lesions?

The KTP laser is an Nd:YAG laser that has been frequency-doubled. The Nd:YAG light passes through a potassium (**K**) titanyl (**T**) phosphate (**P**) crystal to double the frequency and halve the wavelength to 532 nm. These continuous-wave lasers deliver long pulses in the range of 1–50 msec. Spot sizes of 1, 2, and 4 mm usually are available.

These lasers are touted as effectively treating facial telangiectasias, port-wine stains, and leg veins. Long-term clinical studies are still pending. After a pulse of KTP laser impacts on a vessel, there is immediate clearing of the blood from this area. One theory is that the longer pulse generates an intravascular steam bubble without rupturing the vessel wall. This clears the lumen while damaging the wall. In this way, there is essentially no purpura after the treatment.

PIGMENTED LESION LASERS

31. Which lasers are used to treat pigmented lesions?

Pigment Lesion Lasers

LASER TYPE	WAVELENGTH	USE
Flashlamp pulsed dye	520 nm	Epidermal pigmented lesions, some red tattoos
Copper vapor, green	511 nm	Epidermal pigmented lesions
Krypton, green	521 nm, 531 nm	Epidermal pigmented lesions
Frequency-doubled Nd: YAG	532 nm	Epidermal pigmented lesions, red tattoos

32. Discuss the basics of the flashlamp pulsed dye pigment lesion laser.

Pulsed Dye Pigment Lesion Laser

510 nm (green light) wavelength	Good for epidermal pigmentation
Pulsed mode	High cost
Selective photothermolysis	

33. In which clinical conditions is the flashlamp pulsed dye pigment lesion laser most useful?

The green light pulsed dye laser is effective in treating lentigines (age spots), lightly pigmented café-au-lait spots, and freckles. Other deeper or thicker pigmented lesions and larger moles do not respond well to this laser. Some red tattoos have been reported to respond to this laser. This laser is rarely used due to mechanical problems.

34. What other lasers are used to treat pigmented lesions?

The copper vapor laser, krypton laser, and Nd:YAG laser all use a concept similar to selective photothermolysis to target the melanin within the melanosome of the epidermis. The **copper vapor** laser at 511 nm is effective in treating superficial epidermal pigmentation but does not appear to remove deeper dermal pigmentation. The **krypton** laser at 520 nm has a penetration depth of up to 4 mm and therefore might be more effective at treating deeper dermal pigmentation. With higher energy settings, hyperpigmentation and scarring are risks. The Q-switched frequency-doubled Nd:YAG laser at 532 nm may be useful in treating epidermal pigmentation.

35. Are there any problems associated with the pigment lasers?

The pulsed dye pigment lesion lasers have been plagued by mechanical difficulties and are no longer manufactured. The copper vapor, krypton, and Nd:YAG lasers all have some risk of hypopigmentation, hyperpigmentation, and scarring. All of these pigment lasers have the problem of cost justification. The Q-switched Nd:YAG laser is probably the most cost-effective laser to use for brown spots because it also has the 1064-nm wavelength.

HAIR REMOVAL LASERS

36. What lasers are used for hair removal?

Hair Removal Lasers

TYPE	WAVELENGTH	PULSE DURATION
Nd:YAG	1064 nm	5–18 msec
Ruby	694 nm	2 msec
Alexandrite	755 nm	3–20 msec
Diode	810 nm	50–250 msec

37. How is the Nd:YAG laser used to remove hair?

The hair to be removed is waxed and then a carbon suspension is rubbed into the skin. The theory is that the carbon will penetrate into the hair follicles and the Nd:YAG light will be absorbed by the carbon particles. The heat will then be transferred to the hair follicle, causing destruction of the hair. There is little evidence that this theoretical process actually works as described and the hair loss is short-lived. This laser is losing acceptance as an effective method for permanent hair removal.

38. Describe hair removal by other types of lasers.

The ruby, alexandrite, and diode lasers operate on the theory of selective photothermolysis. The wavelength of the laser light will penetrate to the depth of the hair follicle and destroy the hair. There are slight differences in wavelengths that may affect the depth of penetration and the absorption by the melanin within the hair follicle and the hair itself. Lasers with effective surface-cooling devices are better able to destroy the hair without damaging the epidermal surface. These devices are either cryogenic sprays or mechanical devices that the laser will shoot through.

39. How effective are the hair removal lasers?

At this time, the mechanics of the ruby lasers and the alexandrite lasers appear to be the most effective methods of hair removal. The diode lasers are being improved and ultimately may be as effective. The only hair that may be removed is the darkly pigmented hair; blond or gray hair will resist all treatment. The hair is always in various growth phases, so treatments must be repeated several times to catch all hair in the phase of active growth.

40. Are there any risks associated with laser hair removal?

Surface changes of hyper- and hypopigmentation are the greatest risks because all of these lasers have wavelengths of light that are absorbed by the epidermal melanin. Too much heat may lead to scarring in rare cases. Failure of hair to be removed permanently also is a common problem.

41. Why should patients consider using laser to remove hair?

Laser hair removal is by far the most effective method available to remove unwanted dark hair. The only other method is electrolysis, which is time-consuming and painful. Laser is very fast and has minimal side effects.

TATTOO LASERS

42. List the lasers that are used to treat tattoos.

Tattoo Lasers

LASER TYPE	WAVELENGTH	USE
Q-switched ruby	694 nm	Blue, black, and green tattoos
Q-switched Nd:YAG	1064 nm	Blue and black tattoos
Frequency-doubled Nd:YAG	532 nm	Red tattoos
Q-switched alexandrite	755 nm	Blue, black, and green tattoos

43. How do the Q-switched lasers treat tattoos?

Tattoo pigment is in small clusters of pigment. The professional tattoos have smaller clusters (~145 µm) than amateur tattoos (~180 µm). The clusters of pigment absorb the short pulses of high-energy Q-switched laser light, leading to an explosive interaction. The pigment clusters are dispersed into smaller pigment globules that may be removed by the surrounding macrophages.

44. Does the color of the tattoo ink influence the treatment success?

Yes. The Q-switched ruby laser may be effective in treating blue-black and green ink tattoos. The Q-switched Nd:YAG laser at 1064 nm effectively treats black tattoo pigment, and the same laser at 512 nm may be effective at treating red, purple, and orange pigment. The alexandrite laser may be effective at treating blue, black, and green. None of the lasers appears to effectively treat white or yellow tattoo pigment.

45. Are there any complications of treating tattoos with Q-switched lasers?

Some white and yellow tattoo inks form a rust color to a deep black color when treated. This may represent Fe_2O_3 being reduced to FeO.

46. Discuss the ruby laser.

The ruby laser has an active medium of aluminum oxide (Al_2O_3) that has been chromium-doped. This means that some of the aluminum atoms have been replaced with chromium atoms. This laser emits light with a wavelength of 694 nm that is in the red visible light spectrum. The tattoo lasers use Q-switching to generate a high-energy pulse of 25–70 nsec. The red light is well absorbed by black, blue, and green tattoo pigment. The Q-switched ruby lasers have also been used in treating some dermal pigmentation abnormalities. The main problem with the ruby laser is that the light is absorbed by the melanin in the epidermis and may lead to scarring or hypopigmentation.

Ruby Laser

694 nm (red light) wavelength	Black, blue, and green tattoos
Q-switched mode	Moderate to high cost
Selective photothermolysis	

47. Discuss the Nd:YAG laser.

The Nd:YAG laser uses a yttrium-aluminum-garnet crystal in which neodymium has been dispersed into the crystal. The standard wavelength of light emitted is 1064 nm, which is in the near-infrared spectrum. The Q-switched Nd:YAG lasers have a short pulse in the range of 5–10 nsec. There is a frequency doubler that generates a wavelength of 532 nm, in the green spectral region. The 1064-nm light has been useful in treating dark tattoos, and the 532-nm light has been useful in treating red tattoos.

Nd:YAG Laser

1064 nm standard, 532 nm frequency-doubled	Q-switched mode
1064-nm nonselective thermal destruction, dark tattoos	Moderate cost
532-nm selective photothermolysis, red tattoos	

48. Discuss the alexandrite laser.

Alexandrite is a chrysoberyl crystal that has been chromium-doped (replacing some Al^{3+} with Cr^{3+} in the $BeAl_2O_4$ crystal). Both Q-switched and flashlamp-pumped alexandrite lasers are available. The Q-switched lasers have a pulse duration of 10–40 msec and a wavelength of 755 nm. Like the other Q-switched lasers, the alexandrite laser operates on the concept of selective photothermolysis using an optico-acoustic pulse to fragment the tattoo pigment particle. This laser has been good at treating blue, black, and green tattoos. Some use has been found for treatment of epidermal and dermal pigmentation.

Alexandrite Laser

755 nm	Blue, black, and green tattoos
Q-switched mode	High cost
Selective photothermolysis	

49. Why should you use a laser rather than other more conventional therapies?

The foremost concern is cost. A laser should never be used if a less-expensive technique works equally well. In clinical practice, however, a practitioner may use a CO_2 laser for treatments that could be performed with other equipment if the laser is already in the office. This makes economic sense as long as there is no added expense to the patient for this more expensive instrument. This same controversy arises with the treatment of lentigines with liquid nitrogen versus pigment lesion lasers. There may be better results with laser, but at significantly higher cost.

There are many uses for lasers—such as the treatment of congenital vascular disorders, tattoos, and many pigmented lesions—for which laser is either the only treatment or by far the most effective modality. In these cases, laser use is certainly justifiable.

BIBLIOGRAPHY

1. Alster TS: Q-switched alexandrite laser treatment (755 nm) of professional and amateur tattoos. J Am Acad Dermatol 33:69–73, 1995.
2. Anderson RR, Geronemus R, Kilmer SL, et al: Cosmetic tattoo ink darkening: A complication of Q-switched and pulsed-laser treatment. Arch Dermatol 129:1010–1014, 1993.
3. Anderson RR, Parrish JA: Selective photothermolysis: Precise microsurgery by selective absorption of pulsed radiation. Science 220:524–527, 1983.
4. Ash K, Lord J, et al: Hair removal using a long-pulsed alexandrite laser. Dermatol Clin 17:387–399, 1999.
5. Dinehart SM, Waner M, Flock S: The copper vapor laser for the treatment of cutaneous vascular and pigmented lesions. J Dermatol Surg Oncol 19:370–375, 1993.
6. Fitzpatrick RE: Laser resurfacing of rhytides. Dermatol Clin 15:431–447, 1997.
7. Fitzpatrick RE, Lowe NJ, Goldman MP, et al: Flashlamp-pumped pulsed dye laser treatment of port-wine stains. J Dermatol Surg Oncol 20:743–748, 1994.
8. Goldberg DJ, Ahkami R: Evaluation comparing multiple treatments with a 2-msec and 10-msec alexandrite laser for hair removal. Lasers Surg Med 25:223–228, 1999.
9. Goldberg DJ, Cutler KB: The use of the erbium:YAG laser for the treatment of class III rhytids. Dermatol Surg 25:713–715, 1999.
10. Goldberg DJ, Littler CM, Wheeland RG: Topical suspension-assisted Q-switched Nd:YAG laser hair removal. Dermatol Surg 23:741–745, 1997.
11. Goldberg DJ, Meine JG: A comparison of four frequency-doubled Nd:YAG (532 nm) laser systems for treatment of facial telangiectases. Dermatol Surg 25:463–467, 1999.
12. Grekin RC, et al: 510-nm pigmented lesion dye laser. J Dermatol Surg Oncol 19:380–387, 1993.
13. Herd RM, Dover JS, Arndt KA: Basic laser principles. Dermatol Clin 15:355–372, 1997.
14. Hsia J, Lowery JA, Zelickson B: Treatment of leg telangiectasia using a long-pulse dye laser at 595 nm. Lasers Surg Med 20:1–5, 1997.
15. Kilmer SL: Laser treatment of tattoos. Dermatol Clin 15:409–417, 1997.
16. Lask G, et al: Laser-assisted hair removal by selective photothermolysis. Dermatol Surg 23:737–739, 1997.
17. Lowe NJ, et al: Skin resurfacing with the Ultrapulse CO_2 laser. Dermatol Surg 21:1025–1029, 1995.
18. Massey RA, Katz BE: Successful treatment of spider leg veins with a high-energy, long-pulse, frequency-doubled neodymium:YAG laser (HELP-G). Dermatol Surg 25:677–680, 1999.
19. McBurney EI: Clinical usefulness of the argon laser for the 1990s. J Dermatol Surg Oncol 19:358–362, 1993.
20. McDaniel DH, Lord J, Ash K, Newman J: Combined CO_2/erbium:YAG laser resurfacing of peri-oral rhytides and side-by-side comparison with carbon dioxide laser alone. Dermatol Surg 25:285–993, 1999.
21. Olbricht SM: Use of the CO_2 laser in dermatologic surgery. J Dermatol Surg Oncol 19:364–369, 1993.
22. Rendon-Pellerano MI, Lentini J, et al: Laser resurfacing: Usual and unusual complications. Dermatol Surg 25:360, 1999.
23. Spicer MS, Goldberg DJ: Lasers in dermatology. J Am Acad Dermatol 34:1–25, 1996.
24. Taylor CR, et al: Treatment of tattoos by Q-switched ruby laser. Arch Dermatol 126:893–899, 1990.
25. Teikemeier G, Goldberg DJ: Skin resurfacing with the erbium:YAG laser. Dermatol Surg 23:685–687, 1997.
26. Williams RM, et al: Hair removal using the long-pulsed ruby laser. Dermatol Clin 17:367–372, 1999.

54. THERAPEUTIC PHOTOMEDICINE

Paul Thompson, M.D.

1. What is ultraviolet B (UVB) phototherapy?

Phototherapy is the use of nonionizing electromagnetic radiation to treat cutaneous disease. UVB phototherapy utilizes intermediate ultraviolet light with a wavelength of 290–320 nm. Although the Greeks first used sun as a therapeutic light source 3000 years ago, modern phototherapy began in 1923 with the use of quartz-jacketed mercury-discharge lamps to treat patients with psoriasis. UVB may be administered as a monotherapy or in combination with emollients or tar. Recently researchers have attempted to improve UVB phototherapy by the introduction of narrow-band UVB that uses TL-01 fluorescent tubes emitting at 311 nm. Interest in narrow-band UVB relates to its reduced risk of carcinogenicity compared to PUVA and clearing of psoriasis more efficiently with reduced erythema compared to broad-band UVB.

2. What diseases are usually treated with UVB phototherapy?

Psoriasis, various forms of dermatitis such as atopic dermatitis, and pityriasis rosea are the most common indications.

Diseases Treated with UVB Phototherapy

Acne vulgaris	Pityriasis rosea*
Dermatitis (eczema)*	Pruritic eruptions of HIV infection
Lichen planus	Pruritus (especially in renal failure)*
Parapsoriasis	Psoriasis*
Photodermatoses	

*Best indications

3. How is UVB phototherapy administered?

It is usually administered in a physician's office or psoriasis treatment center. Less commonly, patients purchase UVB phototherapy units and treat themselves at home. Patients receive a controlled dose of UVB while standing in a booth lined with high-output UVB bulbs (Fig. 1). While phototherapy regimens vary considerably, treatments are usually given 2–5 times per week.

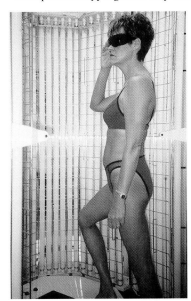

FIGURE 1. Typical ultraviolet booth demonstrating banks of bulbs. Most modern ultraviolet booths deliver both UVA and UVB. Note that the patient is wearing sunglasses with wrap-around eye protection.

The initial UVB exposure is determined by assessing the patient's skin type and historical ease of burning or by establishing the minimal erythema dose (MED). Normally, treatment times are gradually increased until clearing occurs, unless there is an adverse reaction such as itching or burning from previous treatments. An exception is pityriasis rosea, in which patients receive one exposure of an erythemogenic (sunburn-producing) dose of UVB.

4. What is Goeckerman therapy?

Goeckerman therapy, named in honor of Dr. William H. Goeckerman who developed it in 1925, is UVB phototherapy used in combination with topical coal tar to treat psoriasis. The therapy is administered by having patients apply crude coal tar or tar derivatives to the skin and removing the excess tar before exposure to UVB. After treatment, the patient takes a bath or shower to remove any remaining tar or scale. With each visit, the dose of UVB administered is gradually increased, with the treatment being administered three or more times per week for 3–4 weeks or longer. The treatment can be supplemented with topical corticosteroid preparations or descaling agents. Once remission is achieved, patients may stay in remission for 12–18 months or longer. Long remission rates and relative safety have made this the therapy of choice in many psoriasis treatment centers. Disadvantages include its inconvenience, messiness of the tar, and need for numerous office visits.

5. Does UVB phototherapy produce side effects?

The most common acute side effect is a sunburn-like erythema and pain resulting from overexposure to UVB. When this occurs, the amount of UVB administered is usually reduced at the next treatment session. Patients who fail to wear eye protection that blocks UVB may develop corneal burns. Occasionally, patients with psoriasis may experience temporary pustular flares of psoriasis during treatment. Topical preparations used in conjunction with UVB phototherapy, such as emollients and tar, may produce a folliculitis. This complication can be prevented by instructing the patient to apply topical preparations in a downward fashion to prevent follicular irritation.

Long-term side effects include skin cancer and skin aging (dermatoheliosis). The exact risk of skin cancer has not been determined, but it is greater in patients with fair skin, with family history of skin cancer, or who use other therapies associated with a risk of producing skin cancer (e.g., PUVA). Patients with prolonged UVB therapy and other risk factors should have periodic skin examinations to detect early skin cancers.

6. What is PUVA phototherapy?

PUVA is an acronym for **P**soralen and **U**ltra**V**iolet light, type **A**. It involves the combined use of a prescription psoralen (methoxsalen or trioxsalen) and long-wave ultraviolet light (UVA). PUVA therapy for psoriasis was approved by the Food and Drug Administration in 1982 and has since become the treatment of choice for many adult patients with extensive patch- and plaque-type psoriasis. The psoralen usually is administered orally (sometimes topically) and followed by UVA.

7. What are psoralens, and how do they work?

Methoxsalen (8-methoxypsoralen, 8-MOP) is a naturally occurring photoactive plant substance found in the seeds of *Amni majus*, a plant that grows wild along the Nile delta. Methoxsalen is absorbed from the upper gastrointestinal tract and metabolized by the intestine and liver. Ninety percent is excreted within 24 hours, with the major portion being excreted in the urine. **Trioxsalen** is a synthetic psoralen usually reserved for the treatment of vitiligo.

Psoralen compounds by themselves do not affect the skin in the absence of UVA, but in the presence of UVA (320–400 nm), they are potent photosensitizers. Photosensitization selectively inhibits epidermal DNA synthesis without a proportionate inhibition of epidermal-cell function. Ninety minutes after oral ingestion, absorption of UVA photons photochemically links the DNA by forming cylo-additive products between the intercalated psoralen and the pyrimidine bases of cellular DNA. These psoralen–DNA crosslinks cause a decrease in the rate of epidermal DNA synthesis, which is believed to be the primary mechanism of action of these agents. Irradiation of psoralens also induces the formation of reactive oxygen species that can damage both cell membranes and organelles, as well as activate arachidonic acid metabolism. There is also evidence that PUVA therapy has a direct effect on the cutaneous immune system.

8. What diseases are usually treated with PUVA?

Acne vulgaris
Alopecia areata
Chronic graft-versus-host disease
Dermatitis (eczema)
Granuloma annulare
Lichen planus
Mycosis fungoides
Parapsoriasis

Photodermatoses
Pigmented purpuric dermatoses
Psoriasis
Pityriasis lichenoides
Pruritic eruptions of HIV infection
Urticaria pigmentosa
Vitiligo

PUVA is most commonly used to treat psoriasis, various forms of dermatitis such atopic dermatitis and nummular dermatitis, vitiligo, and mycosis fungoides.

9. Which psoriatic patients are good candidates for PUVA phototherapy?

PUVA is usually recommended for patients with >20–30% of the skin involved who have not improved with more conservative treatments, such as topical corticosteroids or UVB phototherapy. In most patients, PUVA therapy is more effective than UVB therapy. Stable plaque-type psoriasis, palmar and plantar psoriasis, and guttate psoriasis are subsets of psoriasis that are particularly responsive to PUVA photochemotherapy.

10. How is oral PUVA photochemotherapy administered?

PUVA photochemotherapy is always administered in a physician's office or psoriasis treatment center. The patient takes 0.5–0.7 mg/kg of methoxsalen with low-fat food or milk 90–120 minutes before receiving UVA radiation. The initial exposure varies from 0.5–3.0 J/cm^2 depending on the skin type or minimal phototoxic dose (MPD). The amount of time spent in each treatment booth varies, and the maximum radiant exposure for each booth must be determined by a calibrated radiometer. The exposure time or total Joules of energy delivered is recorded and increased with each treatment. Following treatment, the patient must wear UV-blocking sunglasses for 24 hours to prevent premature cataracts. Generally, an average of 24–30 treatments are required for clearance of psoriasis. Thereafter, the PUVA treatments may be stopped or continued on a maintenance basis. PUVA photochemotherapy should only be used by physicians with special training and experience with this modality. While UVA is most commonly delivered in booths, special portable units are also available to treat the hands, feet, and scalp (Fig. 2).

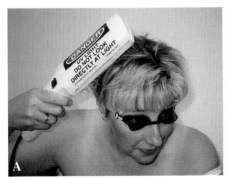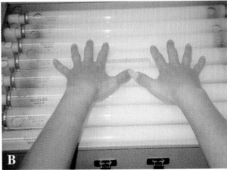

FIGURE 2. Portable UVA units for treating the scalp (A) or the hands and feet (B).

11. Are there contraindications to using PUVA?

Contraindications include a history of psoralen hypersensitivity reactions; photosensitive diseases including lupus erythematosus, porphyria, xeroderma pigmentosum, and albinism; malignant melanoma; pregnancy; and aphakia (absence of a lens may produce retinal damage). PUVA photochemotherapy should be used with caution in patients with fair skin, a history of previous ionizing radiation, history of multiple skin cancers, cataracts, immunosuppression, uremia, or renal failure. Patients with severe myocardial or other diseases that may disallow standing for prolonged periods in the treatment cabinet may not be able to receive photochemotherapy.

12. What is bath PUVA?

The patient is immersed for 15 minutes in a bathtub containing five 10-mg capsules of methoxsalen dissolved in the water. Topical methoxsalen gradually loses its photoactivity, and the patient should ideally be treated with the standard UVA light treatments within 15 minutes after immersion. Bath PUVA therapy using trimethylpsoralen (TMP), which is more hydrophobic than 8-methoxypsoralen (8-MOP), has been used for more than 20 years in Sweden and Finland with no observed increase in the number of skin cancers. It is also useful for patients who are not able to tolerate oral methoxsalen because of nausea and for children under 15 years of age. This technique also may be adapted for use on the palms and soles for hand and foot dermatoses.

13. How effective is PUVA photochemotherapy in the management of "dermatitis"?

While photochemotherapy has approved indications for the treatment of vitiligo and psoriasis, it is also very effective for many inflammatory dermatoses, including seborrheic dermatitis, neurodermatitis, atopic dermatitis, chronic hand and foot dermatitis, and nummular dermatitis. Photochemotherapy for these conditions is indicated when more conservative treatment fails. In atopic dermatitis, controlled trials have demonstrated that 90% of patients will initially clear with PUVA therapy, but only 70% can maintain clearance.

14. Can any photodermatoses be treated with PUVA?

Yes. Paradoxically, polymorphous light eruption, solar urticaria, chronic photosensitive eczema, actinic reticuloid, hydroa vacciniforme, and erythropoietic protoporphyria all have been treated successfully with PUVA. Interestingly, many of these dermatoses are produced by the UVA spectrum.

15. How effective is PUVA in the treatment of vitiligo?

PUVA is considered by most authorities to be the treatment of choice for subtotal vitiligo. It is time-consuming and expensive, typically requiring 100–150 treatments, but retrospective studies have shown that >50% of patients will have "acceptable" repigmentation that lasts for years.

16. What are the side effects of PUVA therapy?

The most common short-term cutaneous side effect is PUVA erythema and burning of the skin, which peaks at 48–72 hours after therapy. Mild erythema is an expected reaction, while severe erythema with marked pain indicates either excessive psoralens or UVA. Psoralens also produce nausea in about 10% of patients and can be severe enough that patients may have to discontinue therapy. Long-term side effects include an increased risk of cutaneous squamous cell carcinomas (especially of the male genitalia), cataracts, and dermatoheliosis (ultraviolet "aging" of the skin). For these reasons, male genitalia should be shielded unless involved with the disease process, and all patients should have yearly ophthalmologic examinations during therapy. Approximately 180 months after the first initial PUVA treatment, the risk of melanoma increases, especially in patients who received 250 or more treatments.

17. What is RePUVA?

RePUVA treatment uses an oral retinoid (usually etretinate) and PUVA in combination. Studies suggest that this therapeutic combination offers a practical way to clear psoriasis with less cumulative UVA exposure than PUVA alone. Patients receiving etretinate plus PUVA clear 40% faster than those treated with PUVA alone, even though the UVA dose is reduced by 50%. Most commonly, the oral etretinate is begun 7–10 days before the first PUVA treatment, and the two therapies are given concurrently until 100% clearing occurs. The etretinate is usually discontinued, and the patient is maintained on PUVA for about 2 months.

18. Can any malignancies be treated with PUVA?

Yes. Mycosis fungoides (cutaneous T-cell lymphoma) is commonly treated with PUVA as monotherapy, or it may be combined with retinoids (RePUVA) or recombinant interferon α-2a.

When PUVA is used alone in patch or plaque stage disease, approximately three-quarters of patients will experience remission. Tumor-stage mycosis fungoides usually does not respond to PUVA.

19. What is photopheresis?

Photopheresis,or **extracorporeal photochemotherapy,** is a relatively new procedure that involves discontinuous leukopheresis by centrifugation, followed by exposure of the buffy coat lymphocytes to UVA light in a special unit about 2 hours after the administration of methoxsalen. Following exposure of the lymphocytes to UVA, the photoirradiated cells are reinfused into the patient. The procedure is done on 2 consecutive days at 4-week intervals. The adverse side effects are minimal; patients may experience nausea and about 10% develop a transient fever after reinfusion.

20. Which diseases have been treated with extracorporeal photopheresis?

Photopheresis is approved for the treatment of cutaneous T-cell lymphoma (mycosis fungoides). It is most effective in the erythrodermic variants (Sézary syndrome) that involve >25% of the body surface. The response rate in this group of patients is about 64%. Photopheresis as a form of immunotherapy has also been tried on other T-cell mediated diseases, such as pemphigus vulgaris, chronic Lyme arthritis, psoriatic arthritis, and progressive systemic sclerosis.

21. What is photodynamic therapy for cancer?

This form of therapy uses light-activated drugs to selectively kill cancer cells. It was first utilized in 1903, when eosin and light were used to treat skin cancer. This therapy fell out of favor, but today there is a revival of interest in this area following the development of more effective photosensitizing compounds. Photodynamic therapy is a two-step process: a photosensitizing agent is topically or systemically administered to the patient followed by illumination with a light source of the proper wavelength. Porphyrins (usually photofrin II) used in combination with red light (600–700 nm) are the most common form of photodynamic therapy. Other sensitizers in use include phthalocyanines, chlorins, purpurins, and porphins.

At present, photodynamic therapy is used primarily for palliation of obstructive malignancies of the esophagus and lung. Less commonly, it has been used for malignancies of the skin, brain, and bladder. More clinical studies and improvement of this technique are required.

22. What is blue-light phototherapy?

Some degree of jaundice is common in newborns and is seen in up to 50% of infants between the second and fourth day of life. Before birth, bilirubin is conjugated and excreted chiefly by the placenta; however, after birth this function shifts to the neonatal liver. Transient neonatal hyperbilirubinemia is the result of insufficient activity of the conjugative hepatic enzyme glucuronyl transferase. Phototherapy with blue light (400–460 nm) is an effective means of preventing hyperbilirubinemia by producing a photoproduct called photobilirubin which is nontoxic.

BIBLIOGRAPHY

1. Abdullah AN, Keczkes K: Cutaneous and ocular side-effects of PUVA photochemotherapy: A 10-year follow-up study. Clin Exp Dermatol 14:421–424, 1989.
2. Armus S, Keyes B, Cahill C, et al: Photophoresis for the treatment of cutaneous T cell lymphoma. J Am Acad Dermatol 23:898–902, 1990.
3. Coven TR, Murphy FP, Gilleaudeau P, et al: Trimethylpsoralen bath PUVA is a remittive treatment for psoriasis vulgaris. Evidence that epidermal immunocytes are direct therapeutic targets. Arch Dermatol 134:1263–1268, 1998.
4. Honig B, Morrison WL, Karp D: Phototherapy beyond psoriasis. J Am Acad Dermatol 31:775–790, 1994.
5. Stern RS, Members of the Photochemotherapy Follow-up Study: Genital tumors among men with psoriasis exposed to psoralens and ultraviolet A radiation (PUVA) and ultraviolet B radiation. N Engl J Med 322:1093–1097, 1990.
6. Thomsen K, Hammar H, Molin L, Volden G: Retinoids plus PUVA (RePUVA) and PUVA in mycosis fungoides, plaque stage: A report from the Scandinavian Mycosis Fungoides Group. Acta Derm Venereol (Stockh) 69:536–538, 1989.
7. Wildfiang IL, Jacobsen FK, Thestrup-Pedersen K: PUVA treatment of vitiligo: A retrospective study of 59 patients. Acta Derm Venereol (Stockh) 72:305–306, 1992.

55. RETINOIDS

James E. Fitzpatrick, M.D.

1. What are retinoids?

Retinoids are structural analogs of vitamin A (retinol). Vitamin A is a fat-soluble vitamin that was first extracted from egg yolk in 1909. It can be obtained directly from the diet (e.g., liver) or produced from carotenoids, a pigmented precursor that is found in abundance in yellow vegetables such as carrots. Beta-carotene, the primary carotenoid found in carrots, is particularly efficient in its ability to be converted to vitamin A. The physiologic effects of vitamin A are broad, but the most important functions include tissue differentiation (especially epithelial tissues), general growth, visual function, and reproduction. Retinoids may be produced naturally during vitamin A metabolism, but most retinoids are synthetic. Synthetic retinoids are produced by changing either the polar end group, polyene side chain, or cyclic group of vitamin A. More than 1,500 retinoids have been synthesized and tested for their biologic properties since 1968.

2. How do vitamin A and retinoids exert their effect at a molecular level?

Vitamin A exerts its effect on cells by a mechanism similar to corticosteroids; some authorities have suggested that it should be classified as a hormone. Vitamin A acts on cells by binding to retinoic acid receptors (RAR) and/or other retinoid X receptors (RXR) that are found in the nucleus. Each of these receptors demonstrates three distinct receptor subtypes, which have been named α, β, and γ. Retinoids vary in their affinity for these six receptors, which partially accounts for the different pharmacologic effects produced by different retinoids. Another important factor is that different tissues appear to vary in the expression of receptor subtypes. In human keratinocytes, RAR-γ is the major retinoid receptor expressed. Tissues appear to regulate their requirement for vitamin A and retinoids by changing the concentration of the binding proteins.

3. Which retinoids are clinically used in dermatology?

Retinoids may be used topically or orally. Topical retinoids approved for use in the United States include tretinoin (all-*trans* retinoic acid), a naturally occurring metabolite of vitamin A; tazarotene, a synthetic retinoid; and alitretinoin (9-*cis*-retinoic acid). Tretinoin is available as a cream (0.025%, 0.05%, and 0.1% strengths), gel (0.01% and 0.025% strengths), and liquid (0.05% strength) and is sold under the trade name Retin-A. Adapelene is a retinoid-like drug that is also available topically.

The two oral synthetic retinoids available in the United States are isotretinoin and acitretin. Etretinate was formerly available but it has been pulled from the market and replaced by acitretin. Isotretinoin (13-*cis*-retinoic acid) is available as capsules (10 mg, 20 mg, 40 mg) and is sold under the trade name of Accutane. Acitretin is also available as capsules (10 mg, 25 mg) and is sold under the trade name of Soriatane.

Prescription Retinoids

TOPICAL PREPARATIONS	ORAL PREPARATIONS
Tretinoin (all-*trans* retinoic acid)	**Isotretinoin** (13-*cis*-retinoic acid)
Retin-A cream (0.025%, 0.05%, 0.1%;	Accutane (10- and 40-mg capsules)
gel 0.01% and 0.025%; liquid 0.05%)	**Acitretin**
Retin-A Mico (gel microsphere 0.1%)	Soriatane (10- and 25-mg capsules)
Renova (emollient cream 0.05%)	
Avita (0.025% cream and gel)	
Tazarotene	
Tazorac (gel 0.05% and 0.1% gel)	
Alitretinoin (9-*cis*-retinoic acid)	
Panretin (0.1% gel)	
Adapalene (retinoid-like drug)	
Differin (0.1% gel)	

4. What are the clinical indications for using topical tretinoin?

Topical tretinoin has received FDA approval only for treatment of acne and dermatoheliosis (sun-induced skin aging); however, it has been used in many other dermatologic conditions.

Therapeutic Applications of Topical Tretinoin

FDA-APPROVED INDICATION	SELECTED NONAPPROVED APPLICATIONS	
Acne vulgaris	Acanthosis nigricans	Linear epidermal nevus
Dermatoheliosis	Actinic keratoses	Melasma (chloasma)
(photodamaged skin)	Fox-Fordyce disease	Nevus comedonicus
	Ichthyoses (e.g., ichthyosis vulgaris, lamellar ichthyosis)	Porokeratosis Postinflammatory hyperpigmentation
	Keloids and hypertrophic scars	Psoriasis
	Keratosis follicularis (Darier's disease)	Reactive perforating collagenosis
	Lichen planus (cutaneous and oral)	Verruca plana (flat warts)

5. What is the mechanism of action of tretinoin in acne vulgaris?

The precise mechanism of action is not proved but tretinoin is believed to exert its therapeutic effect by decreasing the cohesiveness of follicular epithelial cells that are responsible for producing microcomedones. Microcomedones are the earliest recognizable abnormality in acne vulgaris. Tretinoin also stimulates mitotic activity of follicular keratinocytes, promotes extrusion of comedones by rapid cell turnover, and decreases the production of sebum, although this effect is minimal.

6. How should topical tretinoin be used to treat acne vulgaris?

Tretinoin is applied once per day to affected areas. It should be applied in the evening to minimize photodegradation. The strength and formulation depend on the severity of the acne and the tolerance of the individual patient. After washing the face, the patient should wait 20–30 minutes before applying the medication or use a hair dryer to blow dry the face before application. The periocular skin, mouth, and angles of the nose should be avoided since these are more susceptible to irritant reactions. The medication should be applied sparingly to dry skin. Care should be taken when using other topical preparations such as benzoyl peroxide or antibiotics in conjunction with tretinoin since the irritant effect of these medications is additive.

Patients should be advised that an apparent exacerbation of acne vulgaris during the first month of therapy represents externalization of deep-seated acne lesions. Patients should not discontinue therapy and should understand that beneficial effects may not be seen for 6 weeks. Maximum improvement may take up to 6 months or more with continued therapy. The most common reasons for tretinoin failures are failure of the health care provider to instruct patients thoroughly about proper application and failure to provide an accurate assessment about expected results. Patients often discontinue therapy after failing to see improvement during the first month.

7. Is topical tretinoin cream really useful in treating photoinduced wrinkles?

Yes. Several vehicle-controlled studies have clearly demonstrated that topical tretinoin improves the wrinkling and irregular pigmentation of photoaged skin. It does not make the skin normal but it does increase both the thickness of the epidermis and the synthesis of anchoring fibrils and collagen. New blood vessels form and cutaneous blood flow increases. Topical tretinoin is not a panacea; prevention of dermatoheliosis by reducing sun exposure and using sunscreens is still preferable.

8. What are the side effects of topical tretinoin?

The most common side effect is an irritant reaction that manifests as erythema and scaling. Severe irritant reactions may require decreasing the concentration or frequency of application. True allergic contact dermatitis to topical tretinoin preparations has been reported but is rare. An unusual potential problem is that the topical tretinoin gels are flammable. At least one dermatologist has reported that it is useful during hunting trips for starting camp fires! Patients who are not able to tolerate tretinoin gel or cream may be able to tolerate tretinoin gel with microspheres (Retin-A Micro) and adapalene gel, since they are less irritating.

9. Is topical tretinoin safe to use during pregnancy or nursing?

Topical tretinoin is classified as a pregnancy category C drug, which means that a risk to the fetus cannot be ruled out. Prospective human studies are lacking but studies on animals using doses up to 320 times those used in humans did not produce teratogenic effects. A retrospective British study on pregnant women who had received topical tretinoin did not demonstrate teratogenic effects. However, because high-dose (1000 times the topical human dose) oral tretinoin has been demonstrated to be teratogenic in rats, many dermatologists do not use this drug in pregnant women to avoid litigation in the event congenital abnormality occurs. Other dermatologists continue to use topical tretinoin in pregnant women because the benefit outweighs the unproved risk. It is not known whether topical tretinoin is secreted in human milk, but the manufacturer recommends that caution be exercised when this drug is administered to nursing mothers.

10. What are the clinical indications for tazarotene?

Tazarotene is a recently introduced synthetic retinoid. It is a prodrug that is rapidly converted in vitro by skin esterases to tazarotenic acid. Tazarotenic acid has a high affinity for RAR-γ, which is the primary retinoid receptor in keratinocytes. Tazarotene is approved for the treatment of psoriasis and acne vulgaris. Dermatologists typically use a topical corticosteroid in conjunction with tazarotene when treating psoriasis.

11. What are the clinical indications for alitretinoin?

Alitretinoin (9-*cis*-retinoic acid) is a retinoid that binds to all six retinoid receptors. It is indicated for the topical treatment of Kaposi's sarcoma. It is formulated in a 0.1% gel that is applied to individual lesions. Irritant dermatitis is seen in approximately 75% of patients and severe irritant dermatitis is seen in about 10% of patients. In two different studies, 35% and 36% of patients, respectively, demonstrated significant responses.

12. What are the clinical indications for oral isotretinoin?

Oral isotretinoin is FDA-approved for the treatment of severe recalcitrant cystic or nodular acne vulgaris. It is the most effective form of therapy for acne vulgaris; however, it is not a first-line drug and should be reserved for patients with cystic acne who are not responsive to conventional therapies such as oral antibiotics. Isotretinoin produces wide-ranging biologic effects and is used in many other diseases. Many authorities consider it to be the drug of choice for pityriasis rubra pilaris, severe lichen planus, Darier's disease, and the ichthyoses. A partial list of clinical indications is presented below:

Therapeutic Applications of Topical Tretinoin

FDA-APPROVED INDICATION	SELECTED NONAPPROVED APPLICATIONS	
Severe recalcitrant acne vulgaris	Hidradenitis suppurativa	Nevoid basal cell carcinoma— prevention of basal cell carcinomas
	Ichthyoses	Pityriasis rubra pilaris
	Keratosis follicularis (Darier's disease)	Rosacea
	Lichen planus	Xeroderma pigmentosum— prevention of skin cancers
	Lupus erythematosus, cutaneous	
	Mycosis fungoides (cutaneous T-cell lymphoma)	

Oral isotretinoin also has nondermatologic uses in oncology. It may be used as a monotherapy, but most studies have demonstrated better results when it is used with other agents such as cytokines. Oral retinoids have been used in experimental studies for the treatment of myelocytic leukemias, head and neck squamous cell carcinoma, breast carcinoma, cervical intraepithelial dysplasia, cervical cancer, and renal cell carcinoma.

13. What is the mechanism of action of oral isotretinoin in acne vulgaris?

Like tretinoin, the mechanism of action has not been precisely determined. Isotretinoin is the most effective known inhibitor of sebum production (up to 90% inhibition). Since clinical improvement in acne vulgaris appears to correlate with a reduction of sebum production, this is believed to be the most important mechanism of action. Isotretinoin also markedly affects keratinization and probably exerts an effect on the cohesiveness of the follicular keratinocytes, thus reducing microcomedone formation. Less important actions include anti-inflammatory effects, antibacterial effects, and inhibition of microbial enzyme activity.

14. Are there any contraindications to the use of oral isotretinoin?

Isotretinoin is classified as a pregnancy category X drug, which means that it is absolutely contraindicated for patients who are pregnant. Between 1982 and 1989, the manufacturer received 151 reports of patients who carried their fetuses to term. In 47% there were significant congenital malformations, with most being cardiovascular, craniofacial, or central nervous system in nature. Isotretinoin is considered very teratogenic, and the manufacturer suggests that women of child-bearing age use at least two reliable forms of birth control while taking the drug. Patients who become pregnant while taking the drug should consider the desirability of continuing the pregnancy. **Health care providers who are not knowledgeable about the proper way to administer and monitor oral retinoids should never use this class of drugs.**

Relative contraindications for oral retinoid therapy include patients with pseudotumor cerebri, inflammatory bowel disease, hyperlipidemia, or hepatitis, and children.

15. How is oral isotretinoin administered for the treatment of acne vulgaris?

Patients should initially have comprehensive counseling about the potential side effects of this drug. At a minimum, all patients should have pretreatment blood lipid and liver function studies. Some dermatologists also obtain complete blood counts. Women of child-bearing age should receive extensive counseling and require a serum pregnancy test within 2 weeks of starting isotretinoin.

Oral isotretinoin is taken with food in a dose range of 0.5–2.0 mg/kg given in two divided doses for 15–20 weeks. It is better absorbed if taken with a fatty meal. Women of child-bearing age should start therapy on the second or third day of their next normal menstrual period after having had a negative serum pregnancy test. After 20–24 weeks, therapy should be stopped. If significant acne is still present after a 2-month period, a second course of isotretinoin therapy may be considered.

16. What are the side effects of oral retinoid therapy?

More than 50 different acute and chronic adverse reactions of oral retinoid therapy have been documented in the literature. More than 90% of patients receiving oral isotretinoin at therapeutic levels demonstrate cheilitis or xerosis to some degree.

Oral Retinoid Toxicity

Acute Adverse Reactions

Mucocutaneous
Alopecia (<10%)
Cheilitis (>90%)
Dermatitis (50%)
Pruritus (<20%)
Pyogenic granuloma–like lesions in acne
  vulgaris (rare)
Xerosis (>50%)

Laboratory
Elevated liver function tests (<10%)
Hyperlipidemia (25%)
Leukopenia (<10%)

Systemic
Arthralgias (16%)
Impaired night vision
Mental depression (uncommon)
Pancreatitis (rare)
Pseudotumor cerebri (rare)
Spontaneous abortion
Teratogenicity (cardiac, head and neck, CNS)

Chronic Adverse Reactions

Mucocutaneous
Alopecia, persistent (rare)
Dry eyes (rare)

Systemic
Osteoporosis
Premature epiphyseal closure
Skeletal hyperostosis

17. Are there any strategies or treatments that reduce the dry skin and lips associated with retinoid therapy?

Yes. The most common adjunctive treatment is lip balm for the lips and moisturizers for the skin. There are recent reports that taking 800 IU of vitamin E (α-tocopherol) is effective in reducing the cheilitis and to a lesser extent the dry skin. Many dermatologists use this benign treatment, but some do not, since there are no studies that have been done to see if there is a reduction in the effectiveness of this therapy on acne.

18. Are the clinical indications for acitretin the same as for isotretinoin?

No. While both drugs are orally administered retinoids and they have many of the same therapeutic effects, they also demonstrate significant differences. As a general rule, isotretinoin is more effective in follicular disorders (e.g., acne vulgaris, rosacea, gram-negative folliculitis) and acitretin is more effective in pustular psoriasis and chronic pustular eruptions of the palms and soles. They appear to be of equal efficacy in disorders of keratinization such as the ichthyoses and pytiriasis rubra pilaris, although good comparative studies are lacking.

Acitretin is FDA-approved only for the treatment of severe recalcitrant psoriasis. It is especially effective for pustular and erythrodermic psoriasis. It is often used as monotherapy in these variants but also may be used in conjunction with other forms of therapy such as PUVA in plaque-type psoriasis. Like isotretinoin, acitretin has been used in many other cutaneous diseases:

Therapeutic Applications of Oral Acitretin

FDA-APPROVED INDICATION	SELECTED NONAPPROVED APPLICATIONS	
Severe recalcitrant psoriasis	Granuloma annulare, generalized	Palmar/plantar pustulosis
	Ichthyoses (e.g., ichthyosis vulgaris)	Pityriasis rubra pilaris
	Keratosis follicularis (Darier's disease)	Porokeratosis
	Mycosis fungoides (cutaneous T-cell lymphoma)	Subcorneal pustular dermatosis

19. What is the mechanism of action of acitretin?

As with the other retinoids, the mechanism of action is not known. Acitretin's clinical and histologic effect on psoriasis and disorders of keratinization suggests normalization of keratinization. The therapeutic response of pustular psoriasis, pustular eruptions of the palms and soles, and subcorneal pustular dermatosis suggests that this drug also modifies neutrophil function.

20. How is acitretin administered for the treatment of psoriasis?

After appropriate counseling and laboratory tests (liver function tests, serum lipid tests), oral acitretin is initially taken with food twice per day in a dosage range of 25–50 mg/day. Studies have shown that higher doses are only marginally more effective but the dose-related side effects are much more common and severe. After the initial response to therapy, which usually takes 8–16 weeks, the maintenance dose can often be lowered to 25 mg/day or every other day.

21. What are the contraindications for using oral acitretin?

The contraindications are the same as for oral isotretinoin (previously discussed). As for isotretinoin, acitretin is a pregnancy category X drug and is absolutely contraindicated in pregnant patients. In contrast to isotretinoin, which has a terminal elimination half-life of 10–20 hours, acitretin has a longer half-life of 2–4 days. Acitretin should not be taken with alcohol, since the alcohol induces esterification of acitretin to etretinate, which has a terminal half-life of 120 days. Women of childbearing age should begin effective contraception for at least 1 month before starting therapy and continue for at least 3 years after discontinuation of therapy.

BIBLIOGRAPHY

1. Borok M, Lowe NJ: Pityriasis rubra pilaris: Further observations of systemic retinoid therapy. J Am Acad Dermatol 22:792–795, 1990.
2. Dai WS, LaBracio JM, Stern RS: Epidemiology of isotretinoin exposure during pregnancy. J Am Acad Dermatol 26:599–606, 1992.

3. Katz HI, Waalen J, Leach EE: Acitretin in psoriasis: An overview of adverse effects. J Am Acad Dermatol 41:S7–S12, 1999.
4. Olsen EA, Katz I, Levine N, et al: Tretinoin emollient cream: A new therapy for photodamaged skin. J Am Acad Dermatol 26:215–224, 1992.
5. Peck GL, Coats-Walton DA: Retinoids in dermatology: Current usage. In Sober AJ, Fitzpatrick TB (eds): Yearbook of Dermatology, St. Louis, Mosby, 1995, pp. 1–32.
6. Salasche SJ, Lebwohl M: Clinical pearl: Vitamin E (alpha-tocopherol), 800 IU daily, may reduce retinoid toxicity. J Am Acad Dermatol 41:260, 1999.
7. Saurat JH: Retinoids and psoriasis: Novel issues in retinoid pharmacology and implications for psoriasis treatment. J Am Acad Dermatol 41:S2–S6, 1999.
8. Shornick JK, Formica N, Parke AL: Isotretinoin for refractory lupus erythematosus. J Am Acad Dermatol 24:49–52, 1991.
9. Tangrea JA, Kilcoyne RF, Taylor PR, et al: Skeletal hyperostosis in patients receiving chronic, very-low dose isotretinoin. Arch Dermatol 128:921–925, 1992.

IX. Special Patient Populations

56. NEONATAL INFECTIONS
Elizabeth Shurnas, M.D.

1. What are the TORCHES infections in a neonate?

This acronym stands for several etiologic agents of congenital infections: **TO**xoplasmosis, **R**ubella, **C**ytomegalovirus, **H**erpes, and **S**yphilis. (It might also include HIV, hepatitis, Epstein-Barr virus, and parvovirus B19 infections.) Cytomegalovirus is the most common cause of neonatal infections in the United States.

2. Describe the cutaneous findings in neonatal herpes simplex viral (HSV) infections.

HSV infection usually presents as grouped vesicles on an erythematous base. These lesions can be present on any part of the skin but are more common on the face, scalp, or buttocks (Fig. 1). They may also be generalized or disseminated or occur in the perianal region in a breech-delivered baby. In the intrauterine-exposed baby, they may present as atrophic areas with scarring.

3. Is neonatal herpes simplex dangerous?

Neonatal herpetic infections are usually severe (especially if lesions are disseminated or the CNS is involved) and require immediate diagnosis and treatment. The majority of infants with HSV infection acquire it in the intrapartum period or postnatally. Even with adequate treatment, the mortality rate is 54% in infants with disseminated disease, and the incidence of long-term morbidity is significant.

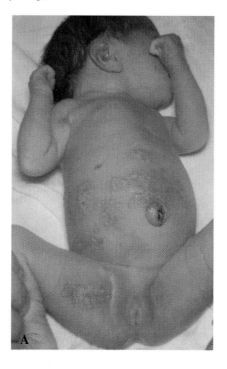
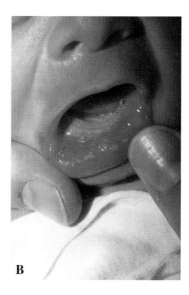

FIGURE 1. *A*, Congenital herpes simplex virus infection. *B*, Congenital mucosal herpes simplex virus infection. (Courtesy of William L. Weston, MD.)

4. **What percentage of herpes-infected neonates display skin or mucosal lesions?**

About 65% of infected infants display lesions shortly after birth, with disseminated disease occurring during the first 2 weeks of life. This includes infants with skin, eye, and mouth lesions (40%) as well as those with disseminated disease (25%) that includes the skin. If intrauterine exposure has occurred, lesions are usually present at birth. Fortunately, intrauterine transmission of HSV occurs in less than 5% of cases.

5. **What percentage of these lesions are HSV-1 versus HSV-2?**

Eighty percent of neonatal infections are due to perinatally acquired HSV-2 infection.

6. **What tests can be done to diagnose herpes infections? How should material be obtained for these tests?**

To obtain specimens for diagnostic testing, scrape the base of a blister and smear the material on a microscope slide. Stain (e.g., Wright stain) and look for multinucleated giant cells. If available, send another slide for HSV-fluorescein antibody test. Confirmation of a cytopathic effect can be made by immunofluorescence using antibodies specific to HSV-1 and HSV-2. Material from the blister base as well as aspirated blister fluid can be sent for viral culture. The sensitivity of culture is 95% for vesicles, 70% for ulcers, and 30% for crusts. It is also advisable to culture urine, nasopharynx, conjunctiva, and cerebrospinal fluid if indicated. The polymerase chain reaction (PCR) detects viral DNA and can be important in diagnosing HSV encephalitis.

7. **What is congenital varicella syndrome?**

Intrauterine infection with varicella virus that occurs in the first trimester may result in congenital varicella syndrome. These infants are born with hypoplasia of the limbs and exhibit cutaneous zosteriform scars and atrophy. Interestingly, there have been reports of neonates developing herpes zoster, which implies that they must have had chickenpox in utero.

8. **What is the average age of onset of lesions in a neonate exposed to varicella perinatally? When is there an increased risk of mortality?**

The average age of onset of varicella lesions is usually within the first 10 days of life. Congenital varicella is fatal in about 30% of patients whose mothers developed lesions from 5 days before to 2 days after delivery.

9. **What is the treatment of neonatal HSV and varicella infection?**

Early identification of infection and initiation of therapy are the most important aspects of treatment. Intravenous acyclovir or vidarabine is recommended for either infection. The usual course is 14–21 days. Ophthalmologic examination may be necessary and adequate isolation precautions must be instituted. For varicella infection, varicella-zoster immune globulin (VZIG) is recommended for cases with evidence of maternal infection 5 days before to 2 days after delivery (given within 48–96 hours after exposure). VZIG is not indicated for infants born to mothers with herpes zoster.

10. **What is a "blueberry muffin baby"? What is the significance of this diagnosis?**

This term applies to babies exhibiting blue-red indurated macules or papules on the face, trunk, or scalp present at birth or within the first 2 days of life. These lesions represent extramedullary dermal erythropoiesis and are seen in congenital rubella syndrome, toxoplasmosis, cytomegalovirus infection, neuroblastoma, leukemia, erythroblastosis fetalis, and twin transfusion syndrome.

11. **At what time during pregnancy is there the highest risk of congenital rubella following maternal infection?**

The risk is highest if maternal exposure occurs during the first 20 weeks of pregnancy. The risk of fetal infection is 90% during the first trimester and the majority of these infants suffer from congenital defects. Between the 12th and 20th weeks of gestation, the infection risk drops to 50% and about one-third of these infants have sequelae.

12. List the classic triad of congenital rubella syndrome (CRS).

Congenital cataracts

Deafness

Congenital heart malformations

The syndrome also includes microcephaly, microphthalmia, and intrauterine growth retardation. It is important to follow at-risk infants as two-thirds of infants with CRS may be asymptomatic at birth. Most will develop sequelae within the first 5 years of life.

13. Are any precautions necessary for infants with congenital rubella syndrome at the time of hospital discharge?

Yes. These infants represent potential risks to other pregnant women, as 5–10% of affected infants may shed virus for 12–18 months.

14. Why is human parvovirus infection important to a pregnant woman?

Human parvovirus B19, the etiologic agent of erythema infectiosum, readily infects erythroblasts and may therefore result in hydrops fetalis and fetal death. This risk is small, with current studies showing a 2–9% risk after infection during the first 16–28 weeks of pregnancy. Fortunately, about 50% of pregnant women have serologic evidence of prior exposure to parvovirus B19.

15. Are most infants with congenital cytomegalovirus (CMV) infection symptomatic?

No. Ninety percent of congenitally CMV-infected infants are asymptomatic. The other 5–10% usually have disease manifested by hepatosplenomegaly, hemorrhagic diatheses, and jaundice. The mortality rate in overtly symptomatic infants is almost 30%.

16. What cutaneous findings are seen in congenital CMV infection?

Petechiae

Purpura

Maculopapular rash

Papulonodular eruptions (with blueberry muffin lesions)

Vesicular eruption (rarely)

17. What clinical findings are seen in congenital Epstein-Barr virus infection?

Micrognathia	Scaly erythematous rash
Cryptorchidism	Hepatosplenomegaly
Cataracts	Persistent atypical lymphocytosis
Hypotonia	Hemolytic anemia

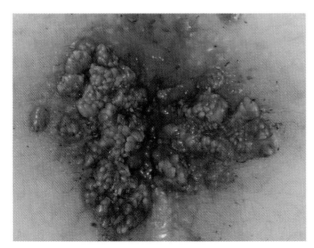

FIGURE 2. An infant with perianal warts. (Courtesy of William L. Weston, MD.)

18. Describe a clinical presentation of congenital human papillomavirus infection.

The infant can present with voice changes or a persistent abnormal hoarse cry, due to laryngeal papillomas thought to be acquired during passage through the infected birth canal. The time between rupture of the amnion and delivery seems to be a critical factor in vertical transmission rate. These signs of infection may not be evident for several months to several years of age.

Anogenital warts in young children can also be acquired as a congenital infection, through sexual abuse, or by other postnatal, nonsexual contact with affected adults (Fig. 2).

19. What percentage of infants born to HIV-positive mothers are born infected with HIV?

Most pediatric (80%) AIDS cases result from perinatal transmission. The rate of vertical transmission of HIV from infected mothers to their babies is 7–40%. This figure represents the actual infection rate, not the presence of antibody alone, as these infants can be seropositive at birth due to transplacentally acquired maternal antibody; this antibody can persist for 15–18 months. Infected and uninfected infants usually cannot be distinguished clinically at birth:

OB/GYN PROFILE	INFECTED INFANTS	UNINFECTED INFANTS
Maternal HIV risks		
IV drug use	59%	39%
Transfusion history	0%	2.7%
High-risk partner	4.5%	18%
No known risk	27.2%	29%
Birth weight	2786 gm	1842 gm
Birth length	47 cm	47.8 cm
Head circumference	33.5 cm	33.4 cm
Gestational age	39.2 wks	38.1 wks
Delivery type		
Cesarian	14%	15%
Vaginal	86%	85%

20. What is Hutchinson's triad?

Interstitial keratitis, Hutchinson's teeth, and eighth nerve deafness. These are common findings in late congenital syphilis. **Interstitial keratitis** is the most common lesion in this triad. It is rare before age 8 and after age 40. Both eyes are usually affected and the corneal clouding may be spotty or diffuse. **Hutchinson's teeth** are due to deficient development of the permanent teeth buds and are characterized by conical central incisors with notching of the distal free margin. **Eighth nerve deafness** usually occurs after interstitial keratitis, is usually bilateral, and is often preceded by tinnitus and vertigo.

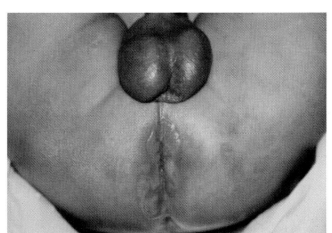

FIGURE 3. Congenital syphilis demonstrating perianal erosions.

21. Are there any other stigmata of late congenital syphilis?
Bone involvement is common with periostitis of long bones resulting in thickened and bent tibias (saber shins) and other bony abnormalities. Other stigmata include scarring and wrinkling at the corners of the mouth (rhagades), saddle nose, dish facies, Parrot's nodes on the skull, and salt-and-pepper fundi.

22. What are the physical findings of early congenital syphilis?
Syphilitic rhinitis is the most important and frequent physical finding in early congenital syphilis. It is characterized by a profuse serous nasal discharge (**snuffles**) that is teeming with spirochetes. The inflammatory process leads to eventual cartilage and bone deformity. Other findings include papulosquamous skin lesions, perianal erosions (Fig. 3), blistering of the hands and feet, hepatosplenomegaly, meningitis, meningoencephilitis, and osteochondritis. Congenital syphilis is a serious infection which, if untreated, has significant mortality.

BIBLIOGRAPHY

1. Behrman RE (ed): Nelson Textbook of Pediatrics. Philadelphia, W.B. Saunders, 1992.
2. Champion RH, Burton JL, Ebling FJG (eds): Rook/Wilkinson/Ebling Textbook of Dermatology. London, Blackwell Science, 1993.
3. Donley DK: TORCH infections in the newborn. Semin Neurol 13:106–114, 1993.
4. Gray J: HIV in the neonate. J Hosp Infect 37:181–198, 1997.
5. Hurwitz S: Clinical Pediatric Dermatology, 2nd ed. Philadelphia, W.B. Saunders, 1993, pp 28–32.
6. Jacobs RF: Neonatal herpes simplex virus infections. Semin Perinatol 22:64-71, 1998.
7. Johnson RA: Infectious disease update. Fitzpatrick's J Clin Dermatol (Suppl):49–66, 1994.
8. Nesheim SR, et al: A prospective population-based study of HIV perinatal transmission. AIDS 8:1293–1298, 1994.
9. Newton ER: Diagnosis of perinatal TORCH infections. Clin Obstet Gynecol 42:59–70, 1999.
10. Peter G (ed): 1994 Red Book: Report of the Committee on Infectious Diseases. Elk Grove Village, IL, American Academy of Pediatrics, 1994.
11. Rawlinson WD: Diagnosis of human cytomegalovirus infection and disease. Pathology 31:109–115, 1999.
12. Rodis JF: Parvovirus infection. Clin Obstet Gynecol 42:107–120, 1999.
13. Stamos JK, Rowley AH: Timely diagnosis of congenital infections. Pediatr Clin North Am 4:1017, 1994.
14. Tenti P, Zappatore R, Migliora P, et al: Perinatal transmission of human papillomavirus from gravidas with latent infections. Obstet Gynecol 93:475–479, 1999.
15. Weintrub PS, et al: Use of PCR for the early detection of HIV infection in the infants of HIV-seropositive women. AIDS 5:881–884, 1991.
16. Weston WL, Lane AT: Color Textbook of Pediatric Dermatology. St. Louis, Mosby, 1991.

57. PEDIATRIC DERMATOLOGY

Joseph G. Morelli, M.D.

1. What is the most common skin disease seen in children?

Acne vulgaris is the most prevalent skin condition observed in the pediatric age group, with two peaks of onset being noted. The first is in the neonatal period, and the second is during adolescence.

2. Name the papulopustular facial eruption often associated with inappropriate topical steroid use?

Perioral dermatitis is a perioral, periorbital, and perinasal, erythematous, slightly scaling papulopustular eruption seen most commonly in preschool children. Treatment of this condition is the discontinuation of topical steroids and the use of the same oral or topical antibiotics that are used for acne vulgaris.

3. At what age does atopic dermatitis typically begin?

Atopic dermatitis generally first appears between 1 and 4 months of age. By adolescence, over 90% of people who will get atopic dermatitis will have manifested the disease.

4. What is the natural history of atopic dermatitis?

By grade school, only one-third of children who had atopic dermatitis will continue to have difficulties with the disease. By adolescence, 90% will no longer have symptoms of atopic dermatitis.

5. What organism complicates irritant diaper dermatitis?

Candida albicans. It can be expected to superinfect any diaper dermatitis that has been present for 3 or more days.

6. Red, scaly, itchy weight-bearing surfaces of the feet in children are usually not due to tinea pedis, but what?

Juvenile plantar dermatosis. This is a nonspecific dermatitis, with a debatable relationship to atopic dermatitis.

7. Plant dermatitis, such as poison ivy, is the most prevalent cause of allergic contact dermatitis in children. What are some others?

Neomycin, nickel, and potassium dichromate.

8. One to 2 mm keratotic papules located on the face, outer upper arms, and thighs are frequently misdiagnosed as folliculitis. What are they really?

Keratosis pilaris. It may be inherited as an autosomal dominant disease or be associated with xerosis and/or atopy. The keratotic plugs are composed of corneocytes and sebum. Keratosis pilaris often spontaneously clears in adulthood.

9. What is the most common cutaneous bacterial infection in children?

Impetigo. This common, contagious, superficial infection is due to streptococci, staphylococci, or a combination of the two organisms.

10. What two organisms are most often responsible for tinea capitis?

Trichophyton tonsurans and *Microsporum canis.*

11. How is tinea capitis treated?

Oral griseofulvin is the treatment of choice. Topical antifungals have no role in the treatment of tinea capitis. Some authorities recommend twice-weekly shampooing with 2% selenium sulfide as a useful adjunctive therapy to griseofulvin, since it is sporicidal and may prevent spread to other children and family members.

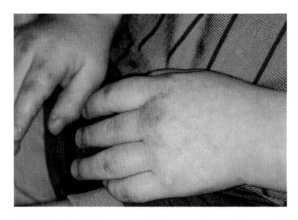

FIGURE 1. Dermatomyositis. Note Gottron's papules, that present as purple papules over the finger joints.

12. What is the hypersensitivity reaction to tinea capitis that is commonly mistaken for a bacterial superinfection?

A kerion. Kerions present as inflammatory plaques and abcesses and may be associated with regional adenopathy and fever. Some patients may have residual scarring and permanent alopecia.

13. Name the three conditions most often misdiagnosed as tinea corporis.

The herald patch of pityriasis rosea, nummular dermatitis, and granuloma annulare.

14. What percentage of children with psoriasis will have guttate psoriasis?

Although psoriasis vulgaris is still the most common type of psoriasis in childhood, up to one-third of children with psoriasis will have guttate flares. Guttate psoriasis is most often associated with streptococcal pharyngitis but may also be seen following perianal streptococcal infections.

15. Describe the rash associated with childhood dermatomyositis.

A malar photosensitive rash, with red flat-topped papules on the knuckles (Gottron's papules) and edematous plaques on the elbows and knees, is often seen in childhood dermatomyositis (Fig. 1). Unlike adult disease, childhood dermatomyositis is not related to internal malignancies.

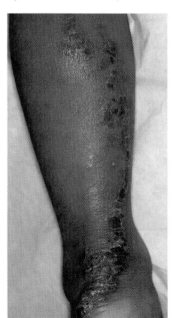

FIGURE 2. Lichen striatus presenting as hyperkeratotic linear plaque on the lower leg of a child.

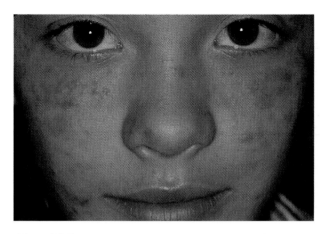

FIGURE 3. Polymorphous light eruption presenting as erythematous photodistributed papules.

16. A child's mother tells you that the rash started at one end of her child's extremity and has now progressed to form a line the entire length of the limb. What is your diagnosis?

Lichen striatus. It occurs in children aged 2–12 years and characteristically begins at one end of an extremity and slowly progresses the length of the extremity. The nature of the rash may vary from hypopigmented and macular to thickened and scaly (Fig. 2). No treatment is effective, and the lesions disappear spontaneously. The pathogenesis of this unusual dermatoses is unknown.

17. Name the most common sun-induced disease of childhood.

Sunburn. Excessive exposure to ultraviolet radiation causes sunburn. It is now known that excessive sun exposure and frequent sunburns in childhood are important in the development of skin cancers in adulthood.

18. If it's not sunburn, but a photosensitive eruption is suspected, what is it?

Polymorphous light eruption (Fig. 3), erythropoietic protoporphyria, and systemic lupus erythematosus are the three most common causes of a non-sunburn photoeruption in childhood.

19. Name the mildly inflammatory tongue eruption with day-to-day changes in appearance.

Geographic tongue (Fig. 4) is the name given to this usually asymptomatic childhood disorder.

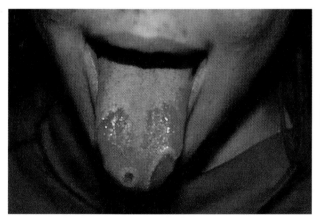

FIGURE 4. Geographic tongue presenting as migrating annular lesions on the tongue.

20. Which disease should be considered in a child with easy blistering of the skin?

A child with skin that blisters with minimal trauma should be evaluated for one of the mechanobullous diseases, also known as **epidermolysis bullosa.** There are 17 subtypes, but clinically there are three important variants: epidermal and junctional, which are both nonscarring, and dermal, which is scarring (see Chapter 6).

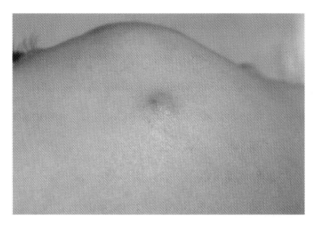

FIGURE 5. Pilomatrichoma pre-senting as firm nodule on the cheek of a child.

21. Two common nodules are seen in childhood. Name them.

Epithelial (epidermoid) cysts comprise 60% of the nodules seen in children, and **piloma-tricomas** (Fig. 5) account for another 10%. The other 30% of nodules in children are caused by many relatively uncommon problems.

22. Crusted purpuric papules and a scaly seborrheic-like eruption in the scalp and groin are seen in what serious disease of childhood?

This constellation of findings should suggest Langerhans cell histiocytosis (formerly called his-tiocytosis-X) (Fig. 6). Most recent evidence relates Langerhans cell histiocytosis to infection with hu-man herpesvirus type 6. The disease can vary from a mild cutaneous-only eruption to a severe, life-threatening, systemic disease. Traditionally, this disease has been treated by pediatric oncologists.

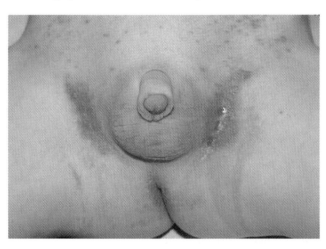

FIGURE   6. Langerhans cell   histiocytosis demon-strating erythematous scale and   crusted papule in the groin of a child.

23. Name the skin nodule in childhood that is characterized by frequent bleeding.

Pyogenic granulomas are <1-cm, dull red, firm nodules that bleed easily when traumatized. They are neither pyogenic nor granulomatous, but are thought to be the result of excessive blood vessel formation in response to minor trauma.

24. Flesh-colored to brown macules and papules that hive when stroked (Darier's sign) are diagnostic of what eruption?

Mastocytosis. Mastocytosis is due to an excess of normal-appearing mast cells in the skin. There are three forms, with solitary mastocytomas and urticaria pigmentosa (Fig. 7) being the most common. Diffuse cutaneous mastocytosis is the third type.

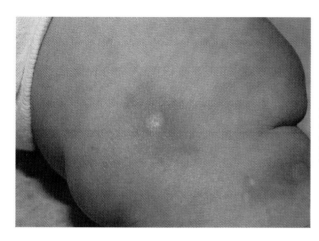

FIGURE 7. Urticaria pigmentosa demonstrating positive Darier's sign (wheal and flare of a brown papule after stroking) in a child with multiple lesions.

25. The onset of annular erythema in sun-exposed areas in children less than 6 months of age should make you want to do what test on the infant's mother?

This eruption is consistent with neonatal lupus erythematosus and is associated with maternal autoantibodies to SS-A/Ro and/or SS-B/La. The mothers are often asymptomatic or have only mild symptoms of Sjögren's syndrome at the time of delivery. Neonatal lupus can also cause complete heart block.

26. Which is the most common type of vasculitis seen in children?

Henoch-Schönlein or anaphylactoid purpura. This type of vasculitis frequently follows upper respiratory tract infections and is characterized by the finding of IgA depositions in the blood vessels. The disease may affect only skin, but arthritis, gastrointestinal pain and bleeding, and kidney and CNS disease may occur.

27. What is a spider telangiectasia (nevus araneus)?

It is a small telangiectatic macule radiating from a central arteriole. They are commonly seen on the faces of children aged 2–6 years. Contrary to popular belief, they rarely disappear spontaneously. Pulsed dye laser treatment is simple and very effective.

28. Outline the major classes of hair loss in children.

A simple classification of hair loss makes it easier for one to reach a diagnosis.

Classes of Hair Loss in Children

Congenital circumscribed
Acquired circumscribed
Congenital diffuse
Acquired diffuse

29. List the three most common types of acquired circumscribed hair loss in children.

Alopecia areata, tinea capitis, and trichotillomania. Alopecia areata is thought to be an autoimmune disorder, whereas tinea capitis is a fungal infection of the scalp hairs. Trichotillomania is self-inflicted.

Common Types of Hair Loss in Childhood

TYPE	PATTERN	SCALP APPEARANCE
Alopecia areata	Circumscribed	Normal
Tinea capitis	Circumscribed	Scaly
Trichotillomania	Irregular	Petechiae

30. What are the two most common causes of congenital circumscribed hair loss?

Sebaceous nevus (organoid nevus) and aplasia cutis congenita. **Sebaceous nevus** is a birthmark of sebaceous glands. It presents as a yellow-orange plaque on the scalp, face, and upper chest. **Aplasia cutis congenita** is a localized absence of skin. It presents as either an open ulceration or a scar. The scalp is the most common location, but areas of aplasia cutis congenita may be seen anywhere on the body. When either of these lesions is present on the scalp, no hair grows in the affected area.

31. What should you think of in a 3-year-old who has never required a hair cut?

Such a child is likely to have either a hair shaft defect or a type of epidermal dysplasia. **Hair shaft defects** are structural abnormalities that cause hair to be fragile and easily breakable. The defects can be recognized by microscopic evaluation. The **ectodermal dysplasias** may affect not only hair but also nails, teeth, and sweat glands.

32. What are the cutaneous findings seen in tuberous sclerosis?

Two congenital lesions may be seen: hypopigmented macules and connective tissue nevi (shagreen patch). The acquired lesions are facial angiofibromas and periungual fibromas.

33. How many café-au-lait macules must be present on a child to make you worry about neurofibromatosis type 1 (von Recklinghausen's disease)?

Six or more café-au-lait macules > 5 mm in diameter in a prepubertal child are one of the major diagnostic criteria for neurofibromatosis type 1.

34. What is a mongolian spot?

This is a blue-black macule found in up to 90% of black and Asian newborns. The most common location is the sacral region, but they may be seen on any portion of the body.

35. What are congenital pigmented nevi, and who cares?

Congenital pigmented nevi are developmental errors of pigment cells (melanocytes). They should be defined as small (<2 cm), medium (2–20 cm), and large (>20 cm) in their largest diameter at birth. Small congenital pigmented nevi are quite common (1/100), whereas large congenital pigmented nevi are rare (1/20,000). The controversy surrounding these lesions concerns their malignant potential. Estimates of 4–10% lifetime risk for the development of melanoma in large congenital pigmented nevi have been made, but this rate seems high when compared to clinical practice. On-going prospective studies will eventually resolve this issue.

36. Child abuse is often incorrectly suspected when a young girl presents with what disease?

Lichen sclerosus et atrophicus. This problem frequently presents as hypopigmented perianal and perivaginal plaques. The epidermis is thinned, and the dermis is sclerotic. Purpura, telangiectasias, ulcerations, and excoriations may also be present. Itching and burning of the genital area are often the complaints that bring the child to the physician.

BIBLIOGRAPHY

1. Aly R: Ecology, epidemiology and diagnosis of tinea capitis. Pediatr Infect Dis J 18:180–185, 1999.
2. Chamlin SL, Williams ML: Moles and melanoma. Curr Opin Pediatr 10:398–404, 1998.
3. DeGroot HE, Friedlander SF: Update on acne. Curr Opin Pediatr 10:381–386, 1998.
4. Hensley DR, Hebert AA: Pediatric photosensitivity disorders. Dermatol Clin 16:571–578, 1998.
5. Krafchik BR: Treatment of atopic dermatitis. J Cutan Med Surg 3(Suppl 2):16–23, 1999.
6. North KN: Neurofibromatosis 1 in childhood. Semin Pediatr Neurol 5:231–242, 1998.
7. Roach ES, Gomez MR, Northrup H: Tuberous sclerosis complex consensus conference: Revised clinical diagnostic criteria. J Child Neurol 13:624–648, 1998.
8. Sadick NS: Current aspects of bacterial infections of the skin. Dermatol Clin 15:341–349, 1997.

58. GERIATRIC DERMATOLOGY

James E. Fitzpatrick, M.D.

1. How common are skin disorders in the elderly population?

Survey studies have demonstrated that skin diseases are more common in the geriatric population than in the general population. One study revealed that 40% of Americans between the ages of 65 and 74 years had a cutaneous disease significant enough to warrant treatment by a physician. Patients older than 74 years are even more likely to develop significant skin diseases.

2. What is intrinsic aging of the skin?

Aging of the skin may be divided into that due to intrinsic aging and that secondary to extrinsic aging. **Intrinsic aging** includes those changes that are due to normal maturity and senescence and thus occurs in all individuals. Classically, intrinsic aging has not been considered to be preventable, but there is renewed interest in the role of antioxidants, such as vitamins C and E, in preventing intrinsic aging. Despite numerous articles in the lay literature, there is no proof that these treatments are effective.

Age-Related Changes in the Skin

Intrinsic Aging	Extrinsic Aging (Primarily UV Light)
Decrease in corneocyte adhesion	Altered keratinocyte maturation (xerosis)
Slight decrease in epidermal thickness with flattening of rete pegs	Freckles (ephelides)
	Solar lentigo
Decreased number of eccrine sweat glands	Guttate hypomelanosis
Decreased numbers of hair follicles	Wrinkling
Canities (gray hair)	Elastosis (yellowish skin)
Thinning and ridging of nails	Telangiectasia
Decreased dermal collagen (decreases 1% per year)	Senile purpura
Decreased number of dermal elastic fibers	Venous lakes
Decreased dermal ground substance	Comedones
Loss or increase in subcutaneous fat (site-dependent)	

3. What is extrinsic aging of the skin?

Extrinsic aging of the skin consists of those changes produced by external agents. The most important extrinsic factor is cumulative ultraviolet (UV) light exposure, and the cutaneous changes produced by sunlight are collectively referred to as **dermatoheliosis.** Most of the changes associated with aging of the skin, such as wrinkles, yellow leathery skin, thin skin, hyperpigmentation, hypopigmentation, lentigo senilis (liver spots), telangiectasias, and senile (solar) purpura, are all secondary to damage from the sun or other UV light sources such as tanning booths. Less important extrinsic agents that accelerate aging of the skin include smoking and possibly environmental pollutants.

4. How does intrinsically aging human skin vary from young skin under the microscope?

Microscopically, the epidermis in aged skin demonstrates flattening of the dermoepidermal junction (loss of the normal rete ridge pattern) with fewer melanocytes and Langerhans cells. The dermis demonstrates atrophy with fewer fibroblasts, mast cells, and blood vessels associated with depigmentation of hair, loss of hair follicles, and fewer sweat glands. The amount of collagen, elastin, and ground substance also decrease.

5. Why does skin wrinkle as we age?

The answer is complicated since some authorities recognize as many as five different subtypes of wrinkles. The most common type of wrinkles on non–sun-exposed skin are fine wrinkles (glyphic wrinkles) that represent accentuation of normal skin markings. Microscopically this is due to focal thinning and decreased numbers of keratinocytes. This appears to be intrinsic to aging (Fig. 1). The deeper wrinkles in photo-damaged skin demonstrate a groove in the epidermis associated with solar elastosis that protrudes on both sides of the groove. These deeper wrinkles are due to extrinsic aging, primarily resulting from ultraviolet light.

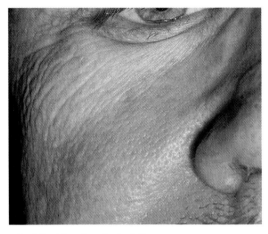

FIGURE 1. Large coarse wrinkles primarily due to photo aging. Some of the fine wrinkles near the eye are glyphic wrinkles and are intrinsic to aging.

6. What is solar elastosis?

Solar (actinic) elastosis refers to the changes due to abnormal elastotic fibers produced by fibroblasts in the papillary and superficial reticular dermis in response to UV light exposure. The precise nature of these fibers is not established, but they stain with elastic tissue stains and are susceptible to elastase digestion. Electron microscopy demonstrates that these fibers are similar, but not identical, to normal elastic fibers. Large aggregates of these fibers impart a yellowish color and account for the yellow leathery appearance of sun-exposed skin in geriatric individuals. Solar elastosis is often most easily appreciated in the posterior neck, where it is termed **cutis rhomboidalis nuchae** (Fig. 2).

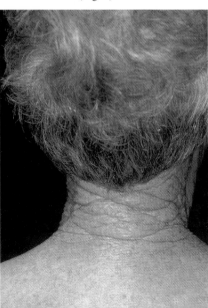

FIGURE 2. Cutis rhomboidalis nuchae. Severe solar elastosis and wrinkling of the posterior neck secondary to sun exposure that clearly demarcates from more normal-appearing skin that is less sun-damaged.

7. What is nodular elastosis with cysts and comedones?

Nodular elastosis with cysts and comedones, also known as Favre-Racouchot syndrome, is characterized by the presence of marked solar elastosis and comedones on the lateral and inferior periorbital areas (Fig. 3). Severe cases may demonstrate cysts. The reason for this regional presentation is not understood, but it has been suggested that the fibroblasts around the hair follicles are damaged by UV light and no longer produce normal elastic tissue. This predisposes to dilatation of the hair follicles, resulting in comedones and cysts. Most cases can be successfully treated with topical tretinoin cream and comedonal extraction.

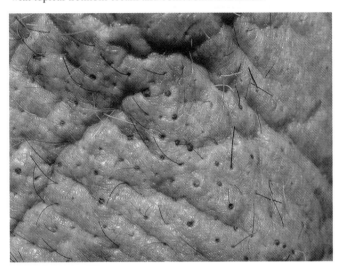

FIGURE 3. Nodular elastosis with comedones. Numerous comedones in characteristic location associated with background of solar elastotic skin.

8. How do liver spots, solar lentigo, and lentigo senilis differ?

Liver spots, age spots, and the more proper dermatologic terms solar lentigo and lentigo senilis, all refer to the same entity. More than one-half of all patients over age 64 will have at least one solar lentigo, and most patients have more than one. Clinically, they are flat to slightly raised, tan to brown lesions on sun-exposed skin, most commonly on the dorsum of the hands, forearms, and face where they are the result of excessive cumulative UV light exposure. Microscopically, solar lentigos demonstrate elongation of the rete ridges (lentiginous hyperplasia) and increased numbers of melanocytes that produce more than the normal amount of melanin. They may be removed with a light freeze of liquid nitrogen, various types of peels, or special lasers. They may also be temporarily bleached with over-the-counter (1–2% concentration) or prescription (3–4% concentration) hydroquinone creams.

9. Why do elderly patients frequently develop bleeding into the skin on the dorsum of their hands and arms?

These lesions, referred to as senile purpura (solar purpura, Bateman's purpura, purpura senilis), are common. One study of patients over age 64 years found them in 9% of those examined. The lesions are characterized by sharply demarcated areas of purpura that typically measure 1–5 cm (Fig. 4). The associated skin is atrophic and inelastic. Patients typically report that these lesions are brought on by minor trauma. It is believed that they are secondary to UV damage to the fibroblasts surrounding the blood vessels, which results in the loss of normal supporting collagen.

10. Advertisements in newspapers and magazines frequently tout products that "rejuvenate" the skin or make the skin younger. Is there truth to these claims?

No. There are no known therapies or products that rejuvenate the skin or make it younger. There are therapies that make the skin appear less wrinkled and thus appear younger. Topical

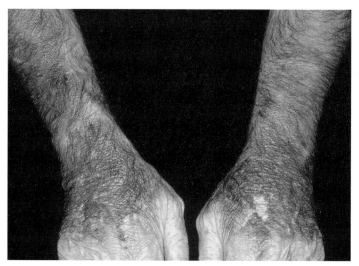

FIGURE 4. Severe senile purpura on the dorsum of the hands and forearms of an elderly patient.

applications of isotretinoin cream and lactic acid-containing moisturizers both have been shown in controlled scientific studies to thicken the skin and make wrinkles less noticeable, but the results of these topical treatments vary from almost imperceptible to moderate. More dramatic results can be achieved by chemical facial peels (phenol, trichloroacetic acid, α-hydroxy acids), laser therapy (laser skin resurfacing), injection of bovine collagen into wrinkles, and facelifts. The best treatment for extrinsic aging of the skin is prevention, by minimizing sun exposure with avoidance, appropriate clothing, and sunscreens. Abstinence from the use of tobacco products also helps.

11. Are some sunscreens better than others in preventing wrinkles due to photo damage?
Probably. The definitive study has not been done but most of the UV-induced deep wrinkles are believed to be primarily a UVB effect, although UVA contributes. Based on this, sunscreens with both UVB and UVA protection should be the most efficient in preventing wrinkling.

12. Which are the most common inflammatory skin diseases in the elderly?
- Xerosis (dry skin)
- Dermatophytosis (see Chapter 31)
- Contact dermatitis (see Chapter 9)
- Stasis dermatitis
- Seborrheic dermatitis (see Chapter 8)
- Rosacea

13. Why are elderly patients prone to develop xerosis?
Xerosis (dry skin, asteatosis, dermatitis hiemalis) is the most common geriatric dermatosis and the most frequent cause of pruritus. Xerosis is believed to be more common in the elderly because of abnormal maturation and adhesion of keratinocytes, which results in rough skin characterized by fine white scale. Diminished eccrine function and sebaceous gland lipids may also play a role but do not represent the primary defect. Asteatosis, which means "without oil," is really a misnomer since this is not the cause of dry skin.

14. What is the best way to treat xerosis?
Xerosis is aggravated by low ambient humidity, especially in dry climates and heated homes, and irritants such as soaps. Xerosis can be improved by increasing the ambient humidity (with a

humidifier) and by using soaps that are mild, such as Dove or Oil of Olay. Most patients also require treatment with an emollient. The most effective emollients contain lactic acid or a lactate salt, but these are expensive and the best ones require a prescription. The effectiveness of all emollients is improved by applying them immediately to the skin after bathing, when the skin is hydrated.

15. How common is chronic venous insufficiency in the geriatric population?

Epidemiologic studies show an incidence in the geriatric population that approaches 6%. The economic impact of this condition is enormous; the estimated total cost in the United States for the treatment of venous ulcers is $665 million per year.

16. Explain the pathogenesis of chronic venous insufficiency.

Chronic venous insufficiency is due to venous hypertension secondary to valvular incompetence in the superficial, perforator, or deep veins, with many patients having defects in two or more valve systems. The most severe disease is produced by deep valvular insufficiency. Valvular insufficiency may be the consequence of hereditary factors (absent or congenitally incompetent valves), prolonged standing, and venous thrombosis that may damage valves. Chronic venous hypertension, depending on the degree of severity, may manifest as edema, varicosities, brown pigmentation secondary to hemosiderin, superficial neovascularization, dermatitis, and venous ulcers (Fig. 5).

17. How should you manage chronic venous insufficiency?

Treatment is primarily directed toward reducing venous pressure. This end can be achieved with elevation of the legs, active exercise, supportive stockings, sclerotherapy of selected perforator veins, or surgical treatment. Surgical options are dependent on the site involved but include ligation and stripping of the saphenous vein, ligation of incompetent perforators, or valve replacement. Dermatitis (stasis dermatitis), if present, may be treated with mild to moderate corticosteroids, and oral antibiotics may be used if secondary infection is present. Venous ulcers are treated with these options but also require wound management.

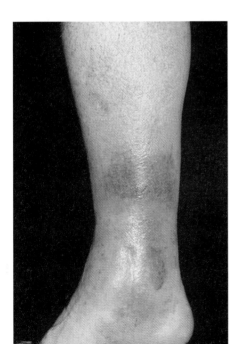

FIGURE 5. Chronic venous insufficiency manifesting as marked erythema and edema, which is often called stasis dermatitis.

18. What is rosacea? How does it present?

Rosacea, or acne rosacea, is a common skin condition that may affect up to 12% of the geriatric population. The pathogenesis is not understood, but it is known that patients with rosacea have increased blood flow to the skin and are more likely to demonstrate infestation with *Demodex folliculorum,* the human hair follicle mite (although its relevance to the pathogenesis of rosacea is unclear). Rosacea primarily affects the forehead, cheeks, nose, and chin. The three primary lesions are telangiectasis, sebaceous gland hyperplasia, and acneiform papules and pustules (see also Chapter 21). One or more of these primary lesions may predominate in a particular patient.

19. Is rhinophyma related to alcohol abuse?

Rhinophyma is a clinical variant of rosacea that presents as severe sebaceous gland hyperplasia of the nose, which may distort the contour of the nose. The lay public often assumes that people with rhinophyma are alcohol abusers. This is not true, although patients with rosacea demonstrate prominent flushing following the consumption of alcohol. This flushing is perceived as being the cause of rhinophyma.

20. Name the most common types of skin tumors seen in the elderly.

- Benign tumors: seborrheic keratoses, cherry hemangiomas, nevi, acrochordons, sebaceous hyperplasia
- Premalignant tumors: actinic keratoses, Bowen's disease
- Malignancies: basal cell carcinoma, squamous cell carcinoma

21. What are seborrheic keratoses?

Seborrheic keratoses are common, benign epidermal growths of the skin. In patients over age 64 years, the incidence of these growths is 88%. The pathogenesis is uncertain, but they are believed to arise from either the epidermal basal cell layer or keratinocytes of the most superficial part of the hair follicle. They typically begin appearing during middle-age or later. They may be located on any cutaneous surface other than the palms and soles but are most commonly found on the face and trunk. Clinically, they present as tan, brown, gray, or black, sharply demarcated, exophytic papules that appear to be "stuck on" the skin. The surface often has an irregular contour or pebbly surface but may be verrucous or smooth (Fig. 6).

22. What are stucco keratoses?

Stucco keratoses are a variant of seborrheic keratoses that present as 1–4-mm gray to white scaly papules. These are most commonly located on the arms and lower legs (Fig. 7).

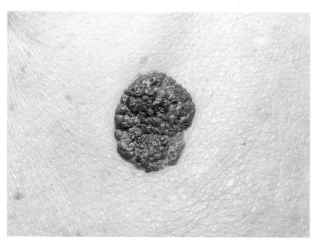

FIGURE 6. Seborrheic keratosis. Typical, deep-brown to black exophytic seborrheic keratosis with a "stuck on" appearance. This is the most common benign cutaneous growth of the elderly.

23. A 70-year-old man presents to your clinic with the sudden onset of hundreds of seborrheic keratoses. Is there any reason for concern?

Yes. This patient may have the sign of Leser-Trélat, which is characterized by the sudden appearance of numerous seborrheic keratoses associated with an underlying malignancy. About one-third of patients with this sign may also present with acanthosis nigricans, another potential cutaneous marker of internal malignancy. The most common associated malignancy is an abdominal adenocarcinoma.

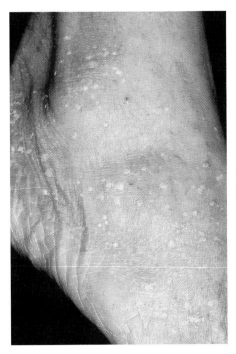

FIGURE 7. Typical stucco kerotosis manifesting as small white or white-gray scaly papules with "stuck on" appearance.

24. Describe the methods for treating seborrheic keratoses.

First of all, not all seborrheic keratoses need to be treated, and many health plans do not pay for their treatment since they are benign lesions. Patients frequently want them removed for cosmetic reasons or because they are pruritic. The most common treatment is **cryotherapy** with liquid nitrogen since it is quick and effective. Seborrheic keratoses can also be removed by **curetting** or **shave biopsy.** Shave biopsies are usually done when the lesion has an atypical clinical appearance and a malignancy, such as squamous cell or basal cell carcinoma, is in the differential diagnosis. Seborrheic keratoses can also be treated with the topical application of **α-hydroxy acids.**

25. An elderly man presents with a soft blue papule on the helix of his cheek and is concerned about malignant melanoma. What is the most likely diagnosis?

The differential diagnosis includes a blue nevus, malignant melanoma, tattoo, and venous lake. In this case, the diagnosis of a venous lake can be established by compression of the papule, which will cause collapse of the lesion (Fig. 8). Venous lakes, like hemorrhoids, are dilated veins that have lost elasticity of their walls. They are usually 1–5 mm in diameter and are typically located on sun-exposed surfaces, such as the lips, ears, and face of the elderly. They are very common, with one epidemiologic study of elderly patients finding venous lakes in 12% of those examined. They are of no clinical significance except that they may mimic malignant melanoma and occasionally become painful or thrombosed. They are easily removed by simple excision.

26. Is there a future in geriatric dermatology?

One hundred years ago, only 2% of the U.S. population was over 65 years old. By 1980, this percentage was 11% and by the year 2030 it will be 20%. Given the high incidence of significant dermatologic diseases in the elderly, it is clear that all health care providers need to familiarize themselves with the diagnosis, prevention, and treatment of skin diseases seen in this population.

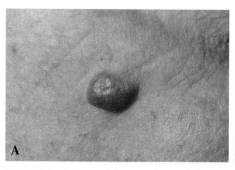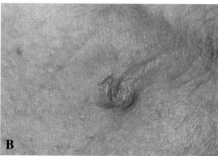

FIGURE 8. *A*, Venous lake presenting as dark blue-violaceous papule on the cheek. *B*, Same venous lake demonstrating collapse after compression.

BIBLIOGRAPHY

1. Beauregard SA, Gilchrest BA: Survey of skin problems and skin care regimens in the elderly. Arch Dermotol 123:1638, 1987.
2. Fitzpatrick JE: Common inflammatory skin diseases of the elderly. Geriatrics 44:40–46, 1989.
3. Fitzpatrick JE: Stasis ulcers: Update on a common geriatric problem. Geriatrics 44:19–31, 1989.
4. Fitzpatrick JE, Mellette JR Jr: Geriatric dermatology. In Schrier RW (ed): Geriatric Medicine. Philadelphia, W.B. Saunders, 1990, pp 138–148.
5. Gilchrest BA: Age associated changes in the skin: Overview and clinical relevance. J Am Geriatr Soc 30:139–142, 1982.
6. Gilchrest BA: Skin and Aging Processes. Boca Raton, FL, CRC Press, 1984, pp 1–120.
7. Long CC, Marks R: Stratum corneum changes in patients with senile pruritus. J Am Acad Dermatol 27:560–564, 1992.
8. Sibenge S, Gawkrodger DJ: Rosacea: A study of clinical patterns, blood flow, and the role of *Demodex folliculorum*. J Am Acad Dermatol 26:590–593, 1992.
9. Uitto J, Brown DB, Gasparro FP, et al: Molecular aspects of photoaging. Eur J Dermatol 7:210–214, 1997.

59. DERMATOSES OF PREGNANCY

Lisa M. Cohen, M.D., and James E. Fitzpatrick, M.D.

SPECIFIC DERMATOSES OF PREGNANCY

1. Name the four well-defined dermatoses of pregnancy.

Herpes gestationis
Pruritic urticarial papules and plaques of pregnancy (PUPPP)
Cholestasis of pregnancy
Impetigo herpetiformis
There are also other inflammatory skin conditions associated with pregnancy, but these are poorly defined.

2. Are the dermatoses of pregnancy confined to the pregnant state?

No. These diseases are also produced by situations such as oral contraceptive therapy and choriocarcinomas that hormonally mimic the pregnant state.

3. What is herpes gestationis? Is it caused by the herpes virus?

Herpes gestationis is an autoimmune bullous disease of pregnancy that typically begins in the late second trimester with a mean onset of 21 weeks. The disease is associated with a circulating antibody that binds to the basement membrane of the skin. Although blisters are the predominant primary lesion (Fig. 1), urticarial papules and plaques, target lesions and polycyclic erythema may be present. The eruption most often begins around the umbilicus but may become generalized. The name "herpes gestationis" is confusing since there is no relationship to herpes virus infection.

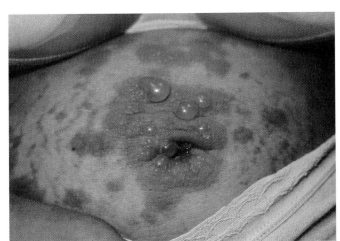

FIGURE 1. Umbilical urticarial plaques and tense blisters in a woman with herpes gestationis.

4. If herpes gestationis is not caused by herpes virus, why is it called "herpes"?

Herpes is a latin word taken from Greek that literally means "to creep." Thus, herpetology, which is the study of reptiles, is literally the study of creeping things (e.g., snakes). In medicine, the term *herpes* is used to describe vesicular processes that cluster. It is usually associated with viral infections, such as herpes simplex and herpes zoster, but can be used to describe noninfectious vesiculobullous disorders such as herpes gestationis.

5. What is pruritic urticarial papules and plaques of pregnancy?

Pruritic urticarial papules and plaques of pregnancy (PUPPP) is a pruritic eruption that characteristically begins in the third trimester with a mean onset at 35 weeks of gestation. The lesions appear initially on the lower abdomen, particularly in the striae (stretch marks), and often spread to involve the chest, extremities, back, and breasts (Fig. 2). Lesions above the breasts are uncommon and the face is almost universally spared. Morphologically, the lesion is of erythematous, urticarial papules and plaques without blisters, although pinpoint vesicles may be present.

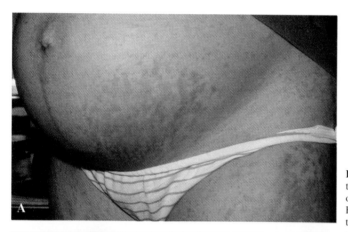

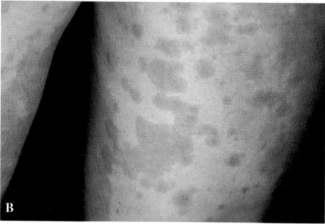

FIGURE 2. Pruritic urticarial papules and plaques of pregnancy (PUPPP). *A*, Erythematous papules in the striae of a 21-year-old primigravida woman. *B*, Urticarial papules and plaques that are not associated with striae on the thighs of a woman with PUPPP.

6. Compare the incidence and prognosis of herpes gestationis (HG) and PUPPP.

	HG	PUPPP
Incidence	1/40,000 pregnancies	1/240 pregnancies
Maternal prognosis	Postpartum flare in 75%; recurrence in subsequent pregnancy common	Rare postpartum flare; rare recurrence in subsequent pregnancy
Fetal prognosis	3–5% have blisters at birth; increased risk of prematurity	No skin lesions; increased twin rate and neonatal birthweight

Older textbooks and papers indicate an increased incidence of fetal mortality and morbidity in herpes gestationis, but more recent information suggests that this is not the case.

7. What is "HG factor"?

HG factor, seen in patients with herpes gestationis, is a circulating IgG_1 antibody that binds to an antigen (180 kD) in the basement membrane zone. This same antigen is found in the human amnion, which may be the reason that this disease is associated with pregnancy. This factor stimulates the classic complement pathway, which results in the deposition of complement (C3) along the basement membrane zone. This deposition produces chemotaxis of inflammatory cells (particularly eosinophils). The inflammatory cells degranulate and release proteolytic enzymes that lead to epidermal/dermal separation. The titer of HG factor is not related to disease activity.

8. Which HLA types have been associated with herpes gestationis?

HLA-DR3 and particularly the combination of HLA-DR3 and HLA-DR4 are associated with this condition (the relative risk for the combination being 23.5). A weaker association has been found for HLA-B8.

9. Is topical therapy adequate for herpes gestationis?

No. Only mild cases will respond to topical corticosteroids and oral antihistamines. Most patients require systemic corticosteroids (20–80 mg/day). Dapsone and plasmapheresis also have been reported to be efficacious.

10. Do the usual direct or indirect immunofluorescence findings in herpes gestationis and PUPPP differ?

Herpes gestationis: Direct immunofluorescence (IF) shows linear C3 along the basement membrane zone in nearly 100% of cases and linear IgG in 25%. Indirect IF is usually negative or demonstrates low titers for IgG, unless indirect complement-added IF techniques are employed. Indirect IF can detect C3 in about 90% of cases.

PUPPP: Immunofluorescence studies are negative.

11. List six factors that link abdominal distention to the development of PUPPP.

Third trimester onset
Occurrence in primigravidas
Initial site on the abdomen, particularly the striae
Increased maternal weight gain
Increased neonatal birthweight
Increased twin rate

12. What is chlolestasis of pregnancy?

Cholestasis of pregnancy is an intensely pruritic condition that begins after the sixth week of pregnancy, progresses throughout the pregnancy, and subsides soon after delivery. Despite the absence of primary lesions, the pruritus is generalized, and patients often present with generalized excoriations. About 50% of patients have an associated icterus due to hyperbilirubinemia. In the absence of hyperbilirubinemia, the disease is often called **pruritus gravidarum.** Both diseases have elevated serum and skin bile acids (predominantly cholic acid).

13. Does the degree of pruritus correlate with serum bile acid levels?

Yes. There is a strong correlation between the two. Serum bile acids in cholestasis of pregnancy range from 150–4000 μg/100 ml (normal, < 60). The degree of pruritus also correlates with bile acid levels in the skin.

14. What is the usual prognosis in patients with cholestasis of pregnancy?

There is little if any response to treatment, and symptoms resolve within 48 hours of delivery. In about 40% of patients, the disease recurs in a subsequent pregnancy. Use of oral contraceptives has been associated with a recurrence of the disease. Postpartum hemorrhage and cholelithiasis may occur with increased frequency. There is a tendency for low birthweight babies and prematurity.

15. How is cholestasis of pregnancy treated?

The disease usually resolves within several days of delivery. During pregnancy, mild cases can be treated with topical emollients. Severe cases may respond to oral antihistamines. Anecdotal reports have suggested that oral cholestyramine or ursodeoxycholic acid may be effective. Many authorities recommend induction or delivery at 38 weeks to improve fetal outcome.

16. Which disease does impetigo herpetiformis mimic?

Impetigo herpetiformis occurs in the third trimester of pregnancy as generalized pustules on an erythematous base with associated fever. The disease is clinically and histologically identical to **pustular psoriasis,** except that it occurs in pregnancy.

The two diseases also share laboratory abnormalities, including an elevated sedimentation rate, leukocytosis, and hypocalcemia. Impetigo herpetiformis occurs in patients without a previous history of psoriasis and may recur with subsequent pregnancy. The risks include tetany, seizures, delirium (secondary to hypocalcemia), sepsis, and stillbirth. The disease is invariably fatal without treatment, which includes systemic corticosteroids, antibiotics, and calcium.

PHYSIOLOGIC CHANGES IN PREGNANCY

17. List the pigmentary changes that can occur in a normal pregnancy.
1. Hyperpigmentation of the nipples, areolae, anogenital area
2. Pigmentation of the linea alba ("linea nigra")
3. Hyperpigmentation of the axillae and inner thighs
4. Melasma (Fig. 3)
5. Darkening of nevi and ephelides

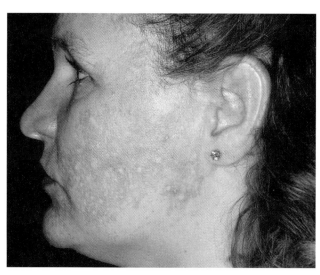

FIGURE 3. Photodistributed macular hyperpigmentation typical of melasma.

18. Since pregnancy is associated with darkening of nevi, does it affect patients with melanoma?

The effect of pregnancy on melanoma is controversial, but most controlled studies show no significant difference in survival in pregnant patients with stage I disease. Furthermore, there appears to be no difference in survival and no increased risk of recurrence in women who become pregnant within 5 years of a diagnosis of melanoma. There have been very few controlled trials to assess the effect of pregnancy on stage II disease, and the results conflict.

19. List the vascular changes that can occur in pregnancy.
1. Palmar erythema (Fig. 4)
2. Spider angiomas
3. Vascular tumors (pyogenic granulomas, cherry hemangiomas, glomus tumors)
4. Varicose veins
5. Hemorrhoids

20. What is "granuloma gravidarum"?
Also known as a pregnancy tumor, this is the name given to a **pyogenic granuloma of the oral cavity** (particularly the gingiva) which occurs with increased frequency in pregnancy. The tumor is associated with gingivitis (gingivitis gravidarum). Pyogenic granulomas are also more common on the skin during pregnancy.

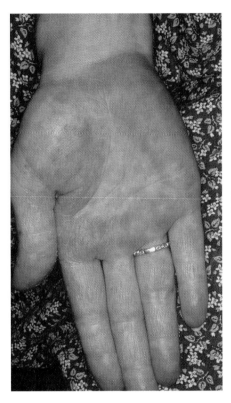

FIGURE 4. Marked palmar erythema in a pregnant woman.

21. Are any mucocutaneous diseases exacerbated in pregnancy?
Yes. Many can be, but not invariably (see table next page).

22. Are any diseases improved during pregnancy?
- Fox-Fordyce disease (possibly due to decreased apocrine gland secretion)
- Hidradenitis suppurativa
- Rheumatoid arthritis
- Psoriasis
- Sarcoidosis
- Atopic dermatitis

Mucocutaneous Diseases Exacerbated by Pregnancy

Infections
    Candida vaginitis
    Trichomoniasis
    Condyloma acuminata
    Pityrosporum folliculitis
    Herpes simplex
    Varicella/zoster
    Leprosy
Diseases of altered immunity
    Lupus erythematosus
    Systemic sclerosis (renal)
    Polymyositis/dermatomyositis
    Pemphigus
Metabolic diseases
    Porphyria cutanea tarda
    Acrodermatitis enteropathica
Connective tissue disorders
    Ehlers-Danlos syndrome (laceration, postpartum hemorrhage)
    Pseudoxanthoma elasticum
Miscellaneous conditions
    Erythrokeratodermia variabilis
    Mycosis fungoides
    Neurofibromatosis
    Acquired immunodeficiency syndrome
    Hereditary hemorrhagic telangiectasia

BIBLIOGRAPHY

1. Aronson IK, Bond S, Fielder VC, et al: Pruritic urticarial papules and plaques of pregnancy: Clinical and immunologic observations in 57 patients. J Am Acad Dermatol 39:933–939, 1998.
2. Breier-Maly J, Ortol B, Breier F, et al: Generalized pustular psoriasis of pregnancy (impetigo herpetiformis). Dermatology 198:61–64, 1999.
3. Cohen LM, Capeless EL, Krusinski PA, Maloney ME: Pruritic urticarial papules and plaques of pregnancy and its relationship to maternal-fetal weight pain and twin pregnancy. Arch Dermatol 125:1534–1536, 1989.
4. Driscoll MS, Grin-Jorgensen CM, Grant-Kels JM: Does pregnancy influence the prognosis of malignant melanoma? J Am Acad Dermatol 29:619–630, 1993.
5. Holmes RC, Black MM, Dann J, et al: A comparative study of toxic erythema of pregnancy and herpes gestationis. Br J Dermatol 106:499–510, 1982.
6. Kelly SE, Black MM: Pemphigoid gestationis: Placental interactions. Semin Dermatol 8:12–17, 1989.
7. McDonald JA: Cholestasis of pregnancy. J Gastroenterol Hepatol 14:515–518, 1999.
8. Ortonne JP, Hsi BL, Verrando P, et al: Herpes gestationis factor reacts with the amniotic epithelial basement membrane. Br J Dermatol 117:147–154, 1987.
9. Shaw D, Frohlich J, Wittmann BAK, Willms M: A prospective study of 18 patients with cholestasis of pregnancy. Am J Obstet Gynecol 142:621–625, 1982.
10. Shornick JK: Herpes gestationis. J Am Acad Dermatol 17:539–556, 1987.
11. Shornick JK, Bangert JL, Freeman RG, Gilliam JN: Herpes gestationis: Clinical and histologic features of 28 cases. J Am Acad Dermatol 8:214–224, 1983.
12. Shornick JK, Black MM: Fetal risks in herpes gestationis. J Am Acad Dermatol 26:63–68, 1992.
13. Vaughn Jones SA, Black MM: Pregnancy dermatoses. J Am Acad Dermatol 40:233–241, 1999.
14. Winton GB: Skin diseases aggravated by pregnancy. J Am Acad Dermatol 20:1–13, 1989.
15. Wong RC, Ellis CN: Physiologic changes in pregnancy. J Am Acad Dermatol 10:929–940, 1984.

60. SPECIAL CONSIDERATIONS IN BLACK SKIN

Nadja Y. Grammer-West, M.D., LTC, MC

1. Besides the obvious difference in color, are there any physiologic differences between black skin and that of other groups?

Yes. Racial differences in skin pathophysiology have been detected although it should be noted that there are more similarities than differences. It is difficult to make generalizations about a heterogeneous group that is comprised of individuals with diverse and complex ethnic backgrounds. As you may have observed, black people range from very dark brown to extremely pale with multiple shades in between.

The stratum corneum has equal thickness in black and white skin. However, it has more layers and is more compact in black skin. Interestingly, there does not appear to be a correlation between the degree of pigmentation and the number of cell layers. This finding may explain why black skin tends to show a decreased susceptibility to cutaneous irritants. It may also explain why some blacks experience a condition commonly referred to as "ashy skin" (not to be confused with "ashy dermatosis"), especially after showering or bathing. This consists of fine white flakes on the skin that gives a dry appearance. Other differences in the barrier function of black skin include increased lipid content, increased electrical resistance, increased desquamation, and a decreased amount of ceramides.

2. Do people with darker skin have more melanocytes per unit area of skin?

No. Although the density of melanocytes in the basal layer of the epidermis varies in different regions of the body, there are no differences in the number of melanocytes in similar sites between black and white individuals. Differences in pigmentation are due to the type of melanin and the shape, size and distribution of melanosomes within the keratinocytes as well as the rate of melanogenesis within melanocytes.

3. What accounts for the differences in color between different ethnic and racial groups?

The two most important factors are the types of melanin produced and the method by which melanin is packaged in melanosomes. The two major groups of melanin that are produced by mammalian melanosomes are eumelanin and pheomelanin. Eumelanin is the tyrosine-derived dark brown to black pigment that is found in most racial and ethnic groups. Pheomelanin has a yellow to reddish-brown color and is also derived from tyrosine by a shunt in the eumelanin pathway. It is the predominant melanin in those individuals with freckles and red hair. Melanosomes are membrane-bound vesicles related to lysosomes that contain tyrosinase and a unique matrix of proteins. There are four stages of melanosome maturation. Stage I melanosomes are spherical and contain melanosomal filaments. Those in stage II are elliptical and contain numerous melanosome filaments. Stage III melanosomes are oval and contain melanin, while those in stage IV have the same shape but the internal structures are obscured by melanin. Blacks have mostly stage IV melanosomes and it accounts for the darker skin color.

4. Are the brown streaks that are sometimes seen on the nails cause for concern?

Nail pigmentation may be a normal variant in blacks as well as Asians. The condition is called melanonychia striata and is characterized by linear, longitudinal stripes that can vary from light brown to dark black. The width can vary and multiple bands may be seen within the same nail. Several or all nails may be involved. The cause is unknown but it has been suggested that the occurrence may be related to repeated trauma since these pigmented bands are rarely seen in children but are present in up to 90% of black adults. Histologic evaluation reveals increased melanin production in the nail matrix underlying the affected area. An acute onset of a solitary nail streak should not automatically be considered normal and the thought of an active junctional nevus or a subungual melanoma should be entertained. Close examination of the nail fold may be helpful, looking

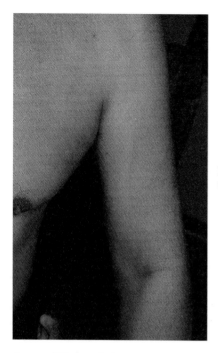

FIGURE 1. Futcher's (Voigt's) line of the upper arm. (Courtesy of James E. Fitzpatrick, MD.)

for any diffusion of pigment. The absence of this sign; however, does not rule out a more serious condition. Other diagnoses that may cause nail pigmentation include drugs such as actinomycin, antimalarials, bleomycin, cyclophosphamide, doxorubicin, 5-fluororuracil, melphalan, methotrexate, minocycline, nitrogen mustard, and zidovudine, to name a few. Some other conditions include Addison's disease, hemochromatosis, Peutz-Jegher's syndrome, and vitamin B_{12} deficiency.

5. True or false: Oral pigmentation may not necessarily be abnormal.
True. Oral pigmentation is common. Melanin deposits within the oral mucosa cause this asymptomatic finding. The gingiva is most frequently affected followed by the hard palate, buccal mucosa, and tongue. The color can vary but most often has a blue or gray appearance. There is no set pattern, but symmetry is often seen. A linear configuration can be seen that° may simulate other entities such as ingestion of drugs or metabolic conditions. As always, history is important, particularly, length of time present and any associated symptoms.

6. Are there any other areas where increased concentrations of pigment may be normal?
The palms and soles can demonstrate increased pigmentation. This is usually observed in darkly pigmented blacks. The lesions are macular and vary from light tan to very dark brown. The density may range from one or two macules to dozens. The findings must be differentiated from other conditions that are manifested by palm and sole involvement. Some include conditions mentioned in previous questions along with trauma, vasculitis, erythema multiforme and secondary syphilis. Any lesion that is changing or has very irregular symmetry, borders or color should be biopsied to rule out acral lentiginous melanoma, the most common form of melanoma occurring in blacks, Asians and Latin Americans. Other areas where increased pigmentation may be found are the sclera, the labia and vaginal mucosa, and the glans penis.

7. What are Futcher's lines?
Also known as Voigt's lines, these pigmentary lines of demarcation between dark and lighter skin can be seen in various regions of the body. They are commonly seen anteriorly on the arms, over the sternum, and on the posterior thighs and legs (Fig. 1). Histologically, there appears to be no difference in melanin concentration between the adjacent dark and lighter areas.

The distribution and symmetry typically allow this finding to be differentiated from other diagnoses that demonstrate linear, alternating pigmentation such as hypomelanosis of Ito, incontentia pigmenti, linear, epidermal nevus, or lichen striatus.

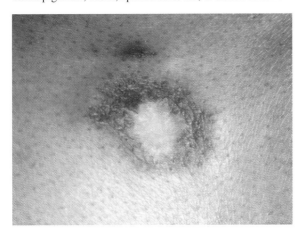

FIGURE 2. Postinflammatory hyperpigmentation in a patient with lupus erythematosus. (Courtesy of James E. Fitzpatrick, MD.)

8. What causes postinflammatory hyperpigmentation?

Postinflammatory hyperpigmentation is the residual darkening of the skin that results from an inflammatory disease such as, lichen planus, lupus crythematosus (Fig. 2), and atopic dermatitis (Fig. 3). Postinflammatory hyperpigmentation is most severe in those diseases (i.e., lichenoid dermatitis) in which there is disruption of the basal layer of the epidermis, which causes melanin to escape into the upper dermis where it is engulfed by macrophages. This is known as pigmentary incontinence and explains why it takes many months to years for the pigment to fade. Treatment of post-inflammatory hyperpigmentation includes bleaching creams such as hydroquinone, tretinoin, and azelaic acid. Hydroquinone, a tyrosinase inhibitor, is formulated in various topical preparations ranging from 2–20%. Those containing greater than 4% should not be used as they may cause **exogenous ochronosis**, which gives the skin a blue-gray discoloration. Monobenzylether of hydroquinone causes permanent, irreversible depigmentation and should never be used for this condition. Patients from countries in Africa and Europe may have access to this without a prescription and should be warned against its use. Disorders such as inflammatory acne should be treated early and aggressively in black patients to prevent this alteration in pigment.

9. What causes postinflammatory hypopigmentation?

Postinflammatory hypopigmentation is thought to be due to impaired transfer of melanosomes from melanocytes to keratinocytes. This occurs more commonly in diseases such as atopic

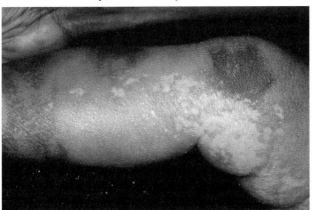

FIGURE 3. Postinflammatory hyperpigmentation and hypopigmentation in a child with atopic dermatitis. (Courtesy of James E. Fitzpatrick, MD.)

dermatitis (Fig. 3) and psoriasis. The increased mitotic rate of keratinocytes and decreased transit time of these cells to the skin surface does not allow sufficient time for pigment transfer. After the inflammatory process that caused the hypopigmentation resolves, pigment usually normalizes after several weeks to months.

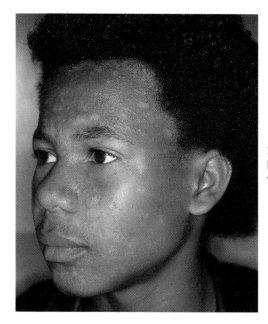

FIGURE 4. Pityriasis alba demonstrating hypopigmented macules of the face. (Courtesy of James E. Fitzpatrick, MD.)

10. Is pityriasis alba the same thing as postinflammatory hypopigmentation?

Pityriasis alba is seen primarily in children and is manifested by hypopigmented patches on the face and upper arms (Fig. 4). The lesions lack a distinct border and may have an overlying fine scale. There is often a history of atopic dermatitis. Although clinically pityriasis alba is probably a form of post-inflammatory hypopigmentation, it is considered a separate entity. This condition resolves with time. Brief treatment with low potency topical corticosteroids may be helpful.

11. Is vitiligo more common in blacks?

Vitiligo is a common disorder, affecting 1–2% of the world's population. There appears to be no racial predisposition for vitiligo; however, since it is more obvious in those with darker skin, more black patients may seek medical attention.

12. Why does tinea versicolor cause hypopigmented spots on dark skin?

Tinea versicolor, also known as pityriasis versicolor, is a common superficial yeast infection caused by the lipophilic organism, *Malassezia furfur* or *Pityrosporum orbiculare*, depending on which name is in current favor. The most common presentation on darker skin is multiple hypopigmented macules with a fine dust-like scale distributed over the upper back, chest, and proximal upper extremities. The cause of the hypopigmentation is unclear; however, extracts from the cultured organisms contain dicarboxylic acids that may competitively inhibit tyrosinase, an enzyme important in melanin production.

13. Why is it more difficult to appreciate erythema in darker skin?

The amount of redness seen in the skin is caused by the percentage of oxyhemoglobin in the capillaries. If the epidermis is deeply melanized, red hues may be difficult if not impossible to detect. Erythema can be caused by vasodilation that leads to an increased amount of blood in the dermis or by physiologic changes in the blood vessels, which is termed **hyperemia**. These reactions

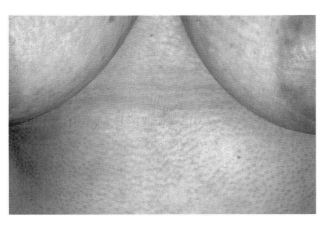

FIGURE 5. Tinea versicolor with follicular accentuation. (Courtesy of William James, MD.)

are also difficult to perceive. Interpretation of patch testing for sensitivity to allergens in black patients is more challenging for this reason. This is an extremely important point to remember, as many diseases that have erythema as a hallmark may not be considered in a black patient if that finding is not observed. Along those same lines, cyanosis is also difficult to perceive in a patient with dark skin for similar reasons.

14. Can any other generalizations be made about common reaction patterns in black skin?
   Besides difficulty perceiving erythema in black skin, there are several other patterns of response that appear more common. Papulosquamous diseases such as psoriasis and nummular eczema tend to exhibit a more violaceous color. Certain diseases such as atopic dermatitis or tinea versicolor may demonstrate follicular origination or accentuation (Fig. 5). In addition, some disorders such as lichen planus and seborrheic dermatitis have the propensity towards forming annular lesions (Fig. 6). Papular manifestations may also be more common as seen in pityriasis rosea and granuloma annulare.

15. What is the significance of the multiple brown papules often seen on the cheeks and nose?
   The condition described is called **dermatosis papulosa nigra**, and is seen very commonly in blacks and mostly frequently in women. They are commonly referred to as "flesh moles." They resemble moles or flat warts but are in fact a variant of seborrheic keratoses. The lesions tend to increase in number over the years and do not have a tendency to resolve on their own. They have no malignant potential and are mainly a cosmetic concern. Removal may be accomplished by light electrodessication and/or curettage. Lesions may be treated with light application of liquid nitrogen but care must be taken to avoid permanent hypopigmentation and scarring.

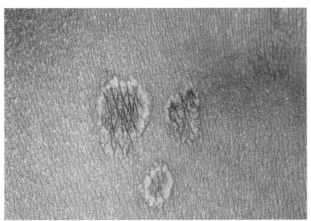

FIGURE 6. Annular lichen planus demonstrating central post-inflammatory hyperpigmentation. (Courtesy of James E. Fitzpatrick, MD.)

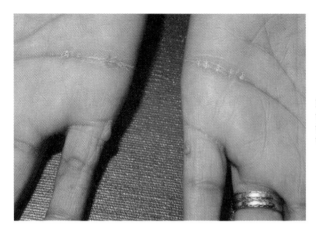

FIGURE 7. Keratosis punctate of the palmer crease. These are sometimes confused with warts. (Courtesy of James E. Fitzpatrick, MD.)

16. Are there any lesions seen more commonly on the palms and soles of blacks?

There is a condition called **keratosis punctata of the palmar crease** that occurs in up to 40% of blacks while it is seen in less than 1% of whites. The primary lesion is a 1–2-mm depression filled with a conical keratinous plug that is confined to the palmer creases (Fig. 7). They are commonly called palmar pits. Lesions are usually multiple and can be seen on the soles as well. The condition is usually asymptomatic. Treatment is not necessary, but the occasional painful lesion can be treated by removal of the cornified plug or punch excision of the entire lesion. This normal variant is distinguished from **hereditary punctate keratoderma** by distribution. The lesions in the former are confined to the creases whereas those in the latter can involve the entire palm diffusely.

17. What causes keloids?

Keloids are benign dermal tumors consisting of thick bundles of collagen that represent an over-response to trauma (Fig. 8). Keloids extend beyond the size of the original wound, as can be seen in earlobes following ear piercing. There are several sites of predilection including the shoulders, mandible, earlobes, presternal area and deltoid region. Any form of trauma can induce keloids such as thermal injuries, insect bites, injections, or surgical incisions. Keloids can occur spontaneously, especially in the central chest area. The exact disruption in the healing process that leads to the development of keloids is not known. It appears, however, that genetically predisposed fibroblasts are stimulated to produce abnormally high levels of procollagen messenger RNA, which leads to excess collagen production and secretion.

18. Why do black men who shave commonly get "razor bumps"?

The hair follicles in blacks are curved. After shaving, as the beard hairs grow, there is a tendency for the sharp end of the hair to curve back into the skin. When the hair pierces the skin it

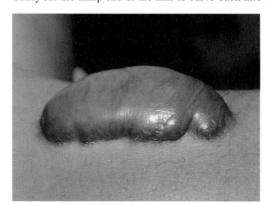

FIGURE 8. Large exophytic keloid of the shoulder. (Courtesy of James E. Fitzpatrick, MD.)

causes an inflammatory, foreign body reaction as one might see with a splinter. This leads to pustule formation that resembles a folliculitis. The condition is called **pseudofolliculitis barbae** (PFB). The condition is not seen in men who grow beards because the hair does not curve back into the skin after it reaches a certain length, usually 3–6 mm. It is common among populations that are required to be clean-shaven, such as in the military.

19. How is pseudofolliculitis barbae treated?

The treatment of choice is growing a beard. If growing a beard is not an option, several techniques may decrease the number of inflamed papules. The beard should be shaved in the direction of growth with a single-edged razor, and the skin should not be stretched while shaving. The ends of beard that have grown into the skin should be released, but the whole hair should not be plucked. Some men with this condition can manage the beard area using barber clippers that leave a short stubble of growth. Others obtain good results with chemical depilatories. If inflammation is severe short-term treatment with a low potency topical corticosteroid may be effective.

20. Are there any racial hair differences that may affect treatment of hair or scalp conditions in blacks?

Although hair from various races is biochemically identical, the structure of hair varies. Blacks have flat, elliptical follicles and spiraled hair with the smallest mean cross-sectional areas, while Asians have round follicles and straight hair with the largest mean cross-sectional area and whites have oval follicles with intermediate mean cross-sectional areas. These are broad generalizations and the racial makeup of the individual must be considered. The great numbers of angles of curvature in the spiral structure of black hair produce multiple vulnerable points along the hair shaft, making it fragile. This structure also inhibits effective transmission of secreted sebum down the shaft, making the hair drier and more brittle and less manageable. This has several significant implications when treating conditions such as psoriasis or seborrheic dermatitis.

Due to the factors mentioned above, black hair cannot be shampooed as often as other racial groups. Daily washing with antiseborrheic shampoos would lead to excessive dryness and hair breakage. A moisturizing conditioner should be recommended after their use. When evaluating alopecia, a thorough history of hair grooming techniques used should be obtained. Specifically, questions about the use of chemical relaxers, permanent hair dyes, curling irons, hot combs, blow driers, braids or weaves should be asked as any of the modalities mentioned could cause damage to the hair shaft or the scalp.

21. Are black patients particularly susceptible to any life-threatening illnesses?

Coccidioidomycosis, also known as San Joaquin Valley fever, is a deep fungal infection caused by *Coccidioides immitis*. It is acquired by the respiratory route and has occasional dissemination to subcutaneous tissues, bone or skin via the hematogenous route. Endemic areas for the disease are in southern California, Arizona, New Mexico, southwestern Texas, northern Mexico, and certain areas in South America. Infection occurs equally in both sexes, all races and ages; however, blacks are 14 times more likely to have severe disseminated disease than Caucasians. Untreated nonmeningeal coccidioidomycosis has a 50% mortality rate; therefore, early aggressive treatment with antifungal chemotherapy is essential.

22. Are there any special considerations when performing surgery on black patients?

Due to the increased risk of pigmentary alterations, hypertrophic scars and keloids, any surgical undertaking should be carefully considered. Liquid nitrogen can cause permanent damage to melanocytes. Treatment of benign growths such as warts or seborrheic keratoses with cryotherapy can therefore result in permanent loss of pigment.

23. List the diseases or conditions that are more common in blacks.

The diseases listed in the following table are seen in higher frequency in blacks. This is by no means an all-inclusive list. Some, such as the tropical infections, may be more common in blacks outside of the United States. These entities may rarely be encountered but are listed for completeness.

Dermatologic Conditions More Common in Blacks

Acne keloidalis nuchae	Lichen nitidus
Acral lentiginous melanoma	Lichen simplex chronicus
Acropustulosis of infancy	Loiasis
African histoplasmosis	Madura foot
Ainhum	Melanonychia striate
Buruli ulcer	Mongolian spots
Chancroid	Nevus of Ito
Dermatitis cruris pustulosa et atrophicans	Nevus of Ota
Dermatosis papulosa nigra	Onchocerciasis
Dissecting cellulitis of the scalp	Papular eruption of blacks
Dracunculiasis (guinea worm)	Pityriasis rotunda
Filariasis	Pomade acne
Granuloma inguinale	Porphyria cutanea tarda (South African Bantus)
Granuloma multiforme	Pseudofolliculitis barbae
Hamartoma moniliformis	Pseudomonas toe web infection
Infundibulofolliculitis	Sarcoidosis
Juxtaclavicular beaded lines	Sickle cell ulceration
Kaposi's sarcoma (endemic)	Traction alopecia
Keloids	Transient neonatal pustular melanosis
Leishmaniasis	Tropical ulcer
Leprosy	Trypanosomiasis

BIBLIOGRAPHY

1. Archer CB, Robertson SJ: Black and White Skin Diseases: An Atlas and Text. Oxford, Blackwell Science, 1995, pp 9–11.
2. Arnold HL, Odom RB, James WD: Epidermal nevi, neoplasms, and cysts. In Andrews' Diseases of the Skin: Clinical Dermatology, Philadelphia, W.B. Saunders, 1990, p 752.
3. Arnold HL, Odom RB, James WD: Seborrheic dermatitis, psoriasis, recalcitrant palmoplantar eruptions and erythroderma. In Andrews' Diseases of the Skin: Clinical Dermatology. Philadelphia, W.B. Saunders, 1990, p 219.
4. Berardesca E, Maibach Hl: Contact dermatitis in blacks. Dermatol Clin 6:363–667, 1988.
5. Berardesca E, Maibach Hl: Racial differences in skin pathophysiology. J Am Acad Dermatol 34:667–670, 1996.
6. From L, Assaad D: Neoplasms, pseudoneoplasms, and hyperplasia of supporting tissue origin. In Fitzpatrick TB, Eisen AZ, Wolff K, et al (eds): Dermatology in General Medicine. New York, McGraw-Hill, 1993, p 1199.
7. Grimes PE, Davis LT: Cosmetics in Blacks. Dermatol Clin 9:60–67, 1991.
8. Jimbow K, Quevedo WC, Fitzpatrick TB, Szabo G: Biology of melanocytes. In Fitzpatrick TB, Eisen AZ, Wolff K, et al (eds): Dermatology in General Medicine. New York, McGraw-Hill, 1993, pp 263–284.
9. Martin AG, Kobayashi GS: Yeast infections: Candidiasis, pityriasis (tinea) versicolor. In Fitzpatrick TB, Eisen AZ, Wolff K, et al (eds): Dermatology in General Medicine. New York, McGraw-Hill, 1993, p 2463.
10. Pathak MA, Fitzpatrick TB: Preventative treatment of sunburn dermatoheliosis and skin cancer with sun-protective agents. In Fitzpatrick TB, Eisen AZ, Wolff K, et al (eds): Dermatology in General Medicine. New York, McGraw-Hill, 1993, pp 1689–1695.
11. Rosen T: Nail pigmentation. In Pietrantonio V (ed): Clinical Dermatology in Black Patients. Bari, Italy, Pigreco, 1995, pp 15–16.
12. Rosen T: Palmar anomalies. In Pietrantonio V (ed): Clinical Dermatology in Black Patients. Bari, Italy, Pigreco, 1995, pp 19–22.
13. Shadomy HJ, Utz JP: Deep fungal infections. In Fitzpatrick TB, Eisen AZ, Wolff K, et al (eds): Dermatology in General Medicine. New York, McGraw-Hill, 1993, pp 2483–2485.

61. CULTURAL DERMATOLOGY

Scott A. Norton, M.D., M.P.H.

1. A child from southern India has had a recent decline in school performance and is noted to be anemic. On examination, the child has an adorable dark mascara-like make-up around her eyes. As an astute cultural dermatologist, you suspect that the make-up is the cause of the difficulties in school and the hematologic profile. What is the name for the traditional Indian eye make-up?

Surma. This is the Punjabi name for the eye make-up and the name that appears most frequently in the medical literature. It is also called *kajal* or *kohl* in other Indian dialects.

2. What is surma made from, and how did it affect the child?

Surma is a fine powder resembling mascara that is applied to the margins of the palpebral conjunctiva. It was originally made from antimony sulfide or from carbon soot, but now it is often adulterated with lead sulfide.

This child has chronic lead toxicity caused by absorption of the lead-based pigments in her surma — **cosmetic plumbism.** Surma usually has lead-based pigments and has created problems with lead toxicity in several Asian communities in the United Kingdom. For that reason, surma is now banned in England.

3. A Vietnamese child is seen in the emergency room with an earache and, on examination, is noted to have several linear ecchymoses on her back. The physician suspects child abuse as the cause of the bruises, but the interpreter says it is not. What caused the marks on the child?

Cao gio, or coin rubbing. This is a traditional Vietnamese medical practice.

The traditional healer massages the patient's skin with a liniment and then rubs a metal object, usually a coin, forcefully over the area. Petechiae and linear ecchymoses often develop. These have been mistaken for stigmata of battering many times by Western providers who are unfamiliar with *cao gio.*

4. An older Chinese man is noted to have dozens of fairly uniform round scars on his back. They resemble self-inflicted cigarette burns, only much larger. The patient is unconcerned about the lesions and indicates that someone like you, a doctor perhaps, did this to him. What ancient Chinese medical practice produces burn scars?

Moxibustion.

5. What is moxibustion?

It is derived from the words *moxa* and *combustion. Moxa* is from *mokusa,* the Japanese word for wormwood (*Artemesia moxa* of the sagebrush and absinthe genus), a commonly used combustible medicinal herb.

Moxibustion is the ancient oriental medical practice of igniting medicinal herbs on the skin. When the healer extinguishes the flame, the herb's therapeutic properties supposedly enter the body. A burn scar is the necessary sequela of properly conducted moxibustion. The sites on which moxibustion is performed are often the same as those used in acupuncture. The practice is still taught in Chinese colleges of traditional medicine.

Note that moxibustion was introduced into Europe by the end of the 17th century. In the movie *The Madness of King George,* there is a scene in which his physicians are treating him with moxibustion to cure his "madness." In actuality, he is believed to have had variegate porphyria.

6. Can acupuncture cause dermatologic problems?

Yes. There have been reports of abundant petechiae (in one case resembling meningococcemia) caused by acupuncture needles. Hematomas and ecchymoses occur frequently. Pyoderma, prolonged anesthesia, needle breakage, burns, itching, foreign-body granuloma, "carcinoma of the skin," and Koebner phenomenon have been reported. Transmission of HIV and hepatitis virus has occurred via acupuncture needles.

7. Do any Western medical practices cause permanent changes in the skin?

Of course, both intentionally and unintentionally. Think of surgical scars and keloids, radiation-port tattoos, radiation dermatitis, amniocentesis pits, hair transplants, *ad infinitum*.

8. Where did the practice of tattooing start?

Archaeologic evidence, such as human remains, shows that tattooing was part of indigenous cultures worldwide. For whatever the reasons, tattoos were used in ancient Europe, the Mediterranean region and Middle East, southern Asia, northern Japan, the Americas, and throughout the Pacific islands.

9. What does the word tattoo mean?

Tattoo comes from the pan-Polynesian word *tatau* meaning "to mark." Polynesian tataus were—and still are—richly symbolic, revealing heritage and status.

10. What culture has the most elaborate tattoos?

The Marquesan Islanders of French Polynesia once applied tattoos to almost the entire body. Hawaiians, Samoans, and New Zealand Maoris also had extensive tattoos. The practice is experiencing a cultural resurgence in many Polynesian groups today. Japanese tattoos (*horimono*) are often regarded as the most skillful and artistically prepared.

11. Why do sailors have tattoos?

European sailors adopted the habit during voyages to the Polynesian islands in the 18th century. The practice is still associated with the occupation of working at sea.

12. Why do bikers have tattoos?

I do not know. It is not in any of my books, and I am afraid to ask.

13. Who is the Ice Man and why are his tattoos so important?

The Ice Man is the name given to 5200-year-old frozen corpse of a Bronze Age hunter found preserved in the ice of a Tyrolean glacier on the border of Austria and Italy. He had 15 groups of tattoos that are noteworthy because they are neither decorative nor on exposed surfaces. Most of the Ice Man's tattoos are on standard acupuncture sites. Subsequent radiographic examinations of the body revealed old trauma at appropriate sites and strengthen the notion that the Ice Man's tattoos served as a form of therapy, akin to acupuncture.

14. A man from rural Nigeria has several sets of small parallel scars on his face. He says that his village doctor made these with a sharp stone when the man was young. What are ritually placed incisions called?

Scarification.

15. Scarification is performed in a number of societies. Why?

Ornamentation and beautification; group identification; protection (from illness or evil); and therapy.

16. What is an omega brand?

It symbolizes the rite of passage by initiates entering the American college fraternity, Omega Psi Phi. Although not officially sanctioned by the fraternity's national office, tens of thousands of men (and many "little sisters") have voluntarily permitted themselves to be branded on the deltoid or pectoral region with hot metal in the shape of the Greek letter Ω.

17. Name the familiar dark-red spot placed on the central forehead of Hindu women.
Bindi, kumkum, or *tilak.*

18. What dermatologic problems can bindi cause?
Allergic contact dermatitis caused by the pigments (mercuric or lead compounds, turmeric); hyperpigmentation that is either postinflammatory or due to a lichenoid eruption; and contact leukoderma.

19. While on a surfing trip to an outer island of Fiji, you notice that many of the men have dry scaly skin. You guess there must be a hyperendemic focus of X-linked ichthyosis. The villagers laugh when you ask if the men are born that way and explain that the skin problem is called *kani* and is caused by drinking too much *yanggona.* What is this?
Kani is the Fijian word for kava dermopathy, which is an acquired ichthyosiform disorder caused by excessive consumption of kava (called *yanggona* in Fiji). The mechanism for the skin disorder is unknown.

20. What is kava?
Kava is a beverage made from the roots of *Piper methysticum,* a true pepper found on many tropical Pacific islands. Kava has psychoactive properties and is used socially and ceremonially throughout Micronesia, Melanesia, and Polynesia.

21. Your favorite professor has invited you to accompany her on an assessment of a refugee camp in southern Africa. In the camp, you see hundreds of children and adults with a strikingly similar shiny, slightly erosive eruption along exposed areas of their clavicular regions and forearms. What is this eruption?
Pellagra.

22. Why is pellagra abundant in the refugee camps?
The inadequate food supplies available in the camps are often heavily reliant on corn-based products that have insufficient levels of nicotinic acid (niacin). This explanation also accounts for the pellagra outbreaks in the southern United States in orphanages, prisons, and among share-croppers in the early 20th century, where the diet was almost exclusively based on corn.

23. What is betel nut? Who chews it?
Betel nut refers to the fruit of the areca palm (*Areca catachu*) that is chewed extensively from Pakistan to Micronesia, a span of over 5,000 miles. Possibly 10–20% of the world's population chews betel, usually mixed with a pepper leaf (*Piper betle*), lime (calcium hydroxide or calcium carbonate, not the citrus), and occasionally tobacco. This compound is chewed by men and women alike, presumably for the mild psychoactive muscarinic properties of the alkaloid, areco-line, found in the palm fruit. Asian and Pacific island immigrants to the United States often continue the practice. (Technically, there is no betel nut; the palm fruit is called areca nut and the entire quid is simply called betel.) Betel leaves have been reported to cause mottled dyschromia of the skin, perhaps as a chemical contact dermatitis.

24. What dermatologic changes are associated with chewing betel?
Betel chewing stains the teeth, gingiva, and oral mucosa. The color ranges from red to black, depending on the preparation used. Chewers regard the color change as cosmetically appealing. More worrisome, however, is the greatly increased risk of oral squamous cell carcinomas in chewers, attributable to both the areca nut and the lime.

25. The visa of a Somali family living in your town has expired. The mother is fighting deportation because she fears that her daughters will be compelled to undergo circumcision if they return to Mogadishu. What is female circumcision?
Female circumcision is the encompassing term that Westerners use for several forms of culturally sanctioned surgical procedures on the female genitalia. It is most commonly performed in

the predominantly Muslim nations of North Africa, where perhaps 100 million women have had the procedure.

There are several forms of female circumcision, ranging from partial clitoridectomy (Sunna circumcision) to total infibulation or pharaonic circumcision (the removal of the clitoris, labia minora, incisions of the labia majora, and partly suturing closed the vaginal orifice).

26. What are the complications of female circumcision?

There can be medical (infections), surgical (hemorrhage), reproductive (fetal death), sexual (dyspareunia), psychological (chronic anxiety), social (peer pressures), and legal (immigration status) complications to the procedure. On the other hand, failure to perform the procedure may also have adverse cultural consequences. An interesting aside is the unsupported hypothesis that infibulation has hastened the spread of HIV infection in Africa by promoting exposure to blood during intercourse.

27. What is the most common culturally sanctioned mutilation in the United States?

Ah, mutilation is such a pejorative term. Let's use "surgical alteration" instead. After all, piercing one's ears is the answer, and we do not want to tag these persons as mutilated.

28. What about culturally sanctioned surgical alterations of male genitalia?

Dozens of these exist, including the religion-associated ritual circumcisions of Judaism, Islam, and the Seventh Day Adventist faith. Many Western societies practice widespread routine circumcision of neonates. Australian aborigines practiced subincision, an incision of the distal ventral penis exposing the urethra. Ancient Pohnpeians practiced hemi-castration (removal of one testicle) as a manhood rite. Many cultures practice the simple release of the ventral frenulum. Occupational castration (eunuchs of the seraglio), punitive castrations, and gender-altering surgery among transsexuals have also received varying degrees of cultural acceptance throughout history.

29. What are artificial penile nodules?

Objects placed permanently under the skin of the prepuce or penile shaft, purportedly to enhance the partner's pleasure during intercourse. Other names include tancho nodules and bulleetus. It is most commonly practiced in east Asian nations (e.g., Thailand and Philippines). In Japan, members of the yakuza, or Japanese criminal underground, often have artificial penis nodules.

30. Your cousin is marrying a woman from Mumbai (Bombay). On the wedding day, the bride's hands are painted with an intricate filigree-like pattern of reddish-brown pigment. What is this form of ornamentation called?

The Indian name for this is mehndi. It is produced by a semi-permanent dye called henna.

31. Describe the use of henna on the skin.

Henna is a natural red-brown pigment obtained from the plant *Lawsonia inermis*. It is used to prepare ceremonial body paint used in many Middle Eastern and south Asian societies. It is most commonly used by women on the palms and soles, especially for celebrations such as weddings. Henna is now commonly used in a deritualized fashion by Western women.

32. Are there any medical problems associated with henna?

Yes, but they are rare. Some people develop irritant contact dermatitis using henna. Henna may also cause hemolysis in G6PD-deficient individuals after percutaneous absorption. Also, some henna preparations contain para-phenylenediamine additives that can induce cutaneous and pulmonary allergic reactions.

33. A patient with a referral to the otolaryngology clinic mistakenly arrives in the dermatology clinic. You see that the consultation is to "rule out congenital absence of the uvula." Sure enough, on your examination, there is no uvula. What gives?

Your patient is missing the uvula not due to a congenital absence but instead due to a perinatal uvulectomy. This procedure is performed in many societies from West Africa to the Middle

East. The usual explanation is that uvulectomy alleviates problems associated with vomiting or cough. It is performed by non-physicians on infants or toddlers. Uvulectomy is also performed by Western physicians as a treatment for obstructive sleep apnea. The name of this procedure, uvulopalatopharyngoplasty, is bigger than the tissue that is removed. (Avoid confusing UPPP with PUPPP—which is a skin disease.)

BIBLIOGRAPHY

 1. Dorfer L, Moser M, Bahr F, et al: A medical report from the stone age? Lancet 354:1023–1025, 1999.
 2. Einterz EM, Einterz RM, Bates ME: Traditional uvulectomy in northern Cameroon. Lancet 343:1644, 1994.
 3. Horowitz CR, Jackson JC: Female "circumcision": African women confront American medicine. J Gen Intern Med 12:491–499, 1997.
 4. Hrdy DB: Cultural practices contributing to the transmission of human immunodeficiency virus in Africa. Rev Infect Dis 9:1109–1119, 1987.
 5. Kumar AS, Pandhi RK, Bhutani LK: Bindi dermatoses. 25:434–435, 1986.
 6. Lestringant GG, Bener A, Frossard PM: Cutaneous reactions to henna and associated additives. Br J Dermatol 141:498–500, 1999.
 7. Levy J, Sewell M, Goldstein N: A short history of tattooing. J Dermatol Surg Oncol 5:851–856, 1979.
 8. Liao YL, Chiang YC, Tsai TF, et al: Contact leukomelanosis induced by the leaves of Piper betle L. (Piperacceae): A clinical and histopathologic survey. J Am Acad Dermatol 40:583–589, 1999.
 9. Look KM, Look RM: Skin scraping, cupping, and moxibustion that may mimic physical abuse. J Forensic Sci 42:103–105, 1997.
10. Mojdehi GM, Gurtner J: Childhood lead poisoning through kohl. Am J Public Health 86:587–578, 1996.
11. Norton SA: Fijian penis marbles: An example of artificial penile nodules. Cutis 51:295–297, 1993.
12. Norton SA, Ruze P: Kava dermopathy. J Am Acad Dermatol 31:89–97, 1994.
13. Norton SA: Betel: consumption and consequences. J Am Acad Dermatol 38:81–88, 1998.
14. Outbreak of pellagra among Mozambican refugees—Malawi, 1990. MMWR 40:209–213, 1991.
15. Yamashita H, Tsukayama H, Taanno Y, Nishijo K: Adverse events in acupuncture and moxibustion treatment: a six-year survey at a national clinic in Japan. J Altern Complement Med 5:229–236, 1999.
16. Yeatman GW, Dang VV: Cao gio (coin rubbing). JAMA 244:2748–2749, 1980.

X. Emergencies and Miscellaneous Problems

62. DERMATOLOGIC EMERGENCIES

Scott Bennion, M.S., M.D., FACP

1. "Dermatologic emergencies" sounds like an oxymoron. Are there dermatologic emergencies?

Yes, several groups of diseases in dermatology are emergencies. In some, the skin is the primary organ affected (e.g., pemphigus vulgaris), and in others, the cutaneous manifestations are an important diagnostic finding of a severe underlying condition (e.g., meningococcemia). Rapid recognition and diagnosis of dermatologic emergencies are important since these conditions are often acutely lethal but can be treated successfully if the diagnosis is made early in the disease course.

2. What are the major groups of dermatologic emergencies?

- Vesiculobullous disorders (e.g., Stevens-Johnson syndrome, toxic epidermal necrolysis, pemphigus vulgaris)
- Infections
- Autoimmune disorders (e.g., acute cutaneous eruption of systemic lupus erythematosus, juvenile rheumatoid arthritis)
- Inflammatory cutaneous disorders (e.g., desquamative erythroderma, acute pustular psoriasis, acute drug eruptions)
- Environmental disorders (e.g., child abuse, heatstroke, electrical burns)

3. How does toxic epidermal necrolysis differ from the Stevens-Johnson syndrome or erythema multiforme major?

Toxic epidermal necrolysis (TEN) and Stevens-Johnson syndrome are commonly confused entities, in part because many clinicians use the two terms interchangeably. Because these two diseases have significantly different prognoses and treatments, it is important to differentiate between them. The diseases can usually be distinguished by their clinical presentation (Fig. 1), histologic findings, and course.

Clinicopathologic Features of Toxic Epidermal Necrolysis (TEN) versus Stevens-Johnson Syndrome (SJS)

	TEN	SJS
Maximal intensity	1–3 days	7–15 days
Skin pain	Severe	Minimal
Mucosal involvement	Mild	Severe
Lesional pattern	Diffuse erythema, desquamation	Annular and targetoid lesions
Skin histology	Few inflammatory cells	Numerous inflammatory cells
Prognosis	Poor	Excellent

The relationship between TEN and Stevens-Johnson syndrome is one of the great controversies in dermatology. Some in vitro research suggests that they are different diseases based on pathogenic mechanisms, but some authorities regard TEN as a more severe form of Stevens-Johnson syndrome. It is universally accepted that Stevens-Johnson syndrome is a more severe form of erythema multiforme.

4. How do you treat TEN and Stevens-Johnson syndrome?

Patients with **TEN** should be treated as burn patients, with supportive care to maintain fluid balance, avoidance of infection, and prevention of the adult respiratory distress syndrome

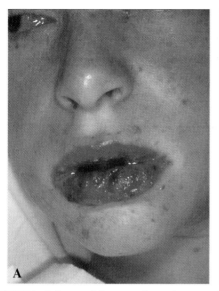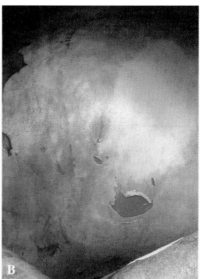

FIGURE 1. *A*, Stevens-Johnson syndrome demonstrating typical mucosal inflammation of the mouth, lips, and conjunctiva. *B*, Fatal case of captopril-induced toxic epidermal necrolysis showing violaceous discoloration with sheets of epidermis peeling away from the skin. (Courtesy of James E. Fitzpatrick, MD.)

(ARDS). In essence, TEN patients should be treated as severe burn victims. There are in vitro data to suggest that this entity may be the result of direct toxicity of drugs or their metabolites to skin cells. Anecdotal reports suggest that systemic corticosteroids are actually detrimental to TEN patients.

Stevens-Johnson syndrome appears to be immunologically mediated and responds to systemic corticosteroids. Patients with severe symptoms, especially involvement of the oral mucosa that interferes with eating and fluid intake, may be treated with a short trial of systemic corticosteroids. Stevens-Johnson syndrome is usually a self-limited disease with a 3-week course, and milder cases may not require systemic corticosteroids. Some authorities consider the use of systemic corticosteroids in this condition as controversial, since there are no good prospective, controlled studies evaluating this treatment. Therefore, an empirical 3–4-day trial of high-dose systemic steroids should be considered. If there is no clinical improvement at that time, the treatment should be discontinued.

5. What is pemphigus vulgaris?

Pemphigus vulgaris is a superficial blistering disease that typically affects middle-aged individuals (Fig. 2). It often presents initially with mouth ulcerations (60% of cases) but can involve blistering on areas above the waist. Pemphigus vulgaris may present acutely and in severe cases may resemble TEN or Stevens-Johnson syndrome. Early diagnosis is important since this condition is usually fatal if untreated, and current therapies are effective.

6. Describe Nikolsky's sign and its relationship to pemphigus vulgaris.

Pemphigus vulgaris involves only the upper layers of the epidermis; therefore, the blisters are very fragile, and typically patients present with only superficial ulcerations. Because of the fragility of the skin, one can apply lateral pressure with a finger to the intact skin around a lesion, causing the upper layer of the skin to become detached. This is called the **Nikolsky's sign,** and it occurs in pemphigus and other superficial blistering diseases. This clinical sign can be helpful in differentiating superficial from deeper blistering diseases (e.g., bullous pemphigoid, bullous lupus erythematosus) in which Nikolsky's sign is usually absent.

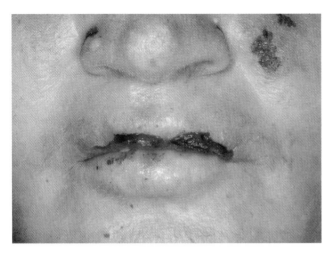

FIGURE 2. Pemphigus vulgaris demonstrating erosive lesions of the lips and left cheek. (Courtesy of James E. Fitzpatrick, MD.)

7. How is pemphigus vulgaris treated?

Therapy is designed to decrease the production of the anti-desmosomal antibodies or to reduce the inflammatory response. Because pemphigus can be deadly, corticosteroids in high doses are used initially, despite their serious side effects. Prednisone is given in daily oral doses of 120 mg as an initial dose, which is then adjusted lower or higher depending on the patient response. Other immunosuppressive drugs, such as azathioprine and cyclophosphamide, have been used in conjunction with corticosteroids because of their steroid-sparing effect.

INFECTIOUS DISEASES

8. Are any dermatologic emergencies infectious in origin?

Yes. These are most commonly bacterial (e.g., necrotizing fasciitis, tularemia) but also include viral infections (e.g., hemorrhagic fevers, neonatal herpes simplex infection), rickettsial infections (e.g., Rocky Mountain spotted fever), and fungal infections (e.g., mucormycosis).

9. Can emergent infections be differentiated by their cutaneous presentations?

Yes, although few cutaneous findings in emergent infections are pathognomonic. Infections that involve the skin can be organized generally by the appearance of the primary lesion. Major cutaneous patterns of presentation include:

- Petechial (e.g., chronic gonococcal septicemia, Rocky Mountain spotted fever)
- Vesicular (e.g., neonatal herpes simplex, Kaposi's varicelliform eruption)
- Pustular (e.g., disseminated candidiasis)
- Maculopapular (e.g., hepatitis B, Lyme disease)
- Diffusely erythematous (e.g., staphylococcal scalded skin syndrome)

Diagnostic Signs in Dermatologic Infectious Emergencies

Petechial/palpable purpura
  Neisseria gonorrhoeae septicemia
  Neisseria meningitidis septicemia
  Acute/subacute bacterial endocarditis (*Staphylococcus aureus,* streptococci)
  Rickettsia rickettsii (Rocky Mountain spotted fever)
  Rickettsia prowazekii (louse-borne typhus)
  Borrelia sp. (relapsing fever)
  Hemorrhagic fevers (Dengue, Rift Valley, Congo-Crimean, Korean)
  Cytomegalovirus (viral hepatitis)

Table continued on facing page.

Diagnostic Signs in Dermatologic Infectious Emergencies (Cont.)

Hepatitis B virus
Yellow fever
Rubella
Plasmodium falciparum (malaria)
Trichinosis
Violaceous skin discoloration
  Infectious gangrene
  Necrotizing fasciitis
  Mucormycosis
Purpura Fulminans (purpura secondary to disseminated intravascular coagulation)
  Neisseria meningitidis
  Streptococcus spp.
  Escherichia coli
  Salmonella typhi
  Bacteroides fragilis
  Other enteric gram-negative organisms
  Hemorrhagic fevers
  Vibrio vulnificus
Vesicular
  Neonatal herpes simplex virus
  Disseminated vaccinia
Pustular
  Staphylococcal endocarditis/sepsis
  Disseminated candidiasis
  Herpes simplex virus
  Corynebacterium diptheriae
Diffuse erythema
  Toxic shock syndrome
Maculopapular eruptions
  Viral infections
  Rickettsial infections
  Spirillum minor (rat-bite fever)
  Disseminated fungal infections
  Toxoplasma gondii
  Tularemia
  Leptospirosis
Annular erythema
  Lyme disease (*Borrelia burgdorferi*)

10. What is the differential to consider in hemorrhagic lesions other than infection?

- Coagulation abnormalities, such as idiopathic thrombocytopenia, disseminated intravascular coagulation, and clotting factor deficiencies
- Toxic epidermal necrolysis, which initially can present with petechial lesions
- Vasculitides, such as leukocytoclastic vasculitis secondary to an underlying collagen vascular disease, or periarteritis nodosa
- Raynaud's syndrome or disease
- Ergot poisoning

11. What causes necrotizing fasciitis?

Necrotizing fasciitis has been well-described for years but has recently received much attention in the lay press as the "flesh-eating bacteria." It is a bacterial infection that is rapidly progressive, often over hours, destroying muscle and subcutaneous tissues. Death or loss of a limb may occur if it is not diagnosed and treated early in its course. It is most commonly associated with β-hemo-lytic streptococci but may also be due to other gram-positive or gram-negative organisms, or it may be polymicrobial.

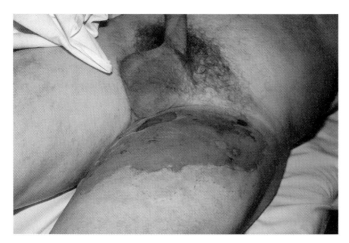

FIGURE 3. Necrotizing fasciitis. The typical well-demarcated dusky purpuric lesion is caused by thrombosis of the involved vessels.

12. Describe the clinical presentation of necrotizing fasciitis.

The bacteria usually enter through a surgical or traumatic wound and quickly move along fascial planes destroying vessels and tissue. Within the first 48 hours, the involved area that is initially erythematous, indurated, and painful becomes a dusky blue, indicating lack of circulation in the area (Fig. 3). Because there is significant vessel thrombosis, a biopsy usually results in little or no bleeding, and this is a useful diagnostic sign if present. Surgical debridement in addition to systemic antibiotics is necessary and often reveals extensive covert tissue necrosis.

13. Can other cutaneous infections look like necrotizing fasciitis?

Actually, necrotizing fasciitis is a type of infectious gangrene or cellulitis that rapidly progresses to destroy skin, subcutaneous tissue, and muscle. There are other types of gangrene, all of which have cutaneous findings similar to those of necrotizing fasciitis.

- *Staphylococcus aureus* and occasionally gram-negative organisms can cause **progressive bacterial synergistic gangrene.** This disease presents with a dusky erythematous discoloration of the skin followed by deep ulceration.
- In **gas gangrene** or **clostridial gangrene,** caused by the anaerobe *Clostridium perfringens,* patients typically present after a penetrating or crush wound with a tender, painful, edematous, white area that often becomes bronze with cutaneous blistering. Occasionally, when one palpates the area, crepitation or a crackling sensation is noted secondary to gas formation in the tissue. As with necrotizing fasciitis, timely diagnosis and treatment are necessary to minimize morbidity and mortality.

14. Are there any parasitic disease "emergencies" that have cutaneous manifestations?

Trichinosis and cysticercosis cutis. Both of these diseases are relatively rare in the United States, but cases are seen every year.

Trichinosis is caused by the small parasitic worm *Trichinella spiralis,* which is ingested in inadequately cooked meat containing its cysts. Common sources of encysted meat include bears and other carnivores or omnivores. Ingestion of pork, once a common source of trichinosis, is extremely rare today. The cutaneous signs include a macular or petechial eruption, splinter hemorrhages, periorbital edema, and conjunctivitis. The systemic signs and symptoms begin 1–4 weeks after ingestion and consist of eosinophilia, fever, headache, myalgias, and brain hemorrhage, which can lead to death.

Cysticercosis cutis is a cestodal infection due to the larval form of the pork tapeworm, *Taenia solium.* Typically, *Taenia* eggs enter the stomach from the intestine via reverse peristalsis, and they develop into oncospheres that penetrate the stomach wall and enter the circulation. They become lodged in internal organs such as the heart, brain, muscles, lungs, and eye. They also move to the subcutaneous tissues and develop into cysts that contain cysticercus larvae. They are usually numerous and can become calcified as evidenced by x-ray. With the presentation of either multiple subcutaneous cysts in a patient with unexplained neurologic signs or symptoms, one must keep this diagnosis in mind.

15. Do mycobacterial infections cause any dermatologic emergencies?

Most mycobacterial infections are relatively chronic and do not constitute emergencies. However, when patients with Hansen's disease (leprosy) are treated, they may undergo a "reversal reaction" that is secondary to a change in their immune status, resulting in acute inflammation of the involved areas. This may produce mild erythema and swelling of the skin and subcutaneous tissue. The apparent benignity of the situation belies its seriousness. The involved nerves are completely destroyed, resulting in permanent motor and sensory damage to the area. The lack of sensory input and resultant trauma over years lead to severe disfigurement of the extremities. Treatment consists of high-dose prednisone tapered over weeks.

AUTOIMMUNE DISORDERS

16. What collagen vascular diseases may become dermatologic emergencies?

Acute cutaneous and bullous systemic lupus erythematosus (SLE)
Dermatomyositis
Leukocytoclastic vasculitis (necrotizing venulitis)
Still's disease
Neonatal lupus erythematosus

17. What are the cutaneous findings in acute and bullous SLE?

The cutaneous findings of **acute SLE** are most common on the sun-exposed areas of the skin. The eruption consists of an evanescent erythema that is especially evident over the malar area of the face, producing the characteristic "butterfly rash." The erythema lasts hours to days and can resolve without residua. In a significant number of patients, the acute erythema can evolve into discoid lupus erythematosus, which is a chronic scaling eruption with scarring.

In **bullous SLE,** the patients present with tense vesicles or bullae, usually in sun-exposed sites. These are important presentations since both may be associated with severe internal disease.

18. How does neonatal lupus present?

It is an acute self-limited disease that gradually improves over 1–2 months. The cutaneous findings include diffuse superficial erythema and scaling that are often most apparent in the malar area of the face but can occur anywhere. Neonates frequently have other systemic findings like those seen in SLE, such as anemia, thrombocytopenia, jaundice, and hepatosplenomegaly with abnormal liver function tests. Another prevalent finding is atrioventricular heart block, which is permanent.

19. Why is prompt recognition and treatment of NLE important?

Frequently NLE eruptions are misdiagnosed as infectious in origin. This subjects the infant to the unnecessary risks of systemic antibiotics, while the presence of heart block may be missed, and appropriate systemic treatment (steroids) for the other NLE problems is delayed.

20. Why is dermatomyositis considered an emergency?

Dermatomyositis can develop rapidly with significant mortality. Skin findings in this disease can predate significant muscle involvement and be quite helpful in early diagnosis and treatment, especially in children. The skin findings that are helpful in diagnosis are:

- Gottron's papules occurring over the dorsa of the DIP and PIP joints of the hands
- Swelling and "heliotrope" erythema of the eyelids
- Periungual erythema (erythema around the proximal nailfold)

21. What is leukocytoclastic vasculitis?

This term is histologically descriptive of a group of diseases that cause acute neutrophilic inflammation and damage to the small vessels of the dermis. This can occur without apparent underlying etiology or as a cutaneous manifestation of a systemic disease such as Henoch-Schönlein purpura, SLE, or cryoglobulinemia. The eruption typically consists of "palpable purpura," varying in size from a few millimeters to several centimeters, mainly on the lower extremities. The cutaneous lesions of this group of diseases usually resolve without sequelae, but the internal organ involvement can be severe.

22. What are the skin signs of Still's disease?

The diagnosis of Still's disease (juvenile rheumatoid arthritis) can be perplexing because a significant number (25–30%) of these patients do not present with arthritis but with an evanescent eruption, spiking fever, leukocytosis, lymphadenopathy, and splenomegaly. The disease can be rapidly progressive, with severe bone and joint destruction and growth retardation. The rash, which occurs in 25–40% of patients, can be present for months to years before the arthritis. The eruption is fleeting, lasting up to 24 hours, and usually occurs in conjunction with fever. The rash may be diffuse with truncal accentuation and consists of coral-salmon red, flat macules to slightly elevated papules. Treatment for this disease usually consists of locally injected or systemic steroids. Other immunosuppressive drugs have also been used successfully.

INFLAMMATORY CUTANEOUS DISORDERS

23. Why is pyoderma gangrenosum a dermatologic emergency?

Pyoderma gangrenosum is one of a group of inflammatory skin diseases called **neutrophilic dermatoses** because histologically they have dermal infiltrates of neutrophils. It is a dermatologic emergency because it is often rapidly progressive, causing severe local tissue destruction. Pyoderma gangrenosum is frequently misdiagnosed as an infectious process or a brown recluse spider bite and is then treated by debridement. However, surgical procedures or any mechanical manipulation of acute lesions induces progression of disease to the normal surrounding skin, enlargement of the lesion, and further tissue destruction. Therefore, it is imperative to recognize and treat these lesions correctly early to avoid massive tissue destruction and loss.

Clinically, the lesions begin as a small papule/pustule that enlarges to form an ulcer. The ulcer has a necrotic center that typically involves the skin and subcutaneous tissues down to muscle, tendons, and fascia (Fig. 4). In older lesions, the intact epidermis at the borders of the lesion is erythematous with a purple hue and has a characteristic undermined edge. Another helpful clinical feature is the extreme pain and tenderness of these lesions. There are few cutaneous diseases that approach pyoderma gangrenosum in the severity of lesional pain and tenderness.

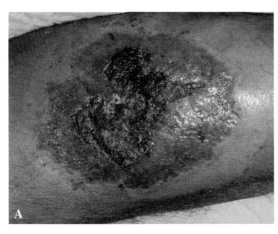
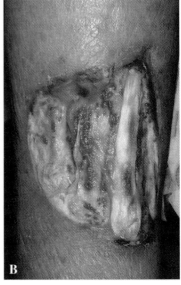

FIGURE 4. Pyoderma gangrenosum. A, Rapidly expanding classic lesion demonstrating characteristic undermined border. B, Older lesion without an active edge. Note that the depth of the ulcer exposes underlying tendons. (Courtesy of James E. Fitzpatrick, MD.)

Most cases of pyoderma gangrenosum occur without an underlying disease (50%), but this condition has been associated with several systemic diseases, most notably Crohn's disease (1–5%), ulcerative colitis (30–60%), leukemias, rheumatoid arthritis, and other collagen vascular disease.

24. Under what circumstances do childhood vascular anomalies become dermatologic emergencies?

The most common vascular anomalies (about 3% of births) that have the potential to become a dermatologic emergency are **capillary hemangiomas** (strawberry nevus). These lesions can be present at birth (approximately 20%) but more often develop over the first several weeks of life. Hemangiomas have a rapid growth phase, during which they rapidly enlarge, and then they regress.

Most commonly, these tumors are only a cosmetic problem, but if they occur around the eyes or in the oral cavity, they can cause significant morbidity and mortality. Some ophthalmalogists suggest that only a few days of obstructed vision in a newborn can inhibit normal visual development. Therefore, a hemangioma that may block an infant's visual fields should be treated aggressively. Likewise, enlarging hemangiomas of the upper respiratory tract and oral cavity can result in acute emergent situations and must be treated early in their course. Hemangiomas can be treated with intralesional steroids, but in lesions involving the facial area, this treatment should be avoided since there have been reports of steroid suspension embolism of the CNS and retinal vessels. In these cases, systemic steroids should be utilized. Rarely, large, rapidly growing hemangiomas have been associated with platelet trapping and acute thrombocytopenia.

25. Is acne fulminans a dermatologic emergency?

Although acne is not usually considered an emergency, this condition, if not treated acutely, can lead to severe cutaneous scarring and its attendant psychological problems. This type of acne usually occurs in teenage males, but there are cases reported in females. The eruption is characterized by rapid suppuration of large, highly inflamed nodules and plaques, resulting in ragged ulcerations and scarring of the chest, back, and, less commonly, face. Often attendant with the cutaneous symptoms are fever, leukocytosis, arthralgias, and myalgias, suggesting a systemic upregulation of the immune system. The treatment for this condition is high-dose oral steroids and early institution of oral retinoids such as 13 cis-retinoic acid.

26. Are there drug eruptions that are dermatologic emergencies?

Most drug eruptions are relatively benign and consist of a morbilliform or macular erythema that occurs without other signs or symptoms. On occasion, drug eruptions can present as diffuse exfoliative erythroderma, or **red man syndrome.** In these cases, patients develop a total body erythroderma with pruritus and scaling. In addition to drugs, other causes of exfoliative erythroderma that must be ruled out include psoriasis, lymphoma, and flares of seborrheic or atopic dermatitis. Other types of drug eruptions that can be dermatologic emergencies include toxic epidermal necrolysis, leukocytoclastic vasculitis, and severe urticaria or angioedema.

27. What are the mucocutaneous findings in Kawasaki's syndrome?

Conjunctival congestion
Oropharyngeal lesions (mucosal injection, strawberry tongue, fissured lips)
Hand and foot erythema
Exanthem

These findings, along with **lymphadenopathy,** constitute the minor criteria for Kawasaki's disease. Four of the five minor plus the major criteria of **fever** >38.3° C are necessary for the diagnosis. The hand and foot erythema may demonstrate variable edema followed by acral desquamation about 2 weeks after the onset. The exanthem is a generalized macular erythema.

28. How do you treat Kawasaki's syndrome?

High-dose aspirin during the febrile phase (100 mg/kg/day) in addition to intravenous gammaglobulin (400 mg/kg/day × 4 days).

ENVIRONMENTAL DISORDERS

29. Is heatstroke considered a dermatologic emergency?

Although heatstroke is not typically considered a "dermatologic problem," it does have characteristic skin findings that are helpful in making a quick diagnosis. In a heatstroke victim, the skin is erythematous, hot, and dry. These findings in association with unconsciousness should alert one to the diagnosis. Therapy needs to be instituted promptly to prevent death or severe CNS damage.

30. What are the cutaneous signs of child abuse?

Because child abuse can lead to acute morbidity and mortality, its recognition should be of paramount importance when evaluating pediatric patients. Cutaneous signs of abuse include:

Bruising and abrasions. These lesions are usually present in patterns or in areas not consistent with the history or trauma from common childhood accidents (Fig. 5).

Burns with unusual patterns. Some examples are cigarette burns that appear randomly over the body or dunking scald injuries, which have distinct borders and occasionally have a "doughnut" pattern around the buttock area when the buttock is pressed against the cooler tub surface.

Generalized wastage and dermatitis due to neglect and malnutrition.

Traumatic alopecia that demonstrates hemorrhage, irregular outlines, or hematoma formation.

Bite marks of adults can be distinguished from a child's by the width, which in adults is >4 cm.

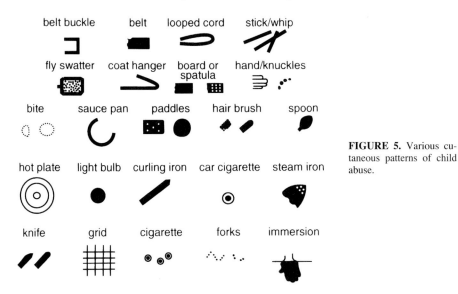

FIGURE 5. Various cutaneous patterns of child abuse.

31. What are the skin signs of a lightning strike?

Lightning strike patients often have very characteristic skin findings. In addition to entry and exit burn wounds, the skin of these patients can often exhibit a swirled or fernlike erythema of the involved area (Fig. 6). If there is any doubt of the etiology, the biopsy findings in the skin are pathognomonic. It is important to diagnose this injury since significant covert injury to the underlying fascia and muscles can occur. The degree of damage must be assessed and the patient treated for arrhythmias, shock, fluid and electrolyte imbalances, peripheral and central neural damage and covert tissue damage to optimize recovery.

32. What is sclerodema neonatorum?

It is typically seen in newborns but has been reported in infants up to 3 months of age. Clinically, it presents as a hardening of the skin with decreased temperature, vascular mottling, and a yellow-white discoloration in a symmetrical distribution, usually over the thighs and trunk. It usually occurs in the setting of an underlying severe illness and is associated with a 50% mortality rate.

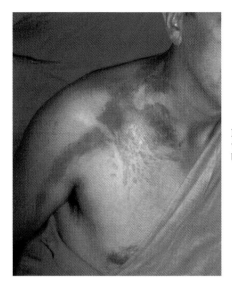

FIGURE 6. Lightning strike skin burn. Note the whorled fern-like pattern characteristic of this type of burn injury.

The pathophysiology of this sign probably is initiated by decreased body temperature that results in the hardening and solidification of the subcutaneous fat. This occurs in newborns because they have increased amounts of saturated lipids in their fatty tissue that solidify at higher temperatures than normal fat. Since this clinical condition often heralds death, it is important to recognize this entity early and aggressively treat the underlying illness.

33. What are the cutaneous findings in cholesterol emboli?

Cholesterol emboli can present anywhere in the body, but cutaneous manifestations most commonly occur on the lower extremities. This condition can occur spontaneously, but often cholesterol emboli to the skin present after angiography when trauma to aortic plaques dislodges cholesterol into the circulation. Clinically, the patient presents acutely with fairly well-demarcated areas of cyanosis or livedo reticularis on the feet and lower legs as a result of emboli blocking arterial circulation. These areas can undergo necrotic changes resulting in painful ulcers.

Cholesterol crystals within the lumina of the vessels on biopsy are diagnostic. The skin biopsy should ideally be an excision, and step sections should be examined because the atheromatous emboli are often focal. It is helpful to auscultate carefully over the major vessels of the abdomen and lower extremities after the patient has exercised to increase the pulse rate.This presentation is important since patients often have involvement of other organ systems, especially the kidneys. Further angiographic studies should be limited and treatment of the underlying hyperlipidemia initiated.

BIBLIOGRAPHY

1. Arnold H, Odom R, James W: Andrew's Diseases of the Skin, 8th ed. Philadelphia, W.B. Saunders, 1990.
2. Bennion SD, Fitzpatrick JE: Sweet's syndrome associated with breast cancer. Cutis 40:434–436 1987.
3. Demis DJ (ed): Clinical Dermatology. Philadelphia, J.B. Lippincott, 1994.
4. Fitzpatrick T, Eisen A, Wolff K, et al (eds): Dermatology in General Medicine, 4th ed. New York, McGraw-Hill, 1993.
5. Johnson R, Jackson R, Bennion SD: The effect of toxic epidermal necrolysis and erythema multiforme major patients' sera on human keratinocyte viability in culture. Clin Res 42:11A, 1994.
6. Krusinski PA, Flowers FP (eds): Life-Threatening Dermatoses. Chicago, Year Book, 1987.
7. Lever W, Schaumburg-Lever G: Histopathology of the Skin, 7th ed. Philadelphia, J.B. Lippincott, 1990.
8. Resnick SD: Staphylococcal toxin-mediated syndromes in childhood. Semin Dermatol 11:11–18, 1992.
9. Sureau P: Firsthand clinical observations of hemorrhagic manifestations in Ebola hemorrhagic fever in Zaire. Rev Infect Dis, 11(suppl 4): S790–793, 1989.
10. Weber D, Gammon W, Cohen M: The acutely ill patient with fever and rash. In Mandell GL, et al (eds): Principles and Practice of Infectious Diseases, 3th ed. New York, Churchill Livingstone, 1990.
11. Wilkins EW, Dineen J, Gross P, et al: Emergency Medicine. Baltimore, Williams & Wilkins, 1989.

63. OCCUPATIONAL DERMATOLOGY

Leslie A. Stewart, M.D.

1. How common is work-related skin disease?

According to the Bureau of Labor and Statistics, in 1996 there were 58,000 cases of skin disease in private industries. Skin disease was the second most common occupational illness of 439,000 cases, behind repetitive trauma cases such as carpal tunnel syndrome. The incidence of skin disease was 69 per 10,000 workers. Over the last decade, skin diseases have accounted for a disproportionately large percentage of all occupational illnesses, ranging from 24–37%. The true number of cases is thought to be 10–50 times higher than what is documented, due to underdiagnosis, under-reporting, and misclassification of cutaneous disease. Interestingly, the epidemiology of occupational skin disease varies from state to state. For example, in South Carolina, skin diseases accounted for 83% of all financially compensated occupational illnesses, whereas in California, they were responsible for 40% of all documented work-related disease.

2. What are the costs of occupational skin disease (OSD)?

Approximately 25% of all patients with OSD lose an average of 11 workdays annually. In addition, calculated total cost attributable to OSD ranged between $222 million and $1 billion based on lost productivity, medical care, and disability payments. Recognizing the impact of OSD, the National Institute of Occupational Safety and Health (NIOSH) has included dermatologic disorders among its list of top 10 work-related diseases for which improved efforts for prevention, surveillance, and research should be directed.

3. What is the most common type of skin disease due to workplace exposures?

Contact dermatitis accounts for >90% of OSD cases. The most common location of job-related contact dermatitis is the workers' hands. It is generally accepted that 80% of the contact dermatitis cases are irritant (Fig. 1), while 20% are allergic (Fig. 2). Recent studies have challenged those figures demonstrating that up to 40% of work related skin diseases were from allergic contact dermatitis. Pure allergic contact dermatitis (ACD) in the occupational setting is uncommon since a component of irritant contact dermatitis (ICD) is frequently present. Hands are the most commonly affected site in occupational skin disease. The "standard" patch test allergens screen for only approximately 75% of common allergens, so additional specialized testing with industrial chemicals to which the worker is exposed is frequently warranted. Testing should only be done with known materials in accepted concentrations.

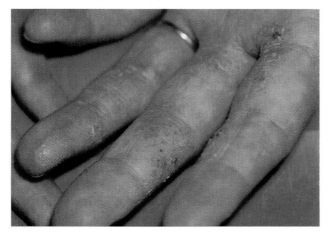

FIGURE 1. Chronic cumulative insult form of irritant contact dermatitis in a hairdresser, due to repeated hand washing with soap and water.

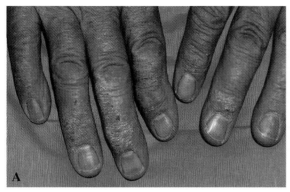

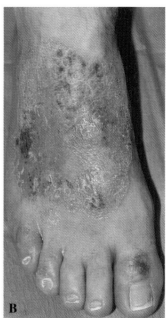

FIGURE 2. Chronic allergic contact dermatitis. *A*, A case in a machinist due to sensitization to preservatives used in cooling fluids. Note how the scaling dermatitis can mimic irritation. *B*, This patient developed sensitization to chromium, which was used to tan the leather in his work boots. The dorsal foot distribution is typical for a shoe contact dermatitis.

4. List some other types of OSDs and give examples of their causes.

Folliculitis or acne (e.g., due to greases and oils)
Chemical-related depigmentation (e.g., due to germicidal phenolic detergents)
Lichen planus (e.g., from photographic developing agents)
Granulomas (e.g., due to silica or beryllium dust)
Infections (e.g., a dentist contracting herpetic whitlow from a patient with oral herpes)
Photodermatoses (e.g., due to celery psoralens in agricultural workers)
Contact urticaria (e.g., due to latex gloves in hospital workers)

The above conditions can result from exposures to other agents in addition to the examples listed. The workplace can also exacerbate underlying conditions such as psoriasis. For example, repeated occupational skin trauma, known as the Koebner phenomenon, can induce a psoriatic lesion.

5. Are there any risk factors for the development of an OSD?

Various investigators have found a personal **history of atopic dermatitis** to be a significant risk factor. A history of childhood eczema has been found to be the most important predictive factor for the development of adult hand dermatitis. Affected individuals have a diminished skin irritation threshold to soaps, detergents, solvents, and chemicals and are more likely to develop irritant contact dermatitis on the job. Other preexisting skin diseases with compromised epidermal barriers, such as xerosis or nummular eczema, can predispose a person to contact dermatitis because of enhanced absorption of irritants and allergens through the skin.

Poor **personal hygiene** plays a role in patients who neglect to wash off irritating and sensitizing chemicals, thereby prolonging contact time. However, **overwashing** is actually the more common problem. The use of harsh soaps and frequent wetting/drying cycles induce chapping and desiccation, which compromises the skin barrier.

Environmental factors are also important. If it's hot and humid, workers may perspire, which can solubilize particulate matter, enhancing its penetration into the skin. Sweat can also leach out allergens such as chromates from leather shoes, inducing an allergic contact dermatitis. Conversely, low temperature and humidity causes chapping of the skin which can lead to irritant contact dermatitis.

6. My patient has a hand dermatitis that appeared to begin at his job. Does this mean he has an occupationally related skin disease?

Not necessarily. Just because a patient has a rash and he or she works does not mean it is job-related. To help make that determination, investigators have outlined seven criteria to be assessed. Four out of the seven should be present for reasonable medical probability:

1. *Is the eruption consistent with a contact dermatitis?* It should look like an eczematous dermatitis and not like other disorders, i.e., vasculitis.

2. *Are there occupational exposures to possible irritants or allergens?* There should be known documented irritating or sensitizing compounds to which the patient has been exposed at work.

3. *Is the anatomic location of the eruption consistent with the exposure a worker would obtain on the job?* For example, a worker may handle a chemical daily and breaks out in a dermatitis only on his back. This is not consistent with an OSD because he should have developed an eruption where he contacted the compound the most, namely his hands.

4. *Is the onset and time course of the eruption consistent with contact dermatitis?* Allergic contact dermatitis is a delayed reaction (occurring 48–72 hours after exposure), while irritant reactions may be immediate or delayed. Contact dermatitis is not, for example, consistent with a worker's one-time exposure to a chemical when a rash occurs 3 months after that one incident.

5. *Are nonoccupational exposures excluded as a possible cause of the dermatitis?* Hobbies, second jobs, and household contactants should be pursued as possible sources of contact dermatitis.

6. *Does the eruption improve away from work?* Work-related eruptions tend to improve when a worker is away from his job, although sometimes the same allergens and irritants may be found at home. Also, approximately 25% of workers with an OSD have a chronic and persistent dermatitis despite leaving their job and therapeutic intervention, and improvement does not occur when the worker is away from his place of employment.

7. *Does patch testing reveal a likely causative agent?* If a positive patch test reveals a likely allergen source with which the worker had contact, it is useful for pointing to the job exposure as the problem. However, patch tests must be interpreted within the context of the patient's history and physical examination. A positive test does not necessarily mean the allergen is responsible for the patient's current dermatitis, because it could be unrelated sensitization. The patch test reaction must always be assessed for its relevance to the present eruption.

7. How do I find out what a worker is exposed to on his job?

By law, employers must provide their employees information regarding all possible workplace exposures. Each of these information sheets, known as **Material Safety Data Sheets,** has information about a particular compound, including hazardous ingredients that it contains in concentrations >1%. They also list the manufacturer's name and phone number, which is useful for the dermatologist to check on other ingredients, since many cutaneous allergens are present in the final product in concentrations <1%. Dermatology and occupational medicine textbooks also provide general lists of allergens and irritants that may be specific to a particular occupation. On occasion, a more in-depth investigation may require a visit to the patient's place of employment. It is a unique opportunity to observe the worker performing his duties, the general working conditions, protective measures used, and other contactants which the patient might have overlooked.

8. What are some typical workplace irritants and allergens?

Irritants: Water, soaps and detergents, solvents, particulate dusts, food products, fiberglass, plastics, resins, oils, greases, agricultural chemicals, and metals. Of note, irritating compounds can be allergenic and allergenic compounds can be irritating.

Allergens: Metals (i.e., nickel), germicides (i.e., formaldehyde, glutaraldehyde), plants (i.e., poison ivy), rubber additives (i.e., thiurams), organic dyes (i.e., *para*-phenylenediamine in hair dye), plastic resins (i.e., acrylics and epoxies), and first-aid medications containing neomycin.

Occupations and Their Possible Contactants

	IRRITANTS	ALLERGENS
Construction workers	Cleansers, solvents, cement, dirt	Chromium (cement, leather boots), rubber chemicals (gloves), epoxy resin (adhesives)
Hairdressers	Shampoo, water, permanent wave solutions	p-Phenylenediamine (hair dyes), formaldehyde (shampoos), fragrances (shampoos and cosmetics), glyceryl monothioglycolate (permanent hair wave solutions)
Housekeepers	Cleansers, disinfectants, water	Rubber chemicals (gloves), fragrances and preservatives (cleaning and disinfectant solutions)
Health care workers	Soap, water, gloves, disinfectants	Rubber chemicals (gloves), glutaraldehyde (cold sterilizer for instruments), preservatives (skin care products)
Photographers	Water, developers, fixers, bleaches	Color developers, black and white developers

9. What is the prognosis of an OSD?

In general, workers with occupational hand dermatitis do not fare well. Approximately 25% have complete remission, 50% have periodic recurrences, and 25% have chronic persistent dermatitis, despite a change in jobs and therapeutic intervention. Some remediable reasons for persistent dermatitis include failure to diagnose and remove the sensitizer responsible for allergic contact dermatitis, continued exposure to nonspecific irritants at home and work, continued inadvertent allergen exposure, and secondary sensitization (e.g., to preservatives contained in moisturizers and topical steroids which physicians give as treatment). Unfortunately, once the hand dermatitis reaches a chronic stage, it is likely to remain chronic despite the best therapeutic efforts.

10. Aren't gloves enough protection for preventing OSD?

No. There is a widespread misconception that gloves guarantee safety. While gloves are recommended on a routine basis to protect against environmental insults, they are also the cause of a great deal of contact dermatitis themselves. Irritant dermatitis occurs because patients sweat underneath their gloves. Allergic contact dermatitis occurs commonly to rubber gloves containing the chemicals thiuram, mercaptobenzothiazole, and carbamates, which are "rubber accelerator" chemicals that speed up the vulcanization process of the final rubber latex product. The latex rubber proteins themselves also have induced type I IgE urticarial and anaphylactic reactions in glove wearers.

Some protective gloves are actually worse than wearing no gloves at all, because certain allergens may penetrate various glove materials and become trapped against the skin. This occlusion against the skin increases its cutaneous absorption, inducing a more severe contact reaction. For example, acrylics, formaldehyde, glutaraldehyde, and epoxies all penetrate latex gloves (Fig. 3). While protective clothing is useful, the proper type of equipment for the specific process must be chosen carefully.

11. How do you treat an occupationally related skin disease?

1. Remove the allergen and as many irritants as possible from both work and home. Allergens need to be substituted with less sensitizing alternatives. For example, vinyl gloves can be used in place of rubber gloves.

2. Patients must be instructed to avoid both excessive water exposure and frequent hand washing. The constant wetting and drying can lead to chapping, which makes all hand dermatitis worse. Hands can be protected from the elements by using cotton glove liners to absorb perspiration inside a proper protective glove for the job. Moisturizers should be used immediately after wetting the hands or whenever they appear dry and scaling.

3. Topical corticosteroids are the mainstay of therapy for occupational contact dermatitis, with systemic steroids reserved for acute, severe situations.

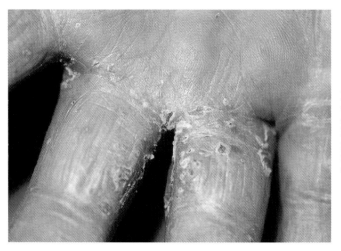

FIGURE 3. Dental assistant with allergic contact dermatitis due to glutaraldehyde. Latex gloves do not provide protection against glutaraldehyde that may penetrate gloves.

With treatment and hand protection, many workers can and do continue to work despite a hand dermatitis. Job change should only be considered in patients whose inadvertent and direct exposure to irritants or an allergen cannot be eliminated adequately. Most workers suffer financial and social consequences from changing occupations and do best with environmental modifications that allow them to remain on their job.

BIBLIOGRAPHY

1. Adams R: Occupational Skin Disease, 3rd ed. Philadelphia, W.B. Saunders, 1999.
2. Bureau of Labor Statistics, U.S. Department of Labor, 1997.
3. California Department of Industrial Relations, Division of Labor Statistics and Research: Occupational Skin Disease in California (with special reference to 1977). Sacramento, CA, California Department of Industrial Relations, 1982.
4. Fowler JF: Occupational dermatology. Curr Probl Dermatol 10:211–246, 1998.
5. Fregert S: Occupational dermatitis in a 10-year material. Contact Derm 1:96–107, 1975.
6. Hogan DJ: The prognosis of occupational contact dermatitis. Occup Med State Art Rev 9:53–58, 1994.
7. Keil JE, Shmunes E: The epidemiology of work-related skin disease in South Carolina. Arch Dermatol 119:650–654, 1983.
8. Marks JG, DeLeo VA: Contact and Occupational Dermatology. St. Louis, Mosby, 1992.
9. Mathias CGT: Contact dermatitis and worker's compensation: Criteria for establishing occupational causation and aggravation. J Am Acad Dermatol 20:842–848, 1989.
10. Mathias CGT: The cost of occupational skin disease. Arch Dermatol 121:332–334, 1985.
11. Mathias CGT: Prevention of occupational contact dermatitis. J Am Acad Dermatol 23:742–748, 1990.
12. National Institute for Occupational Safety and Health, Association of Schools of Public Health: Proposed national strategies for the prevention of leading work-related diseases and injuries: Dermatologic conditions. Washington, DC, NIOSH, 1988. [NIOSH publ no. 89–136.]
13. Rietschel R, Fowler JF: Fisher's Contact Dermatitis, 4th ed. Baltimore, Williams & Wilkins, 1995.
14. Shmunes E, Keil JE: The role of atopy in occupational dermatoses. Contact Derm 11:174–178, 1984.
15. Stewart L: Occupational contact dermatitis. Immunol Allergy Clin North Am 12:831–846, 1992.

64. PSYCHOCUTANEOUS DISEASES

Margaret E. Muldrow, M.D.

1. How do the fields of psychiatry and dermatology overlap?

Many studies confirm that a high percentage of dermatology patients have coexistent psychiatric morbidity. Our understanding of this phenomenon remains limited. We do know that the skin and nervous system have the same embryologic origin and that tactile stimulation is critical for full neuropsychological development, but many questions remain.

Recent biomedical advances have begun to take psychocutaneous disease out of the realm of speculation and myth. As we examine shared symptom complexes and response to pharmacologic intervention, many psychocutaneous disorders can now be thought of in terms of neurotransmitters and their receptors, with all the inherent implications for treatment. This does not negate a role for various modalities of psychotherapy. Instead, our deeper understanding of psychocutaneous disease can only lead to improved patient care.

2. What types of psychocutaneous disease are encountered in dermatology?

Psychocutaneous disease can be classified into several major categories:
1. Primary psychiatric disorders with dermatologic manifestations
2. Primary dermatologic disorders which result in secondary psychiatric problems
3. Primary dermatologic disorders exacerbated by stress

3. What is the differential diagnosis of patients who complain that they are infested with parasites?

True parasitic infestation
Intoxication or withdrawal from alcohol, amphetamines, or cocaine
Drugs such as corticosteroids and methylphenidate
Organic brain syndromes
Systemic disease such as diabetes, renal or hepatic failure, endocrinopathies, multiple
   sclerosis, and lymphoma
Pellagra
Vitamin B_{12} or folate deficiency
Obsessions, phobias, delusions, and hallucinations

4. Define an obsession or compulsion, phobia, delusion, and hallucination.

Obsession/compulsion. An obsession is a persistent preoccupation with an idea or impulse, while a compulsion is a persistent, repetitive behavior performed in response to an obsession.

Phobia. An overwhelming fear that motivates individuals to avoid others or particular situations.

Delusion. A fixed, false idiosyncratic belief.

Hallucination. A perception without a stimulus.

5. What are delusions of parasitosis?

These patients believe that their skin is infested with parasites. They often describe insects mating, laying eggs, and crawling around in their skin. They do not admit to actually seeing the insects themselves, as they are not hallucinating. On presentation, patients may bring in specimens containing hair, lint and even living organisms for examination. They develop elaborate purification rituals and are often well-known to pest control organizations. It is not uncommon for the delusion to be shared by other family members. This is called **folie à deux.**

Of note is the fact that the delusion is often referred to as a **monosymptomatic hypochondriacal psychosis.** It is "circumscribed," and patients tend to function well in other aspects of their lives.

6. How do you diagnose this disorder?

Delusions of parasitosis is a diagnosis of exclusion. One must rule out all other possible reasons that a patient might complain that he or she is infested with parasites.

7. How do you treat this problem?

Delusions, like hallucinations, are psychotic symptoms which are theorized to result from increased levels of dopamine in parts of the brain. Patients with delusions of parasitosis have been shown to respond to neuroleptics, in particular pimozide (Orap), which is a dopamine antagonist.

8. What are the major side effects of pimozide?

Anticholinergic effects—dry eyes, dry mouth, constipation, urinary retention

Extrapyramidal symptoms—dystonia (muscle spasm), akathisia (motor restlessness), parkinsonian-like syndrome (characterized by a pill-rolling tremor, rigidity, stiffened gait, and flattened facial expression)

Antiadrenergic effects—orthostatic hypotension

Tardive dyskinesia (less common)

In addition to having these side effects, pimozide is a **calcium channel blocker** with the potential to alter cardiac conduction and prolong the QT interval. Although the medication is usually used only in small doses, patients should be followed closely for any adverse effects. A baseline ECG should be obtained and repeated after initiation of therapy and periodically with dose increases.

9. What if the patient is noncompliant with pimozide treatment?

It is often difficult to convince a patient with delusions of parasitosis to take medication. Diphenhydramine (Benadryl) is very helpful in relieving extrapyramidal symptoms and often helps prevent patients from discontinuing their medication.

10. What is dysmorphophobia?

In syndromes of dysmorphophobia, patients hold delusional beliefs about the structure or function of their skin. Symptoms range from complaints of excessive facial redness, scarring, or large pores, to olfactory delusions in which patients feel they are passing excessively smelly flatus or emitting body odor that drives people away. Diagnosis and treatment are similar to those for delusions of parasitosis. Prognosis is poor especially in women with facial symptoms, who tend to be severely depressed and even suicidal. Patients with olfactory delusions can be driven to homicide.

11. Name the three major categories of self-inflicted skin lesions. What differentiates them?

1. **Obsessive-compulsive disorders.** Patients acknowledge being driven to self-inflict skin lesions through conscious repetitive action.

2. **Dermatitis artefacta, or factitious dermatitis.** Patients self-inflict skin lesions but adamantly deny doing so. The motive for their actions remains unclear. While they are conscious of what they are doing, patients are unable to change their behavior easily.

3. **Malingering.** Patients consciously and deceitfully self-inflict skin lesions for a goal that is recognizable when circumstances are known. The behavior may or may not eventually be acknowledged, but patients can stop producing the symptoms when they are no longer useful to them.

12. What are the clinical manifestations of dermatitis artefacta?

The self-inflicted lesions vary widely in morphology and distribution. Depending on the method used, it is possible to see blisters from suction cups, burns from caustic chemicals or cigarettes, edema and ulcerations from the use of elastic bands, or deep scars from the use of glass or knives. Lesions are often bizarre and irregularly rectilinear (Figs. 1–4). They are necessarily within reach.

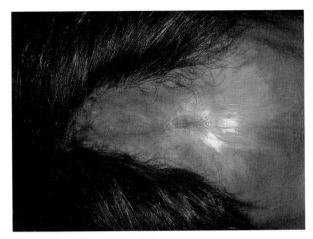

FIGURE 1. Patient-induced ulceration and scars of the scalp.

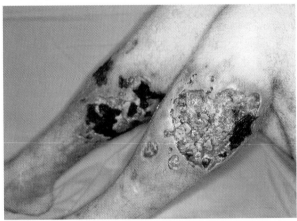

FIGURE 2. Young man with factitial panniculitis. The patient was injecting unknown substances into his legs in an attempt to get doctors to provide him with narcotic agents. (Courtesy of James E. Fitzpatrick, MD.)

13. What is the Gardner-Diamond syndrome?

Also known as **autoerythrocyte sensitization syndrome,** this disorder is characterized by the sudden unexplained appearance of purpura in young and middle-aged women. Skin lesions are associated with times of stress and are often preceded by burning pain. Permanent damage is rare. The exact etiology of the purpura remains controversial. Patients usually deny a history of trauma. Some individuals have been reported to have a positive skin test to their own red blood cell membranes, but laboratory evaluation is usually otherwise unremarkable. Interestingly, similar lesions have been produced by suggestion under hypnosis. Most authors believe that the disorder represents a factitious dermatitis.

14. How do Munchausen syndrome and Munchausen syndrome by proxy differ?

Munchausen syndrome is a chronic factitious disorder in which patients totally fabricate their symptoms, self-inflict lesions, or exaggerate or exacerbate a preexisting physical condition. The motive for the behavior remains unclear. Unfortunately, the disorder often leads to multiple hospital admissions and unnecessary procedures, surgery, and laboratory studies. When confronted with evidence that the symptoms are factitious, patients usually deny the allegations and leave against medical advice, only to repeat their actions in another hospital, city, state, or country.

In **Munchausen syndrome by proxy,** a third party facilitates an illness in another individual, usually a child, and receives some vague secondary gain from the behavior.

15. What is the differential diagnosis of patchy nonscarring alopecia?
Alopecia areata
Tinea capitis
Traction alopecia
Trichotillomania

16. What is the psychiatric diagnosis associated with trichotillomania?
Trichotillomania is an obsessive-compulsive disorder in which patients are driven to pull out their own scalp hair or, less commonly, their eyebrows, eyelashes, and even pubic hair.

17. How do you differentiate between the different forms of nonscarring alopecia?
In **alopecia areata,** there usually are circular areas of noninflammatory, nonscarring alopecia with "exclamation point" hairs at the margins, and there may be associated nail pitting.
Tinea capitis is characterized by patchy alopecia with varying degrees of erythema and scale that is KOH and/or fungal culture positive.
In **trichotillomania** irregular patches of nonscarring, noninflammatory alopecia are covered with broken-off hairs of variable lengths that are scattered randomly between empty hair follicles (Fig. 4). Patients with trichotillomania often pull out their upper lid eyelashes but leave the lower lid eyelashes, as these are more difficult to grasp. Patients with alopecia areata may have eyelash loss on both the upper and lower lids.

18. Can a biopsy help in the differential diagnosis of patchy nonscarring alopecia?
Yes. A biopsy would reveal a nonscarring alopecia with hemorrhage and pigmented follicular casts in trichotillomania. Alopecia areata shows a perifollicular lymphocytic infiltrate and small anagen hairs. Tinea capitis shows fungal elements within hair follicles.

19. What are neurotic excoriations?
In this disorder, patients compulsively pick at their skin. Lesions may be preceded by focal pruritus or insect bites, or they may be generated de novo by rubbing. Once initiated, ritualized picking of all lesions occurs when they catch the patient's attention or at a particular hour or location. On exam, lesions are found in all stages of development, ranging from ulcerations with hyper- or hypopigmented margins to hypertrophic nodules and atrophic scars. They are usually found within easy reach of the dominant hand (Fig. 3).

20. How do you treat this disorder?
Obsessive-compulsive disorders have been theorized to be associated with a deficiency of the neurotransmitter serotonin in the brain. Not surprisingly, patients with neurotic excoriations and trichotillomania who have an underlying obsessive-compulsive disorder have been shown to respond to serotonin reuptake inhibitors such as fluoxetine (Prozac).

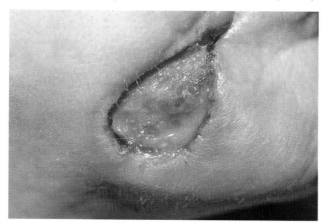

FIGURE 3. Factitial ulcer. (Courtesy of John L. Aeling, MD.)

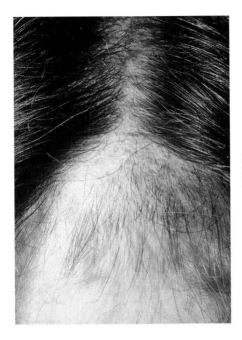

FIGURE 4. A young girl with trichotillomania. Note hairs of varying lengths. (Courtesy of John L. Aeling, MD.)

21. What are the side effects of fluoxetine?

The major side effects include anxiety, insomnia, headache, tremor, dizziness, sweating, and gastrointestinal complaints such as nausea and diarrhea. Although a relatively safe medication, this drug should not be administered to patients on monoamine oxidase inhibitors or to those individuals with a bipolar disorder.

22. What is glossodynia?

Glossodynia, or painful tongue, is one of the many atypical pain syndromes encountered in dermatology. Others include vulvodynia, burning feet syndrome, and atypical facial pain. Patients with these disorders often have underlying depression and respond to antidepressants.

23. Name some primary dermatologic disorders which might result in secondary psychiatric problems. What sort of problems might these patients have?

As an organ of self-expression, the skin plays a key role in emotional development and often defines interaction with others. Major disfiguring conditions, such as cystic acne, can result in a poor self-image and feelings of isolation and anger. Studies reveal that these individuals also suffer from higher rates of substance abuse, unemployment, and mental illness than the general population.

24. Can stress exacerbate a primary dermatologic disorder?

Yes. Psoriasis and atopic dermatitis are two dermatologic disorders that are classically exacerbated by stress. Also, all psychiatric conditions associated with dermatologic disorders will be exacerbated by stress.

BIBLIOGRAPHY

1. American Psychiatric Association: Diagnostic and Statistical Manual of Mental Disorders, 3rd ed.—revised. Washington, DC, American Psychiatric Association, 1987.
2. Farber EM, Nickoloff BJ, Recht B, Fraki JE: Stress, symmetry, and psoriasis: Possible role of neuropeptides. J Am Acad Dermatol 14:305–311, 1986.
3. Gil KM, Sampson HA: Psychological and social factors of atopic dermatitis. Allergy 44:84–89, 1989.

4. Ginsburg IH, Link BG: Feelings of stigmatization in patients with psoriasis. J Am Acad Dermatol 20:53–63, 1989.
5. Gupta MA, Gupta AK: Fluoxetine is an effective treatment for neurotic excoriations: Case report. Cutis 51:386–387, 1993.
6. Gupta MA, Gupta AK, Haberman HF: The self-inflicted dermatoses: A critical review. Gen Hosp Psychiatry 9:45–52, 1987.
7. Gupta MA, Gupta AK, Haberman HF: Psoriasis and psychiatry: An update. Gen Hosp Psychiatry 9:157–166, 1987.
8. Gupta MA, Gupta AK: Psychodermatology: An update. J Am Acad Dermatol 34:1030–1046, 1996.
9. Gupta MA, Gupta AK: Depression and suicidal ideation in dermatology patients with acne, alopecia areata, atopic dermatitis and psoriasis. Br J Dermatol 139:846–850, 1998.
10. Hollander E, Liebowitz MR, Winchel R, et al: Treatment of body-dysmorphic disorder with serotonin reuptake blockers. Am J Psychiatry 146:768–770, 1989.
11. Jankovic J, Sekula S: Dermatological manifestations of Tourette syndrome and obsessive-compulsive disorder. Arch Dermatol 134:113–114, 1998.
12. Joe EK, Li VW, Magro CM, et al: Diagnostic clues to dermatitis artefacta. Cutis 63:209–214, 1999.
13. Koblenzer CS: Stress and the skin: Significance of emotional factors in dermatology. Stress Med 4:21–26, 1988.
14. Koblenzer CS: The broken mirror: Dysmorphic syndrome in the dermatologist's practice. Fitzpatrick's J Clin Dermatol (Mar/Apr):14–19, 1994.
15. Koblenzer CS: Pharmacology of psychotropic drugs useful in dermatologic practice. Int J Dermatol 32:162–168, 1993.
16. Koblenzer CS: Psychologic aspects of skin disease. In Fitzpatrick TE, et al (eds): Dermatology in General Medicine, 4th ed. New York, McGraw-Hill, 1993, pp 14–26.
17. Koo JYM, Pham CT: Psychodermatology: Practical guidelines on pharmacotherapy. Arch Dermatol 128:381–388, 1992.
18. O'Sullivan RL, Lipper G, Lerner EA: The neuro-immuno-cutaneous-endocrine network: Relationship of mind and skin. Arch Dermatol 134:1431–1435, 1998.
19. O'Sullivan RL, Phillips KA, Keuthen NJ, Wilhelm S: Near-fatal skin picking from delusional body dysmorphic disorder responsive to fluvoxamine. Psychosomatics 40:79–81, 1999.
20. Slaughter JR, Zanol K, Rezvani H, Flax J: Psychogenic parasitosis: A case series and literature review. Psychosomatics 39:491-500, 1998.
21. Stein DJ, Hollander E: Dermatology and conditions related to obsessive-compulsive disorder. J Am Acad Dermatol 26:237–242, 1992.
22. Trabert W: Shared psychotic disorder in delusional parasitosis. Psychopathology 32:30–34, 1999.
23. Wang CK, Lee JY: Monosymptomatic hypochondriacal psychosis complicated by self-inflicted skin ulceration, skull defect and brain abscess. Br J Dermatol 137:299–302, 1997.
24. Winsten M: Delusional parasitosis: A practical guide for the family practitioner in evaluation and treatment strategies. J Am Osteopath Assoc 97:95–99, 1997.
25. Wu SF, Kinder BN, Trunnell TN, Fulton JE: Role of anxiety and anger in acne patients: A relationship with the severity of the disorder. J Am Acad Dermatol 18:325–333, 1988.
26. Wykoff RF: Delusions of parasitosis: A review. Rev Infect Dis 9:433–437, 1987.
27. Zomer SF, De Wit RF, Van Bronswijk JE, et al: Delusions of parasitosis: A psychiatric disorder to be treated by dermatologists? An analysis of 33 patients. Br J Dermatol 138:1030–1032, 1998.

65. APPROACHING THE PRURITIC PATIENT

Theresa R. Pacheco, M.D.

1. What is the most common symptom of dermatologic disease?
Pruritus, or "itching."

2. What is an "itch"?
It is an unpleasant sensation that provokes the desire to scratch.

3. Is an itch a separate modality of pain or a submodality of pain?
Although controversial, the general consensus views an itch a separate modality of pain. Though distinguishing between the sensations of pain and pruritus is easy, distinguishing between the neurophysiology of pruritus and pain is not. Pruritus and pain share many neurophysiologic features and pathways. Cutaneous nerve fibers arranged in an arborizing plexus immediately below the epidermis receive itch impulses. Unmyelinated C fibers conduct itch impulses from the skin to the ipsilateral dorsal root ganglia, ascend in the opposite anterolateral spinothalamic tract (closely associated with pain fibers), continue to the thalamus, and proceed through the internal capsule to the sensory cortex.

The following factors support that pain and itching are separate and distinct sensations: Itch leads to the reflex or urge to scratch; pain leads to withdrawal. Itch occurs only in the skin; pain arises from deeper structures as well. Heat may stop itch; heat usually increases pain. Removal of the epidermis eliminates itch; removal of the epidermis causes pain. Analgesics, particularly opioids, relieve pain; analgesics cause itch.

4. What causes an itch in inflamed skin?
A number of mediators for pruritus exist. Histamine, produced by skin mast cells, is the classical pruritus mediator. Pricking the skin with histamine produces pruritus in most individuals; however histamine does not account for all pruritus. Many pruritic diseases do not respond to antihistamine treatment.

Other pruritus mediators include prostaglandin, serotonin, tachykinins, cytokines, and opioid receptors. Prostaglandin E_1 lowers the threshold of the skin to itching provoked by histamine. Serotonin, 5-hydroxytryptamine, may regulate itch by acting on $5HT_3$ receptors. Tachykinins, such as the neuropeptide substance P, cause pruritus for reasons attributable to histamine release from mast cells. Cytokine iterleukin-2 may be an important peripheral mediator of itching. Opioid receptors in the central nervous system regulate the intensity and quality of perceived itch.

5. Describe the difference between localized and generalized pruritus.
Pruritus occurs with a host of dermatologic conditions, or it can mark systemic disease. Some dermatologic conditions that cause pruritus are inconspicuous or nonspecific. Other dermatologic conditions are apparent on physical exam. A physician must differentiate between localized and generalized pruritus and know a variety of skin diseases that cause pruritus.

Localized pruritus is defined as itching focused to certain regions. Localized pruritus usually results from a regional infection or dermatosis. Generalized pruritus typically appears as itching that affects the entire body surface. It implies a dermatologic or systemic disorder.

6. What is the best approach to evaluation of a patient with localized pruritus?
The most important diagnostic tools are the history and physical exam. After obtaining a thorough history, the best clinical approach is to organize the patient regionally. The physician should ask the patient if there are any lesions associated with pruritus. The patient's physical exam should focus on identifying a primary skin lesion or disorder in the affected region. After identifying a primary lesion, the physician can categorize the skin disease based on the lesion's morphology.

7. What are the common causes of localized pruritus?

The differential diagnosis of localized pruritus should include dermatoses that are limited to certain parts of the body and those that are diffuse but have a predilection for these sites.

Differential Diagnosis of Localized Pruritus

Scalp	Psoriasis, seborrheic dermatitis
Trunk	Contact dermatitis (axillae, waistline), erythrasma (axillae), psoriasis (periumbilical), scabies, seborrheic dermatitis, urticaria
Inguinal region	Candida, contact dermatitis, erythrasma, overuse of topical steroids, pediculosis, scabies, tinea cruris
Anal region	Candida, contact dermatitis, gonorrhea, hemorrhoids, pinworm, psoriasis, tinea cruris
Hands	Contact dermatitis, scabies, eczema
Legs	Atopic dermatitis (popliteal fossae); dermatitis herpetiformis (knees), lichen simplex chronicus (malleoli), neurotic excoriations, nummular eczema, stasis dermatitis
Feet	Contact dermatitis, pitted keratolysis, tinea pedis

8. What is the physician's best approach when seeing a patient with generalized pruritus?

The physician's most important diagnostic tools are a thorough and systematic history and physical exam. Laboratory testing for systemic disease may be necessary. Common questions include the following:

- What are the extent, severity and quality of the itch?
- When does the pruritus occur and what is its duration?
- Are there provocative factors, i.e., change in temperature or climate?
- Does the patient have a history of previous skin disorders or allergies?
- What are the patient's current medications?
- Has the patient taken any new oral medications or ingested any new foods?
- How often does the patient bathe?
- What products does the patient use on his/her skin?
- Has the patient used any new skin products?
- Is there a history of systemic illness?
- Is health maintenance up-to-date?
- Is there a history of psychiatric illness?
- What is the home environment?
- Are there pets at home?
- Does any other family member experience itching?
- Is there any recent travel?
- Is there any emotional stress?

In examining the skin, the physician should focus on whether it is normal or abnormal. If the physician identifies a primary skin lesion, the physician should rely on the lesion's morphology to categorize the skin. If the physician cannot identify a skin disease, the physician should perform a directed physical exam for icteric sclera indicative of hepatic cholestasis, unexplained adenopathy suggestive of an occult malignancy or oral candidiasis often seen in occult HIV infection.

9. List the laboratory tests a physician should order for a patient with generalized pruritus in whom a dermatologic disease cannot be identified.

- Complete blood count and differential
- Liver function tests, including alkaline phosphatase for obstructive liver disease
- Renal function testing; including blood urea nitrogen, creatinine, and urinalysis
- Optional tests include thyroid function tests and chest x-ray

The laboratory evaluation of the pruritic patient can be expensive. In addition to the suggested tests, some authors recommend a fasting glucose, stool exams for occult blood, Papanicolaou smear, serum iron, and serum protein electrophoresis. The laboratory tests the physician should order depend on the duration of the disease, the patient's health plan, and the philosophy of the health care provider.

10. What are common causes of generalized pruritus?

The numerous causes of generalized pruritus include:

Dermatologic disease	Systemic disease
Xerosis (dry skin)	Chronic renal failure
Atopic dermatitis	Hepatic cholestasis
Contact dermatitis	Primary biliary cirrhosis
Urticaria	Pregnancy
Bullous pemphigoid	Drugs
Dermatitis herpetiformis	Hematopoietic disorders
Infectious disease	Polycythemia rubra vera
Scabies	Hodgkin's lymphoma
Pediculosis	Iron deficiency anemia
HIV	Endocrine disorders
Psychiatric disease	Hyperthyroidism
Delusion of parasitosis	Diabetes mellitus
Depression	Carcinoid syndrome

11. How prevalent is an underlying systemic disease in a patient who seeks medical attention for pruritus?

Medical literature reports suggest that the prevalence of an underlying systemic disease in a patient who seeks medical attention for pruritus has been reported to be between 10–50%. Therefore, most causes of pruritus are secondary to a dermatologic disease. The following dermatoses are among the most severely pruritic: xerosis, atopic dermatitis, contact dermatitis, urticaria, pediculosis, scabies, bullous pemphigoid, and dermatitis herpetiformis.

12. What is "winter itch"? In which patient population is it common?

Winter itch is the term applied to xerosis (dry skin) which is aggravated by the low ambient humidity that occurs in many homes during the winter months. Xerosis occurs with great frequency in elderly patients and is the most common cause of pruritus for this age group. Xerosis is also aggravated by repeated water exposure due to excessive bathing, swimming, or hot tub use and strong soaps. The physical exam often shows dry, cracked, scaly skin on the lower legs. Treatment includes limiting frequency, duration, and water temperature of bathing, use of superfatted soaps, and use of emollients immediately after bath or shower. Use of oral antihistamines may help treat "winter itch."

13. The patient complains that "wool makes me itch" or "I am allergic to wool." What disease does this patient probably have?

Pruritus is such an integral part of atopic dermatitis that no diagnosis of active atopic dermatitis can be made without a history of itching. External factors such as irritating clothing (like wool), dry air, and emotional stress exacerbate atopic dermatitis. Patients tend to have a personal or family history of asthma, rhinitis and various allergies. Primary skin lesions are not typically seen, but lichenification (an exaggeration of the skin folds) is common because of constant rubbing by the patient. Therapy involves avoiding wool or other irritating clothing. Antihistamines are used to treat pruritus in atopic dermatitis, although some physicians attribute their beneficial effects to their sedative properties.

14. What treatment should the physician consider if a patient presents with pruritus and "hives"?

Urticaria occurs as a consequence of histamine release. A history of wheals is usually associated with pruritus. A physical exam may reveal dermatographism, even if wheals are not present. Therapy includes antihistamines that have a peripheral antipruritic action when itch is due to histamine release.

15. What disease should the physician consider if the patient volunteers that his spouse also suffers from itching?

This history suggests an arthropod reaction such as scabies or pediculosis pubis. Scabies commonly infects the entire family, especially if young children are present. The characteristic primary lesion is a burrow. Burrows may be difficult to visualize but are most commonly located on the flexor wrists, fingerwebs, and glans penis. Vesicles, papules, pustules, and excoriations are other skin lesions that may be present. Women often complain of pruritus about the nipples. Nocturnal itching is also characteristic of scabies.

If both members of the family have genital itching, the patient should be examined for pubic lice (*Phthirus pubis*) and nits attached to pubic hairs. Pediculosis pubis is one of the most infectious sexually transmitted diseases. Individuals have a 95% chance of becoming infected after a single exposure to an infected partner.

16. Is pruritus in HIV-infected patients common? What are the common causes of pruritus in these patients?

Pruritus is common in HIV-infected patients and is experienced with increasing frequency as the disease progresses. Occult HIV infection can present with generalized pruritus. Causes of pruritus secondary to skin disease in HIV-infected patients include (1) xerosis; (2) infectious etiologies like scabies; and (3) noninfectious etiologies like photoeruptions, eosinophilic pustular folliculitis or pruritic papular eruption. Pruritus unassociated with skin disease is probably secondary to immune dysregulation of HIV disease. The physical exam will help identify specific causes of skin disease, but a significant number of HIV-infected patients have no demonstrable skin lesions.

17. Which psychiatric disorder often presents with intractable pruritus?

Delusions of parasitosis is the fixed belief that a patient is infested with living organisms in the absence of evidence of such infestation. Delusions of parasitosis often occurs as a sole psychological disturbance, but it may be associated with an underlying personality disorder, such as the obsessive-compulsive type. A physician must take care not to miss a true infestation. A careful history; thorough examination of the skin; microscopic review of "bugs" brought in by the patient; and, occasionally, a biopsy of the "bite" sites is needed. Establishing a dermatology-psychiatry liaison is helpful in establishing a diagnosis and selecting therapy. The neuroleptic, pimozide, a blocker of dopamine receptors, is considered an effective treatment, but requires careful monitoring because of several potentially serious side effects.

18. Which patients with renal failure experience "renal itch"?

Pruritus reportedly affects 50-90% of patients undergoing peritoneal dialysis or hemodialysis. Pruritus usually starts six months after the start of dialysis and can be episodic, mild, and localized or generalized, intractable, and severe. The etiology of uremic pruritus is poorly understood. Possibilities include secondary hyperparathyroidism, histamine release by mast cells, hypervitaminosis A, iron deficiency anemia or some combination of these. The cornerstone of treatment is regular, intensive, efficient dialysis. Dietary restrictions, phosphate-binding therapy, and phototherapy (UVB) are alternative therapies.

19. Which patients with liver disease are most likely to experience pruritus? What is the best screening laboratory test?

Cholestasis, or biliary obstruction, is the common denominator in pruritus due to liver disease. Although alanine aminotransferase, cholesterol, and bilirubin are usually elevated, the single best screening test for this is a serum alkaline phosphatase measurement.

20. What are the common causes of cholestic pruritus?

The three most common causes of cholestic pruritus are primary biliary cirrhosis, cholestasis of pregnancy, and cholestasis from drugs. Pruritus affects virtually 100% of all patients with primary biliary cirrhosis and is the initial symptom in 50%. PBC is a disease of unknown etiology characterized by the destruction of small intrahepatic bile ducts by a granulomatous reaction.

Approximately 90% of the patients are female. The serum antimitochondrial antibody test against M2, a component of the pyruvate dehydrogenase complex of mitochondrial enzymes, is 88% sensitive and 96% specific for PBC. Treatment is hepatic transplantation and completely eliminates the pruritus. Benign cholestatic jaundice of pregnancy is a frequent cause of pruritus in pregnancy. The pruritus is most severe in the third trimester. The pruritus disappears and elevated liver function tests return to normal after delivery. Pruritus secondary to cholestasis frequency occurs with drug therapy. Common culprits includes oral contraceptives, anabolic steroids, cephalosporins, chlorpropamide, cimetidine, erythromycin estolate, gold, NSAIDs, nicotinic acid, penicillin, phenothiazine, phenytoin, progestin, and tolbutamide. Removal of the offending drug usually leads to resolution of symptoms. Other causes of cholestatic pruritus include primary sclerosing cholangitis, obstructive choledocholithiasis, carcinoma blocking the biliary tree, or chronic hepatitis C.

21. Which hematologic disorders are known to present with pruritus?

Polycythemia rubra vera and Hodgkin's lymphoma are the two most common hematologic disorders known to cause pruritus. Between 14%-52% of patients with polycythemia rubra vera suffer from pruritus. Pruritus is classically triggered by a sudden decrease in temperature, i.e., sudden cooling off after emerging from a warm bath. Treatment of the underlying disease is necessary to treat this symptom. A patient suffering from Hodgkin's lymphoma may present with a pruritus that precedes the diagnosis by as many as 5 years. The pruritus can be intolerably severe and continuous, or, less commonly, the patient may complain of a burning sensation. A review of 10 studies on Hodgkin's disease noted that 35% of patients suffered from pruritus sometime during the disease course, 15% presented with pruritus along with other symptoms, and 7% presented only with the symptom of pruritus. The significance of pruritus as a prognostic sign in Hodgkin's disease is unknown. Treatment of the lymphoma is the best therapy for pruritus of Hodgkin's disease.

22. Is generalized pruritus a common symptom of endocrine disorders?

Generalized pruritus occurs in 4% to 11% of patients with thyrotoxicosis and occurs more commonly in patients with long-standing disease. No recent publications on the incidence of pruritus in patients with diabetes mellitus exist. Notwithstanding, patients are more likely to experience pruritus vulvae and pruritus ani secondary to candidiasis, dermatophyte infection, and bacterial infection.

23. Can itching cause skin disease?

Tissue damage caused by scratching may lead to chronic skin conditions like lichen simplex chronicus, or prurigo nodularis. Lichen simplex chronicus results from repeated scratching which leads to a patch of chronic dermatitis that subsequently becomes lichenified, later becomes intensely pruritic, and leads to a perpetuation of the itch-scratch cycle. Lichen simplex chronicus seems to be precipitated by stress, depression, and frustration. Prurigo nodularis, rather than lichenification, may result from persistent localized itching and scratching. Postinflammatory hypopigmentation and hyperpigmentation is often seen with chronic skin conditions and is a result of repeated scratching and associated inflammation.

24. What is the best symptomatic treatment for a patient with pruritus?

The best treatment for a patient with pruritus involves identifying an underlying dermatosis or systemic disorder responsible for the pruritus and treating that disease. Various topical or systemic pharmacological agents should also be considered. Topical agents containing menthol produce a cooling sensation. Topical agents containing phenol or camphor have local anesthetic effects. Pramoxine, another topical anesthetic, can provide relief. If appropriate, topical corticosteroids can be used for local control. Oral antihistamines, like hydroxyzine or doxepin, are commonly used and often provide the first-line treatment for pruritus with no identifiable cause.

BIBLIOGRAPHY

1. Bernard JD: Itching in the nineties. J Am Acad Dermatol 24:309–310, 1991.
2. Bernard JD (ed): Itch: Mechanisms and Management of Pruritus. New York, McGraw-Hill, 1994.

3. Denman ST: A review of pruritus. J Am Acad Dermatol 14:375–392, 1986.
4. Driscoll MS: Delusional parasitosis: A dermatologic, psychiatric and pharmacologic approach. J Am Acad Dermatol 29:1023–1033, 1993.
5. Gilchrest BA: Pruritus: Pathogenesis, therapy, and significance in systemic disease states. Arch Intern Med 142:101–105,1982.
6. Greaves MW, Wall PD: Pathophysiology of itching. Lancet 348:938–940, 1996.
7. Greaves MW, Wall PD: Pathophysiology and clinical aspects of pruritus. In Freedberg IM, et al (eds): Dermatology in General Medicine, 5th ed. New York, McGraw-Hill, 1999, pp 487–494.
8. Greece PJ, Ende J: Pruritus: A practical approach. J Gen Intern Med 7:340–349, 1992
9. Robertson KB, Meuller BA: Uremic pruritus. Am J Health Syst Pharm 53:2159–2170, 1996.

66. NAIL DISORDERS

Brian J. Gerondale, M.D.

1. What functions do nails serve?

1. Nails protect the terminal phalanx and fingertip from traumatic impact.

2. They increase our discriminatory ability and, hence, manual dexterity.

3. They are unparalleled in their ability to relieve itching and represent to many people an extension of their esthetic beauty.

2. Why are nails important in medicine?

Nails are important because they are easily observable and often the first clue that an underlying disorder may be present. Furthermore, nails are commonly affected by numerous internal and external factors, including infectious agents, trauma, drugs, and various habits or tics. Lastly, nail changes may help differentiate between two closely related dermatologic disorders.

3. Do any systemic diseases have specific nail findings?

Many systemic diseases have characteristic but not mutually exclusive nail findings. Most nail changes are part of a symptom complex or a reaction pattern that may be extremely helpful in making a particular diagnosis.

Nail Disorders in Systemic Disease

NAIL ABNORMALITY	AREA INVOLVED	ASSOCIATED DISEASE
Splinter hemorrhages	Bed	Bacterial endocarditis
Mees' lines	Plate	Arsenic exposure
Muehrcke's lines	Bed	Nephrotic syndrome
Terry's nails	Bed	Cirrhosis
Half-and-half nails	Bed	Chronic renal failure
Blue lunulae	Matrix	Wilson's disease
Red lunulae	Matrix	Rheumatoid arthritis
Clubbing	Plate/matrix	Pulmonary disorders
Spoon nails	Plate/matrix	Iron deficiency
Nailfold telangiectases	Nailfold	Scleroderma, SLE

4. What are Beau's lines? How are they formed?

Beau's lines represent the most common but least specific nail changes seen with systemic diseases. They are a forward-pointing, wedge-shaped depression in the nail plate of variable depth and obliquity. They occur when there is temporary cessation of nail growth or decreased deposition of nail plate by part of the nail-forming unit. Any moderate to severe systemic upset remains a recognized standard precipitant of generalized Beau's lines, while localized events (trauma) produce isolated lines.

5. What is a splinter hemorrhage?

A splinter hemorrhage is due to the extravasation of blood from the longitudinally oriented vessels of the nailbed. The blood usually attaches to the overlying nail plate and moves distally with it. The occurrence close to the lunula and in multiple nails simultaneously correlates more directly with systemic disease.

6. Are splinter hemorrhages always associated with subacute bacterial endocarditis?

A commonly held, almost "sacred teaching" in medical school but rarely true. There is a myriad of causes, with subacute bacterial endocarditis representing only a small portion. Trauma is much more common. Drug reactions, psoriasis, general illness, vasculitis, and trichinosis are all associated causes, to name a few.

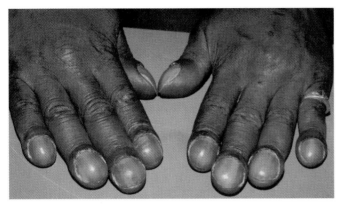

FIGURE 1. Benign clubbing of the nails inherited in an autosomal dominant fashion.

7. What is the difference between Mees' lines and Muehrcke's lines?

Mees' lines represent single or multiple transverse white lines that occur in the nail plate and move distally as the nail grows out. They are classically felt to be caused by arsenic intoxication, but many severe systemic insults may initiate them. **Muehrcke's lines** were described in 1956 by Robert C. Muehrcke in an article entitled "The Fingernails in Chronic Hypoalbuminaemia." These represent transverse double white lines that are an abnormality of the **vascular bed,** probably a localized edematous state secondary to the hypoalbuminemia. The underlying causes of these lines include the nephrotic syndrome, liver disease, and malnutrition.

8. What is nailfold capillaroscopy, and what is it used for?

It is the in vivo examination of nailfold and cuticle finger capillaries with magnification to detect variations in capillary patterns. It is quite useful in predicting which patients with Raynaud's syndrome will likely develop scleroderma. In those with scleroderma, the severity of capillary lesions may correlate with the degree of multisystem organ disease. While lupus erythematosus has a distinctive pattern, dermatomyositis is more a combination of lupus and scleroderma patterns.

9. What is clubbing?

Clubbing refers to the increased bilateral curvature of the nails with proliferation of the soft tissues restricted to the distal phalanges (Fig. 1). It causes a change in the emergence angle of the nail that becomes >180° (normally <180°). There are diverse causes of clubbing, including congenital or genetic factors, but 80% of clubbing is associated with respiratory ailments.

10. How is hypertrophic osteoarthropathy related to clubbing?

Clubbing may occur in association with hypertrophic osteoarthropathy, an uncommon but important entity. It consists of simple clubbing (including the toes), hypertrophy of the upper and lower extremities, peripheral neurovascular disease, acute burning bone pain, joint problems, and muscle weakness. More importantly, when complete, it is associated 90% of the time with malignant tumors of the chest.

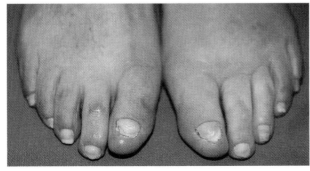

FIGURE 2. Yellow nail syndrome, demonstrating typical thick, yellow, and curved nails. (Courtesy of James E. Fitzpatrick, MD.)

11. What is the yellow nail syndrome?

The yellow nail syndrome consists of the classic triad of lymphedema of the lower extremity, nail changes, and pleural effusion. The nails are thickened, yellowish, and curved side to side with absent lunulae and cuticles (Fig. 2). It is associated with a multitude of pulmonary diseases including tuberculosis, asthma, and respiratory tract cancers.

12. Are there any characteristic nail changes in primarily dermatologic diseases?

Unfortunately, because the nail unit has only limited ways of responding to pathologic insults, pathognomonic changes are rarely encountered. However, examination of the nails is imperative because there are characteristic changes that, viewed in context with the entire clinical picture, can help establish a diagnosis.

Dermatologic Disorders with Nail Changes

DISEASE	INCIDENCE	FINDINGS
Psoriasis	10–50%	Pits, "oil spots"
Alopecia areata	10%	Pits
Lichen planus	10%	Pterygium
Scleroderma	Frequent	Pterygium inversus unguium
Darier's disease	High	Wedge-shaped, hyperkeratosis
Pityriasis rubra pilaris	Majority	Yellow-brown, hyperkeratotic

13. What are nail pits?

Nail pits are shallow depressions in the nail plate that are the result of abnormally retained nuclei of the keratin-forming cells which shed with growth (see figure on page 44).

14. Are there any differences in the nail pits of psoriasis and alopecia areata?

Nail pits are the most common finding in **psoriasis** and are generally deep, large, and randomly placed. The nail pits in **alopecia areata** tend to be small and uniform and classically arranged in a "cross-hatched" pattern.

15. What are the other nail findings seen in psoriasis?

Psoriasis can affect all parts of the nail unit and hence causes a wide variety of changes in the nail that are characteristic and helpful diagnostic aids. In descending order of frequency, the nail findings in psoriasis are:

Nail pits   Subungual hyperkeratosis
Oil spots (brownish-yellowish discolorations) (Fig. 3)   Nail plate abnormalities
Onycholysis (separation of the distal nail plate)   Splinter hemorrhages

16. How does a pterygium differ from pterygium inversus unguium?

A **pterygium,** which is Greek for *wing,* is classically associated with **lichen planus.** Lichen planus attacks the nail-forming unit, the matrix, and causes permanent scarring. Since the nail plate at that site is no longer made, the proximal nailfold attaches to the nailbed directly, and both grow out distally. This produces the "wing-like" appearance.

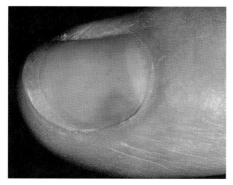

FIGURE 3. Typical "oil spot" on the nails of a patient with psoriasis. (Courtesy of James E. Fitzpatrick, MD.)

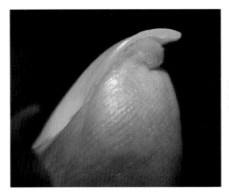

FIGURE 4. Lack of distal separation in a patient with scleroderma and pterygium inversus unguium. (Courtesy of James E. Fitzpatrick, MD.)

Pterygium inversus unguium occurs when the nail plate distally does not separate from the underlying digital bed skin. The fingertip ulcerations and scarring also seen in scleroderma contribute to the inability of the nail to separate (Fig. 4).

17. What is the most common cause and sequela of onychohemia?

First, you have to know that onychohemia is another name for a **subungual hematoma.** By far, the most common cause is **trauma to the nailbed.** Most subungual hematomas are accompanied by a throbbing pain secondary to the accumulation of blood below the nail plate that exerts pressure on the underlying bed. An effective and simple treatment for even the most unskilled practitioner is simply to pass the tip of a heated paper clip through the nail into the hematoma. Pressure relief and lessening of pain rapidly ensue, making you an instant hero!

18. Do malignant melanomas occur in the nails?

Yes, although subungual melanomas account for only 1–4% of all melanomas in light-skinned individuals. However, they account for 25% of melanomas occurring in black individuals.

19. How do you tell the difference between a subungual hematoma and a malignant melanoma?

This is a very important distinction to make because a melanoma can have a high mortality rate if diagnosed late. A high suspicion for melanoma would occur if pigment developed in a single nail of a person aged 50–80 years old. Also, any band in the nail that is wider at the base or darkening is worrisome. Hutchinson's sign, the leaching of pigment into the surrounding nailfold, is considered pathognomonic. Hematoma pigment remains confined to the nailbed and gradually grows out with the nail.

20. What causes the pigmentary changes in the nails of AIDS patients?

Patients with AIDS may develop acromelanosis, in which hyperpigmented macules occur on the fingers, palms, soles, and nails. In the nails, they appear as longitudinal pigmentary bands (melanonychia). A more common cause of nail pigmentation is the nail pigmentary changes due to treatment with zidovudine.

21. What is onychocryptosis, and why does it occur?

By far the most common condition affecting the toenails, onychocryptosis represents an **ingrown toenail**. It occurs when the free edge of the nail plate penetrates through the soft tissue of the nailfold. Factors that are known to precipitate or secondarily cause this condition are excessive rotation of the toe, onycholysis along the nail margin, ill-fitting shoes, hyperhidrosis, and poor cutting (rounding the edges) of the nails. Infection is a secondary complication.

22. What is a paronychia?

A paronychia is an inflammation of the nailfold surrounding the nail plate, which may occur in either an acute or chronic form. Acute forms are precipitated by some form of trauma or chemical

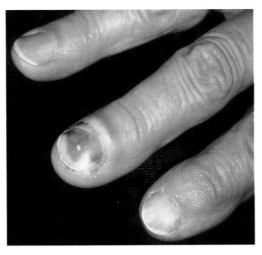

FIGURE 5. Acute paronychia demonstrating swelling, pus, and hemorrhage.

damage and usually present as painful infections (Fig. 5). Chronic paronychias tend to occur in several fingers simultaneously and result from repeated wet activities. An exception to this rule is the chronic paronychia caused by the habitual sucking of a finger, which tends to favor only one finger! Primary skin conditions, eczema, and atypical infectious organisms may also contribute to chronic paronychias.

23. Which infectious organisms cause paronychia?

Typically, acute lesions are caused by bacteria such as *Staphylococcus, Streptococcus,* and *Escherichia coli.* Chronic infectious paronychia is more commonly due to *Candida* sp., molds (*Scytalidium* sp.), syphilis, tuberculosis, and leprosy.

24. How do you treat an acute paronychia?

A quick and easy method to relieve pain and hasten healing is to stab the purulent area with a no. 11 scalpel blade and discharge the pus. A topical refrigerant spray to temporarily numb the area prior to incision will make for a grateful patient. Antibiotics and soaks should then be instituted, starting with coverage for *Staphylococcus aureus* (usually dicloxacillin) until the culture is back.

25. What is the most common cause of green nails?

The most common cause is *Pseudomonas aeruginosa,* which can colonize nail plates that are abnormally lifted up. This bacterium produces a pyocyanin pigment that imparts the green discoloration. After the nail is cut away, local therapy with a topical antiseptic or antibiotics is all that is needed for a cure.

26. A rampant epidemic of scabies is running through your ward despite adequate treatment. What might you suggest to stop it?

Since this question is in the nail chapter, you may have guessed that nails may play a role! Although not usually a site of infestation, subungual debris may harbor the *Sarcoptes scabiei* mite (secondary to scratching). This site has been known to cause persistent infestation or epidemics. Patients should be instructed to cut their nails short and brush the fingertips with the scabicide.

27. What organisms most commonly cause tinea unguium? Where does the infection typically start?

Tinea unguium refers specifically to dermatophyte infection of the nail. The most common organisms are *Trichophyton rubrum* (most common), *Trichophyton mentagrophytes,* and *Epidermophyton floccosum.* The vast majority of infections start at the distal end of the nail. Proximal subungual infections are quite rare in people with normal immune system.

28. List the newer antifungal medications used in the treatment of onychomycosis.

DRUG	BRAND NAME	DOSE
Itraconazole	Sporanox	Continuous: 200 mg qd for 12 weeks
		Pulse: 200 mg bid 1 week per month for 12 weeks
Terbinafine	Lamisil	Continuous: 250 mg qd for 12 weeks
		Pulse: 250 mg bid 1 week per month for 12 weeks
Fluconazole	Diflucan	300 mg every week for 12 months or until nails clear

29. What is "habit tic" disorder?

This is a common self-induced nail condition characterized by horizontal parallel ridges in the nail plate induced by constant manipulation of the cuticle and proximal nailfold. A closely related idiopathic condition, median nail dystrophy, can be easily confused with the above. Median nail dystrophy is marked by a normal cuticle and a fir tree appearance to the nail plate.

30. List the common benign "tumors" that occur in and around the nail unit.
- Acquired digital fibrokeratoma
- Exostosis
- Glomus tumor
- Periungual fibroma
- Pyogenic granuloma
- Myxoid (mucous) cyst

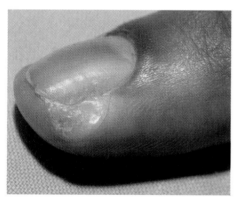

FIGURE 6. Subungual exostosis. (Courtesy of James E. Fitzpatrick, MD.)

31. What is an exostosis?

An exostosis is a common benign bony growth that occurs on the distal phalanx, usually of the great toe. It involves the bone first and secondarily the nail. Trauma is thought to play a role in its development, and it most commonly affects adolescent women. It presents as a slow growing painful mass under the nail with frequent secondary infection (Fig. 6). Plain x-rays will easily delineate the pathology.

32. Name the four most common malignant tumors of the nail unit.

Squamous cell carcinoma (including Bowen's disease) is by far the most common malignant tumor of the nail unit and entire digit. The next common is malignant melanoma, followed by basal cell carcinoma and keratoacanthoma.

BIBLIOGRAPHY

1. Baran R, Dawber R, Haneke E, Tosti A: A Text Atlas of Nail Disorders. St. Louis, Mosby, 1996.
2. Cohen PR, Scher RK: Geriatric nail disorders: Diagnosis and treatment. J Am Acad Dermatol 26:521–531, 1992.

3. Daniel CR, Sams WM, Scher RK: Nails in systemic disease. Dermatol Clin 3:465–483, 1985.

4. Jebson PJL: Infections of the fingertip: Paronychias and felons. Hand Clin 14:547–555, 1998.

5. Mantoura A, Bryant H: Nail disorders due to trauma and other acquired conditions of the nail. Clin Podiatr Med Surg 6:347-354, 1989.

6. Muehrcke RC: The finger-nails in chronic hypoalbuminaemia. BMJ Jun:1327–1328, 1956.

7. Nzuzi SM: Common nail disorders. Clin Podiatr Med Surg 6:273–294, 1989.

8. Pappert AS, Scher RK, Cohen JL: Nail disorders in children. Pediatr Clin North Am 38:921–937, 1991.

9. Rich P: Nail disorders: Diagnosis and treatment of infectious, inflammatory and neoplastic nail conditions. Med Clin North Am 82:1171–1182, 1998.

10. Salasche SJ, Orengo IF: Tumors of the nail unit. J Dermatol Surg Oncol 18:691–700, 1992.

11. Scher RK, Daniel CR: Nails: Therapy, Diagnosis, Surgery. Philadelphia, W.B. Saunders, 1990.

12. Sher RK: Onychomycosis: Therapeutic update. J Am Acad Dermatol 40: S21–S26, 1999.

13. Tosti A: The nail apparatus in collagen disorders. Semin Dermatol 10:71–76, 1991.

67. DERMATOLOGIC TRIVIA

Scott A. Norton, M.D., M.P.H

There are three levels of knowledge: trivia, significa, and necessaria. Information that you consider to be trivial, your attending physician may regard as necessary.

1. What does the X in histiocytosis X mean?

It expresses the common etiologic link among the three clinical forms of the disease: eosinophilic granuloma, Hand-Schüller-Christian disease, and Letterer-Siwe disease. When Louis Lichtenstein coined the name histiocytosis X in 1953, he chose the X to represent the then-undetermined cause of the disorders. He wrote that the suffix X "has the advantage of brevity and, by implication, emphasizes the necessity for an intensive search for the etiologic agent." We now know that the common link is a proliferation of macrophages that are ultrastructurally and immunologically similar to Langerhans cells. Indeed, they probably are Langerhans cells, as reflected in the current name for histiocytosis X—Langerhans cell histiocytosis. Much about the disorder is still unknown, so perhaps Langerhans cell histiocytosis deserves to keep an X-designation.

2. The suffix *itis* has come to mean *inflammation*. What is inflamed in "pruritis"?

Nothing. The word is prur*itus*, not prur*itis*. It is derived from the Latin *prurire*, "to itch." Pruritus is commonly misspelled; please learn how to spell it correctly.

3. What is the difference between pruritus and itch?

Nothing; the words are clinically interchangeable. Their ICD-9 codes are the same (698.9), so they are reimbursably equal, too.

4. Several names are used for the disease caused by *Bartonella bacilliformis*. These include bartonellosis, verruga peruana, Peruvian warts, Oroya fever, and Carrión's disease. Who was Carrión?

Daniel Carrión studied the relationship between the disfiguring but seemingly benign cutaneous disease, verruca peruana, and the often-deadly disease, Oroya fever. As part of a student research competition in 1885, the 26-year-old medical student inoculated himself with the blood of a patient with verruga peruana. Carrión soon developed the malignant form of *Bartonella* infection, Oroya fever, characterized by high fevers, severe myalgias, and profound hemolytic anemia. He postulated that the two conditions were related, but his experiment ended fatally. A few decades later, his theory was proved correct, and now Carrión is the hero of the Peruvian medical profession.

5. What other illnesses are caused by *Bartonella* species?

Cat-scratch disease is caused by *B. henselae* and trench fever is caused by *B. quintana*. Other conditions caused by various *Bartonella* species (including *B. henselae* and *B. quintana*) are most common in immunocompromised individuals, particularly those with HIV infection. These conditions include bacillary angiomatosis, peliosis hepatis, and a form of culture-negative endocarditis.

6. There are many types of Ehlers-Danlos syndrome (EDS) based on clinical and biochemical differences. Textbooks list them as EDS I through EDS XI but never describe EDS IX. What happened to EDS IX?

Ehlers-Danlos syndrome is a group of diseases characterized by inheritable defects in collagen synthesis. EDS IX, or the occipital horn syndrome, is not a fundamental disorder of collagen or connective tissue; it is a disorder of **copper transport.** Copper is a necessary cofactor in a number of biosynthetic pathways, one of which is the formation of collagen. Nosologists (disease taxonomists) have reclassified the occipital horn syndrome as a primary disorder of copper transport. Menkes' syndrome is another disorder of copper transport with dermatologic findings.

7. What is the difference between Klippel-Trénaunay-Weber syndrome and Klippel-Trénaunay-Parkes-Weber syndrome?

There is no difference. They are examples of eponymy with synonymy; both refer to osteohypertrophic nevus flammeus or angio-osteohypertrophy syndrome. The medical literature contains many reports, erroneous but oft-perpetuated, that distinguish the two as different syndromes on the basis of limb-length discrepancies. Weber and Parkes-Weber refer to the same person: Frederick Parkes Weber (1863–1962), an Englishman who was a consummate physician and erudite collector of unusual medical cases.

8. Which other eponymous dermatologic conditions include the name Weber?

• Rendu-Osler-Weber disease, or hereditary hemorrhagic telangiectasia
• Sturge-Weber syndrome (aka Sturge-Weber-Dimitri), or encephalomeningeal angiomatosis
• Weber-Cockayne syndrome, or epidermolysis bullosa (mild epidermal variant)
• Weber-Christian disease (nodular nonsuppurative panniculitis)

9. What is ciguatera poisoning?

Ciguatera poisoning is caused by ingestion of ciguatoxin, a tasteless toxin produced by dinoflagellates *(Gambierdiscus toxicus)*. Humans are affected by eating carnivorous fish, such as barracuda or red snapper, that have accumulated the toxin as it is passed along the oceanic food chain. Ciguatera occurs along coral reefs in tropical or warm subtropical waters. Ciguatoxin interferes with sodium channels in mammalian cell membranes. There are a number of gastrointestinal symptoms, but the occasional fatality is usually due to cardiorespiratory involvement.

10. What are the neurocutaneous manifestations of ciguatera poisoning?

Pruritus is noted in about half of the cases, often confined to palms and soles, and is exacerbated by exercise or alcohol consumption. There are often perioral and acral dysesthesias, which most distinctively demonstrate a heat-cold reversal phenomenon. Dry mouth may also occur.

11. From what is cantharidin made?

Cantharidin ($C_{10}H_{12}O_4$), a vesicant therapy for molluscum contagiosum and warts, is a semi-purified extract from blister beetles. The compound induces a blister at the epidermal-dermal junction. Blister beetles, mostly in the family Meloidae, have been used in Asian folk medicine for millennia. In the southern United States, horses are often afflicted with cantharidin toxicity after inadvertently eating the blister beetles that live in mowed alfalfa.

12. What is Spanish fly?

It is the legendary aphrodisiac powder made from crushed blister beetles *[Lytta* (syn. *Cantharis) vesicatoria]*. Supposedly, it served as an excitatory rubifacient when applied to an uncooperative male appendage.

13. Seriously now, cantharidin has been confirmed as an aphrodisiac. Who uses it and how does it work?

Male beetles of the species *Neopyrochroa flabellata* secrete cantharidin from a gland on their heads as a courtship or prenuptial offering. Females prefer to mate with males who offer cantharidin, which the female then uses to protect her eggs from predacious grubs.

14. Who is generally considered the father of modern dermatology?

Robert Willan (1757–1812), a Yorkshireman, was awarded the Fothergillian Gold Medal in 1790 for establishing a classification of skin disease that is still used today.

15. Name the eight orders in which Willan classified cutaneous disease.

Papules, scaling disorders, rashes (exanthems), bullae, vesicles, pustules, tubercles, and maculae. The terms are retained today in the daily parlance of the dermatologist.

16. What were Willan's four subtypes of pustules?

Phlyzacium, psydracium, achor, and cerion. Willan distinguished pustules by differences in size, characteristics of the pus, and quality of the scab. These terms have been abandoned. (Now this is trivia.)

17. What is a hunterian chancre?

It is the ulcer of primary syphilis, a syphilitic chancre.

18. Why does Jonathan Hunter's name grace this ulcer?

Jonathan Hunter was one of medicine's most influential practitioners. Among his works is the treatise *On the Venereal Disease* that addressed the then-unanswered question of whether gonorrhea and syphilis were different expressions of the same disease. Hunter attempted to settle the issue by inoculating himself in this manner: "Two punctures were made on [my] penis with a lancet dipped in venereal matter from a gonorrhea." Unfortunately, the donor of the "venereal matter" had both gonorrhea and syphilis. Hunter soon developed a chancre on his penis and later developed secondary syphilis. The mistaken conclusion of his little experiment was that gonorrhea and syphilis were the same disease. Incidentally, Dr. Hunter died 26 years after his self-inoculation from classic syphilitic heart disease.

19. Mucicarmine is a histologic stain used to detect mucin. From what natural source is mucicarmine obtained?

Cochineal, which is produced by a mealybug-like insect *(Dactylopius coccus)* that lives on several species of cacti. The pigment's chemical properties serve as deterrents against predation by other insects. Cochineal dye is crimson and has long been used as a traditional textile dye in Mexico. Emily Dickinson described the colors of a ruby-throated hummingbird as "A resonance of Emerald/A rush of Cochineal." Check the ingredients on bottles of pink grapefruit juice and you're likely to discover that the pinkish-red color is conferred by cochineal-laden bug poop.

20. How does the Food and Drug Administration differentiate between an underarm deodorant and an underarm antiperspirant?

Deodorants are cosmetics that control, obscure, or mask body odor. As a cosmetic, it has no claim to alter the body's physiologic process of perspiring. **Antiperspirants** alter the natural process of sweating and are therefore considered an over-the-counter drug. Antiperspirants are often deodorants, too.

21. What is Compound 606?

Also called salvarsan, Compound 606 was introduced to clinical medicine by future Nobel-laureate Paul Ehrlich in 1909. It was long considered the drug of choice for treponemal infections such as syphilis and yaws. The name reflects its place as the 606th compound tested by Ehrlich and his partner Sahachiro Hata. Ironically, salvarsan was developed not as a treatment for human syphilis but as part of an experiment on murine trypanosomiasis.

22. Who was James Lind?

James Lind (1716–1794), British naval surgeon, has received an inordinate share of credit in establishing the preventive and curative role of citrus products in the management of scurvy. Although Lind believed scurvy was caused by clogged skin pores, he conducted several shipboard trials of alleged antiscorbutic substances, leading to the use of citrus products (limes) by the Royal Navy during long voyages, hence the moniker "limeys" for British sailors.

23. If citrus products prevent scurvy, why did the Royal Navy suffer from so many scurvy outbreaks a century after Lind?

Not all citrus fruits have high amounts of vitamin C. In the mid-1800s, long before Casimir Funk's theory of vital amines (vitamins), the Royal Navy changed its fruit supplier and started receiving a strain of Caribbean lime that has very little vitamin C. Several polar exploring expeditions used the nonprotective limes and suffered severe losses from scurvy. This led many to doubt the efficacy of citrus fruit in the management of scurvy. After the discoveries of Pasteur and Koch, a paradigm swept through medicine that most diseases were caused by bacteria, either by direct infection or by ptomaine, a bacteria-induced food poisoning. Indeed, several nutritional diseases had their "offending bacteria" identified—including scurvy, pellagra, and beriberi.

24. Hansen's disease (leprosy) is generally considered a tropical condition. Where was G.H. Armauer Hansen working when he discovered the causative bacillus of leprosy?

Norway. Leprosy was abundant in coastal Norway in the mid-1800s, so Hansen did not leave his country to study this "tropical" disease. Bergen, Norway, was the world's center for leprosy research. Leprosy may have been carried to Norway by Viking voyagers a millennium earlier.

25. In the United States, most persons with newly diagnosed Hansen's disease are immigrants from southeast Asia, but in one region of the country, Hansen's disease is endemic. Where is this region of endemic Hansen's disease?

Louisiana and eastern Texas. Individuals there can acquire the disease autochthonously, apparently with no contact with any other infected persons.

26. What seems to be the natural reservoir of Hansen's disease in these states?

In the last several decades, the nine-banded armadillo *(Dasypus novemcinctus)* has been found naturally infected with *Mycobacterium leprae*. The disease manifests itself similar to lepromatous leprosy. Persons who handle armadillos for work or sport are at increased risk for acquiring Hansen's disease. Curiously, the first reports of naturally occurring armadillo leprosy appeared several years after the animals started being used for experimental infections.

27. Urology textbooks list about 50 causes of discolored urine. Several inherited metabolic disorders with cutaneous manifestations can cause discolored urine. If an infant's diapers have a black discoloration, what genodermatosis should you include in your differential diagnosis?

Alkaptonuria or hereditary ochronosis. This is a rare, autosomal recessive disorder due to the absence of an enzyme, homogentisic acid oxidase, that normally helps metabolize tyrosine and phenylalanine. Much of the excess metabolite, homogentisic acid, is excreted in the urine. The urine turns dark on oxidation; hence a freshly removed, urine-soaked diaper may have a normal color, but will quickly turn black upon exposure to air. Homogentisic acid is also accumulated in cartilage, leading to arthritis and to characteristic darkening of the sclera and pinnae.

28. If an infant's diapers have a reddish discoloration, what genodermatosis should you include in your differential diagnosis?

Erythropoietic porphyria. This is another very rare autosomal recessive disorder due to an absence in uroporphyrinogen III cosynthase, an enzyme required early in the heme synthesis pathway. Much of the excess substrate is excreted in the urine and may give diapers a distinctive reddish color. Patients develop a destructive, scarring photodermatitis and a variety of hematologic abnormalities. In acute intermittent porphyria, the urine of adolescents and adults may turn red upon standing also.

29. What is the eponymic name for erythropoietic porphyria?

Günther's disease. Some authorities believe that people with this disease are the basis for reports of "werewolves" in Europe. Individuals afflicted with this disorder avoid light, since it produces burning, and they demonstrate marked diffuse hypertrichosis, scarrring, and erythrodontia (red-stained teeth).

30. What is North Carolina spotless fever?

The tick-borne disease caused by *Rickettsia rickettsii* is usually called Rocky Mountain spotted fever. However, this name is often a misnomer, because the disease rarely occurs today in the Rocky Mountain states but is common in the vicinity of North Carolina. Perhaps 20% of cases lack the petechial eruption at presentation. Each year, there are more cases of North Carolina spotless fever than there are of Rocky Mountain spotted fever, hence the proposed name change.

31. What is the carrier protein of a hapten called?

Schlepper, from the German word for "drag" or "haul." The molecular weight of a hapten is too low to induce an allergenic response. The schlepper protein provides the molecular muscle to allow the hapten to serve as an antigen.

32. Do hair removal techniques (shaving, plucking, depilatories, waxing, electrolysis) cause new hair growth to be increasingly dark, coarse, or thick?

No, there is no scientific evidence to support this commonly held belief. The new growth is often sharp-tipped and stubbly, depending on the removal technique, and gives the illusion of bristliness.

33. Fifth disease is the common childhood exanthem also known as erythema infectiosum and is caused by parvovirus B19. (Everyone knows that.) But what is fourth disease?

It was a childhood exanthem described around 1900 that has been abandoned as a nosologic entity. A century ago, common childhood exanthems were assigned numbers one through six for ease of classification. Only fifth disease retains its numeric name. Fourth disease, also called Dukes' disease or Filatow-Dukes' disease, purportedly consisted of a nonspecific febrile illness accompanied by a cutaneous eruption. It may have been a streptococcal toxin-mediated disease, but it is not considered a precise or specific disease description.

34. Onchocerciasis is found in both Africa and South America. Where did the disease originate, and how did it cross the Atlantic?

It appears that disease caused by *Onchocerca volvulus* was originally endemic to tropical West Africa. The human cargo of the slave trade carried the disease to the Americas, where there were already native black flies and an awaiting ecological niche.

BIBLIOGRAPHY

 1. Beighton P, et al: International nosology of heritable disorders of connective tissue, Berlin, 1986. Am J Med Genet 29:581–594, 1988.
 2. Bernhard JD: Itch: Mechanisms and Management of Pruritus. New York, McGraw-Hill, 1994.
 3. Bialecki C, Feder HM, Grant-Kels JM: The six classic childhood exanthems: A review and update. J Am Acad Dermatol 21:891–903, 1989.
 4. Blythe WB: Lest we forget—spring is here: North Carolina spotless fever in adults. North Carolina Med J 46: 347–348, 1985.
 5. Carpenter KJ: The History of Scurvy and Vitamin C. Cambridge, Cambridge University Press, 1986.
 6. Clendening L: Robert Willan. In Source Book of Medical History. New York, Dover, 1960, pp 560–563.
 7. Eisner T, Smedley SR, Young DK, et al: Chemical basis of courtship in a beetle (*Neopyrochroa flabellata*): Cantharidin as "nuptial gift". Proc Natl Acad Sci USA 93:6499–6503, 1996.
 8. Gibbs DD: Rendu-Osler-Weber disease: A triple eponymous title lives on. J R Soc Med 79:742–743, 1986.
 9. Hoeppli R: Parasitic Disease in Africa and the Western Hemisphere: Early Documentation and Transmission by the Slave Trade. Basel, Verlag, 1969.
10. Irgens LM: The discovery of *Mycobaterium leprae*. Am J Dermatopathol 6:337–343, 1984.
11. Lange WR: Ciguatera fish poisoning. Am Fam Physician 50:579–584, 1994.
12. Leonard J: Daniel Carrión and Carrión's disease. Bull Pan Am Health Organ 25:258–266, 1991.
13. Lichtenstein L: Histiocytosis X. Arch Pathol 56:84–102, 1953.
14. Nicholls DSH, Christmas TI, Grieg DE: Oedermid blister beetle dermatosis: A review. J Am Acad Dermatol 22:815–819, 1990.
15. Schoen LA, Lazar P: The Look You Like. New York, Marcel Dekker, 1990.

INDEX

Page numbers in **boldface type** indicate complete chapters.